GERIATRIC MEDICINE

ROBERT W. SCHRIER, M.D.

Professor and Chairman
Department of Medicine
University of Colorado
School of Medicine
Denver, Colorado

1990
W.B. SAUNDERS COMPANY
Harcourt Brace Jovanovich, Inc.
Philadelphia ■ London ■ Toronto ■ Montreal ■ Sydney ■ Tokyo

W. B. SAUNDERS COMPANY
Harcourt Brace Jovanovich, Inc.

The Curtis Center
Independence Square West
Philadelphia, PA 19106

Library of Congress Cataloging-in-Publication Data

Geriatric medicine / [edited by] Robert W. Schrier.

p.   cm.

ISBN 0-7216-3031-6

1. Geriatrics.   I. Schrier, Robert W.
   [DNLM: 1. Geriatrics.   WT 100 G36632]

RC952.G393   1990b

618.97—dc20

DNLM/DLC   89-70197

for Library of Congress   CIP

Editor: John Dyson

Designer: Maureen Sweeney

Production Manager: Bill Preston

Manuscript Editor: Stephanie Mangum

Illustration Coordinator: Lisa Lambert

Indexer: Dorothy Stade

GERIATRIC MEDICINE   ISBN 0–7216–3031–6

Last digit is the print number: 9   8   7   6   5   4   3   2   1

To our senior citizens,
whose courage, wisdom, and humanity
have enriched our lives.

It is too late! Ah, nothing is too late
Till the tired heart shall cease to palpitate.
Cato learned Greek at eighty; Sophocles
Wrote his grand Œdipus, and Simonides
Bore off the prize of verse from his compeers,
When each had numbered more than four-score years, . . .
Chaucer, at Woodstock with the nightingales,
At sixty wrote the Canterbury Tales;
Goethe at Weimar, toiling to the last,
Completed Faust when eighty years were past.
These are indeed exceptions; but they show
How far the gulf-stream of our youth may flow
Into the arctic regions of our lives. . . .
For age is opportunity no less
Than youth itself, though in another dress,
And as the evening twilight fades away
The sky is filled with stars, invisible by day.

LONGFELLOW, Morituri Salutamus, 1. 238.

CONTRIBUTORS

Stephen F. Albert, D.P.M.
Assistant Clinical Professor, Department of Family Medicine, University of Colorado Health Sciences Center School of Medicine; Chief, Podiatric Section, Department of Surgery, Veterans Administration Medical Center, Denver, Colorado.
Skin Problems Associated with Pressure
Foot Disorders

William P. Arend, M.D.
Professor of Medicine, University of Colorado Health Sciences Center School of Medicine; Head, Division of Rheumatology, University Hospital, Denver, Colorado.
Musculoskeletal Diseases

Richard R. Augspurger, M.D.
Associate Clinical Professor of Surgery, Urology, University of Colorado Health Sciences Center School of Medicine, Denver; Lutheran Medical Center, St. Anthony Hospital Systems, Children's Hospital, University Hospital, Veterans Administration Medical Center, Denver; Humana Mountain View Hospital, Aurora, Colorado.
Urinary Incontinence and Catheters in the Elderly Male and Female

Eric P. Brass, M.D., Ph.D.
Associate Professor of Medicine and Pharmacology, Division of Clinical Pharmacology, Case Western Reserve University School of Medicine; University Hospitals, Cleveland, Ohio.
Drug Use

William R. Brown, M.D.
Professor of Medicine, University of Colorado Health Sciences Center School of Medicine; Head, Gastroenterology Division, University of Colorado Health Sciences Center School of Medicine; Medical Investigator, Veterans Administration Medical Center, Denver, Colorado.
Common Gastrointestinal Diseases

Ronni Chernoff, Ph.D., R.D.
Professor, Nutrition and Dietetics, College of Health Related Professions, University of Arkansas for Medical Sciences; Associate Director, Geriatric

Research Education and Clinical Center, John L. McClellan Memorial Veterans Hospital, Little Rock, Arkansas.
Nutrition

Jeffrey A. Cohen, M.D.
Assistant Professor, Department of Neurology, University of Colorado Health Sciences Center School of Medicine; Neurologist, Denver Health and Hospitals; University Hospital; Denver, Colorado.
Cerebrovascular Disease

David H. Collier, M.D.
Assistant Professor of Medicine, University of Colorado Health Sciences Center School of Medicine; Chief, Rheumatology Section, Denver Health and Hospitals, Denver, Colorado.
Musculoskeletal Diseases

E. David Crawford, M.D.
Professor and Head, Division of Urology, University of Colorado Health Sciences Center School of Medicine; University Hospital, Veterans Administration Medical Center, Denver, Colorado.
Diseases of the Prostate

Michael D. Cressman, D.O.
The Cleveland Clinic Foundation, Cleveland, Ohio.
Hypertension

Marilyn A. Davis, R.N., M.S.
Senior Instructor, Department of Surgery, University of Colorado Health Sciences Center School of Medicine, Denver, Colorado.
Diseases of the Prostate

Robert E. Donohue, M.D.
Associate Professor of Surgery (Urology), University of Colorado Health Sciences Center School of Medicine; Chief, Urology, Veterans Administration Medical Center, Denver, Colorado.
Diseases of the Prostate

Michael P. Earnest, M.D.
Professor of Neurology and Preventive Medicine, University of Colorado Health Sciences Center School of Medicine; Director of Neurology, Denver Health and Hospitals, Denver, Colorado.
Cerebrovascular Disease

Christopher M. Filley, M.D.
Assistant Professor of Neurology and Psychiatry, University of Colorado Health Sciences Center School of Medicine; Attending Neurologist, University Hospital and Veterans Administration Medical Center, Denver, Colorado.
Alzheimer's Disease and Other Dementia States

James E. Fitzpatrick, M.D.
Assistant Chief, Dermatology Service, Fitzsimons Army Medical Center, Aurora; Clinical Assistant Professor, Department of Dermatology, University of Colorado Health Sciences Center School of Medicine, Denver, Colorado.
Geriatric Dermatology

John G. Gerber, M.D.
Professor of Medicine and Pharmacology, Division of Clinical Pharmacology, University of Colorado Health Sciences Center School of Medicine; University Hospital, Denver, Colorado.
Drug Use

Ray W. Gifford, Jr., M.D.
Senior Physician, Hypertension and Nephrology; Director of Regional Health Affairs; Director, Cleveland Clinic CompreCare Affiliate Program; The Cleveland Clinic Foundation, Cleveland, Ohio.
Hypertension

Steven R. Gordon, D.M.D.
Assistant Professor, Department of Prosthodontics, Harvard School of Dental Medicine, Boston; Director of Geriatric Dentistry, Veterans Administration Medical Center, West Roxbury/Brockton, Massachusetts.
Oral and Dental Problems

Catherine E. Harmon, M.D.
Associate Professor of Medicine, Medical College of Ohio at Toledo; Acting Head, Division of Rheumatology, Medical College of Ohio at Toledo; Toledo, Ohio.
Musculoskeletal Diseases

William R. Hiatt, M.D.
Associate Professor of Medicine, Divisions of General Internal Medicine and Clinical Pharmacology, University of Colorado Health Sciences Center School of Medicine; University Hospital, Rose Medical Center, Denver, Colorado.
Peripheral Vascular Disease

Fred D. Hofeldt, M.D.
Professor of Medicine, University of Colorado Health Sciences Center School of Medicine; Chief, Endocrine Division, Denver Health and Hospitals, Denver, Colorado.
Diabetes Mellitus and Hyperlipidemic Disorders

Dennis W. Jahnigen, M.D.
Head, Section of Geriatric Medicine, Department of Internal Medicine, The Cleveland Clinic Foundation, Cleveland, Ohio.
The Physician-Patient Relationship

Palmi V. Jonsson, M.D.
Research Fellow in Geriatric Medicine, Harvard Medical School; Beth Israel Hospital, Brigham and Women's Hospital, Hebrew Rehabilitation Center for the Aged, Boston, Massachusetts.
Syncope

Abraham J. Kauvar, M.D.
Goodstein Professor of Medicine, University of Colorado Health Sciences Center School of Medicine; University Hospital, Denver, Colorado.
Preventive Medicine

Marguerite M. B. Kay
Director, Division of Geriatric Medicine, Professor of Medicine, Professor of Medical Biochemistry and Genetics, Professor of Microbiology and Immunology, Texas A & M University College of Medicine, College Station; Associate Chief of Staff for Research and Development, Olin E. Teague Veterans' Center, Temple, Texas.
Immunologic Problems

Talmadge E. King, Jr., M.D.
Associate Professor of Medicine, University of Colorado Health Sciences Center School of Medicine; Director, Cohen Clinic, National Jewish Center for Immunology and Respiratory Medicine, Denver, Colorado.
Acute and Chronic Pulmonary Disease

Andrew M. Kramer, M.D.
Associate Professor of Medicine, Associate Director, Center for Health Services Research, University of Colorado Health Sciences Center School of Medicine, Denver, Colorado.
Demographic, Social, and Economic Issues

F. Marc LaForce, M.D.
Professor of Medicine, University of Rochester School of Medicine and Dentistry; Physician-in-Chief, Genesee Hospital; Associate Attending Physician, The Strong Memorial Hospital, Rochester, New York.
Infections, Chemoprophylaxis, and Immunoprophylaxis

Roger H. S. Langston, M.D., C.M.
Program Director, Department of Ophthalmology; Cornea Service, The Cleveland Clinic Foundation, Cleveland, Ohio.
The Aging Eye

Alan E. Lazaroff, M.D.
Assistant Clinical Professor of Medicine, University of Colorado Health Sciences Center School of Medicine; Medical Director, Senior Citizens Health Center; AMI & St. Luke's Hospital, Denver, Colorado.
Ethical Issues

Moshe Levi, M.D.
Assistant Professor of Internal Medicine, University of Texas Health Science Center at Dallas Southwestern Medical School; Chief, Hemodialysis, Dallas Veterans Administration Hospital, Dallas, Texas.
Renal Disease

JoAnn Lindenfeld, M.D.
Director, Coronary Care Unit, Associate Professor of Medicine, University of Colorado Health Sciences Center School of Medicine, Denver, Colorado.
Congestive Heart Failure

David A. Lipschitz, M.D., Ph.D.
Professor of Medicine, Department of Medicine, University of Arkansas for Medical Sciences; Director, Geriatric Research Education and Clinical Center, John L. McClellan Memorial Veterans Hospital; Head, Division on Aging, University of Arkansas for Medical Sciences, Little Rock, Arkansas.
Nutrition

Lewis A. Lipsitz, M.D.
Assistant Professor of Medicine, Harvard Medical School; Director of Education and Clinical Research, Hebrew Rehabilitation Center for the Aged, Boston, Massachusetts.
Syncope

David E. Mann, M.D.
Associate Professor of Medicine, University of Colorado Health Sciences Center School of Medicine; University Hospital, Denver, Colorado.
Cardiac Arrhythmias

Frank H. Marsh, J.D., Ph.D.
Professor, Medical Ethics, University of Colorado Health Sciences Center School of Medicine; Professor of Philosophy, University of Colorado, Denver, Colorado.
Legal Issues

L. Mary Mathew, M.D.
Associate Professor of Medicine, University of Colorado Health Sciences Center School of Medicine; Director, Hospice Program, Veterans Administration Medical Center, Denver, Colorado.
Living Conditions

Robert H. Meier, III, M.D.
Associate Professor and Chairman, Department of Rehabilitation Medicine, University of Colorado Health Sciences Center School of Medicine; Chief, Rehabilitation Medicine, University Hospital, Denver, Colorado.
Mobility, Exercise, Muscular Problems, and Rehabilitation

Gordon Meiklejohn, M.D.
Professor Emeritus of Medicine, University of Colorado Health Sciences Center School of Medicine; University Hospital, Veterans Administration Medical Center, Denver Health and Hospitals, Denver, Colorado.
Infections, Chemoprophylaxis, and Immunoprophylaxis

J. Ramsey Mellette, Jr., M.D.
Chief, Dermatology Service, Fitzsimons Army Medical Center, Aurora; Clinical Assistant Professor, Department of Dermatology, University of Colorado Health Sciences Center School of Medicine, Denver, Colorado.
Geriatric Dermatology

Paul D. Miller, M.D.
Associate Clinical Professor of Medicine, University of Colorado Health Sciences Center School of Medicine, Denver, Colorado.
Osteoporosis and Other Metabolic Bone Diseases

Michael G. Moran, M.D.
Assistant Professor of Psychiatry and Medicine, University of Colorado Health Sciences Center School of Medicine; Head, Adult Psychiatry, National Jewish Center for Immunology and Respiratory Medicine, Denver, Colorado.
Depression, Suicide, and Paranoia

Gerit D. Mulder, D.P.M., M.S.
Clinical Instructor, Family Medicine, University of Colorado Health Sciences Center School of Medicine. Clinical Professor, Departments of Orthopedics and Surgery, University of Colorado Health Sciences Center School of Medicine; Assistant Chief, Podiatry; Director, Dermal Ulcer Clinic, Veterans Administration Medical Center, Denver, Colorado.
Skin Problems Associated with Pressure
Foot Disorders

Richard H. Nodar, Ph.D.
Adjunct Professor, Purdue University, Lafayette, Indiana; Kent State University, Kent, Ohio; Case Western Reserve University, School of Medicine, Cleveland, Ohio; Head, Section of Communicative Disorders, Department of Otolaryngology and Communicative Disorders, The Cleveland Clinic Foundation, Cleveland, Ohio.
Hearing Problems

Sylvia K. Oboler, M.D.
Assistant Professor of Medicine, University of Colorado Health Sciences Center School of Medicine; Assistant Chief, Ambulatory Care, Veterans Administration Medical Center, Denver, Colorado.
The Hospitalized Elderly Patient

Nancy L. Peters, M.D.
Assistant Professor of Medicine, University of Colorado Health Sciences Center School of Medicine; Medical Director, Nursing Home Care Unit, Veterans Administration Medical Center, Denver, Colorado.
Living Conditions

Judith G. Regensteiner, Ph.D.
Assistant Professor of Medicine, Division of General Internal Medicine, University of Colorado Health Sciences Center School of Medicine, Denver, Colorado.
Peripheral Vascular Disease

Laurence J. Robbins, M.D.
Associate Professor of Medicine, University of Colorado Health Sciences Center School of Medicine; Chief, Geriatrics and Associate Chief of Staff, Extended Care, Veterans Administration Medical Center, Denver, Colorado.
The Hospitalized Elderly Patient

Leonard R. Sanders, M.D.
Clinical Associate Professor, Department of Internal Medicine, Texas Tech University Health Sciences Center; Assistant Chief, Department of Medicine, William Beaumont Army Medical Center; Attending Physician, Endocrinology, R. E. Thomason General Hospital, El Paso, Texas.
Pituitary, Thyroid, Adrenal, and Parathyroid Diseases in the Elderly

Robert W. Schrier, M.D.
Professor and Chairman, Department of Medicine, University of Colorado Health Sciences Center School of Medicine, Denver, Colorado.
Demographic, Social, and Economic Issues
The Physician-Patient Relationship
Renal Disease

Paul A. Seligman, M.D.
Associate Professor of Medicine, University of Colorado Health Sciences Center School of Medicine; University Hospital, Denver, Colorado.
Hematologic and Oncologic Problems

John W. Singleton, M.D.
Professor of Medicine, University of Colorado Health Sciences Center School of Medicine, Denver, Colorado.
Management of Constipation and Diarrhea

John F. Steiner, M.D., M.P.H.
Assistant Professor of Medicine, University of Colorado Health Sciences Center School of Medicine; Attending Physician, University Hospital, Denver, Colorado.
Preventive Medicine

Earl W. Sutherland, III, M.D., Ph.D.
Associate Professor of Medicine, University of Colorado Health Sciences Center School of Medicine; Clinical Chief of Geriatrics, Denver Health and Hospitals, Denver, Colorado.
Parkinson's Disease and Other Movement Disorders

Troy L. Thompson II, M.D.
Professor and Chairman, Department of Psychiatry and Human Behavior, Jefferson Medical College of Thomas Jefferson University; Senior Attending Physician and Psychiatrist-in-Chief, Thomas Jefferson University Hospital, Philadelphia, Pennsylvania.
Depression, Suicide, and Paranoia
Sexual Disturbances

Wendy L. Thompson, M.D.
Associate Professor of Psychiatry, Jefferson Medical College of Thomas Jefferson University; Medical Staff, Thomas Jefferson University Hospital, Philadelphia, Pennsylvania.
Sexual Disturbances

John M. Vierling, M.D.
Associate Professor of Medicine, Director, Transplantation Hepatology, University of Colorado Health Sciences Center School of Medicine, Veterans Administration Medical Center, Denver, Colorado.
Hepatobiliary Disease

Eugene E. Wolfel, M.D.
Assistant Professor of Medicine, University of Colorado Health Sciences Center School of Medicine; Staff Cardiologist, Denver Health and Hospitals; Co-medical Director, Cardiovascular Rehabilitation Unit, University Hospital, Denver, Colorado.
Coronary Artery Disease

PREFACE

My wife's grandmother was virtually blind for the last several years of her life prior to her death at age 104; yet, she enjoyed flowers, trees, and all of nature in a manner as to enrich the lives of those around her. In such a relationship, it is clear that there are strengths in many of our aged population that we must strive to reveal and nurture. Our society has become so enamored of youth and physical beauty that old age is feared by many. This fear must not allow us to forget the grace, wisdom, and humanity that can only be imbued in our spirits by the experiences accrued from the passing of the years. It is likely that these spiritual qualities of older age allowed Grandma Moses to paint her famous "Christmas Eve" at the age of 100 and Michelangelo to finish his "Last Judgment" in the Sistine Chapel at age 66. George Bernard Shaw continued to write when he was in his eighties, and one of his inspirational quotations from "Back to Methuselah," which has meant much to me, is "You see things; and you say, 'Why?' But I dream things that never were; and I say 'Why not?'" The old as well as the young have the spiritual gift to dream and ask why not. As physicians, we must commit ourselves to preserve the function and health of our older citizens so that their dreams can enrich future generations.

In the play "The Elephant Man," the physician, Mr. Frederick Treves, tells John Merrick, the patient suffering from neurofibromatosis, "We cannot cure you but we can care for you." Out of that caring emerged a kindly and creative spirit that endeared John Merrick to London society, although physical beauty and good health were not his to possess. As physicians, we may be able to cure the diseases of our elderly only infrequently, but we can always project a feeling of caring to our aged patients. We must encourage our aged citizens to share with us their wisdom, courage, and spiritual strength, since these should be ingredients of the basic moral fiber of any society.

A lesson that physicians and nonphysicians alike must remember was stated by Samuel Johnson in "The Rambler": "He that would pass the latter part of life with honor and decency, must when he is young, consider that he shall one day be old and remember when he is old that he was once young."

ROBERT W. SCHRIER, M.D.

ACKNOWLEDGMENT

I want to acknowledge the excellent support of Jennifer Weber in the preparation of the manuscript. The quotations throughout the book were chosen by my wife, Barbara. In this endeavor, as in everything I undertake, her support and love have been a constant inspiration to me.

Contents

SOCIAL, ECONOMIC, AND ETHICAL ISSUES

CHAPTER 1

Demographic, Social, and Economic Issues

Andrew M. Kramer
Robert W. Schrier

It is abundantly apparent that we are not only wasting the talents of our unemployed adults and the potential of our young, but neglecting the continuing contribution of our elderly as well. And, in doing so, we are not only losing the people's faith in society's institutions, we are wasting the very life of this nation.

HUBERT HUMPHREY

Health care practitioners are confronted with unique challenges in providing care to an increasing number of older patients. For physicians in the present and even more so for those in the future, this will require greater understanding of social and economic changes that typically accompany aging in our society. This chapter considers these demographic, social, and economic issues, with particular attention given to the functional attributes of health that should be evaluated and emphasized in caring for the elderly. In addition, the chapter discusses the influence of public policy on the utilization of health care services by the elderly as well as trends for the future.

WHO ARE THE ELDERLY?

Defined in terms of chronological age the elderly usually include individuals 65 years of age and older, a group that is characterized by considerable variation in physiologic, mental, and functional capacity. It has become common to distinguish subgroups of the elderly, such as the "young old" (age 65 to 74), the "old old," "frail elderly," or "aged" (age 75 and older), and the "oldest old" or "extreme aged" (85 years of age and older), as differences in terms of demographics, health status, and utilization of health services among these subgroups have become apparent.[1-3] Dissimilarities among subgroups are often so pronounced that it can be misleading to consider the elderly as a single group. For example, approximately 5 percent of the elderly reside in nursing homes, but this includes only 2 percent of the young old, close to 7 percent of those 75 to 84 years of age, and approximately 22 percent of the oldest old.[4]

Twenty-nine million people, or 12.1 percent of the total population, were 65 years of age or older in 1986.[5] Approximately 60 percent of this group were 65 to 74, 30 percent were 75 to 84, and 10 percent were 85 years of age and older (Table 1–1). There were 50 percent more women in the over-65 age group as a whole and more than twice as many women in the over-85 age group.

This gap between the number of men and women widens in the older age groups because the average life expectancy for men who reach the age of 65 is about 4 years less than the average life expectancy for women who reach age 65 (i.e., 14.4 years and 18.8 years, respectively, in 1982).[6] One result of this widening gender differential is that approximately 79 percent of elderly men are married, in contrast to only 39 percent of elderly women.[7] More than 50 percent of elderly women are widowed. In the over-85 age group, close to half of the men are married compared with approximately 10 percent of the women.[8]

A central issue that emerges from this demographic profile is the availability of support in the home for elderly patients. Among the noninstitutionalized elderly, 39 percent of women and 14 percent of men lived alone in 1981 (Table 1–2).[7] Research suggests that there is a greater risk of institutionalization and long-term care services for the elderly living alone, and concerns exist about the potential for loneliness and isolation among these elderly persons.[9, 10] Recent surveys indicate that the majority of the elderly living at home do have children or siblings with whom they visit or have telephone contact.[11] In the 2 weeks prior to the aforementioned surveys, 73 percent of the elderly living alone had visited with relatives, 84 percent had talked with relatives on the telephone, and only 12 percent had done neither.

As suggested by the proportion of elderly who are married, 74 percent of elderly men and 36 percent of elderly women live with their spouses.[7] It is quite possible, however, that elderly spouses have limitations that hamper their ability to provide care to one another, particularly over an extended period of illness. Children, if accessible and not too elderly or disabled themselves, can provide some types of additional assistance. It has been found that among the elderly living in the community, three quarters lived within 30 minutes of the nearest child and had been visited within the previous week.[12] The remaining 12 percent of men and 25 percent of women who did not live alone or with a spouse generally lived with other relatives, most often with their children.

This demographic profile underscores the variation that exists in the social networks available to most elderly, most notably in relation to age and sex. Women predominate in all elderly age groups, particularly the oldest old, and are far more likely to be living alone. Contrary to a common concern, it appears that the majority of the elderly, including those living alone, have relatively regular contact with relatives. Whether these contacts are sufficient to provide assistance to the elderly who are infirmed or disabled, however, is uncertain. Thus, functional capacity is a major consideration in whether someone can continue to live in the community either on his or her own or with the support of a spouse or family member.

FUNCTIONAL ABILITIES OF THE ELDERLY POPULATION

Functional capacity has been increasingly recognized as an important marker

TABLE 1–1. U.S. Elderly Population by Age and Sex, 1986

Age (Years)	Population (× 1,000,000)	Percent of Elderly	Percent of Males
65+	29.3	100	40
65–74	17.2	59	44
75–84	9.2	31	31
85+	2.9	10	27

(From US Bureau of Census: Estimates of the population of the United States, by age, sex, and, race. Series P-25, No 1000. Washington, US GPO, 1987.)

TABLE 1–2. Living Arrangements of the Elderly by Age and Sex, 1981

	Male (%)	Female (%)
Living Alone		
65 and over	13.8	38.8
75 and over	19.0	45.1
Living with Spouse		
65 and over	74.1	35.5
75 and over	64.8	19.3
Living with Others		
65 and over	8.3	19.4
75 and over	9.1	23.8
Not in Household		
65 and over	3.8	6.3
75 and over	7.1	11.7

(From US Bureau of Census: Marital status and living arrangement: March 1981. Series P-20, No 372. Washington, US GPO, June 1982.)

of health status in the elderly and as an essential measure of the success of treatment for elderly patients.[13, 14] Functioning is generally measured in terms of ability to perform personal-care activities including, at a minimum, bathing, dressing, toileting, transferring, eating, and maintaining continence. These are commonly referred to as activities of daily living (ADL). Among the noninstitutionalized elderly, home-management activities (e.g., ability to perform housework, do laundry, prepare meals, shop, make telephone calls, and take medications) are also used to measure functioning and are referred to as instrumental activities of daily living (IADL).

Estimates of the proportion of elderly with ADL and IADL limitations tend to vary based on the definition of a functional limitation and to the amount of time that a functional limitation needs to exist to classify it as such. One survey of the elderly in the community in 1982 found that 19 percent of aged Medicare enrollees had one or more ADL or IADL limitations that either had lasted for 3 months or was expected to last for at least 3 months.[15] A previous national survey found functional impairment in only 9 percent of the elderly living in the community but screened only for problems that had existed for the prior 3 months.[16] In a more recent survey, it was found that 23 percent of the elderly had difficulty performing personal-care ac-

tivities, but only 10 percent received help for personal care.[17] For home management, 27 percent had difficulty performing an IADL, and 22 percent received help with one or more IADLs.

It is evident from all of these survey results that the proportion of functionally impaired elderly increases with age. For example, approximately 17 percent of the young old and 49 percent of the oldest old report having difficulty with one or more personal-care activities. Only 6 percent of the young old were receiving help for one or more personal-care activities, whereas 31 percent of the 85-year-and-older group received help with one or more personal-care activities (Fig. 1–1).

Among those with some functional impairment, approximately one fifth had only one ADL limitation (which was generally bathing, whereas eating was usually the last activity to be affected). This is consistent with Katz's original concept of the ADL index as hierarchical in that functional abilities are generally lost in a sequence of how basic the activities are to daily life.[18] Continence, which is one of the more basic activities—along with eating—was a problem in approximately one quarter of the functionally impaired elderly. Incontinence is one of the more difficult functional problems for family caregivers to manage over an extended period.

Reliance on special equipment, rather than the need for personal assistance, was the extent of the functional limitation for a large percentage of individuals dependent in bathing, toileting, transferring, and getting around inside the home.[15] Special equipment in combination with personal help was the next most frequent form of assistance in the activities related to mobility. Thus, access to and use of special equipment among functionally impaired elderly are extremely important in maintaining functional effectiveness.

Cognitive impairment can result in functional problems in activities and is also an important domain of functioning to assess in the elderly. Common indicators of cognitive functioning include awareness of time and place, knowledge of personal information, awareness of events outside of personal interaction, memory of recent past, and ability to maintain attention span. Several instruments for measuring

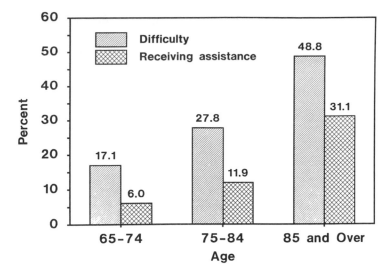

FIGURE 1–1. Percentage of elderly, by age group, having difficulty with and receiving assistance with personal care activities (bathing, dressing, eating, transferring, walking, getting outside, using toilet) because of health and physical problem, 1984. (From National Center for Health Statistics: Aging in the 80s; functional limitations of individuals age 65 years and over. Pub No (PHS) 87-1250. Hyattsville, MD, 1987.)

mental status in the elderly are available and can be administered quite easily.[14, 19] Using one such instrument, it was found that 34 percent of the elderly in the community with functional impairments had minor mental-status impairment, approximately 6 percent had moderate impairment, and less than 1 percent had severe impairment.[15] Cognitive impairment at all levels was much more common in the over-85 age group.

The elderly who reside in nursing homes are much more likely to have cognitive and functional impairments in ADLs. A 1977 national survey of nursing home residents found that 86 percent of the young old and 96 percent of the oldest old had one or more ADL impairments.[20] Approximately half of the nursing home residents were incontinent. Over 60 percent of elderly nursing home residents suffered either chronic brain syndrome or senility, both of which are probably similar to cognitive impairment.[20, 21]

Functional capacity is an important measure of health status in the elderly and a useful indicator of utilization of health care services. Maximizing functional abilities by treating specific conditions and with the use of special devices is an extremely important consideration in caring for the elderly because of the potential benefits that can accrue from enhanced functioning. Often, a small change in functional capacity can have a major impact on whether an elderly person can function effectively in a more independent living situation. At least three quarters of the

elderly in the community do not have functional limitations, and a similar proportion considers their health to be good or excellent rather than fair or poor.[6] These are cross-sectional estimates, however, that do not indicate the likelihood of whether functional disability will occur during their remaining years of life. A recent study of the elderly in Massachusetts suggested that people 65 to 69 years of age can expect to remain independent in functioning for only 10 of an expected 16.5 years of life: Those independent at 85 years of age can expect to be dependent in functioning for about half of their estimated remaining 7.5 years of life.[10] Thus, maintenance of function is an important consideration for all elderly patients.

HEALTH CARE UTILIZATION AMONG THE ELDERLY

The average person over 65 years of age uses more health care services than nonelderly individuals. Personal health care expenditures per capita (i.e., per-person average over a 1-year period) among the elderly in 1984 were $4202.[22] This level of expenditure contrasts sharply with per capita health care expenditures of $1394 for the population as a whole in 1984.[23] A substantial proportion of these expenditures is used by a relatively small percentage of the elderly population; most are more moderate users.

As indicated in Figure 1–2, close to half of the expenditures for the elderly is for

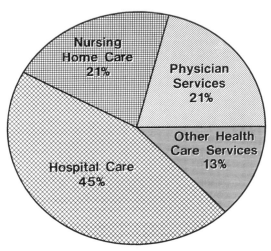

FIGURE 1–2. Percent Distribution of Personal Health Care Expenditures for the Elderly by Type of Care, 1984. (From Waldo DR, Lazenby HC: Demographic characteristics and health care use and expenditures by the aged in the United States: 1977–1984. Health Care Finan Rev, 1984.)

hospital care, which is comparable to that for the population as a whole. Physician services and nursing home care each account for approximately 20 percent of the expenditures, whereas the remaining expenditures are for dental services, for services provided by other health care practitioners, and for durable and nondurable goods. Nursing home care is a greater expense for the elderly than for younger individuals, whereas other health care services account for a larger proportion of expenditures in younger age groups.

Despite the chronicity of many of the medical conditions from which the elderly suffer, the hospital is the setting where most health care resources are consumed. In 1985, there were approximately 369 hospitalizations per thousand elderly, which was more than twice the number of hospitalizations for all ages.[24] The young old were hospitalized at a rate close to 300 admissions per thousand, whereas the 75-year-and-over age group were hospitalized at a rate close to 500 admissions per thousand. In addition, hospital stays lasted 2 to 3 days longer for elderly patients, averaging just under 9 days in 1985.

Average length of stay in the hospital, which was gradually decreasing during the 1970s, declined further following the implementation of Medicare's reimbursement system for hospital care using diagnosis-related groups (DRG). Hospital stays for the elderly averaged over 13 days in

1970, approximately 10 days in the early 1980s, and less than 9 days in 1985.[24] Since 1983, the number of hospital admissions per thousand elderly has also declined by more than 10 percent. It is too soon to determine whether declining rates of hospitalization and briefer hospital stays have had a negative effect on the quality of care received by the elderly. However, the risk of developing iatrogenic problems during hospitalization is well documented in this age group.[25, 26] In addition, if inactivity occurs during an extended hospitalization, it can delay recovery of function and strength in the elderly. Thus, fewer hospital days at the margins may prove to be beneficial if and when the hospital is not the only alternative for treating or monitoring a patient.

Nursing homes provide an important modality of care for the elderly both as a short-term transition facility for rehabilitation and subacute nursing care and as a long-term residental alternative for individuals with pronounced functional and chronic care needs. The length of stay for those admitted to nursing homes forms a bimodal distribution. The short-stay group, which accounts for about half of nursing home admissions, are those in residence for up to 90 days. The long-stay group has an average length of stay of well over a year.[27, 28] These two groups represent the two uses of nursing homes, with short-stay patients much more likely to be discharged than long-stay patients.[29] It is important to remember that although approximately 5 percent of the elderly population reside in nursing homes at this time, a much larger percentage will spend some portion of their lifetime in an institution.[30] Those 65 years of age and older can expect to average about 1 year in an institution during their remaining lifetime, and more if they are currently residing in a nursing home.

The term nursing home is used to describe a range of facilities. Some focus on short-term care, which may be covered by Medicare under the skilled nursing facility (SNF) benefit. Such care is often provided in hospital-based facilities (i.e., those affiliated with an acute care hospital) as well as in more typical community-based nursing homes. In rural areas, acute care hospitals can provide nursing home care in hospital beds, called swing beds, which generally are used for short-stay patients requiring transitional care. The majority of nursing homes, however, provide services for chronic care. As discussed below, such care is generally funded out-of-pocket, unless the individual is eligible for Medicaid. Other facilities that may be considered nursing homes also exist and provide residential care, with nursing care available to varying degrees.

Physician care is one of the more rapidly expanding components of care for the elderly. A relatively large percentage of physician visits occur in the hospital, including those related to surgery and daily patient rounds. However, in 1986, the average patient 65 to 74 years old had over eight contacts with a physician in an ambulatory care setting, and the average patient 75 years old and older had over 10.[31] Multiple diagnoses were given for over half of the office visits among those 75 years of age and older.[32] The most common were essential hypertension, chronic ischemic heart disease, diabetes mellitus, osteoarthritis, and cataracts.

Other health care expenditures included dental care provided to approximately 30 percent of the elderly over a 1-year period.[22] Prescribed medications, used by 75 percent of the elderly over a 1-year period, were also a significant portion of these other expenditures, with an average of 10 prescriptions per person. Home health care, which is probably the most rapidly expanding health service for the elderly, is also a major expenditure. Generally, home care is provided on a short-term basis (i.e., less than 12 visits per episode on average). Owing to the nature of reimbursement for home care, it is focused on skilled nursing and rehabilitation services. Medical equipment was also an important component of other health care expenditures, with close to 15 percent of the elderly making at least one purchase or rental over a 1-year period.

PAYMENT FOR THE ELDERLY'S HEALTH CARE

Public policy has more control over health care for the elderly than for other age groups because public payers cover approximately two thirds of their personal health care costs (Fig. 1–3). This propor-

tion of publicly funded health care for the elderly exists largely because of the Medicare program, which covers almost half of their health care costs. Medicaid, a program designed to cover health care for the poor, pays for another 13 percent of the elderly's care because many of the elderly are also poor. Private funding for health care is mainly an out-of-pocket expense because private insurance coverage for the elderly is limited.

The Medicare program was enacted into law in 1965 as Tittle XVIII of the Social Security Act to cover health care costs for the elderly and physically disabled. The hospital insurance part of the Medicare program covers inpatient hospital care, post-hospital skilled nursing facility (SNF) care, and home health care. The supplemental medical insurance portion covers medical services and supplies furnished by physicians, outpatient hospital clinics, and other health care professionals (e.g., physical therapists, speech therapists). Approximately 97 percent of the elderly are enrolled in Medicare, excluding only those who did not pay into the Social Security program and those who receive Veterans' Administration benefits (see further on). A monthly premium of about $25, however, is required to receive the supplemental medical insurance benefits and is paid by a majority of Medicare enrollees.

Although two thirds of Medicare enrollees used some type of services in 1984, approximately 2 percent of enrollees accounted for one third of the reimbursements, and 8 per cent accounted for two thirds of the reimbursements.[22] Thus, the use of Medicare funds is concentrated among a relatively few beneficiaries. The oldest old had higher use rates (73 percent) and average costs per user ($2960) than did younger age groups (use rate of 60 percent and average cost per user of $2172 among those aged 65 to 74).

It is not surprising that a significant portion of Medicare expenditures for the elderly occur in the last year of life. In 1978, the elderly who died that year represented 6 percent of Medicare enrollees, but consumed 28 percent of Medicare expenditures.[33] Another way of looking at this is that Medicare reimbursements for users who died were 4 times as high on average as Medicare reimbursements for

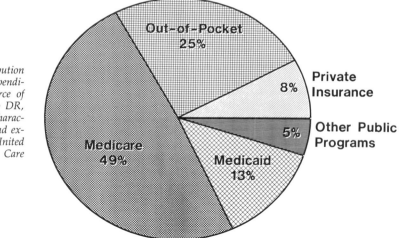

FIGURE 1–3. Percent Distribution of Personal Health Care Expenditures for the Elderly by Source of Payment, 1984. (From Waldo DR, Lazenby HC: Demographic characteristics and health care use and expenditures by the aged in the United States: 1977–1984. Health Care Finan Rev, 1984.)

users who survived. Almost half of the expenditures used in the last year of life occurred in the last 60 days of life. These expenditure patterns and other quality-of-life concerns about treatment for dying patients prompted Medicare to cover hospice care under the Supplemental Medical Insurance benefit in the early 1980s.

Hospital insurance benefits under Medicare are tied to a benefit period that begins with hospital admission and ends after the beneficiary has been out of the hospital or nursing home for 60 consecutive days. The most dramatic change in the Medicare program since its inception occurred in 1983, when reimbursement according to DRGs was initiated for hospital care, in contrast to reimbursement based on hospital reported costs. The amount of payment under the DRG system is determined by the DRG into which a patient is classified, and to a lesser extent, by the hospital's cost per admission and other hospital characteristics (e.g., location and type of hospital). Under this system, the same payment is provided to the hospital regardless of the length or cost of stay, resulting in a clear incentive for hospitals to contain costs and discharge patients as soon as medically possible.

Medicare covers only approximately 2 percent of total nursing home care costs because of both the relatively short benefit period for SNF care (150 days) and the restrictions on eligibility. Medicare's home health benefit now accounts for three times as much Medicare funding as the SNF benefit owing to its rapid growth in

the past several years. The Medicare home health benefit emphasizes skilled care, with the resulting home health care population including patients with pronounced subacute care needs but fewer functional and personal care needs than the nursing home population.[34] The implementation of the DRG system has stimulated the growth of home health care and SNF care and increased the intensity of needs among patients receiving these services.[35]

Supplemental medical insurance benefits are available after an annual deductible of $75 is paid. Medicare pays physicians an amount equal to 80 percent of reasonable and customary charges. Beneficiaries are responsible for the remaining 20 percent of the allowed charge as well as the difference between the total charges and the Medicare-allowed charges, unless the physician accepts Medicare assignment. Medicare beneficiaries are also liable for the cost of goods and services not covered by the program, such as long-term care, routine or preventive medical and dental care, and eye glasses.

Medicaid covers a number of health care costs for the elderly that are not covered by Medicare, if an individual meets the income eligibility requirements. Medicaid was established in 1966 as Title XIX of the Social Security Act and is administered by each state under broad federal guidelines. The program provides health care to the poor, with the elderly representing slightly more than 15 percent of all Medicaid recipients but accounting for 40 percent of program payments. This is largely because Medicaid is the major payer for long-term nursing home care, covering 42 percent of nursing home expenses.

The elderly who do not qualify for Medicaid must pay Medicare copayments, reasonable charge reductions, and care not covered by Medicare. Although private health insurance, called "medi-gap" insurance, is available largely to cover deductible and coinsurance costs, it generally has the same limits on service and length of stay as Medicare. Thus, most of the other expenses for the elderly are paid out-of-pocket, although over half of the aged population has private insurance coverage. Owing to the limitations of Medicare, Congress recently enacted an expansion of medical benefits in the Catastrophic Coverage Act of 1988. This increased the SNF benefit and provides coverage for prescribed medications, among other changes.

The Veterans' Administration provides care through VA Medical Centers, including 172 hospitals, associated outpatient clinics, and over 100 nursing home units. The average age of veterans is increasing more rapidly than for the population as a whole, so geriatrics is a major consideration in VA health care.

Because of Social Security and Medicare, there has been considerable improvement in the past two decades in the financial well-being of the elderly and their access to health care services. In 1982, the median income in households headed by an elderly person was $11,000, and 17 percent of such households had incomes under $5000.[22] Third-party reimbursement (e.g., Medicare, Medicaid, private insurance) has reduced the relationship between income and use of health care services to such an extent that cost of service is generally not a consideration for the elderly in health care use. Thus, providers and health care policy play the major role in determining the types of services and amount of services that the elderly receive.

TRENDS FOR THE FUTURE

Over the next 50 years, the elderly population is expected to double, whereas the total population is expected to increase by about only 35 percent.[36] Thus, the elderly

are expected to make up close to 20 percent of the total population by the year 2030 (Fig. 1–4). Growth will be moderate until approximately 2010, when the "baby boom" generation will become seniors. At this point, an increase in the proportion of young old will begin, followed by an increase in the proportion of the old old in the 2020s, and an increase in the proportion of the oldest old in the 2030s.

Such projections are obviously based on assumptions about trends in fertility, immigration rates, and mortality extrapolated from historical data that may not necessarily prove to be true. All estimates suggest that there will be a constant increase in life expectancy for both men and women through the year 2050, resulting in a greater percentage of the elderly reaching advanced ages in the future. There is considerable variation, however, in the rate at which life expectancy is projected to increase, leading the Social Security Administration to provide three series of figures, with a wide range as an uncertainty interval.[36] According to the second of the three series, a 65-year-old man is expected to live 3 years longer, and a 65-year-old women is expected to live about 4 years longer by the year 2050 (i.e., average life expectancy of 82 years and 88 years, respectively). Past projections have generally underestimated the rate of increase in life expectancy, so these projections or even the higher projections made in the other series are most probable.

Although life expectancy has increased substantially during this century and is projected to continue to increase more gradually in the future, controversy exists over whether the human life span (i.e., maximum survival potential) is actually increasing. It has been suggested that the human life span is fixed, and that as morbidity is postponed until the very end of the life span, we are approaching a time when the elderly will be living more vigorous and less dependent lives until the point of natural death.[37] The evidence in recent years, however, challenges this theory. Mortality rates among the oldest old are declining significantly, but the incidence of chronic illness and disability in the aged does not appear to be declining.[38, 39] Hence, although we should continue to work toward preventing or postponing the onset of disabling chronic

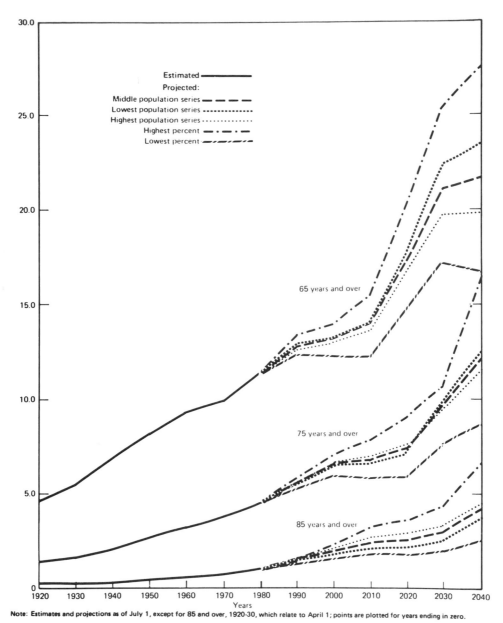

Note: Estimates and projections as of July 1, except for 85 and over, 1920-30, which relate to April 1; points are plotted for years ending in zero.

FIGURE 1–4. Percent of the total population in the older ages: 1920–2040. (From US Bureau of the Census: Demographics and socioeconomic aspects of the aging in the United States. Series P–23 No 138. Washington DC, 1984.)

disease, society must be prepared to meet the long-term health care needs of a growing number of disabled elderly.[40, 41]

What are the implications of this change in demographics for the health care system and health care costs? If the age and gender mix projected for the year 2026 were imposed on the 1986 health care system, total expenditures for health care would increase by about 25 percent over current levels.[42] Although an increasing percentage of health care dollars will be spent on

the elderly, the projected demographic change does not necessarily mean that the United States will spend an increasing share of the gross national product (GNP) on health. Using different scenarios for economic growth and change in intensity of service use, it was found that demographics is not the most important factor in determining health care expenditures and that GNP growth is projected to offset any rise in spending. Thus, if health care expenditures rise as a share of the GNP, it will be a result of other factors as well as demographics.

In view of the influence of service use patterns on costs of health care, in recent years there has been an emphasis on cost containment, particularly in publicly funded health care programs. Reform of Medicare reimbursement for hospital care was intended as a first step. Other modifications in Medicare reimbursement are under consideration for both nursing home care and physician services, with an emphasis on capitation (i.e., fixed payment for a period of health care provision).

As the elderly population increases, however, emphasis must be given to programs that integrate health care services and expand alternatives to institutional care. Hospice programs, noninstitutional long-term care, and various types of residential care are gradually being investigated through demonstration programs or are being implemented in larger statewide or national programs. Optimal care for geriatric patients, particularly those with chronic conditions and disabilities, requires the involvement of all health care providers. Physicians will have to play an active role if new approaches to old problems are to be used.

SUMMARY AND CONCLUSIONS

- The elderly are a heterogeneous group in terms of availability of social supports, health status, and use of services.
- Functioning is one of the more critical issues for the elderly because it has a profound influence on where individuals can live, the amount of support that they require, and their quality of life.
- As a group, the elderly are the largest users of health care services, although high use is concentrated in a relatively small proportion of the elderly population.
- Payment for most health care services for the elderly is provided through public programs, particularly Medicare, with the result that providers and policies have a major influence on the amount and type of health care service use.

- Although the number and proportion of the elderly are expected to increase dramatically over the next 50 years, demographics is only one of several factors influencing health care costs and will not necessarily require health care to consume an increasing share of the GNP.
- Demographic trends, growing knowledge of geriatric care, and policy changes intended to contain health care costs are gradually stimulating necessary consideration and development of alternative delivery systems for the elderly.

REFERENCES

1. Suzman R, Riley MW: Introducing the "oldest old." Milbank Q 63:2 1985.
2. US Bureau of the Census: America in transition: an aging society. Series P-23, No 128. Washington, US GPO, 1983.
3. Streib GF: The frail elderly: research dilemmas and research opportunities. Gerontologist 23:40, 1983.
4. National Center for Health Statistics: the national nursing home survey: 1977 Summary for the United States. Series 13, No 43. Washington, US GPO, 1979.
5. US Bureau of Census: estimates of the population of the United States, by age, sex, and race: 1980 to 1986. Series P-25, No 1000. Washington, US GPO, 1987.
6. National Center for Health Statistics: Health, United States, 1983. (PHS)84-1232. Washington, US GPO 1983.
7. US Bureau of Census: Marital status and living arrangements: March 1981. Series P-20, No 372. Washington, US GPO, June 1982.
8. Rosenwaike I: A demographic portrait of the oldest old. Milbank Q 63:2, 1985.
9. Branch LG, Jette AM: A prospective study of long-term care institutionalization among the aged. Am J Public Health 72:1373, 1982.
10. Katz S, Branch LG, Branson MH, et al: Active life expectancy. N Engl J Med 309:1218, 1983.
11. National Center for Health Statistics, Kovar MG, ed: Aging in the 80s, age 65 years and over and living alone, contact with family, friends, and neighbors. (PHS)86-1250. Hyattsville, MD, Public Health Service, May 1986.
12. Shanas E. National survey of the aged: final report. Chicago, University of Illinois at Chicago Circle, 1977, pp 24–26.
13. Rowe JW: Health care of the elderly. N Engl J Med 312:827, 1985.
14. Kane RA, Kane RL: Assessing the elderly: a practical guide to measurement. Lexington, MA, Lexington Books, 1981, pp 25–67.
15. Macken CL: A profile of functionally impaired elderly persons living in the community. Health Care Finan Rev 7:33, Summer 1986.
16. Feller BA: Americans needing help to function at

home. (PHS)83-1250. Public Health Services, September 1983.

17. National Center for Health Statistics, Dawson D, Hendershot G, Fulton J, eds: Aging in the 80s: functional limitations of individuals age 65 years and over. (PHS)87-1250. Hyattsville, MD, Public Health Service, June 1987.

18. Katz S, Ford AB, Moskowitz RW: Studies of illness in the aged: the index of ADL: a standardized measure of biological and psychosocial function. JAMA 184:914, 1963.

19. Pfeiffer E: A short portable mental status questionnaire for the assessment of organic brain deficit in elderly patients. J Am Geriatr Soc 23:433, 1975.

20. National Center for Health Statistics: Characteristics of nursing home residents, health status, and care received: national nursing home survey United States, May–December 1977. Series 13, No 51. (PHS)81–1712. Hyattsville, MD, Public Health Service, 1981.

21. Reisberg B: Alzheimer's Disease: the standard reference. New York, Free Press, 1983, p 8.

22. Waldo DR, Lazenby HC; Demographic characteristics and health care use and expenditures by the aged in the United States: 1977–1984. Health Care Finan Rev 6:1, 1984.

23. Levit KR, Lazenby H, Waldo D: National health expenditures, 1984. Health Care Finan Rev 7:1, 1985.

24. National Center for Health Statistics, Moss AJ, Moien MA, eds: Recent declines in hospitalization, United States, 1982–1986. (PHS)87-1250. Hyattsville, MD, Public Health Service, September 1987.

25. Jahnigen D, Hannon C, Laxon L, et al: Iatrogenic disease in hospitalized elderly veterans. J Am Geriatr Soc 30:387, 1982.

26. Reichel W: Complications in the care of five hundred elderly hospitalized patients. J Am Geriatric Soc 13:973, 1965.

27. Keeler EB, Kane RL, Solomon DH: Short- and long-term residents of nursing homes. Med Care 19:363, 1981.

28. Liu K, Mento KG: The characteristics and utilization pattern of an admission cohort of nursing home patients (11). Gerontologist 24:70, 1984.

29. National Center for Health Statistics, Sekscenski ES, ed: Discharges from nursing homes: preliminary data from the 1985 National Nursing Home Survey. (PHS)87-1250. Hyattsville, MD, Public Health Service, September 1987.

30. Kastenbaum R, Candy SE: The 4-percent following: a methodological and empirical critique of extended care facility population statistics. Int J Aging Hum Dev 4:15, 1973.

31. National Center for Health Statistics, Dawson DA, Adams PF, eds: Current estimates from the National Health Interview Survey, United States, 1986. Series 10, No 164. (PHS)86-1592. Washington, US GPO, October 1987.

32. National Center for Health Statistics, Koch H, Smith MC, eds: Office-based ambulatory care for patients 75 years old and over, national ambulatory medical care survey, 1980 and 1981. (PHS)85-1250. Hyattsville, MD, Public Health Service, August 1985.

33. Lubitz J, Prihoda R; The use and costs of Medicare services in the last two years of life. Health Care Finan Rev 5:117, 1984.

34. Kramer AM, Shaughnessy PW, Pettigrew ML: Cost effectiveness implications based on a comparison of nursing home and home health case mix. Health Serv Res 20:387, 1985.

35. Shaughnessy PW, Kramer AM, Pettigrew ML: Case mix and quality of care in nursing homes and home health agencies. Denver, University of Colorado, 1987, p 111.1–111.26.

36. US Bureau of the Census: Demographics and socioeconomic aspects of aging in the United States. Series P-23, No 138. Washington, US GPO 1984.

37. Fries JF: Aging, natural death, and the compression of morbidity. N Engl J Med 303:130, 1980.

38. Schneider EL, Brody JA: Aging, natural death and the compression of morbidity: another view. N Engl J Med 309:854, 1983.

39. Manton KG: Changing concepts of morbidity and mortality in the elderly population. Milbank Q 60:183, 1982.

40. Schatzken A: How long can we live?: a more optimistic view of potential gians in life expectancy. Am J Public Health 70:1199, 1980.

41. New York State Office for the Aging: Family caregiving and the elderly, policy recommendations and research findings. Albany, New York State Office for the Aging, March 1983.

42. Office of the Actuary, Health Care Financing Administration: National health expenditures, 1986–2000. Health Care Finan Rev 8:1, 1987.

CHAPTER 2
Ethical Issues

Alan E. Lazaroff

What makes old age so sad is, not that our joys but that our hopes cease.

JEAN PAUL RICHTER, *Titan*

Modern scientific medicine offers great benefits to the elderly, but its application to this group is especially problematic. The prevalence of chronic illness and functional impairment, the proximity of inevitable death, and the variable prognosis of chronic disease are factors that complicate decision making about the elderly. Often, the benefits of treatment are relatively modest and the burdens relatively great. Although a high degree of skill in diagnosis and therapy remains the prerequisite for excellent medical care, such skill alone is not sufficient to guide the decision making of everyday geriatric practice.

MEDICAL DECISION MAKING

Medical decision making incorporates two complementary basic principles.[1] The principle of *beneficence* obliges the physician to act at all times to promote the well-being of his patient and to cause no harm. Well-being can be promoted, for example, by treatment that prolongs life, prevents or relieves suffering, or preserves or improves function. Except as constrained by law and by realities such as cost containment, the physician's obligation is to each individual patient, precluding actions that sacrifice the patient's interests for any reason, including the goals of science and society. Since the results of any medical intervention are uncertain, and since an intervention may promote one goal (such as prolonging life) while frustrating the achievement of another (e.g., relieving suffering), it is often difficult to meet the obligation of beneficence.

Beneficence provided the ethical basis for the paternalistic model that historically described the relationship between physician and patient. Because medical decisions are so complex, it was held that only the physician possessed the knowledge and judgment required to make them. The patient placed himself in the hands of the wise and beneficent physician, reserving for himself little, if any, decision-making authority. In the prescientific era, when the physician had little ability to influence the course of disease, such empowerment may have been a crucial element of the therapeutic relationship.

An infusion of ideas from outside the field of medicine, derived in part from the writings of social philosophers such as Kant and Mill, has contributed to a more balanced model of decision making. The principle of *autonomy* asserts the value of permitting each person to exercise control over his own life, and embodies respect for his values and preferences. Both legal doctrine and ethical thought place ultimate decision-making authority with the patient and not with the physician. Patient autonomy is not without limits, however. The physician is not obliged to provide useless or dangerous treatment demanded by a patient, or to act illegally or unethically in other ways. Also, when resources are limited, no patient has an absolute claim on their use.

Patients lack the factual knowledge that they need to make decisions and must rely upon physicians to provide it. Physicians lack a knowledge of the beliefs and preferences of patients; such factors may influence profoundly the relative merits of treatment alternatives for the individual. Good decision making, therefore, is a shared responsibility, requiring the participation of both the beneficent physician and the autonomous patient.

INFORMED CONSENT

The doctrine of informed consent provides for shared decision making, incorporating both beneficence and autonomy.[2] The patient decides whether to be a patient, chooses the physician, and accepts or rejects a course of action proposed by the physician. The physician assesses the patient and his problems, explains the medical facts, makes recommendations, describes alternatives, and estimates benefits and risks.

Believing his advice to be sound, the physician will urge his patient to accept it, but consent must be voluntary, not coerced. With few exceptions, legally, an individual cannot be forced to accept medical advice, no matter how strong the indications or how dire the anticipated consequences of refusal. (Cases in which legal intervention to force involuntary treatment may be appropriate include patients with communicable diseases whose refusal of treatment would endanger others; possibly, patients whose refusal would pose an undue burden on society or dependents; patients who lack decision-making capacity.)

The doctrine of informed consent is a valuable standard for decision making. Unfortunately, most attention has been directed toward minimal technical requirements, such as consent forms for surgical procedures. Many physicians express appropriate skepticism about the value of this limited version of informed consent.

DECISION-MAKING INCAPACITY

Patient participation in decision making requires the ability to comprehend information, to reason, and to communicate preferences.[3] The elderly patient may lack such capacity because of dementia, delirium, stroke, coma, or severe psychiatric illness. Such incapacity is invariably a consequence of disease, not an attribute of age.

The need to assess decision-making capacity is frequent in geriatric practice. The fact that the patient is uncooperative or makes a "bad" decision is not evidence of incapacity. Such a determination should be made only in the demonstrable absence of "the *ability* to make decisions that promote his well-being in conformity with his own values and preferences" (emphasis added).[3] Thus it is the integrity of the decision-making "machinery," rather than the content of decisions, that must be evaluated. A thorough medical assessment, including careful mental status examination, is mandatory, but ultimately decision-making capacity must be judged by a common sense standard focused on the patient's ability to make the particular decision at issue.

Except in the comatose patient, incapacity is seldom absolute. Patient participation may be possible to varying degrees in some, if not all, decisions and should be respected and encouraged.

SURROGATE DECISION MAKING

When incapacity precludes patient participation in decision making, autonomy should be respected by identifying a surrogate who can represent the patient. In most cases, the most appropriate surrogate will be found among family members, who are more likely than others to be familiar with the patient's attitudes and to promote his interests. However, family members may disagree, may be unfamiliar with or unsympathetic to the patient's values, or may be motivated by self-interest. Thus, although consultation with family members is the usual recourse in the event of patient incapacity, this informal approach is sometimes inadequate.[4]

More formal methods, such as the living will or the durable power of attorney, permit a measure of advance direction by the patient.[5-7] Finally, the courts may appoint a guardian to act as surrogate decision maker.

Surrogate decision makers must act in a principled fashion.[3] Under the preferred "substituted judgment" standard, the surrogate will decide to act as the patient would, were he able to do so. Adherence to this standard is possible only when the patient's wishes are known, preferably explicitly and in writing. If such evidence is absent, as is common, a "best interests" standard must be used, whereby the surrogate will act as the "average person" would. Surrogate decisions cannot carry the same ethical force as contemporaneous decisions made by an informed competent adult. Highly idiosyncratic decisions by a surrogate may require mediation by an institutional ethics committee or even recourse to the judicial system.

SPECIAL SITUATIONS

The aforementioned methods of decision making are applicable to most clinical circumstances. A few special situations have been the subject of exceptional interest and controversy, and so are given further attention.

Cardiopulmonary Resuscitation

Cardiopulmonary resuscitation (CPR) was developed in the 1960s for use in sudden, unexpected life-threatening emergencies, but increasingly, its subsequent clinical application has reflected a "positive obligation" to employ it in all cases, unless a decision not to do so has been reached in advance.[8] The presumption in favor of CPR is consistent with respect for life in circumstances in which it is impossible for the patient to give (or refuse) consent. The presumption is unique in that medical judgment is not consulted as to the advisability of administering the treatment. Many physicians and lay persons believe that CPR is attempted too often in settings where it is not in the patient's best interest.

Cardiopulmonary resuscitation usually fails, especially outside of defined circumstances such as ventricular fibrillation in the coronary care unit.[9] Survivors may experience serious morbidity, including hypoxic encephalopathy, fractured ribs, and cardiac contusions. For many who survive initially, death is postponed for only hours or days, in an intensive care unit, encumbered by resuscitators, catheters, and monitors.

Since CPR fails to promote well-being in many patients, we are obliged to define the circumstances in which it will not be attempted. The balancing principles of beneficence and autonomy are applicable, but because contemporaneous decision making is impossible, discussions must be carried out in advance. Many patients appreciate the opportunity to deal with the issue before the development of serious illness; such discussions can promote a bond of trust with the physician and serve to allay patient fears. In the event of approaching death, discussions about CPR are more difficult for both patient and physician but generally should be attempted within the context of a supportive relationship. A surrogate decision maker should be consulted when incapacity precludes patient participation, as frequently occurs. Relevant issues include the nature of the underlying disease, its prognosis and effect on function and quality of life, the likelihood of successful resuscitation, and the anticipated quality of survival should CPR succeed.

Many institutions have adopted policies and procedures for CPR decisions.[10] In general, orders not to administer CPR should be written, should be given only after discussion with the patient or surrogate and documented in the medical record, and should be unambiguous. An order not to resuscitate carries no implication regarding the appropriateness of other treatment measures.

Artificial Feeding and Hydration

The provision of food and water to avoid hunger and thirst is a basic obligation that transcends specifically medical responsibility. The use of artificial techniques to treat transient and reversible loss of the ability to eat and drink generates little controversy. When such loss is permanent, a difficult ethical dilemma is encountered. Few physicians would insist that technological interventions such as CPR, assisted ventilation, dialysis, and transplantation be provided to every patient who may "need" them, but some view artificial feeding as fundamentally different.[11]

Artificial feeding is invasive and involves risk, discomfort, and cost.[12, 13] Parenteral nutrition requires insertion and maintenance of central venous catheters, with attendant risks such as pneumothorax and sepsis. Nasogastric feeding often leads to aspiration. Nasogastric tubes are uncomfortable (although smaller tubes are less so) and are frequently removed by patients, necessitating reinsertion, possibly by inadequately trained personnel, especially in long-term care facilities. We prefer gastrostomy tubes, but these require surgical or endoscopic placement and can be complicated by leakage, infection, or aspiration.

Elderly patients for whom permanent artificial feeding is a consideration usually suffer from neurologic disorders, including advanced dementia or Parkinson's disease, coma, or the residua of stroke. Though artificial feeding may prolong survival in such patients, few regain any semblance of good health and most will succumb to other complications such as pneumonia, pressure sores, or urosepsis. It is also far from clear that suffering resulting from hunger and thirst is experienced by such patients.

A consensus is emerging, supported by court decisions, that artificial feeding does not differ in any fundamental respect from other medical treatment and can be addressed according to the same ethical principles.[13, 14] Consultation with a surrogate decision maker is nearly always needed, since such patients usually lack decision-making capacity. Relevant issues are similar to those involved in resuscitation decisions.

Dementia and Intercurrent Illness

Advanced dementia is characterized by the loss of functional abilities such as walking and eating, lack of self-awareness, loss of recognition of family members, markedly impaired or absent communication skills, and the inability to interact with and influence the external environment. Intercurrent illnesses (e.g., pneumonia or urosepsis) often occur. Although readily treatable, sometimes such episodes are not treated because intervention may not be felt to offer meaningful benefit. Such non-treatment decisions usually have not been reached by careful ethical analysis.

When treatment cannot relieve suffering or enhance function, prolonging life is the remaining rationale for intervention. Few would argue that the obligation to sustain life is absolute, for to do so would demand administering any treatment with the remotest chance of success, whatever the cost in human suffering. It is therefore necessary to develop principles that can identify circumstances in which the prolongation of life is no longer an ethical obligation.[15]

Assessing the quality of life of another person is difficult, and decisions based on such a standard may be capricious, particularly when made by the young and healthy. Human beings, including physicians, are capable of egregious violations of humane behavior in making such assessments, when not guided by carefully articulated ethical principles.[16]

Loewy has proposed that we view life not as an intrinsic "good" but as a necessary but not sufficient condition for experience.[17] The capacity for self-awareness, thought, and social interaction are the characteristics that give meaning to our biologic existence. When such characteristics are irretrievably lost, the primary obligation to sustain life ceases.

Decisions not to intervene in readily treatable intercurrent illness should be made very cautiously, after careful consideration of the benefits and burdens of treatment in consultation with a surrogate decision maker, and only in the case of a very severely and permanently impaired patient.

CONCLUSION

Before the era of scientific medicine, the physician had little of a tangible nature to offer patients. His ministrations had little ability to produce either benefit or harm. Near mystical faith in the healer was perhaps central to the effectiveness of "treatment." Paternalism was not only appropriate, but necessary.

Science has given the physician the power to influence events. The physician must accept the burden of the judicious use of such power. Respect for the rights of patients and careful consideration of the effects of proposed intervention are important now as never before.

Ethics can never order that particular decisions be made, but only provide tools for making them. By use of a rational and ethical decision-making process, we can enhance our ability to further the humane goals of our profession.

REFERENCES

1. President's Commission for the Study of Ethical Problems in Medicine and Biomedical and Behavioral Research: Making health care decisions. Washington, US GPO, 1982.
2. Marsh FH: Informed consent and the elderly patient: Clin Geriatr Med 2:3, 1986.
3. President's Commission for the Study of Ethical Problems in Medicine and Biomedical and Behavioral Research: Deciding to forego life-sustaining treatment. Chap 4. Washington, US GPO 1983.
4. Areen J: The legal status of consent obtained from families of adult patients to withhold or withdraw treatment. JAMA 258:2, 1987.
5. Society for the Right to Die: The physician and the hopelessly ill patient. New York, Society for the Right Die, 1985.
6. Lazaroff AE, Orr WF: Living wills and other advance directives. Clin Geriatr Med 2:3, 1986.
7. Steinbrook R, Lo B: Decision making for incompetent patients by designating proxy. N Engl J Med 310:24, 1984.
8. National Conference on Cardiopulmonary Resuscitation and Emergency Cardiac Care: Standards and guidelines for cardiopulmonary resuscitation and emergency cardiac care. JAMA, 244:504, 1980.
9. Bedell SE, Delbanco TL, Cook EF, et al: Survival after cardiopulmonary resuscitation in the hospital. New Engl J Med 309:10, 1983.
10. President's Commission for the Study of Ethical Problems in Medicine and Biomedical and Behavioral Research: Deciding to forego life-sustaining treatment, Appendix I. Washington, US GPO, 1983.
11. Siegler M, Weisbard AJ: Against the emerging stream: Should fluids and nutritional support be discontinued? Arch Intern Med 145:129, 1985.
12. Ciocon JO, Silverstone FA, Graver LM, et al: Tube feedings in elderly patients: indications, benefits, and complications. Arch Intern Med 148:429, 1988.
13. Dresser RS, Boisaubin EV Jr: Ethics, law and nutritional support. Arch Intern Med 145:122, 1985.
14. Lo B, Dornebrand L: Guiding the hand that feeds: caring for the demented elderly. New Engl J Med 311:6, 1984.
15. Braithwaite S, Thomasma DC: New guidelines on foregoing life-sustaining treatment in incompetent patients: an anti-cruelty policy. Ann Intern Med 104:711, 1986.
16. Lifton RJ: The Nazi Doctors. New York, Basic Books Inc, 1986.
17. Loewy EH: Treatment decisions in the mentally impaired: limiting but not abandoning treatment. New Engl Med 317:23, 1987.

CHAPTER 3

Legal Issues

Frank H. Marsh

When the body is assailed by the force of time,
And the limbs weaken from exhausted strength,
The mind breaks down, and thought and speech fail.
(Ubi jam validis quassatum est viribus ævi
Corpus et obtusis ceciderunt viribus artus,
Claudicat ingenium delirat lingua, labat mens.)
　　　　　　　　LUCRETIUS, *de Rerum Natura*

A major concern of most elderly people is the loss of independence and control over matters they deem important in their lives. This is particularly true in cases involving the sick and disabled elderly patient. In these situations, there is a tendency on the part of some physicians to use advanced age as a qualifying factor in determining the ability to participate in the decision-making process and to give an effective, informed consent or refusal to treatment. Whereas the right of autonomy in medical decision-making exists with the elderly patient, exercising that right is often difficult because of the "presumed" incompetence by the physician. Often, there is a general failure on the part of the physician to significantly understand the concept of patient competency and the weight assigned to it by law.

DETERMINING PATIENT COMPETENCY

The physician should recognize in his approach to decisions regarding the appropriate course of action for the patient that the elderly patient is vested with a "presumption of competency."[11] This presumption is conferred by law and undergirds the principle of patient autonomy. Unfortunately, some physicians start from a qualified position that the elderly patient may or may not be competent. This approach commits the physician to the task of ascertaining if the patient is, in fact,

competent. In doing so, the physician needlessly assumes the burden of overcoming the patient's presumption of competency and demonstrating that the patient is incompetent. However, by accepting the legal principle, the physician can avoid the difficult and time-consuming task, which often includes an unpleasant confrontation with the patient and his family.

Only after the physician has been alerted by a "warning flag" should the presumption of competency be seriously questioned and, perhaps, challenged. For example, whereas a patient's refusal to accept recommended treatment that is necessary for his well-being is *not* evidence of incompetence, it would support an inquiry by the physician into the extent of the patient's capacity to understand the particular information being disclosed to him. Such an inquiry may then lead to the conclusion that the patient is, in fact, unable to comprehend in any informed sense the nature of his illness, the prognosis, and the appropriateness of the proposed course of action.

The physician should also move cautiously in those cases in which the patient simply agrees to go along with the treatment being proposed. A consent to treatment here may very well be a consent, but one that is uninformed. Such a situation may occur, for example, when the patient is depressed or feels helpless, and the physician and family are in accord as to the proposed treatment. The patient may simply agree with the family, yet, if questioned, would be unable to give informed reasons for his consent. This sort of consent in most cases would fall short of the required standard of care.[4]

The primary responsibility for determining if a patient is incompetent and lacks the capacity to make an informed decision rests solely with the physician.[10] This is an extension of the legal dictate that the sole responsibility for obtaining informed consent from a patient is that of the attending physician.[6] Thus, if a physician has been alerted by a "warning flag," it becomes his responsibility to pursue the matter further and to determine if, in fact, the patient is incompetent. It should be noted here that because the patient is presumed to be competent, no proof of competency is necessary. The physician is required to start from the premise that the patient is competent and then to consider only evidence that the patient may be incompetent.

The question then is: How does the physician determine whether or not his patient is incompetent, and, more critically, how does he override the patient's presumption of competency? Fundamentally, patient competency does not describe a continuous, 24-hour capacity to make a decision. It is, for the most part, an isolated mental state, applicable only to the particular moment the patient's decision is to be rendered. Because the law recognizes the presumption of competency in every adult, it is erroneous to assign to the elderly patient a general incapacity to decide based on isolated areas of irrationality.[10] The law requires, instead, that judgments associated with a patient's capacity or incapacity to enter into the decision-making process be restricted to the particular medical decision being sought at the time.

This principle is very important to the physician for whom incapacitation and forgetfulness of the elderly patient often are interpreted as incapacity to decide. For example, the fact that a guardian has been appointed to manage the affairs of an elderly patient does not render the patient incompetent in any total sense, nor should it be relied upon as a controlling factor by the physician. Only the circumstances connected to the particular decision to be made should be considered. It should be pointed out that some guardianships do carry with them a court finding of incompetency. In these cases, the guardian generally has been given the authority to make decisions regarding medical treatment for the patient. It is incumbent then upon the attending physician to inquire into the nature and dimensions of every guardianship before the final decision to treat the patient has been made.

The decision-making capacity of an elderly patient is not in itself a diagnostic category, as is so often assumed. It rests, instead, on the type of judgment that an informed layperson would use, which a patient who lacks the ability to understand the situation and to make a choice in light of that understanding does not possess.[10] The attending physician should take comfort in the fact that his role in determining the patient's incapacity to decide is not as a medical expert but as a layperson. Ultimately, the assessment of an individual's incapacity to decide is largely a matter of common sense.[10] Thus, determination of whether a patient lacks capacity to make a particular decision requires the following:

1. An assessment of the patient's capability to understand information relevant to the decision.

2. An assessment of whether the patient is able to communicate with the physician regarding the information relevant to the decision.

3. An assessment of whether the patient can reason about relevant alternatives against a background of rational personal values and goals.[1, 10]

Finally, it is important to note that an elderly patient who essentially feels powerless in the decision-making process may very well not hear what is being communicated to him by the physician. This should not be interpreted as evidence of incompetence but a condition that is conducive to an uninformed decision.

THE INCOMPETENT PATIENT

The two values that guide decision making for competent patients—promoting patient welfare and respecting patient self-determination—are not denied to the incompetent patient simply because of his inability to enter into the decision-making process. Only the implementation of these values during the process differs. The physician's goal should be to determine with as much accuracy as possible the wants and needs of the incompetent individual before making a decision. The urgency of many life-threatening conditions and the fact that patients may be decisionally incapable at the time a treatment decision must be made emphasizes the importance of determining patients' wishes about life-sustaining treatment before a life-threatening emergency occurs. One way is for the physician to discuss with the patient, whenever possible and appropriate, the use of an advanced written directive such as a "living will" or "durable power of attorney." These advanced directives protect the rights of patients to participate in health care decisions even after they become decisionally incapable. In addition to clarifying the patient's treatment preference, they offer physicians a measure of protection as well. Physicians and others attending elderly patients should be aware of their need to execute advanced directives as an expression of the right of self-determination. Both the living will and the durable power of attorney are recognized by most states, and physicians should become knowledgeable about the procedures and policies for implementing them.

The Living Will

Through 1987, 38 states and the District of Columbia had enacted "living wills" legislation. In terms of overall population, two of every three citizens have access to a recognized means of deciding in advance the extent and under what conditions they desire their life to be prolonged by artificial life-support measures.[5] All are based on the concept that a competent patient may execute in advance a declaration directing the physician to withdraw life-sustaining procedures in circumstances in which the patient has a terminal condition.[5]

At its most basic level, a living will requires the attending physician to make a determination that the patient satisfies criteria specified by statute and, if so, to put in motion steps for certifying the will and implementing its provisions. The procedures for doing this may be found in the particular state statutes that establish the living will.

A form for the patient's declaration is included in all but three (Alabama, Arkansas, and New Mexico) of the 38 state statutes.[13] The provisions of this form, however, do not have to be followed verbatim in the majority of the states with living will legislation (Fig. 3–1). Only four states (California, Georgia, Idaho, and Oregon) have laws that prevent individual

additions or modifications to the specific form specified in the state statute.

Although no two state statutes are identical, the following characteristics are shared by all: (1) criteria for determining a "qualified patient," (2) requirements for certifying and implementing the will, and (3) specific immunity from liability.

A *qualified patient* refers to a patient who has executed a declaration in accordance with the state statute where he resides and who has been certified to have injury, disease, or illness that is not curable or reversible and who is in a terminal condition.[13]

Terminal condition is usually described as an irreversible condition from which death will ensue, whether or not life-sustaining procedures are utilized.[13] In turn, *life-sustaining procedures* are usually defined as any medical interventions that will only prolong the dying process.[13]

The patient initiating the living will must be an adult (18 years or older) and competent when he executed the document. All but three states require that the will be witnessed by two disinterested adult parties (i.e., parties not related by blood or marriage to the patient or heirs or claimants to any part of the declarant's estate). The latter provision excludes the patient's physician or his employees as well as the hospital staff treating the patient.

Once a physician is notified of the patient's living will, he is responsible for its *certification* and *implementation* by way of the following steps: (a) determining if the patient is suffering from a terminal condition as defined by law; (b) confirming the diagnosis by a second physician and recording the certification in the medical record; and (c) exercising reasonable steps to advise the patient's immediate family, if any, of the existence of the patient's will and the subsequent diagnosis and certification of a terminal condition.

This last step is extremely important. After the diagnosis has been certified, most states require a 48-hour waiting period before the patient's requests can be carried out. During this waiting period, the family may contest the validity of the patient's declaration in an appropriate court.[3] The attending physician should be aware that simple objections by the family to the patient's declaration are insufficient

DECLARATION AS TO MEDICAL OR SURGICAL TREATMENT

I, _____, being of sound mind and at least eighteen years of
(name of declarant)
age, direct that my life shall not be artificially prolonged under the circumstances set forth below and hereby
declare that:

1. If at any time my attending physician and one other physician certify in writing that:
   a. I have an injury, disease, or illness which is not curable or reversible and which, in their judgment, is
   a terminal condition; and
   b. For a period of seven consecutive days or more, I have been unconscious, comatose, or otherwise
   incompetent so as to be unable to make or communicate responsible decisions concerning my person;
   then

I direct that in accordance with Colorado law, life-sustaining procedures shall be withdrawn and withheld
pursuant to the terms of this declaration, it being understood that life-sustaining procedures shall not include
any medical procedure or intervention for nourishment considered necessary by the attending physician to
provide comfort or alleviate pain. However, I may specifically direct, in accordance with Colorado law, that
artificial nourishment be withdrawn or withheld pursuant to the terms of this declaration.

2. In the event that the only procedure I am being provided is artificial nourishment, I direct that one of the
   following actions be taken:

_____ a. Artificial nourishment shall not be continued when it is the only procedure
(initials of declarant)   being provided; or

_____ b. Artificial nourishment shall be continued for _____ days when it is the only
(initials of declarant)   procedure being provided; or

_____ c. Artificial nourishment shall be continued when it is the only procedure being
(initials of declarant)   provided

3. I execute this declaration, as my free and voluntary act this _____ day of _____, 19_____

By: _____
                                                      Declarant

The foregoing instrument was signed and declared by _____ to
be his/her declaration, in the presence of us, who in his/her presence, in the presence of each other, and at
his/her request, have signed our names below as witnesses, and we declare that, at the time of the execution
of this instrument, the declarant, according to our best knowledge and belief, was of sound mind and under
no constraint or undue influence.

Dated at _____, Colorado, this day of _____ , 19_____.

_____
Name and Address

_____
Name and Address

FIGURE 3–1. Living Will Declaration in the Colorado Natural Death Act.

grounds to delay the obligation to carry out the terms of the will in accordance with state law when the waiting period has ended. The parties objecting to the will must seek a court order enjoining the physician from proceeding until the matter has been properly adjudicated.

All 38 states provide *immunity* from civil and criminal prosecution to physicians who comply with the patient's declaration.[3, 13] However, to be protected under this immunity, the physician must either comply with the patient's declaration or transfer the patient to another physician; failure to do so may subject the physician

to a penalty. In most states, adherence to the provisions of the patient's living will is a legal obligation.

Finally, the physician caring for the elderly patient should familiarize himself with the provisions of the living will statutes in the state in which he practices. In Table 3–1 are summarized the key points that each state provides for a living will.

The Durable Power of Attorney

Another aid to decision making in which the patient cannot participate effectively is

TABLE 3–1. Natural Death Acts in the United States (Living Wills)

State	Form	Restrictions	Physician's Responsibility†
Alabama	Must be substantially as written in act	Pregnancy, entire term; nutrition not considered life-sustaining procedure	"Must permit transfer"
Arizona	Must be substantially as written	Pregnancy, if fetus is viable	"Reasonable effort"
Arkansas*	Any form; form allows for statement for maximal treatment		Not mentioned
California*	Form is mandated; form must be signed subsequent to diagnosis of terminal illness	Pregnancy, entire term; nutrition not considered life-sustaining procedure; time limit; procedure different for nursing home residents	Nonbinding
Colorado	Must be substantially as written	Pregnancy, if fetus is viable or can become viable	Unprofessional conduct
Connecticut*	Must be substantially as written	Pregnancy, entire term	Not mentioned
Delaware	Must be substantially as written	Nutrition not considered life-sustaining procedure; procedure different for nursing home residents	Unprofessional conduct
District of Columbia	Must be substantially as written	Procedure different for nursing home residents	Unprofessional conduct
Florida	Any form; form must be signed subsequent to diagnosis of terminal illness	Pregnancy; entire term	"Reasonable effort"
Georgia	Form is mandated	Pregnancy, entire term; procedure different for nursing home residents	"Reasonable effort"
Idaho	Form is mandated; form must be signed subsequent to diagnosis of terminal illness	Time limit	Not mentioned
Illinois	Must be substantially as written	Nutrition not considered life-sustaining procedure; only attending physician needs to certify terminal illness	"Must permit transfer"
Indiana	Must be substantially as written; form allows for statement of maximal treatment	Pregnancy, entire term	"Must permit transfer"
Iowa	Any form	Pregnancy, if fetus is viable or can become viable	"Reasonable effort"
Kansas	Any form	Pregnancy, entire term; nutrition not considered life-sustaining procedure	Unprofessional conduct
Louisiana	Any form	Nutrition not considered life-sustaining procedure	"Reasonable effort"
Maine	Any form	Only attending physician needs to certify	"Reasonable effort," "must permit transfer"
Maryland	Must be substantially as written; form allows for statement for maximal treatment	Pregnancy, entire term	"Reasonable effort"

Table continued on following page

TABLE 3–1. Natural Death Acts in the United States (Living Wills) *Continued*

State	Form	Restrictions	Physician's Responsibility†
Mississippi*	Any form	Pregnancy, entire term; cannot withhold therapy; two other physicians must certify terminal illness	Not mentioned
Missouri	Any form	Pregnancy, entire term	Unprofessional conduct
Montana	Any form	Nutrition not considered life-sustaining procedure	Criminal offense
Nevada	Form is mandated	Pregnancy, entire term; nutrition not considered life-sustaining procedure	Nonbinding
New Hampshire	Any form	Pregnancy, entire term	"Must permit transfer"
New Mexico	Any form	Pregnancy, entire term; nutrition not considered life-sustaining procedure	None
North Carolina*	Form is mandated		
Oklahoma	Must be substantially as written; form must be signed subsequent to diagnosis of terminal illness	Pregnancy, entire term	Unprofessional conduct
Oregon	Form is mandated	Time limit; procedure is different for nursing home residents	"Reasonable effort"
South Carolina	Must be substantially as written	Three witnesses; pregnancy, entire term	Unprofessional conduct
Tennessee	Must be substantially as written	Nutrition not considered life-sustaining procedure	Unprofessional conduct
Texas	Any form; oral contract only in presence of M.D.	Pregnancy, entire term	"Reasonable effort"
Utah	Must be substantially as written	Pregnancy, entire term	Unprofessional conduct
Vermont	Form is mandated	Nutrition not considered life-sustaining procedure	"Must permit transfer"
Virginia	Any form		"Must permit transfer"
Washington	Must be substantially as written	Pregnancy, entire term	"Reasonable effort"
West Virginia	Must be substantially as written	Nutrition not considered life-sustaining procedure	"Must permit transfer"
Wisconsin	Form is mandated	Pregnancy, entire term; nutrition not considered life-sustaining procedure	
Wyoming	Must be substantially as written	Pregnancy, entire term	"Reasonable effort"

*Unique status

†The references to the physician's responsibility under the Natural Death Acts denote the following meaning: "must permit transfer" means that the physician must comply with a qualified patient's directive or transfer the patient to another physician. "Reasonable effort" means that a physician who cannot comply with the provisions of a living will shall tell the patient or family, and at their option, make every reasonable effort to assist in the transfer of the patient to another physician. "Not mentioned" means that no reference is made to any physician's responsibility in the statutory act. "Nonbinding" means that the provisions of the statutory act are not obligatory and the physician may exercise his own discretion in following the act. "Unprofessional conduct" provides for penalties against the physician for failure to follow the provisions of a qualified patient's living will. These penalties do not carry criminal sanctions against the physician but rather the possibility of censure by the state medical board as in the case of unprofessional conduct: "Criminal offense" means that a physician who refuses to comply with a qualified patient's living will, will be subject to criminal prosecution by the state.

a proxy designated in advance by the patient to speak on his behalf.[9] Since the clinical circumstances of a future illness and available treatment options are unpredictable, a proxy chosen by the patient offers the advantage of decision making based on both an intimate knowledge of the patient's wishes and the physician's recommendation. Because the living will cannot predict all the various alternatives that can arise as acute illnesses develop and is not applicable except in cases involving a terminal condition, a proxy can be of real assistance to the physician trying to decide the best course of treatment for the patient.

All 50 states have durable power of attorney statutes. However, there is some question as to whether health care decisions can be made by a proxy under a "standard" durable power of attorney statute. Basically, these statutes permit a person to designate another to act in his behalf in the event of his future incompetence.

Several states have approved the use of durable powers for health care decisions.[5, 9, 13] In 15 states, the living will statutes specifically provide for appointment of a proxy whose role is to authorize medical treatment that is consistent with the advanced directive executed by the patient. In addition, the proxy may make necessary decisions when no directive has been executed by the patient or when the directives appear ambiguous as to the patient's intent. Three states (California, Pennsylvania, and Colorado) have enacted special durable power statutes that expressly include and designate health care decisions (Fig. 3–2).

Although the durable power of attorney for health care decisions has the advantages of broad scope and flexibility, the potential for abuse should be recognized by the physician. For example, a proxy may have a conflict of interest, either emotionally or legally. If the proxy's decision appears to be contrary to the patient's best interests and cannot be resolved, the physician should seek the intervention of a court.

Finally, it should be recognized that neither the living will nor the durable power of attorney is a perfect mechanism for projecting a patient's wishes into a period of future incompetency. Neverthe-

less, in spite of imperfections, the living will and the proxy can be of real assistance to the physician trying to decide the best course of treatment for the incompetent patient.

DRIVER'S LICENSES FOR THE ELDERLY

The subject of driver impairment and the risks this presents not only to the driver but also to the general public is of increasing concern today. Along with this concern are questions about the specific role and obligation of physicians caring for the elderly driver.

Studies show that there is a sharp increase in the rate of accidents involving drivers over age 65, with the rate for the driver over age 70 double that of drivers in the middle years. In addition, not only do older drivers have an increased accident rate, but they also are at an increased risk of dying in the accident.[7] The fatal accident frequency rate per 100,000 drivers over age 75 is 55, compared with only 38 for the total driver average.[7] Even though individuals over 70 years of age drive fewer miles, the chance of an accident per mile is considerably higher because of the many changes related to aging.[7]

Along with our concern for the safety of the driver and general public are questions regarding the specific role and obligation of physicians to prevent or deter the impaired elderly patient from driving. For example, what are the legal obligations of the physician for reporting an impaired driver? Currently, only two states, California and Oregon, specifically provide for statutory liability on the part of the physician for not reporting a potentially unsafe driver to the Department of Motor Vehicles.

In states without the mandatory reporting statute, physicians may face liability under common law when some reasonable attempt is not made to keep the impaired elderly driver off the highways. The rationale behind this rule is sound. Generally, a person does not have a duty to control the conduct of a second person so as to prevent that person from harming a third person, unless a special relationship

I, _____, hereby appoint: _____
name/address

as my agent to make health care decisions for me if and when I am unable to make my own health care decisions. This gives my agent the power to consent to giving, withholding or stopping any health care, treatment, service, or diagnostic procedure. My agent also has the authority to talk with health care personnel, get information, and sign forms necessary to carry out those decisions.

If the person named as my agent is not available or is unable to act as my agent, then I appoint the following person(s) to serve in the order listed below:

1. _____   2. _____
       name   address   name   address

By this document I intend to create a power of attorney for health care which shall take effect upon my incapacity to make my own health care decisions and shall continue during that incapacity.

My agent shall make health care decisions as I direct below or as I make known to him or her in some other way.

(a) Statement of Desires Concerning Life-Prolonging Care, Treatment Services and Procedures:

(b) Special Provisions and Limitations:

By signing here I indicate that I understand the purpose and effect of this document.

I sign my name on this form on _____

My current home address _____
(you sign here)

Witnesses:
I declare that the person(s) who signed or acknowledged this document is personally known to me, that he/she signed or acknowledged this durable power of attorney in my presence, and that he/she appears to be of sound mind and under no duress, fraud, or undue influence. I am not the person appointed as agent by this document, nor am I the patient's health care provider, or an employee of the patient's health care provider.

First Witness: _____ Second Witness: _____
            name/address   name/address
(At least one of the above witnesses must also sign the following declaration.)

I further declare that I am not related to the patient by blood, marriage, or adoption, and to the best of my knowledge, I am not entitled to any part of his/her estate under a will now existing or by operation of law.

_____
            name/address

FIGURE 3–2. Sample of a General Form for Creating a Durable Power of Attorney for Health Care.

imposing such a duty exists between the first and second persons, or between the first and third persons that gives the latter a right to protection.[8] The courts have recognized a "special relationship" between a physician and his patient.[8, 12] Because of this, physicians are in a unique position to evaluate general health problems of the elderly, including their ability to drive. If the physician knows, or should have known, that his patient is potentially an unsafe driver, he must take reasonable steps to protect the patient as well as the general public. A physician with such knowledge cannot simply remain silent under the guise of patient confidentiality. Confidentiality of the patient gives way when it is necessary to protect the welfare of the individual or the community.[1, 12]

Several options are available to the physician to exercise reasonable care. Certainly, he should have a frank discussion with the patient and explain to him the increased risk of accidents. He should strongly suggest that the patient voluntarily stop driving and surrender his license. An alternative would be to suggest a license renewal examination with specific emphasis on vision and motor performance. If the state authorities renew the individual's license, the physician will have fulfilled his responsibility. In taking these steps, the physician should enlist family support if possible. Thus, even though all states except California and Oregon do not require physicians to report an impaired driver, it still should be done. Careful records of the report should be maintained by the physician.

In conclusion, because to many elderly patients, a driver's license represents the last vestige of personal autonomy and independence, the physician should explain why he is compelled to breach confidentiality, when appropriate, and to take the aforementioned steps. Because the elderly patient's expectations are extremely fragile, the primary expectation of patient advocacy must not be compromised. The care and attention given to the elderly patient over his safety in driving should strengthen the bonds of the physician/patient relationship.

REFERENCES

1. Beauchamp TL, Childress JE: Principles of Biomedical Ethics. Oxford, Oxford University Press, 1983, pp 66–88.
2. Brennon RE: Duty to warn third parties. JAMA 249:191, 1983.
3. Handbook of Living Wills. New York, Society for the Right to Die, 1985.
4. King J: The Law of Medical Malpractice. Saint Paul, West Publishing Co, 1982, p 153.
5. Office of Technology Assessment: Life-sustaining technologies and the elderly. Washington, U.S. GPO, 1987.
6. Magna v Elie, 439 NE 2d.1319, 1982.
7. Malfetti J, ed: Drivers Fifty-Five Plus. Folk Church, Virginia, AAA Foundation for Traffic Safety, 1985, pp 32–33.
8. McIntosh v Milano, 403 A 2d 500, 1979.
9. Peters DA: Advance medical directives. J Leg Med 8:3, 1987.
10. President's Commission for Study of Biomedical Ethics and Behavioral Research: Making health care decisions. Washington, U.S. GPO, 1982.
11. Rosoff A, Gottlieb G: Preserving personal autonomy for the elderly. J Leg Med 8:1, 1987.
12. Tarsoff v Regents of California, 551 P 2d 334, 1976.
13. The Physician and the Hopelessly Ill Patient: Legal, Medical and Ethical Guidelines. New York, Society for the Right to Die, 1985.
14. Walker JA: Chronic medical conditions and traffic safety. N Engl J Med 273:1413, 1965.

GENERAL CARE OF THE ELDERLY

CHAPTER 4

The Physician-Patient Relationship

Dennis W. Jahnigen
Robert W. Schrier

A physician can sometimes parry the scythe of death, but has no power over the sand in the hourglass.
    HESTER LYNCH PIOZZI, *Letter to Fanny Burney*

Caring for older persons can be a challenging yet satisfying experience for physicians. The growth in numbers of older patients means that the medical student or house officer of the 1990s must be prepared to provide adequate care. It is estimated that by the year 2000, 30 percent of all office visits to family physicians and well over 50 percent of visits to internists will be made by geriatric patients.[1] Physicians in practice during the next 30 years must be skillful in caring for elderly persons in the outpatient setting, the acute care environment, and the nursing home. They must be knowledgeable about the range of emerging alternative community care sites such as home care, day care, and hospice programs as well.

The physician caring for older patients must also be a capable diagnostician, since diseases of the elderly often have an atypical presentation, a confusing course, and a variable response to therapy. Thoughtful sifting of available information is critical because alternative hypotheses for a patient's problems are often possible. Diagnostic parsimony—the principle whereby all of the patient's signs and symptoms are explained by a single disease process—rarely applies in the treatment of older individuals. This is because the older patient usually has several illnesses, and acute events may represent two or more ongoing disease processes.

In addition, physicians who care for older patients must be rigorous in their efforts to keep up with the rapidly growing body of information relevant to aging. Many long-established dogmas concerning the aging process have been found to be incorrect. For example, many of the changes commonly associated with aging have been shown to be the result of disuse.[2] Significant loss of mental function, for example, is now understood to be distinctly abnormal with old age and thus merits careful attention for possible reversibility and treatment. Information about many other aspects of geriatric care is emerging at a brisk pace in both general and subspecialty literature.

To physicians who see the elderly as

worthy recipients of their best efforts, these challenges are not insurmountable. They provide an opportunity to enhance the quality of life for the older individual in a way that can be very satisfying to patient and physician alike.

Until recently, most physicians had chosen not to spend much of their professional time with older persons.[3] This is partly the result of a number of negative perceptions concerning geriatric care. One is the view that the application of medical skills is not likely to be of much use to the older patient. Achieving a cure is also uncommon, although occasionally possible. Today, one must be willing to define success of treatment in somewhat different terms. It can be in the form of helping an older individual remain independent or retain a degree of physical or emotional function, despite the inability to effect a cure of the underlying illness. Another reason is the difficulty in making an accurate diagnosis. The history and physical findings about older persons may be voluminous and the data obtained quite confusing. Frequently, several different plausible explanations can account for a patient's symptoms. These may range from an innocuous process to a very serious disease. However, it is often much more challenging and exacting to collect, organize, and analyze this information than it is for information about single system diseases associated with younger patients. Diagnostic error is more likely, even with conscientious attention by the physician.

Furthermore, less physician time had been devoted to older persons because of the erroneous perception within the medical profession that geriatric care was not as rigorous as some of the other subspecialties. All too often in the past, care of older patients had been relegated to physicians of borderline capabilities, with the benefits derived by older persons equally marginal. Yet, few disciplines in medicine are more demanding that the physician have knowledge of medical science, decision-making skills in the presence of uncertainty, skill in resolving ethical conflicts, and interpersonal communications abilities than is geriatric medicine.

A final, yet important, reason why elderly persons attracted less attention concerns the issue of reimbursement. Nearly three quarters of the health care expenses for the elderly are paid by federal government or private insurance coverage. The reimbursement schemes all emphasize reimbursement for highly technical procedures, with limited reimbursement for the cognitive services that the elderly commonly require. Furthermore, most reimbursement favors hospitalization over medical services provided in other settings. Geriatric care does take more time than similar services administered to younger individuals; however, at present it is not well remunerated. Changes in the reimbursement schemes of the future will almost certainly encourage greater physician involvement in geriatric care.

PROVIDING OPTIMAL CARE

The most important prerequisite to providing the best care for older patients is a belief that even the very old can benefit from the skills of a well-trained physician. Only with such an attitude are physicians likely to exert their best efforts. They also must be willing to define success less in terms of a cure than in terms of achieving the patient's own objectives. This may be a modest outcome such as ameliorating a disabling physical symptom in order to allow the person to remain active. Few older persons fear death as much as they do the loss of autonomy and independence that accompanies disability. Thus, one can view as successful the medical encounter that reduces dependence without necessarily increasing life span.

APPROACH TO THE PATIENT

Older persons customarily see physicians several times each year. This is quite different than for younger persons, who are not likely to see a physician over a period of years. A primary care relationship for older persons is an essential foundation of providing health care services through the later years of life. In this setting, a baseline of information about the person's medical condition, level of mental function, social support, living environment, and value system can be obtained. This information can be invaluable in making recommendations for diagnosis and treatment throughout the course of the relationship. Such comprehensive geriatric assessment can be best accomplished by a physician with the assistance of a social worker and nurse with expertise in caring for the elderly.

Although some important information is obtained from the family, patients should have the option of private discussion with their physicians. Well-meaning family members may answer questions on behalf of frail spouses or parents when they are quite able to do this for themselves. In such circumstances, the physician must ensure that patients have the opportunity to speak on their own behalf.

A number of adjustments are advisable in interviewing and examining older patients.[4, 5] The pace of the questioning and the physical examination must be slow enough so as to not frighten or intimidate the patient. The environment should be a comfortable one that allows for some of the limitations of the elderly. The room should be comfortably warm, well lit, and free from distracting noises. The patient should be treated with courtesy and dignity. It is inappropriate to address patients who are much older than the physician by their first names unless they request that this be done. The physician needs to appreciate the anxiety present in many patients and the dependent feeling that being in a hospital or office setting may produce. Patients should be addressed at eye level, if possible, rather than from the position of the physician standing and the patient recumbent. Since this is the usual position for social interaction, communicating at eye level helps preserve the equality of both parties.

In the outpatient setting, electrical tables that can be lowered to aid in the older person's examination are useful. The patient should be permitted to undress and dress himself, even if it takes a bit longer than with physician or nurse assistance. This simple act helps the individual maintain dignity, as we usually think only of children as needing to be dressed. In addition, firsthand observation can provide knowledge about how much difficulty the individual has with buttons, zippers, and laces. One should monitor nonverbal cues, such as facial expression and body language, to see how the older patient feels about the examination.

When talking to an older patient, the physician should speak clearly, without shouting. Speaking too loudly may exceed the threshold of the hearing deficit and may be painful. One should face the patient, making eye contact, to ensure that the older person understands what is being said as well as to obtain a sense of his emotional response to the discussion.

Most elderly individuals have an extensive medical history. Few physicians or patients could endure the 2 to 3 hours necessary to obtain an exhaustive history and physical examination. For this reason, the encounter should be modified to take place over several 30-minute periods. During these intervals, the physician can focus on the most pressing issues. It is extremely important to address what the patient considers to be his major problem, regardless of how minor it may seem to the physician compared with more serious illnesses that are discovered. If a patient comes to the physician complaining of a painful toenail and the physician should detect a large abdominal aneurysm, the foot discomfort must be dealt with in addition to the more detailed assessment of the aneurysm that may be indicated. Many patients will provide unnecessary details or make frequent, lengthy digressions. When time permits, these discussions can be used to learn more about the patient, but often, the examiner needs to gently direct the conversation and help the patient focus his comments. The comprehensive assessment of an older person can occur during 2 to 4 visits rather than during the traditional single session. In this way, a thorough evaluation can be conducted, and the physician has the opportunity to see the older person and family members in different circumstances.

It is important to utilize the valuable information that can be obtained from family members or close friends. Many older patients tend to minimize disability or problems, such as falls, since they may be fearful that others may decide that they are incapable of living alone. Many patients with dementing illnesses are unable to remember important details, and only information provided by family members or close friends can be considered reliable.

COMPREHENSIVE GERIATRIC ASSESSMENT

This methodology is emerging to help gather and utilize the large volume of important medical, psychological, environmental, and social information about the elderly patient. The process is multidisciplinary, and in addition to a physician, it involves at a minimum a nurse and a social worker, all with expertise in geriatric care issues. The assessment consists of screening interviews and observations of the older patient's strengths, deficits, and functional abilities. In areas in which problems are suspected, more detailed analyses are undertaken. Professionals in many other health care disciplines may participate, if circumstances warrant. These may include specialists in audiology, clinical psychology, dentistry, nutrition, occupational therapy, pharmacy, physical therapy, podiatry, and others. Frequently, consultants in fields such as orthopedics, ophthalmology, neurology, psychiatry, and urology have important contributions to make.

Physical health information is obtained regarding medical history, current problems, prescription and nonprescription medication use, nutritional state, and presence of common geriatric syndromes such as falling, incontinence, immobility, and confusion. Information needed to make health promotion suggestions is obtained about exercise, smoking, alcohol use, and immunization status. Screening assessments of dentition, nutritional status, ambulation and balance, hearing, vision, and cognitive function should also be part of the evaluation.

Information obtained regarding the patient's social support network provides clues to the relative strength of current and potential caregiver support for the patient. Measures of the patient's ability to perform basic activities, called Activities of Daily Living (ADL), are gathered, which include bathing, dressing, toileting, transferring, continence, and feeding. The ability to perform more complex tasks, called Instrumental Activities of Daily Living (IADL), is assessed, which include meal preparation, shopping, light housework, financial management, medication management, use of transportation, and use of the telephone. An attempt is made to evaluate the patient's home environment. Threats to safety, adequacy of basic utilities, and access to services such as shopping and transportation are reviewed.

The comprehensive geriatric assessment is conducted during several encounters with the patient, depending on the urgency and complexity of the problems uncovered and the patient's tolerance of the examinations. At the conclusion, the team meets to develop a plan of interventions and desired outcomes that incorporates patient and family preferences.

DEVELOPING A THERAPEUTIC PLAN FOR THE OLDER PATIENT

A systematic 5-step process (described below) can individualize medical care for older persons.[6, 7] It can be employed in the context of a primary care relationship and is ideally conducted in an outpatient setting, although it can be modified for the inpatient environment as well. The process includes important questions to help the physician make the most reasonable recommendations and to help define what shall represent "success" for the individual patient. It consists of discussions that take place at critical junctures in the older person's life. For example, one could be on admission to a long-term care facility. Another could occur when a major surgical intervention is contemplated. It certainly should occur in the presence of advanced progressive illness and could also be undertaken in the presence of advanced age alone.

Few older persons have not considered their own possible disability and eventual death. Many older persons are quite comfortable discussing some of these issues, if they are handled in a sensitive manner. For those above age 80, each year brings an increasing likelihood of serious morbidity or death. The annual mortality rate for 80-year-olds is approximately 15 percent and increases to 50 percent for those who approach 100 years of age.[8] For these persons, it is not a question of whether some serious threat to health will occur; it is a question of when.

Step 1: Determine the Patient's Expectations from the Encounter

One common assumption is that the older patient desires to be totally cured of a disability or illness. This is often not a reasonable goal, and many other objectives may be more important. These may include controlling disturbing symptoms or reducing disability, understanding what is occurring and what to expect, or simply being informed that a serious illness does or does not exist. Even sympathy, in which the physician both explains and expresses understanding of the patient's fears, is a legitimate objective. A final objective is seeking validation of worth as a human being by virtue of gaining the physician's full attention. The therapeutic value provided by physicians and other health professionals offering this reassurance should not be underestimated.

Step 2: Obtain a Value Inventory

At the onset of the relationship, the physician should seek to obtain an understanding of the person's value scheme. This includes information as to where the person views himself in the course of his own existence. This is likely to be very different for a 90-year-old than for a 20-year-old. The physician can also learn how the patient views life and the source of his values. Does he consider himself to be religious? How high a value does he place on autonomy? How does he feel about the prospects of disability and death? What kind of living arrangement does he currently have? What are his important interpersonal relationships? Where does he look to for support? How would he live with certain kinds of disabilities, such as incontinence, nursing home placement, or need of a wheelchair? What things give him pleasure in life? These are simply examples of the type of information the physician attempts to elicit. Although it may seem a burdensome addition to obtaining the history and performing the physical examination, the few minutes spent in such conversation can be most useful in making sensible diagnostic and therapeutic recommendations in the future.

Failure to obtain this kind of information leaves the physician in a very difficult situation when he is faced with an incompetent or critically ill patient for whom important decisions must be made. Hold-

ing such conversations when the person is in relatively good health can help eliminate any confusion and prevent the application of unwanted medical therapies in the setting of an acute illness when he is unable to make their wishes known and when family members may make decisions in a highly emotional state. This is also an appropriate time to discuss whether the patient has made any formal statement regarding his medical care, such as a living will, durable power of attorney, or similar document. (See Chapter 3.)

Step 3: What Are the Medical Facts?

At this point, the physician conducts the traditional history and physical examination. As noted, this should be an abbreviated process, lasting, if possible, no more than 30 minutes. The essential facts about the patient's history and about any associated signs and symptoms are obtained. A working hypothesis with a differential diagnosis list is generated, with assessment of the natural history of the illness (if any) for this patient, viable diagnostic and therapeutic options, and estimate of risks and benefits to the patient. At this time, the physician makes an individualized recommendation to the patient. This may be for additional diagnostic studies or for initiating a therapeutic trial of a medication or performing a surgical procedure.

Step 4: Reconcile Differences Between Patient and Physician

In this important step, the patient responds to the physician's recommendations. There are often differences of opinion between the patient and physician, and these should be reconciled. Physicians must be willing to negotiate or modify and adjust their recommendations to meet what is acceptable to the patient. Patients often have specific limits as to the therapies that they will accept, such as the number of medicines they will take. For some patients, a major surgical procedure is absolutely out of the question, and they will accept only other types of therapy.

The physician should not take an adversarial stance in this event but should be willing to modify his recommendations. Sometimes, the patient's apparent poor decisions reflect insufficient information or misconceptions on the part of the patient, physician, or both, and an attempt should be made to clarify the issues, if possible.

Family members should be included in these discussions, although the wishes of the patient remain paramount. One must be aware of the tendency of well-meaning family members and others to make decisions for the competent, but frail, older patient. Older persons are often quite willing to accept some risk of injury in order to remain alone in familiar surroundings. Concerned adult children often have much difficulty with this prospect and may request the physician to insist on a safer, but less acceptable, living arrangement for the patient. Within large families, there may be disagreement about the best course of action. The physician can consult a counselor or social worker to help resolve these issues.

Step 5: Develop a Strategy

The final step of this process leads to an agreed-upon plan of action. This may be diagnostic or therapeutic. It may be a strategy to achieve a complete cure, such as removal of a lens cataract or joint replacement of an arthritic hip. It may be palliative, such as administration of an anti-inflammatory medication for arthritis pain. It may be a hospice strategy for a terminally ill patient, in which relief of pain and preservation of autonomy are the measures of success, even though the patient will certainly die. In a rehabilitative strategy, the disabling effects of a physical condition are reduced. The important common theme among all of these is for the patient and physician to agree on the realistic objectives of care.

It is particularly important for those involved with older persons during episodes of care, such as emergency room treatment or acute care hospitalization, to seek information from the primary care physician. It is equally important that when older persons return to a primary care physician after such an episode, appropriate information be transferred from the acute care setting.

The information described in these 5 steps can be obtained in a reasonable amount of time and in the course of typical encounters between patients and physicians. To the physician willing to serve reasonable objectives of the older patient, it can provide one approach to minimize confusion and uncertainty, apply medical technology selectively in ways most beneficial to patients, and allow for a more satisfying doctor-patient relationship for all involved.

REFERENCES

1. US Department of Health & Human Services: Health United States 1980. (PHS) 81–1232. Washington, US GPO, 1980.
2. Bortz W: Disuse and aging. JAMA 248:1203, 1982.
3. Wolk RL, Wolk RB: Professional Workers' Attitudes Toward The Aged. J Am Geriatr Soc 19:624, 1971.
4. Jahnigen DW, Taylor S, Benson L, et al: Interviewing the Older Patient in the Medical Student Source Book for Geriatrics. Salt Lake City, University of Utah Intermountain West Long-Term Care Gerontology Center, 1987, p 93.
5. Balzer D: Techniques for communicating with your elderly patient. Geriatrics 11:79, 1978.
6. Jahnigen DW, Schrier RW: The doctor/patient relationship in geriatric care. Clin Geriatr Med 2:457, 1986.
7. Jahnigen DW: The changing doctor patient relationship. Generations 12:54, 1987.
8. Sacher GA: Evolution of longevity and survival characteristics in mammals. In Schneider EL, ed: The Genetics of Aging. New York, Plenum Press, 1978, p 151.
9. NIH Consensus Development Conference Statement: Geriatric assessment for clinical decision making. Vol 6, No 13. Bethesda, 1987, p 8.

CHAPTER 5

Preventive Medicine

John F. Steiner
Abraham J. Kauvar

Prevention is better than cure.
DICKENS, *Martin Chuzzlewit*

An individual aged 65 has a remaining life expectancy of 16.5 years but can expect to live independently for only 10.0 years, or 61 percent of that time span.[1] The primary goal of preventive care for the elderly is to prolong the period of functional independence; prolongation of life is a secondary objective.[2] Although measures such as smoking cessation, breast cancer detection, and hypertension treatment are of benefit, even if begun after the age of 65, the ideal time for the elderly to begin preventive care is when they are young.[3-5] Preventive medicine in later life also requires identification and modification of risk factors unique to the elderly, such as environmental hazards or gait disturbances, that may cause falls. It is important to avoid inappropriate treatment as well as to prevent disease in elderly patients by identifying and correcting dysfunction caused or worsened by medical therapy. This chapter introduces some general principles of preventive care, summarizes current guidelines for preventive care in the elderly, and discusses overprescribing of medication as a cause of functional impairment in older persons.

The goals of preventive medicine are age-specific. Historically, preventive measures were developed for diseases, such as childhood infections and complications of pregnancy, that caused premature death and disability. More recently, efforts have been made to prevent conditions that generally begin later in life, such as malignancies and atherosclerotic cardiovascular diseases. A concern for the impairments of the aged is the most recent consideration in the preventive care agenda. Breslow and Somers have defined a set of general goals for preventive care of the elderly, based on a division of that population into the "young old" (65 to 74 years of age) and the "old old" (75 years and older)[6] (see Table 5–1). Some of these goals apply to younger age groups as well, whereas others, e.g., preparation for retirement and avoidance of institutionalization, are specific to the elderly.

GENERAL PRINCIPLES OF PREVENTIVE MEDICINE

Preventive interventions have traditionally been divided into three classes: *primary prevention*, or activities that reduce the likelihood that disease or functional impairment will develop (a classic example is immunization); *secondary prevention*, or the early detection and treatment of disease in order to forestall its consequences

TABLE 5–1. Goals for Preventive Care of the Elderly*

Age 65–74
Prolong the period of optimum physical, mental, and social activity
Minimize handicapping and discomfort from onset of chronic conditions
Help to prepare in advance for retirement

Age 75 and Over
Prolong the period of effective activity and ability to live independently and to avoid institutionalization, if possible
Minimize inactivity and discomfort from chronic conditions
Ensure as little physical and mental distress as possible and provide emotional support to patient and family in the event of terminal illness.

*(From Breslow L, Somers AR: The lifetime health-monitoring program. N Engl J Med 296:601, 1977; by permission.)

(e.g., treatment of hypertension); and *tertiary prevention*, or the attempt to slow the progression of established disease or to reduce resulting disability (e.g., physical therapy after a cerebrovascular accident.)[7] These categories are not mutually exclusive. For example, secondary prevention of hypertension provides primary prevention for stroke.[8] Although primary and secondary prevention remain significant, tertiary prevention is of increasing importance for the elderly. Many health conditions that threaten independence, such as incontinence or falls, are the cumulative effect of progressive, often subtle, impairments that are not amenable to primary or secondary prevention. If the impairment is recognized, the dysfunction it produces often can be minimized.

There are two forms of preventive care in geriatrics, which are *screening* and *assessment*. *Screening* is defined as "the presumptive identification of unrecognized disease or defect by the application of tests, examinations, or other procedures, which can be applied rapidly."[9] The goal of screening is to separate an asymptomatic population into groups at higher and lower risk for the outcome of concern. A screening test is not designed to make a definitive diagnosis but to identify a subset of individuals for more detailed evaluation. The use of mammography to detect breast cancer in women without a palpable breast mass is an example of screening, since an abnormal mammogram does not prove the diagnosis but identifies patients who require biopsy. Assessment, in contrast, ". . . involves a more detailed review than does screening and leads directly to diagnostic conclusions and assignment to interventive strategies."[10] Screening and assessment may be performed sequentially; a single screening question that reveals a risk factor (such as recent retirement) may prompt an immediate, detailed assessment of its consequences.

Not all health problems are amenable to screening. For example, lung cancer is a common and devastating disease, but screening for lung cancer has not proved effective. Even if lung cancer is detected early, treatment is of too little efficacy to justify the effort and expense of screening for all individuals at risk.[7] Attributes of the health problem itself, the diagnostic

test, and the treatment regimen must be considered in defining target conditions for preventive screening or assessment. In Table 5–2 are listed general characteristics of diseases and functional impairments that are suitable for preventive efforts in any age group.

Screening or assessment should be performed frequently enough to detect impairments before they become irreversible, yet infrequently enough to avoid unnecessary discomfort, effort, and cost. To illustrate the timing of successful screening, Figure 5–1 plots the natural history of two preventable conditions, breast cancer and falls. The two problems are chosen for their contrasts; breast cancer is a disease diagnosed and treated by traditional biomedical measures, whereas falls are a problem with biomedical consequences, such as fractures, but with a complex pathogenesis and treatment that requires evaluation of the patient's environment and functional ability. The onset of both

TABLE 5–2. Criteria for Evaluation of Preventive Measures*

Characteristics of the Disability or Disease

Prevalence of condition in population

Impact on individual (e.g., disability, pain, social disruption, years of life lost)

Impact on society (mortality, morbidity, cost of care)

Sufficiently long subclinical phase to allow effective screening

Characteristics of the Test for Screening or Assessment

Validity of test (likelihood that test is positive in individuals with the condition and negative in those without it)

Acceptability to patient and health care provider

Risk of harm from the test
   Risk, discomfort, and cost of evaluating a "positive" test
   Personal and social disadvantages of being labeled as "diseased" by the test

Likelihood of compliance with the testing procedure by provider and patient

Characteristics of the Treatment Regimen

Efficacy (Does suitable treatment exist?)

Effectiveness (Is treatment actually rendered?)
   Availability of treatment in community
   Adherence of patients to treatment
   Acceptability of costs of treatment

Evidence of benefit when applied in the general population

*(Adapted from references 7, 9, 11, and 12.)

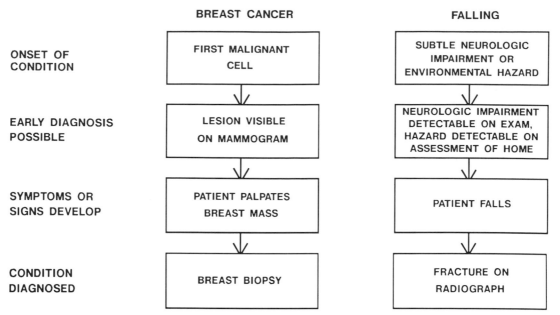

FIGURE 5–1. Natural history of conditions amenable to screening or assessment. Bold arrows denote alteration in natural history due to a successful screening.

conditions is marked by a subclinical event, i.e., the first malignant cell in the breast or the first subtle sign of impaired gait, proprioception, or vision. As they progress, both problems are potentially detectable at a subclinical stage, before symptoms or consequences would bring the patient to medical attention. A useful screening test or assessment instrument should uncover the problem at this stage, when adverse outcomes may be prevented or their impact may be reduced. If the screening test is not administered or is inaccurate, both conditions will progress until the patient discovers a breast mass or suffers a fracture resulting from a fall. At this point, therapeutic interventions are still worthwhile but may be less effective in preserving health.

SPECIAL CONSIDERATIONS IN SCREENING AND ASSESSMENT OF THE ELDERLY

In the elderly, preventive care takes place within a context of interrelated medical, functional, and social factors. Several special considerations should guide decision making about prevention for elderly individuals.

Patients at high risk of losing functional independence, particularly the "frail elderly," should be special targets for preventive efforts. For example, urinary incontinence may be the critical determinant of a family's decision to seek nursing home care for an individual with other disabilities, although the same problem may be only a distressing inconvenience for another, otherwise functional, elderly person. Both patients deserve efforts at prevention and treatment, but the first patient requires particular attention to avoid institutionalization.

Decisions about screening should not be based on age alone; old age does not justify diagnostic nihilism. It may be appropriate to screen a healthy 80-year-old for colorectal carcinoma by testing for occult blood in the stool, yet inappropriate to do so in a 60-year-old patient with end-stage congestive heart failure. Such decisions must be based on the patient's level of function, irrespective of age, as well as on an appraisal of the risks of the screening test and of any further tests required if a screening test is positive.

Therapeutic and diagnostic decisions must be individualized, with the risks of treatment weighed against the potential benefit. In our experience, an 84-year-old woman with congestive heart failure and peripheral vascular disease was scheduled to undergo a lower-extremity amputation after she developed gangrene of three toes. Up to a third of such patients require long-term institutional care after an amputation.[13] After discussion with her, a balloon angioplasty of the common iliac artery was performed, which restored circulation, prevented the loss of her leg, and allowed her to continue to live independently at home. For such patients, high-risk procedures may be justified to prevent an irreversible loss of functional independence.

Screening tests may have different characteristics in elderly patients than in younger individuals. In tuberculosis screening programs, the probability of a positive response to a standard intradermal (5 TU) skin test rises with age into the sixth decade but declines thereafter. A screening program for patients in long-term care facilities found that the rate of positive responses fell from 43 percent in patients aged 65 to 74 to 19 percent in those aged 85 to 94, perhaps resulting from factors such as immunologic senescence, local changes in aging skin, or a decrease in reactivity as the initial infection becomes more remote.[14] Since a single tuberculin skin test is less effective for screening, other strategies, such as a booster dose of tuberculin one week later, may be necessary to diagnose tuberculosis in the elderly.[15]

The effectiveness of preventive treatments may also vary with age. The usefulness of the pneumococcal vaccine was first demonstrated in young men working in South African gold mines.[16] In contrast, a recent randomized clinical trial has raised questions about the benefit of pneumococcal vaccination for older, high-risk patients with chronic illnesses, because of problems in producing and sustaining antibodies to pneumococcal capsular antigens in the vaccine.[16]

In younger adults, screening can be performed during routine visits to health providers.[7] For the elderly, as for pregnant women and for children, visits should be scheduled specifically for preventive care. The proper setting for screening or assessment for many of these problems may be in the patient's home rather than in the provider's office.[7]

No single health professional has either the range of skills or the time necessary to provide comprehensive preventive care for the elderly. An interdisciplinary health care team, typically including a physician, nurse, psychiatrist, physical and occupational therapists, dentist, pharmacist, and social worker, can facilitate thorough assessment. The site of geriatric assessment may be the hospital, an outpatient clinic, or the home; the function of such ambulatory health care teams has been described in several publications.[17, 18]

RECOMMENDATIONS FOR PREVENTIVE CARE OF THE ELDERLY

Comprehensive recommendations for preventive health care in the elderly were first defined in the 1970s with the work of Breslow and Somers and the Canadian Task Force on the Periodic Health Examination.[6, 7] Subsequent authors have recommended additional areas for screening and assessment for these patients.[8, 12, 19] As indicated below, these recommendations are based on a combination of scientific evidence (if available) and clinical judgment. Gaps in the base of scientific information are due, in part, both to the relatively recent interest in preventive care for the elderly and to methodological difficulties in assessing functional endpoints.[20] Table 5–3 lists 16 medical conditions that are generally recommended for preventive care in the elderly. These health problems fall into the following four major categories: (1) immunizations against influenza, tetanus, and pneumococcal disease; (2) diseases amenable to secondary prevention (hypertension control, tests for colorectal, breast, and cervical cancers); (3) functional impairments for which palliative measures exist (dental, podiatric, auditory, visual, and nutritional impairments); and (4) environmental or social risk factors (smoking cessation, accident prevention, alcoholism, and progressive incapacity with aging).

IMMUNIZATIONS

Tetanus

As a result of immunization programs for infants in the United States, tetanus is

TABLE 5–3. Consensus Recommendations for Preventive Care in the Elderly*

Condition	Maneuver	Frequency Age 65–74	Frequency Age 75+
Tetanus	Immunization	10 years	10 years
Influenza	Immunization	1 year	1 year
Pneumonococcal disease	Immunization	†	†
Hypertension	BP recording	2 years	2 years
Breast cancer	Breast examination Mammography	1 year 1–2 years	1 year 1–2 years
Cervical cancer	Pelvic examination Pap smear	1–5 years‡	1–5 years‡
Colorectal cancer	Stool for occult blood	1 year	1 year
Vision loss	Snellen chart Ocular examination	5 years	1 year
Hearing loss	Otologic examination Audiometry	1–2 years	1–2 years
Dental care	Dental examination Radiography	1–2 years	1–2 years
Foot care	Foot examination	1–2 years	1–2 years
Malnutrition	History	2 years	1 year
Smoking	History	§	§
Prevention of falls	History	2–5 years	1 year
Alcoholism	History Questionnaire	5 years	1 year
Progressive incapacity with aging	History	2 years	1 year

*Adapted from references 6, 7, 8, 12, and 20.
†Pneumococcal vaccine should be given one time only after age 65.
‡Recommended screening interval for women who have not had regular Pap smears earlier in life.
§A history of current smoking should be obtained at the initial visit.

now predominantly a disease of older adults; more than 50 percent of cases occur in people over 50 years of age.[21] One survey has shown that only 46 percent of elderly patients have serum levels of antitoxin that protect against tetanus.[21] A number of these patients, especially elderly women, have never been immunized; many men received the vaccine during military service. For those with a prior history of immunization, boosters should be administered every 10 years throughout life.

Influenza

During influenza epidemics, 80 to 90 percent of the excess deaths attributed to pneumonia and influenza occur among persons over age 65.[22] Elderly patients with cardiopulmonary disease and patients in chronic care facilities are at particular risk for influenza-related morbidity, but otherwise healthy elderly individuals are also in increased jeopardy. The influenza vaccine is about 87 percent effective in reducing mortality among chronically ill, elderly individuals, despite their less vigorous immune responses to the vaccine.[23, 24] Based on such information, immunization against influenza is recommended annually for all individuals aged 65 and older.

Pneumococcal Disease

Pneumococcal pneumonia is common in the elderly, with attack rates up to 4 percent per year in patients over age 70.[25] A single immunization with a vaccine containing capsular antigens from 23 bacterial strains has been recommended for prevention in the elderly, based on retrospective evidence that suggests a 60 percent efficacy of the vaccine in reducing episodes of pneumococcal bacteremia.[26] However, a randomized, prospective trial conducted by the Veterans' Administration showed that a 14-valent pneumococcal vaccine did not provide protection for chronically ill men, most of whom were over 55 years of age.[16] Patients who acquired pneumococcal infections despite immunization failed to produce or sustain protective antibodies, although healthy elderly individuals demonstrated excellent immune responses.[16] Because of this evidence, a recommendation for immunization against pneumococcal disease must be based more on minimal cost and reduced potential to cause harm than on proven efficacy in high-risk patients.

DISEASE PREVENTION

The benefits of secondary prevention for common diseases have been difficult to prove in any age group because of the large number of patients and long period of study necessary to prove effectiveness. Even when prevention has been shown to reduce mortality, other relevant issues, such as the optimal frequency and cost-effectiveness of screening and the effect of treatment on functional status, are often overlooked.

Hypertension

The treatment of hypertension in the elderly is discussed at length elsewhere in this volume. Recent findings of the European Working Party on High Blood Pressure suggest that treatment of patients over age 60 with blood pressure greater than 160/90 mmHg reduces cardiovascular mortality by 27 percent.[5] Treatment benefits were not shown to occur in individuals over age 80, most of whom were women.[27] The efficacy of treatment for patients with isolated systolic hypertension (systolic blood pressure greater than 160 but diastolic blood pressure less than 90) is under study at present. Control of hypertension may also improve cognitive function in patients with multi-infarct dementia.[28] Elderly patients should have blood pressure measurements at every office visit to screen for hypertension; those not using

the health care system should be screened in community facilities.

Breast Cancer

The three screening techniques that exist for the early detection of breast cancer are breast self-examination (BSE), clinician breast examination (CBE), and mammography. In general, CBE and mammography are performed in combination. The sensitivity of BSE for detecting breast cancers larger than 1 cm in size is lower in the elderly than in younger individuals; other methods of prevention have more conclusive proof of efficacy and deserve more emphasis in screening programs.[29] The earliest randomized clinical trial of breast cancer prevention using screening mammograms did not include enough women aged 60 to 65 to demonstrate a significant reduction in breast cancer mortality in that age group.[30] More recently, a case-control study of a combination of CBE and mammography has shown a reduction in mortality in women aged 60 to 69.[31] Preliminary results from an ongoing, randomized trial of mammographic screening in Sweden have also shown a reduction (40 percent) in breast cancer mortality in women aged 50 to 74.[4] Based on this evidence, the United States Preventive Services Task Force recommends that yearly CBE and mammography should be continued in women over age 60.[32]

Cervical Cancer

The annual death rate for cervical cancer is 159 per million in women over 65, compared with 44 per million for women aged 35 to 44; 41 percent of all deaths from cervical cancer occur in the elderly.[33] Women under age 65 should be screened for cervical carcinoma with Papanicolaou (Pap) smears at intervals of 1 to 3 years. The rate of cervical cancer is very low in elderly women who had regular Pap smears earlier in life; for these women, continued screening is not warranted. However, 38 percent of women over age 75 and 14 percent of women aged 65 to 74 reported *never* having had a Pap smear, and an additional 28 percent reported that they had not had regular screening.[34] A recent study of a single screening Pap smear in elderly women reported a high prevalence of abnormalities (13.5 per 1000 examinations).[33] Based on such evidence, elderly women who did not receive routine Pap smears earlier in life should be screened at intervals of 1 to 5 years.

Colon Cancer

Colorectal carcinoma is a disease of the elderly; 60 percent of cases occur in patients over age 65.[19] Testing of fecal samples for occult blood is a simple and inexpensive screening procedure used to detect colorectal carcinoma, but its utility is limited by two constraints. First, only 50 to 66 percent of colonic malignancies cause clinically detectable bleeding. In addition, although 13 to 23 percent of patients over age 60 in whom bleeding is detected prove to have colorectal cancer, a positive test requires further evaluation with air-contrast barium enema and flexible sigmoidoscopy or with colonoscopy in many patients who prove not to have the disease.[35] The risk, discomfort, and cost of these procedures must be incorporated into the assessment of screening programs. Large-scale evaluations of screening for colorectal carcinoma are ongoing; to date there is no conclusive evidence that screening reduces mortality associated with the disease.[36]

FUNCTIONAL IMPAIRMENTS

Techniques of clinical assessment and treatment for impairments of vision, hearing, dentition, the foot, and nutrition are discussed elsewhere in this text. To be included in programs of prevention, studies assessing functional impairments should meet the criteria outlined in Table 5–2. By these exacting standards, it is not enough to show, for example, that a program to provide dentures to the elderly enables them to chew their food. To justify the effort and expense of such a program, an evaluation should demonstrate that detection early in the natural history of the impairment improves some measure of overall functional independence or quality of life.

Although most published studies fail to meet these criteria, there are several cogent arguments in favor of screening the elderly for functional impairments. The first argument is the "face validity" of prevention for these ailments; it is hard to imagine, for example, how properly fitting dentures could worsen functional status. Second, elderly patients fail to report many of their significant disabilities to their physicians.[37] As a result, they may live with substantial impairments that would escape detection unless they are specifically sought. Third, even if correction of existing impairments does not improve function immediately, it may prevent future deterioration. Our discussion will emphasize the research that links these disabilities to overall functional deterioration and demonstrates improved function after treatment.

Visual Impairment

Diminished vision restricts independence directly and contributes to other health hazards, such as motor vehicle accidents and falls. Prevention may be as simple as using a 60-watt light bulb; Cullinan and colleagues demonstrated that better lighting in the home improved distant and near vision in 82 percent of visually impaired outpatients.[38] More impressively, a later study showed that surgery to remove cataracts enhanced functional abilities as well as visual acuity.[39] After surgery, 13 percent more patients were able to drive a car, and 6 percent more could read a newspaper. Objective assessments indicated significant improvement of mental status and manual performance. This study serves as a methodological model for the assessment of programs to correct functional impairments in the elderly.

Hearing Loss

Between 30 and 60 percent of elderly patients have impaired hearing. The validity of physical examination as a screening procedure for hearing loss has not been assessed; the "gold standard" for assessment is pure-tone audiometry.[40] Some studies have shown an association between hearing loss and depression or dementia in the elderly, but the findings are inconsistent.[40–42] Hearing aids are of benefit in restoring the loss, but the ability of treatment to reverse broader functional impairment has not been assessed.

Dental Care

Good dentition is important for nutrition, speech, and social function. A screening physical examination of the mouth and teeth can detect oral malignancy and evaluate dental function.[43] The benefits of screening for oral cancer have not been formally assessed. Self-perceived problems with chewing food are associated with poorer nutritional status in elderly males, but studies that demonstrate whether preventive dental care improves nutrition have not been reported.[44]

Foot Care

The goal of preventive foot care is to preserve mobility, which in turn may help preserve social function and independence in activities of daily living.[45] Elderly individuals commonly have foot problems but less commonly report them to their physicians.[37] A direct link between preventive foot care and preservation of function has not been established, except in high-risk patients with diabetes mellitus or peripheral vascular disease.[19]

Malnutrition

Estimates of the prevalence of malnutrition in the elderly vary widely, based on the population studied and on the nutritional indices measured. Malnutrition is more common in individuals who are chronically ill, isolated, or in long-term care facilities.[19] A study of hospitalized veterans showed a 61 percent incidence of malnutrition in patients over age 65 and a 23 percent higher mortality rate among those who were malnourished.[46] However, malnutrition in such individuals may be a consequence of underlying disease, such as the cachexia caused by malignancy; i.e., the disease itself, rather than the malnutrition it produces, may be the cause of death. In cross-sectional surveys of elderly individuals living independently, decreased consumption of vitamins C, B_{12}, riboflavin, or folate has been associated with cognitive impairment, but such studies cannot determine whether the nutritional deficit or the cognitive dysfunction is causal.[47] Nutritional supplementation improved immunologic response to influenza vaccination in malnourished individuals, demonstrating how different modalities of preventive care may be interlinked.[48]

SOCIAL/ENVIRONMENTAL RISK FACTORS

Smoking

A young person's decision to quit smoking cigarettes may be richly rewarded by better health in old age.[49] Until recently, however, there was little evidence to suggest that an elderly, lifelong smoker would benefit from quitting. If the damage already done by cigarettes were irreversible, there would be no point to efforts at prevention. A recent prospective cohort study of patients over age 65 showed that the cardiovascular mortality of elderly individuals who had quit smoking within five years of entering the study was comparable to that of nonsmokers and 45 percent less than the mortality rate for individuals who continued to smoke.[3] Many techniques, from drug therapy to behavior modification, are under investigation to aid individuals who wish to stop smoking.[50] Because of the evidence that smoking cessation is an effective preventive measure, clinicians should continue to persuade their elderly patients to quit.

Alcoholism

Alcoholism affects 1 to 10 percent of the elderly and contributes to 15 to 20 percent of nursing home admissions, yet the problem is commonly overlooked or misdiagnosed.[51] Contrary to earlier teaching, the amount of alcohol consumption remains relatively constant in the elderly, although the incidence of physical and social problems caused by alcohol declines with age.[52] The best available screening tests for alcoholism in younger individuals are structured questionnaires about alcohol-related problems; an optimal method of screening for the elderly has not been defined.[53] Clinicians report that elderly alcoholics respond well to treatment, but the effectiveness of treatment in preserving functional independence (e.g., avoiding nursing home admission) has not been assessed.[54]

Falls

Accidents are the fifth leading cause of death in the elderly; half of these deaths result from falls.[55] Up to 50 percent of elderly patients report episodes of falling, and 8 to 40 percent of these falls result in fractures.[55] Falls in younger, healthier individuals are most often associated with environmental hazards such as stairs, loose rugs, or poor lighting, whereas older, sicker individuals are more likely to fall because of underlying illnesses (neurologic disorders, cardiac arrhythmias producing syncope) or because of the medications used to treat their illnesses.[55–57] As many as two thirds of these falls may be preventable through proper medical diagnosis, cessation of offending medications, or environmental modifications.[56] A patient who falls should have a thorough neurologic assessment, with attention given to impairments in muscle strength, balance, and gait.[57] Prevention or treatment for osteoporosis in postmenopausal women may reduce the morbidity arising from falls. Women who have undergone postmenopausal estrogen therapy have a decreased risk of hip fracture.[58] A randomized trial of treatment with calcium, estrogen, and/or fluoride has shown a decrease in the rate of new vertebral fractures.[59] Other strategies for the prevention of falls, such as assessment of the home for potential hazards, require formal evaluation.

Progressive Incapacity with Aging

The Canadian Task Force defines this type of comprehensive assessment as "enquiry by health care professionals into physical, psychologic, and social competence, conducted in the home, with organ system enquiry and further action if indicated."[7] The perspective of such assessment is ecologic in its attempt to assess the complex interactions of the elderly person with his or her environment and to develop recommendations tailored to the individual. One randomized trial of home visits to elderly individuals in Denmark has shown reductions in overall mortality and in hospital readmissions.[60] In a second trial of comprehensive home care in the United States, no change in overall mortality or functional status was shown, although hospitalizations and nursing home admissions were reduced in the subset of patients in the study who were terminally ill and died within 3 months of enrollment.[18] Thus, there is evidence that comprehensive assessment in the home may benefit some elderly patients, but such programs are costly and require further study.

Additional Conditions Considered for Screening

Many other health problems have been proposed by some authorities for efforts at prevention. Table 5–4 lists 13 additional conditions for which consensus has not been attained. This list is included primarily to identify measures that require further research.

PREVENTION OF IATROGENIC ILLNESS: MEDICATION OVERPRESCRIBING

Any therapy represents a trade-off between benefit and risk; no treatment is without side effects and costs. Iatrogenic illnesses are those that arise as a consequence of medical treatments. In the elderly, they may take many forms including urinary tract infections resulting from prolonged use of catheters, loss of muscle tone or balance after excessive bed rest, and even social dependence fostered by family members concerned about preventing impairments.[2, 8] All iatrogenic conditions are preventable, since they result from actions of health care providers or caregivers. Methods for prevention of many of these problems are discussed

TABLE 5–4. Other Conditions Proposed for Screening or Assessment of Asymptomatic Elderly Patients*

Condition	Screening/Assessment Technique
Hypothyroidism	Physical examination; serum thyroxine
Diabetes mellitus	Blood glucose determination
Hyperlipidemia	Fasting cholesterol; triglyceride
Anemia	Hemoglobin/hematocrit
Prostate cancer	Physical examination
Tuberculosis	Skin test†
Social isolation	Social history; questionnaire
Physical fitness	Medical history
Obesity	Weight
Dementia	Mental status examination
Depression	Mental status examination
Urinary incontinence	Medical history
Elder abuse	Medical history; physical examination

*Conditions recommended in at least one of references 6, 7, 8, 12, 19 but not in more than two sources.

†Screening for tuberculosis may be indicated in nursing home populations but not in individuals living independently.

elsewhere in this text; this chapter focuses on the prevention of dysfunction due to the overprescribing of medications for elderly outpatients.

Between 80 and 90 percent of elderly individuals take medications.[61–63] Medication surveys during home visits have found that the average elderly person takes two to five prescription medications and two to three nonprescription, over-the-counter preparations (generally vitamins and analgesics).[62, 63] Medication "polypharmacy" is common; 18 to 29 percent of these individuals are prescribed four or more different drugs to take each day.[61–64] The medications most often prescribed for the elderly (diuretics, antihypertensive agents, digoxin, antidepressants, hypnotics, and sedatives) are notorious for side effects. As the number of prescribed medications rises, so does the prevalence of adverse effects. Ten to 15 percent of elderly patients taking one medication and 27 to 48 percent of those taking three or more drugs report side effects associated with their therapy.[61, 63, 64] For example, a 75-year-old woman was referred to us with anorexia, nausea, and a recent 20-pound weight loss, which led the referring physician to suspect a gastrointestinal malignancy. A medication history revealed that she was taking digoxin, 0.25 mg a day, despite a serum creatinine level of 2.1. Her serum digoxin level was 2.9 ng/ml, in the toxic range. Cessation of the drug resolved her symptoms.

The elderly face many barriers to the proper consumption of these complex medication regimens such as functional difficulties in reading labels or opening child-proof containers, conceptual problems in understanding treatment regimens or organizing dosage schedules, financial constraints that may preclude buying medications, or transportation limitations that prevent the patient from obtaining them. As a result, noncompliance with treatment is a major problem with the elderly. Pill counts in elderly patients showed that only 47 to 57 percent consumed their medications according to instructions and that the likelihood of compliance fell as the number of medications prescribed increased.[63–65] Such noncompliance is a hindrance to successful therapy but may be an adaptive response (although unsatisfactory from a variety of perspectives) to functional disabilities induced by medications.

Drugs must *always* be considered as a potential cause of functional deterioration in the elderly.[8] Older individuals are susceptible to drug-related dysfunction for several reasons. First, the absorption, distribution, and metabolism of some drugs may change with age, often leading to drug efficacy or toxicity at lower doses than in younger individuals.[66] Furthermore, older individuals are less able to compensate for impairments in homeostasis because of their reduced physiologic reserve.[2, 67] Finally, treatment of one condition in a long list of medical problems may worsen another illness or uncover a latent functional impairment. For example, a nonsteroidal anti-inflammatory drug (NSAID) prescribed for degenerative arthritis may raise blood pressure.[68] If the medication is not recognized as the cause of the hypertension, antihypertensive medications may be administered or increased, exacerbating a tendency to orthostatic hypotension and increasing the risk of falling.

What is the evidence that drugs cause dysfunction in elderly patients and that stopping unnecessary medications can reverse the loss? The following discussion focuses on two common sources of dysfunction: dementia and falls.

Dementia

Medications are a cause of reversible dementia in the elderly. In a case series of 308 elderly patients evaluated for dementia, Larson and colleagues found that cognitive function improved in 35 (11 percent) when an offending drug or drugs were discontinued.[69] Ten of these patients (3 percent of the total) returned to normal mental status, whereas the remaining 8 percent had persistent, but less severe, dementia after cessation of medications. Patients taking more medications were at higher risk of adverse effects. Those whose dementias were caused or worsened by drugs were taking a mean of 3.7 prescription medications, compared with a mean of 1.7 medications for individuals whose dementias were unrelated to medications.

Many medications have been implicated as causes of dementia. In Larson's study, minor tranquilizers (e.g., diazepam), antihypertensives, major tranquilizers (e.g., haloperidol), analgesics, and cimetidine were common offenders. Thus, complete restoration of cognitive function is unusual, but some degree of improvement is possible with reduction of medication regimens in a clinically significant subset of patients with dementia.

Falls

Many different medications may cause falls. Patients suffering from drug-related dementia are three times as likely to fall as those whose dementia is unrelated to

drugs.[69] Hip fractures, most of which result from falls, are more likely to occur in patients who have taken long-acting sedative/hypnotic agents, antidepressants, or major tranquilizers than in patients who have not used these medications.[70] Women who take a wide range of antihypertensive medications report dizziness or syncope more frequently than women who do not take such medications.[71] Vasodilators and barbiturates have also been associated with falls.[72, 73] Finally, the risk of falls rises in proportion to the total number of medications taken.[57] Despite these studies implicating medications as causes of falls, there is not conclusive evidence that stopping such treatment will reduce the subsequent frequency of falls or fractures in the elderly.

The association of polypharmacy with both dementia and falls suggests that clinicians should attempt to reduce the overall intensity of the regimen as well as the administration of specific drugs that place the patient in jeopardy. Of course, the risk of reducing treatment is that the condition for which the drug was originally prescribed will worsen. Patients who undergo drug withdrawal should be monitored closely. In Larson's study of drug-related dementias, drug withdrawal was rarely accompanied by clinical deterioration; patients who required continued therapy could be safely treated with alternative medications or lower doses of the offending agent.[69]

Several studies have demonstrated the effectiveness of attempts to reduce the use of specific drugs or drug classes in the elderly. In two studies, between 85 and 100 percent of nursing home patients who took diuretics were able to stop treatment without clinical consequences. A few individuals reported decreased dizziness or correction of incontinence.[74, 75] About 50 percent of patients taking digoxin who are not in atrial fibrillation may be able to stop the drug without cardiac decompensation.[76, 77] Antihypertensive medications can be withdrawn successfully in up to 40 percent of well-controlled, younger patients without recurrent hypertension; one case series has shown a comparable success rate in the elderly.[78–80] Although specific efforts to reduce psychotropic drugs in the elderly have not been reported, such medications are often overused or misprescribed. Rational evaluation of the need for therapy and the pharmacokinetics of the drug can often lead to discontinuation of unnecessary treatment.[81]

PREVENTION OF FUNCTIONAL IMPAIRMENT DUE TO MEDICATIONS

The foregoing discussion is limited to the effects of the overprescribing of medication on physical function; however, other adverse consequences of overprescribing, such as the cost of medications, the extra visits to health providers who prescribe them, and the evaluations necessary to detect and treat drug-related dysfunction, also argue for efforts at prevention. The following are seven principles for preventing functional impairments caused by medications taken by the elderly.

1. *Think twice before prescribing medications.* It is much easier to initiate treatment than to stop it.

2. *Prescribe lower dosages of fewer drugs for shorter periods of time.* When the patient has fewer drugs to take, compliance can be improved.

3. *Consider pharmacokinetic principles.* Alterations in pharmacokinetics with aging must be taken into account when selecting drugs and dosages to avoid untoward responses.

4. *Consider drug/drug and drug/disease interactions.* Adverse effects can occur when the patient is taking several different drugs or when the patient is taking a particular drug in the presence of other illnesses.

5. *Re-evaluate the need for prescribed medications.* A thorough review of the patient's medical record often identifies drugs that are no longer required or that have no clear clinical indication. This also avoids the possibility that the patient will accumulate medications (and diagnoses) over time.

6. *Consider trials of dosage reduction.* For patients requiring ongoing treatment, a lower dose of a medication may be equally effective and produce fewer side effects.

7. *Consider drugs in differential diagnosis of functional impairments.* Often, it is possible to accomplish more for patients with impairment or deterioration by prescribing less medication.

A home visit may be very helpful in detecting and correcting drug-related problems in the elderly. The patient's home should be assessed for inventories of prescription and over-the-counter medications. It also may be the ideal location to assess barriers to compliance and to devise methods of improving adherence to necessary treatment.

In summary, prevention of disability and disease remains an important part of health care throughout life. The physician must seek a comprehensive understanding of the patient's ability to function in his or her environment and should tailor recommendations for preventive diagnosis and therapy to the needs and constraints of the individual. Finally, the clinician must remain attentive to the potentially adverse consequences of therapy and must be prepared to reverse the harmful effects as well as to enhance the benefits of treatment for the elderly patient.

REFERENCES

1. Katz S, Branch LG, Branson MH, et al: Active life expectancy. N Engl J Med 309:1218, 1983.
2. Kennie DC: Good health for the aged. JAMA 249:770, 1983.
3. Jajich CL, Ostfeld AM, Freeman DH: Smoking and coronary heart disease mortality in the elderly. JAMA 252:2831, 1984.
4. Tabar L, Fagerberg CJG, Gad A, et al: Reduction in mortality from breast cancer after mass screening with mammography. Lancet (i):829, 1985.
5. Amery A, Birkenhager W, Bulpitt C, et al: Mortality and morbidity results from the European Working Party on high blood pressure in the elderly trial. Lancet (i):1349, 1985.
6. Breslow L, Somers AR: The lifetime health-monitoring program. N Engl J Med 296:601, 1977.
7. Canadian Task Force on the Periodic Health Examination: The periodic health examination. Can Med Assoc J 121:1193, 1979.
8. Kane RL, Kane RA, Arnold SB, et al: Prevention and the elderly: risk factors. Health Serv Res 19 (Part II):946, 1985.
9. Fletcher RH, Fletcher SW, Wagner EH, et al: Clinical Epidemiology: The Essentials. Baltimore, Williams and Wilkins, 1982, p 67.
10. Kane RA, Kane RL: Assessing the Elderly: A Practical Guide to Management. Lexington, MA, Lexington Books (DC Health), 1981, p 15.
11. Sackett DL, Haynes RB, Tugwell P, et al: Clinical Epidemiology. Boston, Little, Brown & Co, 1985, p 139.
12. Magenheim MJ: Screening the elderly. In Calkins E., et al., eds: The Practice of Geriatrics. Philadelphia, WB Saunders Co, 1983, p 60.
13. Veith FJ: Limb salvage in the elderly and infirm. J Am Geriatr Soc 32:252, 1984.

14. Dorken E, Grzybowski S, Allen EA: Significance of the tuberculin test in the elderly. Chest 92:237, 1987.

15. Stead WW, To T: The significance of the tuberculin skin test in elderly persons. Ann Intern Med 107:837, 1987.

16. Simberkoff MS, Cross AP, Al-Ibrahim M, et al: Efficacy of pneumococcal vaccine in high-risk patients. N Engl J Med 315:1318, 1986.

17. Tulloch AJ, Moore V: A randomised controlled trial of geriatric screening and surveillance in general practice. J R Coll Gen Pract 29:733, 1979.

18. Zimmer JG, Groth-Juncker A, McCusker J: A randomized controlled study of a home health care team. Am J Public Health 75:134, 1985.

19. Stults BM: Preventive health care for the elderly. West J Med 141:832, 1984.

20. Feinstein AR, Josephy BR, Wells CK: Scientific and clinical problems in indexes of functional disability. Ann Intern Med 105:413, 1986.

21. Weiss BP, Strassburg MA, Feeley JC: Tetanus and diphtheria immunity in an elderly population in Los Angeles County. Am J Public Health 73:802, 1983.

22. Centers for Disease Control: Recommendations for prevention and control of influenza. Ann Intern Med 105:399, 1986.

23. Barker WH, Mullooly JP: Influenza vaccination of elderly persons. JAMA 244:2547, 1980.

24. Howells CHL, Vesselinova-Jenkins CK, Evans AD, et al: Influenza vaccination and mortality from bronchopneumonia in the elderly. Lancet (i):381, 1975.

25. Van Metre TE: Pneumococcal pneumonia treated with antibiotics. N Engl J Med 251:1048, 1954.

26. Bolan G, Broome CV, Facklam RR, et al: Pneumococcal vaccine efficacy in selected populations in the United States. Ann Intern Med 104:1, 1986.

27. Amery A, Birkenhager W, Brixko R, et al: Efficacy of antihypertensive drug treatment according to age, sex, blood pressure, and previous cardiovascular disease in patients over the age of 60. Lancet (ii):589, 1986.

28. Meyer JS, Judd BW, Tawaklna T, et al: Improved cognition after control of risk factors for multi-infarct dementia. JAMA 256:2203, 1986.

29. O'Malley MS, Fletcher SW: Screening for breast cancer with breast self-examination. JAMA 257:2196, 1987.

30. Shapiro S, Strax P, Venet L: Periodic breast cancer screening in reducing mortality from breast cancer. JAMA 215:1777, 1971.

31. Collette HJA, Day NE, Rombach JJ, et al: Evaluation of screening for breast cancer in a non-randomised study (the Dom Project) by means of a case-control study. Lancet (i):1224, 1984.

32. United States Preventive Services Task Force: Recommendations for breast cancer screening. JAMA 257:2196, 1987.

33. Mandelblatt J, Gopaul I, Wistreich M: Gynecological care of elderly women: another look at Papanicolaou smear testing. JAMA 256:367, 1986.

34. Celentano DD, Shapiro S, Weisman CS: Cancer preventive screening behavior among elderly women. Prev Med 11:454, 1982.

35. Winawer SJ: Detection and diagnosis of colorectal cancer. Cancer 51:2519, 1983.

36. Simon JB: Occult blood screening for colorectal carcinoma: a critical review. Gastroenterology 88:820, 1985.

37. Williamson J, Stokoe IH, Gray S, et al: Old people at home: their unreported needs. Lancet i:1117, 1964.

38. Cullinan TR, Silver JH, Gould ES, et al: Visual disability and home lighting. Lancet i:642, 1979.

39. Applegate WB, Miller ST, Elam JT, et al: Impact of cataract surgery with lens implantation on vision and physical function in elderly patients. JAMA 257:1064, 1987.

40. Uhlmann RF, Larson EB, Koepsell TD: Hearing impairment and cognitive decline in senile dementia of the Alzheimer's type. J Am Geriatr Soc 34:207, 1986.

41. Herbst KG, Humphrey C: Hearing impairment and mental state in the elderly living at home. Br Med J 281:903, 1980.

42. Thomas PD, Hunt WC, Garry PJ, et al: Hearing acuity in a healthy elderly population: effects on emotional, cognitive, and social status. J Gerontol 38:321, 1983.

43. Gordon SR, Jahnigan DW: Oral assessment of the dentulous elderly patient. J Am Geriatr Soc 34:276, 1986.

44. Gordon SR, Kelley SL, Sybyl JR, et al: Relationship in very elderly veterans of nutritional status, self-perceived chewing ability, dental status, and social isolation. J Am Geriatr Soc 33:334, 1985.

45. Albert SF, Jahnigan DW: Treating common foot disorders in older patients. Geriatrics 38:42, 1983.

46. Bienia R, Ratcliff S, Barbour GL: Malnutrition in the hospitalized geriatric patient. J Am Geriatr Soc 30:433, 1982.

47. Goodwin JS, Goodwin JM, Garry PJ: Association between nutritional status and cognitive functioning in a healthy elderly population. JAMA 249:2917, 1983.

48. Chandra RK, Puri S: Nutritional support improves antibody response to influenza virus vaccine in the elderly. Br Med J 291:705, 1985.

49. Fielding JE: Smoking: Health effects and control. N Engl J Med 313:491, 555, 1985.

50. Health and Public Policy Committee, American College of Physicians: Methods for stopping cigarette smoking. Ann Intern Med 105:281, 1986.

51. Solomon DH: Alcoholism and aging. In West LJ, moderator: Alcoholism. Ann Intern Med 100:405, 1984.

52. Glynn RJ, Bouchard GR, LoCastro JS: Aging and generational effects on drinking behaviors in men: results from the Normative Aging Study. Am J Public Health 75:1413, 1985.

53. Hays JT, Spickard WA: Alcoholism: early diagnosis and intervention. J Gen Intern Med 2:420, 1987.

54. Brody JA: Aging and alcohol abuse. J Am Geriatr Soc 30:123, 1982.

55. Perry BC: Falls among the elderly. J Am Geriatr Soc 30:367, 1982.

56. Rubenstein LZ: Falls in the elderly: a clinical approach. West J Med 138:273, 1983.

57. Buchner DM, Larson EB: Falls and fractures in patients with Alzheimer-type dementia. JAMA 257:1492, 1987.

58. Kiel DJ, Felson DT, Anderson JJ, et al: Hip fracture and the use of estrogens in postmenopausal women. N Engl J Med 317:1169, 1987.

59. Riggs BL, Seeman E, Hodgson SF, et al: Effect of the fluoride/calcium regimen on vertebral fracture occurrence in postmenopausal osteoporosis. N Engl J Med 306:446, 1982.

60. Hendriksen C, Lund E, Stromgard E: Consequences of assessment and intervention among elderly people: a three-year randomised controlled trial. Br Med J 289:1522, 1984.
61. Klein LE, German PS, Levine DM, et al: Medication problems among outpatients. Arch Intern Med 144:1185, 1984.
62. Ostrom JR, Hammerlund ER, Christensen DB, et al: Medication use in an elderly population. Med Care 23:157, 1985.
63. Darnell JC, Murray MD, Martz BL, et al: Medication use by ambulatory elderly. J Am Geriatr Soc 34:1, 1986.
64. Wandless I, Mucklow JC, Smith A, et al: Compliance with prescribed medications: a study of elderly patients in the community. J R Coll Gen Pract 29:391, 1979.
65. Kendrick R, Bayne JRD: Compliance with prescribed medication by elderly patients. Can Med Assoc J 127:961, 1982.
66. Ouslander J: Drug therapy in the elderly. Ann Intern Med 95:711, 1981.
67. Rowe JW: Health care of the elderly. N Engl J Med 312:827, 1985.
68. Rudack KL, Deck CC, Bloomfield SS: Ibuprofen interferes with the efficacy of antihypertensive drugs. Ann Intern Med 107:628, 1987.
69. Larson EB, Kukull WA, Buchner D, et al: Adverse drug reactions associated with global cognitive impairment in elderly persons. Ann Intern Med 107:169, 1987.
70. Ray WA, Griffin MR, Schaffner W, et al: Psychotropic drug use and the risk of hip fracture. N Engl J Med 316:363, 1987.
71. Hale WE, Stewart RB, Marks RG: Central nervous system symptoms of elderly subjects using antihypertensive drugs. J Am Geriatr Soc 32:5, 1984.
72. Granek E, Baker SP, Abbey H, et al: Medications and diagnoses in relation to falls in a long-term care facility. J Am Geriatr Soc 35:503, 1987.
73. Macdonald JB: The role of drugs in falls in the elderly. Clin Geriatr Med 1:621, 1985.
74. Burr ML, King S, Davies HEF, et al: The effects of discontinuing long-term diuretic therapy in the elderly. Age Ageing 6:638, 1977.
75. Portnoi VA, Pawlson LG: Abuse of diuretic therapy in nursing homes. J Chronic Dis 34:363, 1981.
76. Johnston BD, McDevitt DG: Is maintenance digoxin necessary in patients with sinus rhythm? Lancet (i):567, 1979.
77. Fleg JL, Gottlieb SH, Lakatta EG: Is digoxin really important in treatment of compensated heart failure? Am J Med 73:244, 1982.
78. Langford HG, Blaufox D, Oberman A, et al: Dietary therapy slows the return of hypertension after stopping prolonged medication. JAMA 253:657, 1985.
79. Stamler RA, Stamler J, Grimm R, et al: Nutritional therapy for high blood pressure. JAMA 257:1484, 1987.
80. Hansen AG, Jensen H, Langesen LP, et al: Withdrawal of antihypertensive drugs in the elderly. Acta Med Scand (Suppl 676):178, 1983.
81. Thompson TL, Moran MG, Nies AS, et al: Psychotropic drug use in the elderly. N Engl J Med 308:134, 194, 1983.

CHAPTER 6

Living Conditions

Nancy L. Peters
L. Mary Mathew

Grow old along with me!
The best is yet to be,
The last of life, for which the first was made:
Our times are in his hand
Who saith, "A whole I planned,
Youth shows but half; trust God: see all, nor be
*   afraid!"*

ROBERT BROWNING, *Rabbi Ben Ezra*

Chronic care for the dependent elderly encompasses a variety of formal and informal services. Although many persons, both professionals and laymen, believe that the long-term care system is centered in nursing homes, research has shown that the majority of disabled elderly are cared for in the community. The types of services required by this elderly, noninstitutionalized population range from purely social and financial assistance (e.g., transportation, home repair, legal aid, and money management) to functional assistance (help with bathing, dressing, meal preparation, mobility and transferring, toileting, and so forth) to traditional medical care (disease prevention, diagnosis, treatment, health maintenance, and terminal-stage care). In part, these services may be provided by relatives, friends and neighbors, paid homemakers, nonprofit and home health agencies, case workers, day-care and respite care programs, and health care professionals and institutions. Because individual needs and community resources vary substantially, assistance to the disabled elderly may take many forms.

Case management refers to the evaluation of an individual's needs and the subsequent selection of the appropriate services and environment to help maintain the individual's best level of function, independence, and quality of life. Physicians are often case managers for their elderly patients. It is a role with which many of

them feel uncomfortable, as few traditional medical schools include courses in case management or the use of community resources. This chapter, therefore, describes some of the major community and institutional resources with which the physician may interact to provide quality care to elderly and disabled patients.

FAMILY SUPPORT

In 1982, the National Long-Term Care Survey and Informal Caregivers Survey found that 1.6 million noninstitutionalized, disabled elderly Americans were receiving unpaid assistance from 2.2 million caregivers.[1, 2] The recipients of this care had limitations in performing one or more activities of daily living (ADL); (bathing, 42 percent; dressing, 20 percent; toileting, 21 percent; transferring, 26 percent; and eating, 6 percent). Twenty percent were over age 85, most were female, and 76 percent lived with a spouse, children, or both. Only 11 percent of the group lived alone, in contrast to overall population statistics, which show that one third of the noninstitutionalized elderly live alone.[3] That this population was significantly more disabled than the overall elderly population was confirmed by the 1984 National Health Interview Survey, which indicated that only 6 percent or less of noninstitutionalized Americans over age 65 require assistance with any of the ADLs.[4]

Persons providing informal care to the community-based disabled elderly were predominantly female (72 percent). They were more likely to have incomes below the poverty line and to be unemployed. Caregivers comprised adult daughters (29 percent), wives (23 percent), and husbands (13 percent). One third of caregivers were the sole providers of care, and only 10 percent had paid help. Most (80 percent) provided care 7 days a week, with an average of 4 hours per day devoted specifically to caregiver tasks.

The costs to informal caregivers of providing regular assistance to a dependent elder may be extensive. Sources of stress reported by caregivers include the necessity of giving up or limiting employment, conflicts with childrearing and other family responsibilities, decreased energy and leisure time, and loss of control over their own lives.

The future of this informal home-based care system, which in the past has maintained the majority of disabled elderly outside of institutions, is in jeopardy. Changes in modern family structure are putting pressure on this system. As more and more women join the work force, fewer will be at home to care for elderly relatives. Younger generations may be mobile and not available to provide assistance. High divorce rates and low birth rates decrease the numbers of potential caregivers for elderly relatives. In addition, the increased number of the oldest old (i.e., those 85 years old and over) means that the following generation will be well into their sixties, and perhaps disabled themselves, at a time when the oldest are most frail and at the highest risk of functional decline.

Despite stresses to the system, at the present time, the informal support system is still providing the major portion of care for the elderly. It is estimated that for every resident of a nursing home, there are three equally disabled persons being cared for in the community.[5] Generally, caregivers turn to formal services, programs, and institutions for help only when the burden of care exceeds their capacities or becomes emotionally overwhelming. The following sections describe services and programs available to supplement the informal support system.

HOMECARE

The development of programs to support the elderly living at home received major impetus in 1965 from the passage of the Social Security Amendments (in-

cluding Medicare, Medicaid, and Title XX) and the Older Americans Act. Title XX provided limited federal funding for daycare, protective services, legal services, family counseling, meals, transportation, and home-based services. The costs of these benefits were based on income and, thus, this was predominantly a welfare program. Title III of the Older Americans Act, on the other hand, provided benefits (homemaker services, Meals-on-Wheels, home health aides, senior transportation, legal assistance, and so on) based on age rather than on income. Both Title XX and Title III programs have had limited funding, which explains why these services are not universally available. Local support for such programs is essential; small, rural towns may not have many of these services. Larger communities are more likely to offer a full range of services to the elderly, but the lack of adequate funds may make the resources scarce. Nonprofit organizations, such as the Red Cross, veterans' groups, churches, service clubs, and others, may offer services (transportation, home-delivered meals, home repair, and so on) to the elderly. Fees based on the ability to pay are often charged for such assistance. Physicians may apply to local departments of social services, area councils on aging, American Association of Retired Persons (AARP) organizations, hospital social workers, and others to gain information about local resources available for their dependent elderly patients.

Medically oriented services can also be delivered to the elderly at home. Indeed, the home health care industry has shown dramatic growth over the past decade, with proprietary agencies showing the greatest growth. Most agencies are Medicare-certified. To be eligible for home health care under Medicare regulations, an individual must be home-bound and need part-time skilled nursing care and/or physical, speech, or occupational therapy. If these criteria are met, medical social services and personal-care services provided by a home health aide also may be available. All services must be prescribed by a physician.

Homecare is viewed by some as an alternative to nursing home placement. Indeed, with careful case management, a package of services can be arranged that will prevent institutionalization of some portion of the dependent elderly. However, Medicare-regulated home health care is part-time or intermittent; for those persons requiring round-the-clock assistance or supervision, the 6 to 9 hours a week generally allowed by Medicare is inadequate. As with most programs that attempt to provide community-based services as alternatives to nursing home care, the home health care program depends on the presence of a strong family or informal support structure to provide most of the assistance required by the noninstitutionalized, dependent elderly.

DAYCARE

With the passage of Medicaid and other health care legislation in the 1960s, the nursing home industry became a growth industry, with public expenditure rising more than twenty-fold in 20 years. However, a series of well-publicized nursing home scandals in the 1970s led legislators to look for alternatives to nursing home care. The Health Care Financing Administration (HCFA), which is responsible for administering the Medicare and Medicaid Programs, was authorized to fund home-care research and demonstration projects to find alternatives to nursing home care without increasing government costs. A variety of these were funded during the 1970s, including several adult daycare programs. Although preliminary results did not show significant savings to the government (perhaps owing to high administrative start-up costs and also to the cost of services utilized by the elderly who were not at immediate risk of nursing home placement), the programs were popular and thus politically successful. In 1981, Congress passed the Home and Community-Based Waivers program, which authorized states to initiate programs similar to the earlier research and demonstration projects. Adult daycare is included in the Medicaid Waivers programs.

Adult daycare originated in the 1940s in Great Britain, when hospital outpatient centers for psychiatric patients were set up to decrease the number of hospital inpatients. By the late 1950s, day hospitals for geriatric patients were opened. Such units are now a common feature of British geriatric practice, often closely associated with inpatient geriatric units and sharing the inpatient facilities. In British studies, there is some evidence to suggest that day hospitals reduce the length of inpatient hospital stays and contribute to earlier discharge.

The first geriatric daycare programs in the United States were opened in the 1940s, by both the Menninger Clinic and Yale University. In 1984, over 300 daycare programs were in operation in this country.[9]

Adult daycare is a program for the disabled elderly; federal guidelines specify that daycare should "be provided under health leadership in an ambulatory care setting for adults who do not require 24-hour institutional care and yet, owing to physical and/or mental impairment, are not capable of fulltime independent living."

Daycare programs generally fall into two categories: Model I programs are medically oriented, with physical rehabilitation as a primary goal; Model II programs are socially oriented, with maintenance of function as a primary goal.[10] Model I programs tend to serve more physically disabled clients; to be closely associated with hospitals, rehabilitation units or both; to have a more highly skilled staff; and to be more expensive. These programs are centered around multidisciplinary assessment, with a strong medical presence at the time of admission to the program that emphasizes improvement and eventual discharge from the program. Clients are often referred to these programs after hospitalization.

Model II programs are oriented around such goals as decreasing isolation, maintaining independence, and providing respite for caretakers. They tend to be freestanding and to have a less highly skilled staff. There are often no specific rehabilitative plans or discharge goals, and clients stay in these programs until they die or move into a nursing home. Services offered in these programs may include personal-care assistance (bathing, grooming, nail cutting, exercising), family counseling, legal assistance, help with paying bills or arranging additional financial services, health education, group and leisure activities, and reality orientation. Clients are often referred to Model II programs by social workers, Alzheimer's disease societies, welfare agencies, and friends.

Whether attending Model I or Model II programs, clients characteristically have multiple medical and functional problems, often as severe as those in nursing home patients. The majority of daycare clients do not live alone, in contrast to nursing home patients, the majority of whom previously lived alone, as suggested in the literature. Therefore, it is possible that the major difference between daycare clients and nursing home patients is the amount of family support they have, rather than the degree of functional and medical disability they suffer. Patients with families to care for them can be managed at home with daycare, whereas patients without families must go to nursing homes.

Typical daycare programs are small, serving 15 to 25 clients a day. Staff-to-client ratios average 1:5 to 1:7. Most programs are open from about 9 or 10 A.M. until 3 or 4 P.M. Clients attend 1 to 5 days a week. Obviously, many programs are utilized by caretakers seeking respite, but the shortened day (about 6 hours) of many centers does not allow the caretaker to have a fulltime job. In addition, transportation between home and daycare centers is often a problem.

The cost of daycare is of concern to both state and federal officials as well as to the public, which often has to pay for daycare privately. At the higher end of daycare costs, the per diem rate exceeds that of nursing home care. Even at the lower end of the cost scale, many other factors have to be taken into account before judging the cost-effectiveness of daycare within the long-term care system. Research has shown that many adult daycare clients also receive assistance from other agencies to supply services not available through daycare (i.e., homemaker support, Meals-on-Wheels, and others).[11] In addition, federal and state costs can be expected to increase, not decrease, if daycare becomes widely available and if persons who would not consider nursing home care decide to participate in daycare. Thus far, because of daycare's reputation for being an expensive program with unclear standards and goals, it has not received widespread support.

The major alternative to daycare in preventing institutionalization of the high-risk elderly is home-based care. The number of agencies providing home-based care far exceeds the number of daycare programs. Homecare avoids the investment in transportation and in facility maintenance and upkeep required for daycare. On the other hand, organized group activities and socialization with peers does not occur in home-based programs. It appears that daycare does have a place in the list of long-term care services but issues of cost and benefit will have to be resolved.

NURSING HOME CARE

For most individuals, admission to a nursing home for chronic care occurs only after all other efforts to avoid institutionalization have been exhausted. Nursing homes are viewed as unpleasant places, in which physical and mental capacities decline, bodily functions fail, rights to privacy and self-determination are curtailed, abandonment by friends and family occurs, and imminent death looms. Despite the tremendous amount of money spent in this country on nursing home care, few are satisfied with the result.

According to the National Center for Health Statistics, of 28.5 million Americans age 65 and over, 5 percent were residents of nursing homes on any given day in the 1985–86 National Nursing Home Survey.[13] Specifically, 1,491,400 residents lived in 19,100 nursing homes nationwide. Only 12 percent of the residents were under age 65, and 45 percent were over age 85 (up from 40 percent in the 1977 National Nursing Home Survey). Elderly residents of nursing homes tended to be female (75 percent), white (93 percent), cognitively impaired (63 percent), and without a living spouse (84 percent). Blacks and other minorities were relatively underrepresented. This may be changing, however, as the proportion of elderly blacks residing in nursing homes doubled from 2 to 4 percent between 1973 and 1985.

Residents of nursing homes had significant functional disability. Ninety-nine percent needed assistance with bathing, 78 percent with dressing, 63 percent with toileting, 63 percent with transferring, and 40 percent with eating. Fifty-five percent were incontinent of bowel or bladder, or both. Thirty percent required assistance with all ADLs, and only 8 percent were totally independent in all six categories.

Dependency in ADLs was greater in the 1985 survey than in the 1977 survey, even when age was constant. This perhaps reflects the impact of diagnosis related groups (DRG), instituted in 1983, which possibly led to the earlier discharge of sicker, elderly Medicare patients from hospital beds to nursing home beds.

With this view of a very frail, sick, and disabled population, it is not surprising that nursing homes have significant problems, including (but not limited to):

1. Lack of interest by physicians in providing care to patients in nursing homes
2. High nursing staff turnover rates
3. High incidence of on-the-job injuries
4. Poor staff and patient morale
5. Lack of adequate regulatory standards and quality assurance
6. Infection control problems
7. Cycling of residents back and forth between hospital and nursing home
8. Unresolved ethical issues regarding appropriate and inappropriate treatment for nursing home residents
9. Poor public relations
10. High rate of iatrogenic events

It is the purpose of this section to look at the many ways in which these problems may be—and are being—addressed.

Current geriatric training in medical schools, residencies, and fellowships across the country is aimed at improving the quality of care for the entire aged population. Much of this training will undoubtedly take place in "teaching" nursing homes. Such academically affiliated nursing homes should provide the research and education needed to upgrade the entire nursing home industry. Already, three major initiatives have emerged: The National Institute of Aging Teaching Nursing Home Program, The Robert Wood Johnson Foundation Teaching Nursing Home Program, and the Veterans' Administration Nursing Home Care Unit Program. Research on dementia, incontinence, falls, infections, osteoarthritis, depression, exercise, and functional assessment is being done in such academic nursing home programs. In addition, geriatric physician, nursing, dental, and pharmacy specialists who will be expected to practice in nonacademic nursing homes are now being trained.

Regulatory agencies are attempting to define optimum standards for nursing home care and to enforce compliance with these standards. The Health Care Financing Administration requested that the Institute of Medicine (IOM) of the National Academy of Sciences conduct a study that would "serve as a basis for adjusting federal (and state) policies and regulations governing the certification of nursing homes so as to make those policies and regulations as appropriate and effective as possible." Although there have been critics of the 1986 IOM report, it did serve to summarize the major problems in the nursing home industry and to suggest some directions for change.[14]

In summary, the combination of nursing home research, geriatric education, and progressive legislation should benefit the nursing homes of the future.

HOSPICE CARE

Hospice Evolution

The term hospice was used in the medieval period to denote a way station for travelers. In the 16th century, during the reign of Henry VIII, a hospice was a shelter for the sick, poor, and blind. Over the years, the term has evolved into a philosophy of caring for dying patients. The first modern hospice was established in England in 1905. The recent interest in hospice care stems from the work of a dedicated physician, Dame Cecily Saunders, who fostered, promoted, and expanded the movement in the 1960s in Great Britain. Under her leadership, the hospice has become a viable alternative form of health care that recognizes, addresses, and treats the needs of the dying.[15] In the 1970s, the hospice movement crossed the Atlantic, and today there are over 1300 hospice programs in the United States.

Modern medicine has achieved a level of great technologic sophistication in a highly pressured and competitive environment, focusing almost exclusively on diagnosis and treatment for cure and the prolongation of life. The dying patient suffers progressive dehumanization in such a milieu. Hospice care emphasizes that high-technology medical practices are neither relevant nor appropriate in patients who suffer from terminal illnesses.[16] Indeed, the hospice movement has emerged from dissatisfaction and frustration with the inadequacy of the medical care given to the terminally ill.

The Hospice Philosophy and Principles of Care

Although death is the inevitable and natural conclusion of life, the essence of the hospice philosophy is to optimize the quality of life as death approaches. Hospice care focuses on the special, complex needs of the dying patient and his family. Family members are strongly encouraged to take an active role in the care of their dying relative. Hospices attempt to give dying patients control over their own lives; they are urged to make decisions regarding treatment and care. Perhaps most essential to the philosophy of hospice care is that all possible means are taken to relieve the patient's pain and suffering.

To establish standards of care, the National Hospice Organization has set forth several guidelines; some of the principles of hospice programs are shown in Table 6–1.

Hospice Models

In the United States, there are four basic hospice models to serve the patients and their families. One is the community-

Table 6–1. Principles of Hospice Care

The dying patient and his family are the unit of care.

The program is physician directed.

Care is provided by an interdisciplinary team of physicians, nurses, psychologists, social workers, dieticians, clergy, and volunteers.

Treatment is aimed at symptom and pain control (physical, psychologic, social, and spiritual).

Hospice admission depends on the needs of the patient and family and their expressed request for care.

Services are available 24 hours a day, 7 days a week.

Continuity is maintained between inpatient and home care services.

Bereavement treatment follow-up for the family is mandatory.

based homecare program, in which most hospice care is provided in the home. Although a majority of Americans would prefer to die in familiar surroundings, nearly 70 percent die in institutions. The home hospice approach allows death to occur at home, if the patient and family so desire. The second model is a hospital-based inpatient unit, which includes consultation services and homecare. In this program, an inpatient unit provides patient care when there is no family, when the family is unable to provide homecare, or when intense medical intervention is needed to treat severe symptoms. Such a unit should emulate a caring and comfortable "home-like" environment by allowing for maximum flexibility in room decor, patient visitation, and passes. The third is hospital-based consultative services and homecare. Hospice consultations are provided by physicians who are trained in the principles of palliation and symptom control, but treatment is carried out by the primary care provider. The fourth model is the freestanding hospice program.

Reimbursement for hospice services is approved under Medicare and Medicaid benefits and certain other health insurances. The terms of reimbursement vary with each of these benefit plans and the type of services rendered.[16]

The Physician's Role in Hospice Care

Once the primary physician has determined that a patient has a terminal illness, he must convey this information to the patient and family in a kind, compassionate, and truthful manner. The physician then has the responsibility to help them cope with the poor prognosis.[17] The physician must be willing to devote time and energy to care for the patient from this point. Alternative treatment options, such as hospice care, must be discussed. The physician must explain that cardiopulmonary resuscitation, mechanical ventilation, and other advanced life-support measures merely prolong pain and suffering in the terminally ill patient and that their use is in direct conflict with the hospice concept of care. A "do not resuscitate" order should be established prior to initiating hospice care. The primary focus of treat-

Table 6–2. Narcotic Analgesics in Equivalent Doses

Analgesic (narcotic)	IM (mg)	PO (mg)	Dose Interval
Morphine	10	60	3–4 h
Codeine	130	200	3–4 h
Oxycodone	15	30	3–4 h
Hydromorphone (Dilaudid)	1.5	7.5	3–4 h
Levorphanol (Levo-Dromoran)	2	4	4–6 h
Meperidine (Demerol)	75	300	2–4 h
Methadone (Dolophine)	10	20	6–8 h
Oxymorphone (Numorphan)	1	6	3–6 h
Pentazocine (Talwin)	60	180	2–4 h
Butorphanol (Stadol)	2	—	3–4 h

(Adapted From Foley KM: The treatment of cancer pain. N Engl J Med 313:84, 1985.)

ment is the alleviation of pain and other symptoms that cause suffering as death approaches.

The physician must use his clinical skills at the bedside to diagnose and treat the patient's symptoms; this will help the physician gain the patient's confidence and trust. Most importantly, the physician should both lead and encourage the involvement of the multidisciplinary team members to treat the comprehensive needs of the terminally ill patient.

Pain and Symptom Control

Pain management is the key to successful hospice care. Pain in the dying patient, referred to by Saunders as total pain, has four component parts: physical, psychologic, social, and spiritual pain.[15] These components are so interwoven that the physician and the multidisciplinary team must work cooperatively to diagnose the derivatives of the pain in order to treat it appropriately and effectively.

Physical pain, when severe, is debilitating. It affects the overall functioning of the patient. Therefore, physical pain must be controlled before the other components of pain can be treated. Although cancer accounts for the majority of diagnoses in a hospice, only about 50 percent of cancer patients experience severe physical pain.[18] The principles of pain control in a hospice setting are very different from those used to treat the acutely ill. Pain in the dying patient is a constant reminder of the underlying disease and, therefore, can lead to a vicious circle of apprehension, anxiety, insomnia, loneliness, and depression. Pain must be treated by analgesics, both

non-narcotic and narcotic, given round-the-clock. The dosage of the analgesic is individually titrated to keep the patient pain-free, while allowing him to be awake and alert. Equivalent analgesic dose tables (Table 6–2) are available to help the physician choose the most appropriate narcotic, dose, and route of administration.[19] In most instances, the oral route provides for adequate analgesia. This route produces the least discomfort for the patient and permits greater patient freedom and autonomy in the control of pain. The physician must bear in mind that drug dependence and addiction are of no concern in treating the dying patient. Nonsteroidal, anti-inflammatory agents, corticosteroids, psychotherapeutic agents, nerve blocking agents and radiation therapy may serve as adjuncts to analgesics.

Other distressing symptoms, such as constipation, nausea, vomiting, and oral and decubitus ulcers, should be treated. If a patient is symptomatic with pneumonia, antipyretics, antitussives, and sometimes empirical antibiotic therapy are indicated. Laboratory and other diagnostic tests are not essential to this form of palliative treatment, unless these tests are necessary for symptom relief.

Psychologic symptoms such as anxiety, depression, and insomnia can cause anguish and amplify the patient's perception of physical pain. These symptoms should be carefully considered and aggressively treated. Psychopharmacologic agents, such as anxiolytics, antidepressants, and sedative hypnotics, should be appropriately prescribed. Financial worries also may be distressing to some patients, especially if the patient is young and has a dependent family. Social workers can help with locating sources of financial aid, securing wills and testimonials, overseeing funeral arrangements, and with other neccessitities. Although spiritual pain may be hard to identify, often a clergyman can offer great comfort to the patient and family even if the patient has not been a religious observer through his life.

Research and Education

Considerable information about the care of the dying patient has been gained over the past two decades from research in both Britain and the United States. We have become especially knowledgeable about the physiology and pharmacotherapy of pain.[18, 19] In order to further our ability to care for the terminally ill, clinical research and scientific investigation must continue. More importantly, however, we must incorporate our current knowledge into the educational programs for medical, nursing, and paramedical professionals in order to provide optimal care to the dying patient now and in the years to come.

REFERENCES

FAMILY SUPPORT

1. Stone R, Cafferata GL, Sangl J: Caregivers of the frail elderly: a national profile. Gerontologist 27:616, 1987.
2. Macken C: A profile of functionally impaired elderly persons living in the community. Health Care Finan Rev Vol 7. HCFA Pub No 03223. Office of Research and Demonstrations. Washington, US GPO, 1986.
3. Kovar MG: Aging in the eighties: preliminary data from the Supplement on Aging to the National Health Interview Survey, United States, January-June 1984. DHHS Pub No 86-1250. Hyattsville, MD, Public Health Service, 1986.
4. Dawson D, Hendershot G, Fulton J: Aging in the eighties: Functional limitations of individuals age 65 years and over. DHHS Pub No 87-1250. Hyattsville, MD, Public Health Service, 1987.

5. Kane RL: Long-term care: policy and reimbursement. In Cassel CK, Walsch JR, eds: Geriatric Medicine: Fundamentals of Geriatric Care. New York, Springer-Verlag, 1984, p 383.

HOMECARE

6. American College of Physicians: Home health care. Ann Intern Med 105:454, 1986.
7. Berk ML, Bernstein A: Use of home health services: some findings from the National Medical Care Expenditure Survey. Home Health Care Serv Q 6:13, 1985.
8. General Accounting Office: Determining cost-effectiveness of home and community-based services. Washington, GAO, 1987.

DAYCARE

9. Gelfand DE: Adult daycare. In Gelfand DE: The Aging Network: Programs and Services. New York, Springer Publ Co, 1984, p 189.
10. Weissert WG: Two models of geriatric daycare. Gerontologist 16:420, 1976.
11. Mahoney K: Outside the day care center: additional support for the frail elderly. Hartford, Connecticut Department of Aging, 1978.
12. Brocklehurst JC: Textbook of Geriatric Medicine and Gerontology. New York, Churchill Livingstone, 1985, p 989.

NURSING HOME CARE

13. Hing E: Use of nursing homes by the elderly: preliminary data from the 1985 National Nursing Home Survey. DHHS Pub No 87-1250. Hyattsville, MD, Public Health Service, 1987.
14. Institute of Medicine: Improving the Quality of Care in Nursing Homes. Washington, National Academy Press, 1986, pp 1–44.

HOSPICE CARE

15. Saunders CM: The Management of Terminal Illness. London, Edward Arnold, 1978, pp 193–202.
16. Mathew LM, Scully JH: Hospice care. Clin Geriatr Med 2:617, 1986.
17. Wanzer SH, Adelstein JS, Crawford RE, et al: The physician's responsibility toward hopelessly ill patients. N Engl J Med 310:955, 1984.
18. Twycross RG, Lack SA: Symptom Control in Far Advanced Cancer: Pain Relief. London, Pitman, 1983, pp 3–14
19. Foley KM: The treatment of cancer pain. N Engl J Med 313:84, 1985.

CHAPTER 7

The Hospitalized Elderly Patient

Laurence J. Robbins
Sylvia K. Oboler

It is a grievous illness to preserve one's health by a regimen too strict. (C'est une ennuyeuse maladie que de conserver sa santé par un trop grand régime.)
LA ROCHEPOUCAULD, *Maximes Supprimées*

Hospitalization exposes the elderly patient to problems less often seen among elderly outpatients or young inpatients. This chapter describes two such problems, special considerations of geriatric surgery and iatrogenic complications.

THE ELDERLY SURGICAL PATIENT

Forty percent of the hospitalized elderly undergo surgery.[1] Elderly patients more frequently present with advanced disease and undergo more dangerous emergency operations; thus, delayed diagnosis and emergency treatment contribute to an increase in surgical risk. Since chronic diseases common in elderly individuals increase the likelihood of postoperative complications, advanced age identifies patients at risk of greater postoperative morbidity and mortality. Prolonged postoperative recuperation in the elderly also contributes to rising health care costs. Geriatric surgery and its atttendant complications challenge physicians to diagnose patients sooner and to try to prevent the surgical complications that contribute to increased morbidity, mortality, and expense.

This chapter addresses the demographics of geriatric surgery, diagnoses of geriatric surgical conditions, risks versus benefits of surgical procedures for geriatric patients, preoperative risk assessment, and postoperative complications. Readers should refer to standard surgery and anesthesiology textbooks to review surgical techniques and general perioperative considerations, such as antibiotic prophylaxis, internal cleansing for intestinal surgery, and perioperative diabetes management.[2]

Demographics and Overview

Whereas individuals over 65 years of age represent 11 percent of the United States population, they generate 30 percent of hospital expenditures. Patients over 70 years of age undergo 22 percent of all operations.[3] In the early 1980s, 45 percent of discharged elderly patients in New York had undergone surgery.[4] Elderly individuals were over twice as likely to have had surgery as younger citizens. Because the mean age in this country will increase as the 21st century approaches, the aged will eventually account for 50 percent of all surgical procedures.[5]

Despite more frequent emergency surgery, delayed diagnoses, and increased complication rates, over three quarters of the elderly who survive surgery return to their homes.[6] Although few studies have examined quality-of-life issues following surgery, postoperative elderly patients may remain as functionally independent as age-matched cohorts who were not subjected to surgery.

In 1982, Linn and colleagues exhaustively reviewed the literature on surgical mortality in the elderly from 1940 to 1980.[7] They had difficulty summarizing the data because other authors often failed to define postoperative deaths or to report mortality in a younger comparison group. Elective surgical mortality in the elderly rose gradually from 5 percent in 1940 to 9.5 percent in 1980, which Linn attributed to the willingness of surgeons to operate on elderly patients considered too sick for surgery in prior decades. Therefore, offering surgery to more debilitated elderly patients requires careful preoperative identification and treatment of superimposed medical illnesses if physicians hope to reduce surgical mortality. In Table 7–1 are listed preventive measures that may optimize medical conditions perioperatively and reduce surgical risks.[8-13]

Diagnosis

Conventional differential diagnosis identifies a single disease to explain a patient's subjective complaints, objective physical findings, and laboratory data. This technique may mislead the physician evaluating a geriatric patient. Elderly patients often suffer multiple apparent and occult diseases so that symptoms and signs may reflect more than one diagnosis. These coexisting diseases may obscure surgical diagnosis and hamper perioperative assessment.

Geriatric patients may lack many of the classic signs and symptoms of common surgical conditions. For example, the physician may attribute an elderly patient's elevated alkaline phosphatase activity to Paget's disease and overlook the occult biliary tract common duct stone causing the problem. Thus, failing to confirm the hepatic source rather than the bony source, the physician may delay diagnosis of asymptomatic biliary tract obstruction, which progresses and later requires riskier emergency surgery. Similarly, delirium in the elderly may indicate acute cholecystitis that developed without concomitant abdominal symptoms or signs.[14] If familiar with the unusual presentations of common geriatric surgical diagnoses, physicians may recognize these problems earlier and operate before diseases advance and the patient's surgical fitness deteriorates.

Failing to consider multiple or occult diagnoses may also cause errors during preparation for surgery. Ankle edema in

TABLE 7–1. Principles to Identify and Reduce Risks of Geriatric Surgery

Complete, thorough history and physical examination; observe patient's exercise tolerance (e.g., climbing stairs)

Perform baseline mental status assessment; discontinue unnecessary mind-altering drugs

Complete minimal laboratory assessment including hematocrit, serum creatinine (creatinine clearance is more accurate), serum albumin, blood sugar; other tests as clinically indicated; correct reversible abnormalities

Consider preoperative ECG and chest x-ray (value of routine testing is uncertain); when recent test results are available, repeat only if patient reports new symptoms or examination reveals new findings

Encourage smoking cessation at least 2 weeks prior to surgery

Consider preoperative spirometry and arterial blood gas measurement and treatment of reversible airways disease, particularly if intraperitoneal or thoracic surgery is planned

Begin preoperative chest physiotherapy including incentive spirometry

Treat heart failure; consider right heart catheterization to monitor pulmonary capillary wedge pressure if major abdominal or thoracic surgery is planned, or heart failure responds poorly to preoperative medications

Correct malnutrition if time permits

Prescribe subcutaneous heparin prophylaxis for thrombophlebitis with thoracic or abdominal surgery; prescribe external pneumatic compressive stockings for hip surgery and open prostatectomy

Lower blood pressure if diastolic is > 110 mmHg

Consider less aggressive surgical procedure or nonsurgical management if irreversible severe risks are present

Encourage liberal oxygen use if upper abdominal or thoracic surgery is planned

Mobilize patient as soon as possible postoperatively; this requires attention to adequate postoperative pain relief

the cardiac patient may lead the physician to diagnose fluid overload and to prescribe preoperative diuretics. If coexisting venous insufficiency contributes to the ankle swelling, vigorous diuresis may produce dehydration and complications, including orthostatic falls and renal insufficiency.

Missing or misleading symptoms or signs may also obscure the diagnosis of postoperative complications. Whereas chest pain accompanies 80 to 90 percent of myocardial infarctions occurring out of the hospital, it accompanies less than 50 percent of postoperative infarctions.[15-17] The only clues to acute infarction may be unexplained hypotension, altered mental status, nausea, or congestive heart failure.[16] Similarly, hypoxic postoperative confusion, without accompanying fever or rales, may obscure the diagnosis of pneumonia. Performing routine chest x-rays 3 days postoperatively, Rothfeld and colleagues found 23 cases of pneumonia in 52 geriatric surgical patients. The hospital staff failed to detect pneumonia in 7 of these 23 patients on physical examination. Therefore, postoperative care as well as preoperative diagnosis and assessment requires careful interpretation of all subjective complaints, objective findings, and laboratory data to reduce morbidity and mortality in geriatric surgery.

Decision to Operate

Numerous authors debate whether aging alone contributes to greater surgical risk. Clearly, the elderly patient's increased likelihood of having a complicated surgical diagnosis, emergency surgery, and coexisting life-threatening chronic diseases escalates operative morbidity and mortality. When statistical analysis separates the risk of advanced age from these other risk factors, aging adds little or no risk to various surgical procedures.[3, 18] For example, according to Goldman's criteria for risk of cardiac complications during noncardiac surgery, a healthy 70-year-old patient undergoing an inguinal hernia repair falls into the same low-risk category as a healthy 30-year-old.[19] A similar study has confirmed that advanced age alone does not contribute significantly to overall surgical morbidity associated with cholecystectomy.[18] However, these statistical observations may have limited relevance to the preoperative assessment of an individual elderly surgical candidate. Because the likelihood of having occult disease as well as apparent chronic disease increases with advanced age, the physician must evaluate each elderly surgical candidate carefully to uncover and quantify those additional surgical risks.

Recognizing the frequent presence of occult cardiopulmonary diseases among elderly surgical candidates, the American Society of Anesthesiology classifies healthy

TABLE 7–2. American Society of Anesthesiologists Preoperative Risk Assessment

Class 1	Healthy patients without systemic disease
Class 2	Patients with mild systemic disease; all patients 80 years or older
Class 3	Patients with severe systemic disease but not immediately life threatening
Class 4	Patients with severe systemic disease that is life threatening
Class 5	Patients not expected to live more than 48 hours, with or without surgery

octogenarians in its category 2 risk group rather than its category 1 risk group, as it would for younger patients (Table 7–2).[20, 21] Despite this observation, mortality for healthy octogenarians (category 2) remains as low as 1 percent, whereas mortality among 80-year-old patients with life-threatening disease (category 4) is approximately 25 percent. Therefore, although advanced age alone should not disqualify a patient from surgery, it should lead to careful preoperative identification of confounding risks, particularly unrecognized cardiopulmonary disease.

RISK VERSUS BENEFIT

Any decision to operate on an elderly patient should include an assessment of potential benefits and risks. Curative surgery may justify greater risks than palliative operations. If the surgeon mistakenly believes that a healthy 80-year-old patient may expect to live only a year or two, the surgeon may be reluctant to operate on an 80-year-old patient with a life-threatening surgical disease such as abdominal aortic aneurysm. Since the average 80-year-old may expect to live an additional 6 to 8 years, untreated surgical diseases may significantly shorten life expectancy if the surgeon avoids aggressive curative treatment.[20] Surgeons have recorded an acceptable 4.7 percent mortality rate for abdominal aortic aneurysm repair among octogenarians, whereas nonsurgical management is associated with a 50 percent mortality rate owing to ruptured aneurysms in these potentially curable patients.[22]

Benefits of palliative surgery may also outweigh its risks. While a septuagenarian's hip replacement for incapacitating osteoarthritic pain may not demonstrate the same obvious societal benefit as a 55-year-old who returns to the work force following total hip replacement, the 70-year-old's renewed mobility may prolong independent living and save nursing home care costs for this ambulatory patient.[23] On the other hand, nonsurgical hip fracture management for a demented, nonambulatory nursing home resident may eliminate surgical risks and costs when potential surgical benefit is small. In this setting, conservative measures, including analgesia and traction, rather than surgery may produce better survival and outcome.[20]

In summary, the decision to operate must include a careful risk/benefit analysis. The patient and surgeon may accept greater risks when potential surgical benefits include cure or significant palliation that nonsurgical medical management may not achieve. Uncovering occult chronic diseases and recognizing the long life expectancy of the healthy elderly highlight two aspects of geriatric medicine that the physician must appreciate when determining surgical risks and potential benefits to the patient.

Risk Assessment

As noted, surgery exposes elderly patients to morbidity and mortality often attributable to coexisting medical illness. When postoperative deterioration occurs unexpectedly, it may reflect inadequate preoperative medical assessment and treatment of unrecognized or underestimated chronic diseases. A routine history, physical examination, and laboratory data may not identify patients with a high risk of developing postoperative medical complications.[24] Preoperative stress tests, including cardiac exercise testing and dynamic pulmonary function tests, may be appropriate for patients considering high-risk surgical procedures. Similarly, prolonged or difficult operations may justify intraoperative invasive monitoring to permit a more immediate and accurate assessment of the patient's hemodynamic stability.

PROCEDURE-SPECIFIC RISKS

Surgical and medical literature extensively documents procedure-specific geri-

atric risks. Emergency surgery, a common result of delayed surgical diagnosis, triples the geriatric surgical mortality rate.[1, 25] Intraperitoneal and intrathoracic surgery exposes patients to increased cardiopulmonary complications when compared with surgery performed on more peripheral sites.[5, 15, 17, 20, 26] Table 7–3 ranks the relative risk of various surgical procedures.

Some operations are so safe that they deserve special emphasis. Urologists have successfully performed transurethral prostatectomies on elderly men considered unsuitable for more difficult surgical procedures. In one study, only one death occurred in 104 prostatectomy patients with severe coronary artery disease, including patients with chronic angina and congestive heart failure.[27] In a second study, only one postoperative death occurred in 23 patients who underwent prostatectomy within 6 months of suffering a myocardial infarction, which is usually a strict surgical contraindication.[5] During their attempt to identify risks of cardiac complications for noncardiac surgical procedures, Goldman and colleagues recognized the minimal risk posed by prostatectomy and consequently excluded men undergoing transurethral prostatic resection from their analysis.[19] Similarly, medically ill elderly patients may undergo cataract surgery without systemic complications (one death in 20,000 procedures).[20] In the early 1980s, cataract extraction and cystoscopy or transurethral prostate resection accounted for nearly 20 percent of geriatric operations in New York.[4] Patients with advanced chronic illness should not be rejected for surgery if low-risk procedures, such as prostatectomy and cataract extraction, will improve the quality of their remaining years. However, the safety of these procedures does not relieve the physician from identifying and optimizing modifiable preoperative risks.

TABLE 7–3. Procedure-Specific Risks

Extremely Safe	Transurethral prostatectomy, cataract extraction
Moderately Safe	Peripheral vascular surgery, hip replacement, lower abdominal surgery
Less Safe	Upper abdominal surgery
Least Safe	Intrathoracic surgery

ANESTHESIA RISKS

Anesthesia contributes little to geriatric surgical risk compared with the risk of the specific surgical procedure and the patient's underlying disease.[1, 28–30] Although the anesthesiology literature does not clearly identify a general anesthetic agent that is safer than others for geriatric patients, some anesthesiologists believe that balanced neuroleptic anesthesia eases induction and withdrawal for older patients.[31] Spinal anesthesia may reduce cardiopulmonary risks associated with general anesthesia and intubation; however, urinary retention—requiring bladder catheterization—frequently complicates the postoperative course of elderly patients subjected to spinal anesthesia. Prolonged general anesthesia (over 2 hours) may contribute to geriatric cardiopulmonary problems postoperatively, but this risk cannot be easily isolated from the risk of the prolonged surgical procedure itself.[17, 28] Several publications review geriatric anesthesia in detail.[32, 47]

CARDIAC RISKS

Cardiac complications contribute to many postoperative geriatric deaths. Often, these fatal cardiac events occur in patients with unrecognized or underestimated cardiac disease.[1] Routine preoperative evaluation limited to history, physical examination, chest x-ray, and resting ECG may underestimate occult disease. Goldman and colleagues evaluated more than 40 potential cardiac risk factors and identified 10 that independently predicted postoperative cardiac complications.[19] Goldman's 10-factor cardiac risk index notably excluded hypertension. Diastolic pressure as high as 110 did not increase postoperative cardiac morbidity or mortality.[32] Age over 70 years remained an independent risk, perhaps reflecting the elderly's greater likelihood of having occult coronary disease that the physician may not have identified during routine preoperative examination.[33] Although age over 70 years alone placed an elderly surgical candidate in Goldman's lowest risk group, any additional one of the remaining nine risk factors placed the septuagenarian in a higher risk group (Table 7–4).

Because Goldman's bedside evaluation

TABLE 7–4. Cardiac Risk of Noncardiac Surgery*

Risk Factors	Risk Class	Life Threatening Complication/ Death
Age > 70 years	1 (5 points)	0.9%
Age > 70 years plus 1 other risk†	2 (8 to 12 points)	7%
Age > 70 years plus S₃, JVD, or recent MI	3 (15 to 16 points)	13%

*Adapted from Goldman L, Caldera DL, Nussbaum SR, et al: Multifactorial index of cardiac risk in noncardiac surgical procedures. N Engl J Med 297:845, 1977.
†Except ventricular gallop sound (S_3), jugular venous distension (JVD), or myocardial infarction within 6 months of surgery (recent MI).

may overlook patients risking postoperative cardiac complications, several investigators have extended preoperative geriatric cardiac risk assessment to include more dynamic tests of cardiac reserve, such as exercising testing.[33–37] Using parenteral dipyridamole to induce maximum coronary vasodilation and, thus, to mimic the effect of exercise on coronary blood flow, Boucher and colleagues measured thallium myocardial distribution before and after this pharmacologic exercise in stable candidates for aortic or extensive peripheral vascular surgery.[34] A standard preoperative history and physical examination did not predict thallium scan results, and all patients had low-risk Goldman scores. Fifty percent of patients with dipyridamole-induced thallium redistribution, suggesting potentially ischemic myocardium, suffered postoperative ischemic events. Patients without evidence of thallium redistribution suffered no postoperative ischemic events.

In a similar study, 31 of 96 patients without Goldman risk indicators were unable to raise their pulses to 99 beats per minute or to perform 2 minutes of supine bicycle exercise.[36] Six of these 31 patients suffered postoperative cardiac complications, whereas only one of the 65 who exercised successfully had a postoperative cardiac problem. Finally, Jain used preoperative exercise radionuclide angiography to study candidates for peripheral vascular surgery.[35] Low resting left ventricular ejection fraction and failure to increase ejection fraction by 5 percent or more during exercise predicted patients at risk for postoperative cardiovascular complications. Thus, these three studies suggest that preoperative exercise testing may identify high-risk elderly patients overlooked by conventional bedside assessment. However, no study demonstrates that costly routine preoperative treadmill testing leads to intervention that prevents postoperative complications and reduces surgical expenses.[37] Incorporating exercise testing observations into the bedside examination may improve the sensitivity of the routine preoperative physical examination; the patient unable to walk halls or stairs briskly enough to raise his pulse to 99 beats per minute may deserve more careful preoperative risk assessment. Delaying general surgery until coronary artery bypass grafting is performed may dramatically reduce subsequent operative risks.[32]

Some investigators recommend invasive monitoring to detect hemodynamic compromise that predisposes elderly patients to postoperative complications. Del Guercio and colleagues studied 145 consecutive patients over 65 years old for whom internists had approved major surgery based on conventional preoperative history, physical examination, and laboratory data.[24] Following right heart catheterization, the authors discovered that less than 15 percent of those patients had normal hemodynamics. Attending physicians then treated moderate to severe impairments preoperatively; refractory hemodynamic compromise predicted greater postoperative mortality. In another study, the authors identified 15 of 18 patients who developed serious postoperative complications when their pulmonary capillary wedge pressure fell 4 mm or more intraoperatively.[38] Thus, invasive monitoring may provide its greatest benefit if used not only to assess risk and correct amenable preoperative abnormalities but also to identify and treat intraoperative hemodynamic problems.[28, 39] However, some experts dispute the benefit of catheterization beyond preoperative information obtained less invasively.[40]

Elective right heart catheterization itself has produced few complications in geriatric surgical patients. If contemplating major surgery, physicians should consider invasive hemodynamic monitoring for those with known cardiac disease or those who are unable to exercise.[5]

PULMONARY RISKS

Although cardiac complications are common, they may not produce most postoperative morbidity and mortality. In Goldman's study, noncardiac problems, including respiratory complications, caused three quarters of postoperative deaths.[15] In another study, 14 percent of general surgery patients over age 70 developed pneumonia postoperatively, whereas only 11 percent of Goldman's subjects over age 70 had serious cardiac complications.[6, 19]

Changes in pulmonary function related to age, such as decreased vital capacity, decreased expiratory reserve volume, and increased residual volume, do not predispose elderly patients to postoperative pulmonary complications.[8, 25] However, those who smoke cigarettes, retain carbon dioxide ($P_{CO_2} > 45$ mm), or cough productively (bronchitics) suffer postoperative respiratory problems more frequently.[32, 43] Additional risks include chronic pulmonary diseases, age over 70 years, poor nutrition, and surgery lasting more than 2 hours.[5, 32, 41, 42] Less than 1 percent of geriatric patients undergoing lower abdominal or peripheral surgery may suffer postoperative pulmonary complications, whereas upper abdominal surgery raises this risk to 60 percent.[43] Although numerous reviews cite the use of spirometry to predict postoperative pulmonary complications if the patient's time forced expiratory volume (FEV_1) is less than 2 l or the maximum voluntary ventilation (MVV) is less than 50 percent of predicted values, investigators have made these observations prior to intrathoracic procedures but not prior to other surgical conditions.[8]

Screening patients prior to abdominal surgery, Rothfeld and colleagues noted that a vital capacity less than 80 percent of age-adjusted norms, mid-expiratory flow rate (MEFR) < 200 l/min, and residual volume (RV)/total lung capacity (TLC) > 50 percent predicted respiratory complications more accurately than preoperative chest x-ray.[30] These dynamic measurements may identify limited pulmonary reserve capacity and may, like exercise treadmill testing for cardiac reserve, predict patients who will tolerate surgical stresses poorly. Although supporting literature is scant, simple spirometry is inexpensive, harmless, and will quantify unrecognized reversible airways disease that may respond to aggressive preoperative bronchodilator therapy and chest physical therapy.

Preoperative arterial gas measurements may identify unsuspected hypoxia, leading the anesthesiologist to extubate a patient more cautiously. If blood gas measurements identify unsuspected hypercarbia, anesthesiologists will use oxygen cautiously to avoid exacerbating CO_2 retention and may use local or regional anesthesia to avoid intubating these patients.

OTHER OPERATIVE RISKS

Many diseases that increase surgical risks and require special perioperative attention occur more commonly among elderly patients. Special considerations include warfarin adjustment and antibiotic prophylaxis for patients with valvular heart disease, insulin adjustment for diabetic patients, and prophylactic anticoagulation therapy for postoperative venous thromboembolism in bedridden patients. Perioperative management of these problems is not detailed in this chapter; however, the reference section lists sources that describe them comprehensively.[2, 32] Cognitive impairment and poor nutrition warrant further discussion because they commonly appear in older surgical candidates and rarely in younger patients.

Elderly patients may exhibit acute confusion as the sole sign of acute medical or surgical problems. This disorientation is usually caused by the exacerbation of underlying dementia, although it also afflicts previously rational elderly patients. The patient's incoherence and failure to cooperate during physical examinations or radiologic procedures may delay an accurate surgical diagnosis, which then contributes to postoperative complications. Postoperative mortality in delirious patients may reach 45 percent.[6] Despite the increased surgical mortality associated with dementia and delirium, physicians frequently overlook these problems. Although chart reviews suggest that less than 1 percent of postoperative geriatric patients become confused, routine psychiatric interviews reveal that 22 percent of these patients are cognitively impaired.[44]

When acute cognitive changes begin postoperatively, they interfere with postoperative management. Fifteen percent of elderly surgical patients may suffer acute psychosis postoperatively.[5, 45] Common precipitants of confusion include drug toxicity, metabolic derangements, and infection.[20, 45] The agitated patient's lack of cooperation may necessitate mechanical restraint, leading to exhaustion as the patient struggles against the restraining devices.[46] The medical staff may administer sedatives or tranquilizers to control patient behavior. Because these interventions limit movement, inhibit coughing, and decrease coordination, the patient risks bedsores, aspiration pneumonia, and falls. Although postoperative confusion usually lasts no more than 4 to 5 days, it may persist for 6 weeks.[47] If the staff can identify patients predisposed to postoperative confusion, they should encourage familiar and reassuring family members to remain at the bedside to calm the patient as he awakens from anesthesia, thus reducing the need for mechanical and chemical restraints. Substituting spinal anesthesia for general anesthesia may prevent postoperative disorientation.[20] Eliminating unnecessary mind-altering drugs preoperatively may also reduce the risk of postoperative confusion. Therefore, geriatric surgical candidates deserve routine screening through brief, easily administered mental status questionnaires to identify those at risk for avoidable postoperative confusion.

Malnutrition in geriatric patients may increase postoperative risk, particularly of infectious complications.[9, 48] A serum albumin determination (albumin < 3.0 gm/dl) may indicate surgical risks associated with poor nutrition as accurately as more elaborate investigations.[9] When feasible, delaying surgery to correct nutritional deficiencies may reduce surgical risk.

PREVENTING IATROGENIC DISEASE

Iatrogenic disease is defined as any illness resulting from medical encounters such as diagnostic procedures; therapeutic interventions by physicians, nurses, and other medical personnel; and the medical environment itself. Iatrogenic events can occur in the home, the physician's office, or a nursing home; however, hospitalized elderly patients are especially at risk for iatrogenesis.

Although the concept that physicians cause harm as well as benefit can be found in the Old Testament and in the teachings of Hippocrates, the incidence of iatrogenic events has been studied only recently. For example, adverse drug reactions cause 3 to 4 percent of admissions to teaching hospitals, and contribute to 10 to 25 percent of geriatric patient admissions.[49, 50] Iatrogenic disease also contributes substantially to workloads in intensive care units (ICU); Trunet and coworkers found that 12.6 percent of admissions to an ICU in 1 year were due to iatrogenic disease.[51]

Once hospitalized, elderly patients are at substantial risk of experiencing an untoward event. Several studies in teaching hospitals over a 20-year period are summarized in Table 7–5. In 1964, Schimmel reported that 20 percent of medical inpatients had hospital-induced complications, with adverse drug reactions accounting for more than half.[52] Almost 30 percent of the geriatric patients studied by Reichel experienced iatrogenic complications.[53] More recently, Steel and associates reported iatrogenic illness in 36 percent of 815 patients hospitalized for general medical service, with 9 percent of all patients experiencing a major episode of iatrogenesis.[55] In a study of both medical and surgical patients, Jahnigen and colleagues found that 29 percent of patients under age 65 had an iatrogenic episode compared with 45 percent for those aged 65 and over.[56] In the latter study, despite adjustments made for severity of illness, advanced age independently predicted the likelihood of iatrogenic events.

The following approach to preventing iatrogenic disease focuses on three areas: diagnostic tests, treatment modalities, and patient function in the hospital environment.

Diagnosis

The cornerstone of diagnosis—the history and physical examination—is often difficult to obtain in an elderly patient. Some points requiring more attention with the elderly than with younger patients include:

1. *Awareness of communication problems.* These include patient factors such as decreased hearing or vision, dysarthria, and memory impairment as well as physician factors such as overuse of jargon and information overload.[57] Physician attention to adequate lighting, eye-level contact, clear articulation, avoiding the hemianopic side of a stroke patient, and assessing patient understanding will help ensure adequate communication.

2. *Complete information regarding medications.* A list of medications may require information from family members, other caregivers, and other medical institutions. The list should include prescribed medications, with an estimate of patient compliance, over-the-counter drugs, and medications borrowed from spouses or friends. A home visit may be necessary.

3. *Realistic assessment of the level of function at home.* Attention to actual, and not idealized, activities; current exposures, rather than preretirement occupation; and the role of the spouse or other caregiver in daily activities may help define reasons for deterioration in function.

4. *Importance of continuity of care and communication with other caregivers.* Transfer of elderly patients between acute and chronic care facilities frequently results in miscom-

TABLE 7–5. Iatrogenic Disease in Hospitalized Patients

Author	Date	Group Studied	Sample Size	Incidence of Complications
Schimmel	1964	Medical patients	1014	20%
Reichel	1965	Medical patients > age 65	500	29%
Ogilvie & Ruedy	1967	Medical patients	731	24%
Steel, et al	1981	Medical patients	815	36%
Jahnigen, et al	1982	Medical and surgical Patients < age 65	48	29%
		Medical and surgical Patients ≥ age 65	174	45%

munication of diagnoses and therapies. The telephone is invaluable in maintaining contact and clarifying issues.

Complications related to diagnostic testing include both the risk of performing a diagnostic procedure and the risk of incorrectly interpreting that procedure. Although complications of individual procedures have often been reported, their incidence is hard to determine. In Schimmel's early report, only 29 of 1014 patients (2.9 percent) had adverse reactions to diagnostic procedures, but there were four associated deaths.[52] In a pilot study of invasive diagnostic and therapeutic procedures, Schroeder and associates reported that complications occurred in patients undergoing left heart catheterizations (18 percent), thoracenteses (19 percent), bronchoscopies (25 percent), percutaneous liver biopsies (8 percent), venograms (17 percent), and bone marrow biopsies (5 percent).[58] Although age-specific complication rates were not reported, because older patients are more likely to have conditions requiring diagnostic procedures, they are at high risk for these complications.

Two types of procedures of particular concern for the elderly are gastrointestinal radiography and intravenous contrast radiography.[57] Barium studies to visualize both the upper and the lower gastrointestinal tracts cause increased complications in the elderly. The preparation for barium enemas often involves cathartics and a period of starvation. The elderly tolerate this dehydration poorly because they have reduced total body water and impaired renal concentrating capacity. After the procedure, inadequate evacuation can result in constipation and barium retention. And discomfort during the procedure—especially for a frail, arthritic patient attempting to maintain difficult positions on a hard table—often results in a technically inadequate procedure that the patient is reluctant to repeat. Contrast-induced acute renal failure (ARF) occurs in up to 12 percent of hospitalized patients undergoing angiography.[59] Risk factors for contrast-induced ARF, including paraproteinemias, diabetes mellitus, and pre-existing renal insufficiency, are all more common in the elderly.

Recently, there has been more attention given to interpreting diagnostic tests, but this is often difficult with elderly pa-tients.[65] Sensitivity and specificity of tests are usually established in younger patients with confounding conditions eliminated; the elderly are more likely to have multiple diseases that make clear distinctions less likely. Because of underlying diseases, the elderly are more likely to suffer during further work-up of false positive tests; a laparotomy after a false positive abdominal x-ray is more morbid in a 70-year-old than in a 40-year-old. Therefore, before initiating a diagnostic test, both the risk of the procedure and the risk of misinterpreting the result should be considered.

Treatment

DRUG THERAPY

In several studies, adverse reactions to drugs were noted to be the most common complications of hospitalization. In Table 7–6 are shown the rates of drug reactions during hospitalization in several studies conducted since 1964. Older patients have significantly more reactions than younger patients—2.4 times the rate in Hurwitz's study.[61] Factors contributing to increased risk of drug reactions in the elderly are changes in drug use patterns, changes in drug disposition, and, possibly, changes in drug sensitivity.

Compared with younger patients, patients over age 65 use approximately twice as many prescription medications. Since the incidence of drug reactions increases with the number of medications used, the elderly are at increased risk. Although compliance has not been specifically studied, it is thought that the combination of more complex medication regimens with increased memory impairment in the elderly may lead to poor compliance. In addition, elderly patients use substantially more over-the-counter medications than their younger counterparts.

Multiple drug use in the elderly also increases the chance of drug interactions. A survey in the United Kingdom showed potentially interacting drug combinations in 23.7 percent of geriatric inpatients.[62] Common drug interactions included furosemide with antibiotics, prednisone, and nonsteroidal anti-inflammatory drugs; warfarin with aspirin and co-trimoxazole; heparin with aspirin; antacids with cimetidine,

TABLE 7–6. Adverse Drug Reactions During Hospitalization

Author	Date	Group Studied	Sample Size	Incidence of Drug Reactions
Schimmel	1964	Medical patients	1014	10.2%
Seidl, et al	1966	Medical patients	714	13.6%
Ogilvie & Ruedy	1967	Medical patients	731	18.2%
Hurwitz	1969	Medical patients < age 60	667	6.3%
		Medical patients ≥ age 60	493	15.4%
Jahnigen, et al	1982	Medical and surgical		
		Patients ≥ age 65	148	12.8%

digoxin, tetracycline, and iron; iron with tetracycline; and phenytoin with co-trimoxazole. In the United States, cimetidine and theophylline are commonly implicated in adverse drug interactions.

Pharmacokinetic changes with age have been discussed in recent articles.[63] There is little alteration in drug absorption with age. Important changes include alterations in volume of distribution and impairment of both renal excretion and hepatic metabolism. With age, lean body mass decreases and the fraction of adipose tissue increases. The volume of distribution of fat insoluble drugs such as acetaminophen and ethanol decreases in the elderly, whereas fat-soluble drugs such as diazepam and lidocaine are more extensively distributed. Because glomerular filtration decreases with age, clearance of drugs that depend on renal excretion predictably decreases. Examples of these drugs include digoxin, cimetidine, lithium, procainamide, chlorpropamide, and most antibiotics.

Hepatic metabolism of drugs is not so clearly affected by age. Glucuronidation is not usually altered, whereas oxidation may be reduced. Age-related decline in hepatic oxidative clearance may contribute to the toxicity of diazepam, chlordiazepoxide, quinidine, theophylline, and propranolol. When age affects renal or hepatic drug clearance, dosages need to be reduced to avoid toxicity.

The third area of potential toxicity due to drugs—altered sensitivity—is just beginning to be studied. Increased action of a specific drug level in the elderly has been reported for diazepam and a coumarin anticoagulant; however, these studies are preliminary and cannot be generalized.[63]

In Table 7–7 are lists of medications involved in adverse drug reactions reported for inpatients. Insulin, penicillin, and digitalis—which were so prominent 20 years ago—have been overshadowed in recent years by theophylline, nitrates, and type I antiarrhythmics. Because the list of individual drugs accounting for toxicity is extensive, attention to several types of reactions may minimize their occurrence in the elderly.[57]

Postural hypotension is common, even in the healthy elderly, and can be exacerbated by a number of drugs. Sympatholytic agents, diuretics, and vasodilators used for hypertension treatment can cause orthostatic dizziness, resulting in falls. In addition, many psychotropic drugs, especially phenothiazines and tricyclic antidepressants, frequently cause orthostatic hypotension.

Anticholinergic drugs can precipitate urinary retention, constipation, confusion, and, occasionally, acute narrow angle glaucoma. In addition to drugs prescribed specifically as anticholinergics, including atropine, propantheline, and benztropine, other drugs, especially antihistamines, such as diphenhydramine and tricyclics, such as amitriptyline and doxepin, can have significant anticholinergic side effects. The antiarrhythmic disopyramide is a particular offender that should be used with caution in the elderly male with prostatic hypertrophy.

Delirium can be a side effect of many drugs, both prescription and over-the-counter, used by elderly individuals. A partial list includes analgesics (especially opiates and pentazocine), anticholinergics, tricyclics, antihistamines, anticonvulsants in high doses, antiparkinsonian drugs, benzodiazepines (especially those with long half-lives such as flurazepam), cimetidine, and indomethacin. Whenever an elderly person experiences a change in mental status, the drug list should be carefully reviewed.

Drug-induced renal disease is especially common in the elderly. Nonsteroidal anti-

TABLE 7–7. Drugs Implicated in Adverse Reactions in Hospitalized Patients

	Schimmel (1964)	Reichel (1965)	Seidl (1966)	Ogilvie (1967)	Steel (1981)	Jahnigen (1982)
Number of Episodes	119	54	94	193	208	22
Drug						
Digitalis/Digoxin	7	18	23	41	15	2
Type I antiarrhythmics	—	—	11	2	18	2
Nitrates	—	—	—	—	26	2
Diuretics and antihypertensives	5	9	19	11	10	—
Theophylline	—	2	—	—	15	5
Antibiotics	35	9	28	31	10	6
Sedatives/Tranquilizers	11	4	—	—	—	6
Anticoagulants	9	2	6	—	13	—
Insulin	12	2	—	31	—	—
Prednisone/Steroids	12	1	4	—	—	—
Miscellaneous	28	7	3	77	101	—

inflammatory drugs are frequently implicated as a cause of decreasing renal function in older patients who take diuretics. Renal function, therefore, should be periodically monitored in older patients treated with such antiarthritis agents. Antibiotics that may cause renal dysfunction (particularly aminoglycosides) are frequently used in elderly patients with potential genitourinary or lower gastrointestinal tract infections. Decrease in renal function in an older patient should lead the physician to question the use of possibly offending drugs.

In summary, therapeutic drug use in the elderly should be carefully monitored. Drugs should be prescribed in the lowest effective dose for the individual patient, should be used for the shortest possible time, and should be reviewed regularly to see if withdrawal is feasible.

Therapeutic Devices

In addition to drug treatment, other therapeutic modalities may cause harm to elderly patients. In Steel's study, intravenous lines accounted for 34 of 497 complications, including thrombosis, extravasation, infection, and enforced immobility.[55] About half of the nosocomial infections in this country are caused by medical devices, especially urinary catheters. About 10 percent of all hospitalized patients have urinary catheters inserted. Of these patients, 20 percent will develop bacteriuria, with 0.5 to 2.5 percent experiencing sepsis.[64] Other types of catheters that predispose to infection include arterial lines, parenteral nutrition lines, and subclavian catheters.

Other medical devices that increase the chance of developing iatrogenic diseases include respiratory machines, nasogastric tubes, and implanted prostheses. Intermittent positive pressure breathing and continuous ventilation increase the risk of tracheitis and pneumonia. Nasogastric tubes can be associated with nasal trauma, pulmonary aspiration, and the need for restraints and subsequent immobility.[65] Prosthetic devices such as artificial heart valves and joints are prone to infection following bacteremia, and antibiotic prophylaxis should be used when procedures with significant risk of bacteremia are performed.[57]

Because of their underlying diseases, the elderly are at increased risk of needing multiple treatments. Principles that can help avoid problems include: (1) ensuring that the treatment is necessary, (2) ensuring that the treatment is the safest available, (3) attention to the appropriate route of administration, and (4) constant attention to the benefit/risk ratio for the individual patient.

PATIENT FUNCTION IN THE HOSPITAL ENVIRONMENT

Most of the literature on iatrogenic episodes focuses on adverse drug reactions and complications of procedures; however, a number of other morbid events may affect the hospitalized elderly.

FALLS. A surprisingly high number of hospitalized patients have accidents. A year-long study of the general wards at Bellevue Hospital showed 954 accidents, 41 percent of them experienced by patients over age 65. The accident rate in this age group was 3.5 times greater than that in patients aged 20 to 34. Falls from bed (all with bedrails up) accounted for 36 percent of these accidents, whereas falls from wheelchairs (mostly resulting from failure to set brakes) accounted for 28 percent.[66]

This and other studies have identified the risk factors for falls in hospitalized patients as age, female sex, abnormal mental status (especially Alzheimer's disease), polypharmacy (particularly psychoactive drugs), wandering, use of restraints, vision deficits, musculoskeletal defects, and neurologic deficits (including poor tandem gait, positive Rhomberg sign, and previous stroke).[66, 67] Identification of patients at risk for falls will allow some interventions, such as minimizing drug use, increasing supervision by attendants rather than the use of mechanical restraints, and attention to remediable deficits such as correcting vision (glasses, cataract surgery) and gait (physical therapy, braces, walkers).

DECUBITUS ULCERS. In various studies, 2 to 11 percent of all inpatients have pressure sores. Patients at risk for developing decubitus ulcers can now be identified. Relative risk factors include age greater than 70 years, restricted mobility, incontinence, emaciation, and redness over a bony prominence. Highest risk factors are unconsciousness, dehydration, and paralysis.[68] Attention to prophylaxis, including frequent turning and specialized beds to avoid pressure points, may reduce pressure sores in high-risk patients.

AMBULATION. In addition to bedsores, immobility predisposes a hospitalized patient to atelectasis, pneumonia, deep venous thrombosis, weakness, and prolonged hospital stay. Early ambulation regimens after surgery and medical illnesses, such as myocardial infarction, have decreased the morbidity of hospitalization for these problems. The hospital staff should encourage ambulation as soon as possible and provide the elderly patient with the means to accomplish this through adequate assistance, physical therapy, adequate analgesia with minimal sedation, and avoiding restraints.

NUTRITION. Prior to hospitalization, many chronically ill elderly patients have poor nutritional reserves that are worsened by diagnostic and therapeutic maneuvers. In addition to dietary history and physical examination, total lymphocyte count and serum albumin tests can help establish nutritional state. Measures to improve the nutritional status of the inpatient include diet and medication changes. Since strict adherence to a low-fat or diabetic diet may not be realistic or necessary in an older patient for whom long-term complications are not an issue, the diet often can be relaxed to include more food preferences. Food from home, increased seasoning for patients with a decreased sense of taste, and assistance with eating may be encouraged. Avoiding medications with gastrointestinal side effects such as nonsteroidal anti-inflammatory drugs, theophylline, and narcotics may improve appetite.

ELIMINATION. Urinary retention, or incontinence, or both is a common problem in the hospitalized elderly. As noted, postoperative urinary retention is exacerbated by anticholinergic medications. Incontinence may be precipitated by infection, metabolic abnormalities, or drugs (especially diuretics and central nervous system [CNS] depressants). Often, nocturnal incontinence related to inability to reach the toilet can be improved by simple measures such as a bedside urinal. When bladder catheterization is required, intermittent catheterization may be preferable to an indwelling catheter.[69]

Constipation frequently develops in hospitalized patients who are immobilized, placed on low-fiber diets, and given narcotics and/or anticholinergic drugs. Attention to bowel function including liberal use of fluids, stool softeners, laxatives before fecal impaction occurs, and avoiding constipating drugs can circumvent much patient discomfort.

COGNITION. Various precipitants may cause changes in mental function with hospitalization of the elderly patient. These precipitants include the unfamiliar environment, medications that suppress CNS function either primarily or as a side effect, lack of sensory input when glasses and hearing aids are not available, and unmasked mild dementia (the sundown syndrome). As noted in the discussion on postoperative confusion, the hospital staff should limit offending drugs and encourage socialization with supportive family members. In addition, the staff should increase sensory input and orient the patient frequently, using visual cues such as calendars and repeated auditory cues.

CONCLUSION

Hospitalization exposes elderly patients to special problems including geriatric surgery and iatrogenesis. Judicious use of diagnostic tests, thorough preoperative evaluation and perioperative care, appropriate drug use, and optimizing patient function will help to minimize complications of hospitalization.

REFERENCES

1. Johnson JC: The medical evaluation and management of the elderly surgical patient. J Am Geriatr Soc 31:621, 1983.
2. Goldman DR, et al: A problem-oriented approach to management. In Goldman DR, Brown FH, eds: Medical Care of the Surgical Patient. Philadelphia, JB Lippincott Co, 1982.
3. Johnson JC: Surgery in the elderly. In Goldman DR, Brown FH, eds: Medical Care of the Surgical Patient. Philadelphia, JB Lippincott Co, 1982, p 578.
4. Pasley B, Vernon P, Gibson G, et al: Geographic variations in elderly hospital and surgical discharge rates, New York State. Am J Public Health 77:679, 1987.
5. Keating HJ: Preoperative considerations in the geriatric patient. Med Clin North Am 71:569, 1987.
6. Mohr DN: Estimation of surgical risk in the elderly: a correlative review. J Am Geriatr Soc 31:99, 1983.
7. Linn BS, Linn MW, Wallen N: Evaluation of results of surgical procedures in the elderly. Ann Surg 195:90, 1982.
8. Tisi GM: Preoperative evaluation of pulmonary function. Am Rev Respir Dis 119:293, 1979.
9. Leite JFMS, Antunes CF, Monteiro JCMP, et al: Value of nutritional parameters in the prediction of postoperative complications in elective gastrointestinal surgery. Br J Surg 74:426, 1987.
10. Blery C, Szatan M, Fourgeaux B, et al: Evaluation of a protocol for selective ordering of preoperative tests. Lancet(i) 139, January 1986.
11. Boghosian SG, Mooradian AD: Usefulness of routine preoperative chest roentgenograms in elderly patients. J Am Geriatr Soc 35:142, 1987.
12. Kaplan EB, Sheiner LB, Boeckmann AJ, et al: The usefulness of preoperative laboratory screening. JAMA 253:3576, 1985.
13. McKee RF, Scott EM: The value of routine preoperative investigations. Ann R Coll Surg Engl 69:160, 1987.
14. Cobden I, Venables CW, Lendrum R, et al: Gallstones presenting as mental and physical debility in the elderly. Lancet(i) 1062, May 1984.
15. Goldman L, Caldera DL, Southwick FS, et al: Cardiac risk factors and complications in noncardiac surgery. Medicine 57:357, 1978.
16. Becker RC, Underwood DA: Myocardial infarction in patients undergoing noncardiac surgery. Cleve Clin J Med 54:25, 1987.
17. Steen PA, Tinker JH, Tarhan S: Myocardial reinfarction after anesthesia and surgery. JAMA 239:2566, 1978.
18. Sandler RS, Maule WF, Baltus ME, et al: Biliary tract surgery in the elderly. J Gen Intern Med 2:149, 1987.
19. Goldman L, Caldera DL, Nussbaum SR, et al: Multifactorial index of cardiac risk in noncardiac surgical procedures. N Engl J Med 297:845, 1977.
20. Keating HJ: Preoperative considerations in the geriatric patient. Med Clin North Am 71:569, 1987.
21. Carson JC, Eisenberg JM: The preoperative screening examination. In Goldman DR, Brown FH, eds: Medical Care of the Surgical Patient. Philadelphia, JB Lippincott Co, 1982, p 16.
22. O'Donnell TF, Darling RC, Linton RR: Is 80 years too old for aneurysmectomy? Arch Surg 111:1250, 1976.
23. Wilcock GK: A comparison of total hip replacement in patients aged 69 years or less and 70 years or over. Gerontology 27:85, 1981.
24. Del Guercio LRM, Cohn JD: Monitoring operative risk in the elderly. JAMA 243:1350, 1980.
25. Morrissey K, Schein CJ: Surgical problems in the aged. In Rossman I, ed: Clinical Geriatrics. Philadelphia, JB Lippincott Co, 1986, p 472.
26. Editorial: Postoperative atelectasis. Lancet(i) 965, November 1977.
27. Erlik D, Valero A, Birkham J, Gersh I: Prostatic surgery and the cardiovascular patient. Br J Urol 40:53, 1968.
28. Djokovic JL, Hedley-Whyte J: Prediction of outcome of surgery and anesthesia in patients over 80. JAMA 242:2301, 1979.
29. Hirsh RA: An approach to assessing preoperative risk. In Goldman DR, Brown FH, eds: Medical Care of the Surgical Patient. Philadelphia, JB Lippincott Co, 1982, p 31.
30. Rothfeld EL, Bernstein A, Weiss G, et al: Pulmonary function testing in geriatric surgical patients. Dis Chest 47:20, 1965.
31. Palmberg S, Hirsjarvi E: Mortality in geriatric surgery. Gerontology 25:103, 1979.
32. Elliot DL, Linz DH, Kane JA: Medical evaluation before operation. West J Med 137:351, 1982.
33. Port S, Cobb FR, Coleman RE, et al: Effect of age on the response of the left ventricular ejection fraction to exercise. N Engl J Med 303:1134, 1980.
34. Boucher CA, Brewster DC, Darling RC, et al: Determination of cardiac risk by dipyridamole-thallium imaging before peripheral vascular surgery. N Engl J Med 312:389, 1985.
35. Jain KM, Patil KD, Doctor US, et al: Preoperative cardiac screening before peripheral vascular operations. Am Surg 51:77, 1985.
36. Gerson MC, Hurst JM, Hertzberg VS, et al: Cardiac prognosis in noncardiac geriatric surgery. Ann Intern Med 103:832, 1985.
37. Carliner NH, Fisher ML, Plotnick GD, et al: Routine preoperative exercise testing in patients

undergoing major noncardiac surgery. Am J Cardiol 56:51, 1985.

38. Yang SC, Puri VK: Role of preoperative hemodynamic monitoring in intraoperative fluid management. Am Surg 52:536, 1986.

39. Rao TLK, Jacobs KH, El-Etr AA: Reinfarction following anesthesia in patients with myocardial infarction. Anesthesiology 59:499, 1983.

40. Bille-Brahe NE, Eickhoff JH: Measurement of central haemodynamic parameters during preoperative exercise testing in patients suspected of arteriosclerotic heart disease. Acta Chir Scand 502:38, 1980.

41. Garibaldi RA, Britt MR, Coleman ML, et al: Risk factors for postoperative pneumonia. Am J Med 70:677, 1981.

42. Grodsinsky C, Brush BE, Ponka JL: Postoperative pulmonary complications in the geriatric age group. J Am Geriatr Soc 22:407, 1974.

43. Cebul RD, Kussmaul WG: Preoperative pulmonary evaluation. In Goldman DR, Brown FH, eds: Medical Care of the Surgical Patient. Philadelphia, JB Lippincott Co, 1982, p 356.

44. Thompson TL, Thompson WL: Treating postoperative delirium. Drug Ther Hosp 30:9, October 1983.

45. Millar HR: Psychiatric morbidity in elderly surgical patients. Br J Psychiat 138:17, 1981.

46. Robbins LJ, Boyko E, Lane J, et al: Binding the elderly: a prospective study of the use of mechanical restraints in an acute care hospital. J Am Geriatr Soc 35:290, 1987.

47. Duncalf D, Kepes ER: Geriatric anesthesia. In Rossman I, ed: Clinical Geriatrics. Philadelphia, JB Lippincott Co, 1986, p 494.

48. Barry PA: Primary care evaluation of the elderly for elective surgery. Geriatrics 42:77, 1987.

49. Caranasos GJ, Stewart RB, Cluff LE: Drug-induced illness leading to hospitalization. JAMA 228:713, 1974.

50. Seidl LG, Thornton GF, Smith JW, et al: Studies on the epidemiology of adverse drug reactions, III: reactions in patients on a general medical service. Bull Johns Hopkins Hosp 119:299, 1966.

51. Trunet P, LeGall JR, Lhoste F, et al: The role of iatrogenic disease in admissions to intensive care. JAMA 244:2617, 1980.

52. Schimmel EM: The hazards of hospitalization. Ann Intern Med 60:100, 1964.

53. Reichel W: Complications in the care of five hundred elderly hospitalized patients. J Am Geriatr Soc 13:973, 1965.

54. Ogilvie RI, Ruedy J: Adverse reactions during hospitalization. Can Med Assoc J 97:1445, 1967.

55. Steel K, Gertman PM, Crescenzi C, et al: Iatrogenic illness on a general medical service at a university hospital. N Engl J Med 304:638, 1981.

56. Jahnigen D, Hannon C, Laxson L, et al: Iatrogenic disease in hospitalized elderly veterans. J Am Geriatr Soc 30:387, 1982.

57. Patterson C: Iatrogenic disease in late life. Clin Geriatr Med 2:121, 1986.

58. Schroeder SA, Marton KI, Strom BL: Frequency and morbidity of invasive procedures: report of a pilot study from two teaching hospitals. Arch Intern Med 138:1809, 1978.

59. Hou SH, Bushinsky DA, Wish JB, et al: Hospital-acquired renal insufficiency: a prospective study. Am J Med 74:243, 1983.

60. Ogilvie RI, Ruedy J: Adverse drug reactions during hospitalization. Can Med Assoc J 97:1450, 1967.

61. Hurwitz N: Predisposing factors in adverse reactions to drugs. Br Med J I:536, 1969.

62. Gosney M, Tallis R: Prescription of contraindicated and interacting drugs in elderly patients admitted to hospital. Lancet 2:564, 1984.

63. Greenblatt DJ, Sellers EM, Shader RI: Drug disposition in old age. N Engl J Med 306:1081, 1982.

64. Stamm WE: Infections related to medical devices. Ann Intern Med 89(Part 2):764, 1978.

65. Barry PP: Iatrogenic disorders in the elderly: preventive techniques. Geriatrics 41:42, 1986.

66. Catchen H: Repeaters: inpatient accidents among the hospitalized elderly. Gerontologist 23:273, 1983.

67. Rubenstein LZ: Falls in the elderly: a clinical approach. West J Med 138:273, 1983.

68. Andersen KE, Jensen O, Kvorning SA, et al: Prevention of pressure sores by identifying patients at risk. Br Med J 284:1370, 1982.

69. Kroenke K, Corrie GD: Urinary incontinence. West J Med 146:623, 1987.

CONFUSIONAL AND NEUROPSYCHIATRIC STATES

CHAPTER 8

Depression, Suicide, and Paranoia

Michael G. Moran
Troy L. Thompson

Senile debility, usually called "dotage," is a characteristic, not of all old men, but only of those who are weak in mind and will. (Ista senilis stultitia, quæ deliratio appelari solet, senum levium est, non omnium.)

CICERO, *De Senectute*

Psychiatric illnesses in the elderly present special problems because of their clinical pictures, which are often confusing and atypical. Diagnosis is thus more difficult than in younger persons, and treatment may also be more frequently confounded because of coexisting medical diseases and the potential for adverse interaction with the use of multiple medications.[1, 2] Indeed, medical illnesses and medications can pose as psychiatric illnesses.[3-5] In addition, psychiatric syndromes in the elderly often have significant somatic components.[4, 6] Among the psychiatric diseases associated with the elderly, depression is the most common, and suicide is its most serious conse-

quence.[7, 8] Paranoia is a common symptom of several medical and psychiatric conditions. The increase in the number of elderly persons requires that the physician have a working familiarity with the psychiatric concerns of the aged. These three problems—depression, suicide, and paranoia—deserve special treatment because of the complexity and variety of their presentation to the clinician, the distracting and troublesome reactions that they can produce in the physician trying to make the diagnosis, and their risks to the patient.

DEPRESSION AND SUICIDE

About 15 percent of those over 65 years of age are clinically depressed at any one time, making depression the most common psychiatric disorder in the aged.[4, 8] However, a depressive presentation in an older patient can seem so commonplace as to merit no attention from the physician. After all, with the losses inherent in advancing age, the isolation, the presumed lack of joyful fulfillment in almost every phase of life, shouldn't one *expect* the older person to be at least a little depressed? Such ageism stereotyping can lead the otherwise astute clinician astray.[2, 3] When depressive symptoms are assumed to be normal, they no longer occupy our diagnostic thinking and trigger our curiosity. We no longer ask the empathically probing questions necessary to explore the nature, severity, and origin of the depression. We no longer ask about suicide.

The typical presentation of depression in middle-aged persons is perhaps the best known and easiest to recognize (Table 8–1).[5, 9, 10] Psychomotorically retarded, the patient's posture slumps, and the amplitude of movements decreases. Facial appearance may be consistent with this picture of sadness. The interview and history taking may be difficult or come only from a family member who accompanies the patient. Questions about mood reveal sadness, feeling "down," ruminations that are depressive in character, and hopelessness and helplessness. The mood is often

TABLE 8–1. Diagnostic Criteria for Depression

Depressed mood
Diminished pleasure in most or all activities, most or all of every day
Significant weight loss or gain (change of 5% or greater of body weight)
Insomnia or hypersomnia nearly every day
Psychomotor retardation or agitation nearly every day.
Fatigue or loss of energy nearly every day
Sense of worthlessness or inappropriate guilt nearly every day, which may be delusional
Decreased ability to concentrate nearly every day
Recurrent thoughts of suicide or dying (not just fear of dying)

Five of the above symptoms must be present during a period of at least two weeks. The symptoms must (1) represent a change in function, and (2) include depressed mood or loss of interest or pleasure. There must be no identifiable organic factor causing the symptoms, and symptoms must not be normal, uncomplicated grief reactions to loss.
There must be no superimposed schizophrenia or delusional or psychotic disorder. Psychotic symptoms and symptoms clearly related to a physical condition are excluded.
(Modified from Diagnostic and Statistical Manual of Mental Disorders, 3rd ed, rev. American Psychiatric Association, by permission.)

worst early in the day, coinciding with difficulty arising. The patient may relate to the physician in an inappropriately guilty manner, taking inordinate responsibility and feeling ashamed for reasons that are not apparent. Hopelessness and helplessness may gravitate around a long-standing physical illness or complaint. A renewal of the patient's preoccupation with the medical symptoms and medications, along with a hopeless attitude, frequently emerges with depression in the older patient.

Disturbed sleep, especially with early morning awakening, is a harbinger of other vegetative symptoms and signs. Difficulty falling asleep also may be present. Altered appetite, usually with anorexia, rather than with increased intake, can occur. There may be accompanying weight loss. Weight gain, too, can be a symptom of depression that is often overlooked. Constipation reflects dominance of parasympathetic activity and may even be associated with bradycardia. Overall energy level is low, and the patient tires easily. Hobbies, work, and other activities (including sex) that generally provide pleasure lose their vitality and appeal. Concentration is difficult to sustain. Crying spells and suicidal ideation round out the picture of classic melancholic depression. If the symptoms are of more than two weeks' duration, the diagnosis of depression can be made.

Depression is hard to miss when these symptoms are seen together in one patient during a single office visit, especially if the patient complains of feeling depressed. But the patient may not offer the diagnosis.[3] The atypical picture requires a high index of suspicion for discovery. Agitation may predominate, rather than retardation of motion. The patient may provoke feelings of anger or irritation, rather than of sympathy or compassion. The physician may find himself forgetting the appointment of this patient or even consciously trying to avoid the patient or his phone calls. The patient may complain of weight gain and increased appetite, although this variant is uncommon in the authors' experience. Decreased energy, mild confusion, and the predominance of somatic symptoms without clearly evident physical illness in an elderly patient should alert the physician to atypical depression.

Whatever the clinical picture, the physician must fill in the gaps; complete and classic histories are rarely offered by the patient, and the physician must ask questions that open the interview and allow further exploration. The wish to die, wanting to give up, thinking the family or the world would be better off without the patient are examples of thoughts and ruminations that are usually not offered to the doctor. Probing such areas allows the physician to further fill in the history: Did the patient have a specific plan for suicide? A method? The tools? Inquiry about suicidal ideation is critical, since elderly men (especially widowers who are isolated and medically ill) have the highest rate of completed suicide of any group. The methods they use are notoriously lethal.

Past medical and psychiatric history may reveal repeated depressive episodes or a history of manic episodes that suggest the diagnoses of major depressive disorder and bipolar disorder, respectively. More complex is the life-long story of constant depression, without apparent precipitants or psychosocial stressors. These patients probably have depressive variants such as a dysthymic or cyclothymic disorder. A psychiatrist can be helpful in clarifying the diagnosis and prescribing appropriate treatment.

Family history of psychiatric disorder is also important and relevant. When the history reveals mood disorder or substance use, the physician should be more suspicious of histories that only partially satisfy classic criteria for depression. The physician must remember, however, that he is treating the patient, not the family, and that the diagnosis needs to be made in the patient. None of the diagnostic criteria for depression includes aspects of family history.

Coexistent Medical Illness

The ways in which medical illnesses can coexist with depressive syndromes are several.[1, 5] A medical illness can cause the depressive syndrome directly and may even present as the mood disorder. An example is carcinoma of the head of the pancreas (Table 8–2). Another example is a drug used to treat a medical condition, such as propranolol in the treatment of

TABLE 8–2. Medical Illnesses Associated with Depressive Symptoms

Endocrine Diseases
Hyperthyroidism and hypothyroidism
Adrenal insufficiency and hyperadrenalism
Diabetes and hypoglycemia

Central Nervous System Disorders
Subarachnoid hemorrhage
"Normal pressure" hydrocephalus
Parkinson's disease
Frontal lobe structural lesions

Viral Illnesses
Pneumonia
Hepatitis

Neoplasms
Carcinoma of the pancreas

hypertension or angina. In these examples, the primary medical condition may not demand attention from either the patient or the physician. Timing of the onset of the depressive syndrome and its coincidence with the beginning of the use of the medication are important historical data. The insidious beginning of the depressive symptoms in the patient with carcinoma of the pancreas is a more difficult diagnostic problem for the doctor, especially in the absence of gastrointestinal symptoms, abdominal pain, or evidence of a metastatic process.

The medical illness may cause the depressive syndrome through a less direct route such as the patient's reaction to the illness or its diagnosis.[9] For example, in the diagnosis of myocardial infarction, as the patient becomes aware of the implications of the diagnosis and its associated losses, he could become depressed and may even need psychiatric treatment.

Depression can coexist with medical illness, with no apparent causal relationship. Drugs used to treat the medical illness may produce psychiatric symptoms.[1, 4, 5] The medically ill patient is not immune from acquiring depression, nor is the depressed patient immune from acquiring a medical illness. In fact, dual diagnoses are seen frequently. In the context of chronic illness, a regular finding in the older patient, the coexistence of depression—or at least depressive syndromes—is common. The diagnosis of depression is especially crucial in these settings. Because many of the vegetative symptoms of depression are already present in the sequelae of the chronic medical disease (weight loss, fatigue, loss of pleasure in normally enjoyable activities, and disturbances of sleep and appetite), the diagnosis of depression may be delayed if the vegetative symptoms are attributed to the chronic medical illness alone. The untreated mood disorder can affect the patient's ability to cope with the illness and comply with treatment. In the elderly patient, risk of suicide is increased considerably by the presence of a severe chronic illness.[7]

Some of the mechanisms that cause depression have been elucidated. Cancer may directly affect the brain through primary involvement (e.g., brain tumor) or secondary involvement (e.g., metastatic processes) of the central nervous system. Other intracranial processes, such as subarachnoid hemorrhage, may also directly involve structures that affect mood. Distant cancers such as carcinoma of the pancreas may cause depression through paraneoplastic phenomena, caused by the production of psychoactive substances that affect the brain. Less clear are the routes by which viral diseases and rheumatoid arthritis cause depressive syndromes.

Drugs that cause depression usually affect central mechanisms of storage, release, or production of biogenic amines (probably, norepinephrine and serotonin). In some cases, synaptic reuptake or postsynaptic receptor activity is affected. A classic example of a drug that causes depression is reserpine, which depletes the presynaptic neuron of biogenic amines. Other mechanisms of drug action include direct central nervous system depression, as caused by action of sedative hypnotics and anxiolytics. Alcohol is included in this group.

The older patient is more likely than the younger patient to be taking several medications, a number of which are either psychotropic or psychoactive.[10, 11] A perusal of the medication list of such patients as well as the problem list of diagnoses and symptoms is invaluable in the search for the cause of the depressive syndrome.

Although the coexistence of medical and psychiatric diagnoses is regularly seen, one should remember that depression itself in the elderly is often dominated by complaints of somatic symptoms and hypochondriacal behavior.[7] The tendency to relegate these patients to the realm of "crocks," or hypochondriacs, is a serious error. Elderly patients with somatic symptoms within their depressive presentation have a higher risk for suicide attempts. Indeed, there may be a correlation between their symptoms being incorrectly diagnosed as a medical illness or ignored as hypochondriacal and their attempt at suicide.[3] Obviously, untreated depression is associated with a decreased life expectancy, if only because of the undetected risk of possible suicide. However, untreated depression itself seems to decrease life expectancy by mechanisms not yet clearly understood but possibly involving immune dysfunction. The risk of heart disease is also greater in the population of persons with untreated depression.

Diagnostic Evaluation

As discussed, the merits of a high index of suspicion for the presence of depression in the elderly are clear. Coexisting medical disease, and perhaps especially, coexisting dementia, can make the diagnosis of depression difficult (Table 8–3). An added problem is the cognitive dysfunction that can occur in the depressed patient, which can be mistaken for dementia. The frequency of this error gives rise to the term pseudodementia.[2, 6, 12] If the clinician expects to see a dementing process in all of his elderly patients or has difficulty recognizing depression, he is more likely to mistake the cognitive disturbance of depression for dementia. A thorough history and physical examination, supplemented by data from family, nurses, and previous medical records, can help distinguish between depression and dementia.[7] This in-depth approach also permits the discovery of medical illnesses and drugs that may contribute to the depressive or dementia syndrome.[1, 13]

The history should include a survey of the patient's recent life events and of possible psychosocial stressors. Although almost all patients will try to give a history with causal links to the origins of symptoms, the historical sequence can have a special place in the psychotherapeutic management of the depressed patient. Major changes in the environment, such as a move to a hospital or nursing home, can precede a depressive syndrome.[7]

TABLE 8–3. Differential Diagnosis of Dementia and Pseudodementia

	Dementia	Pseudodementia (Depression)
Presentation	Denies, conceals deficits	Complains of deficits often found in demented patients
Recent Memory	Poor; remote memory intact	Usually normal
Intellect	"Concrete" thinking	Normal if patient motivated
Judgment	Consistently poor, even when trying	Poor secondary to effects of depression
Diurnal Variation	Worse in evening	Worse in morning
Mood	Labile; inappropriate	Hopeless; helpless; sad
Psychotic Symptoms	Content varies; illusions often present	Morbid delusions
Response to Treatment	May improve with low doses of neuroleptics; sedative/hypnotics may cause delirium	Antidepressants may help with vegetative symptoms; symptoms may worsen with CNS depressants

(From Thompson TL II, Psychosocial and psychiatric problems of the aged. In Schrier RW, Clinical Internal Medicine in the Aged. Philadelphia, WB Saunders Co, 1982, by permission.)

Questions about work, income, friends, relatives, hobbies, and physical activity usually provide useful clues to the patient's hedonic state and quality of mentation. Complaints of forgetting (from the patient or accompanying family member), decreased concentration, lack of interest in hobbies, or significant alterations in appetite or sleep may arise during this survey. Recent losses, which are a frequent event for many older persons, may provoke grieving reactions that are similar to or can result in a depressive syndrome. In addition, recent loss is another factor that raises the suicide risk in any depressed patient but perhaps to a greater degree in the elderly medically ill.

A reminder about biases in understanding the history of loss in an older patient: The patient who ruminates, who is preoccupied and obsessed with loss, and whose function is impaired because of mood disturbance, is not normal, no matter how old. Depression is not normal. Geriatric status does not confer acceptability on depression; it remains a treatable and yet a potentially lethal disease.

The mental status examination, which surveys appearance, speech, movement, posture, attention, concentration, mood, form of thought, and orientation, and searches for specific psychotic symptoms, can help the doctor discriminate between depression and dementia. The demented patient (or other historical source) may describe an insidious course of symptom onset, and the patient himself will often try to deny cognitive dysfunction. The depressed patient talks freely of deficits and, often, of mood disturbances. If any memory or concentration disturbances are present, the depressed, pseudodemented patient may discuss the symptoms in detail.[2] Such history from the demented patient is rare; symptoms are obscure and vague. The onset of any apparent mood disturbance and the cognitive dysfunction are found to coincide, and are more easily pinpointed than with the depressed patient. The course of symptoms of the patient with pseudodementia of depression is relatively short; the demented patient reveals symptoms, such as memory deficits, of long duration (often months or years).[6] If the depression is not so severe that the patient has effectively withdrawn from the environment, attention and cognition are found to be effort dependent; the examiner's patience and encouragement reveal a memory and sensorium that are intact.

The depressed patient's mood is often flat and depressed, with hopelessness and helplessness expressed in a distressed manner during the interview. The demented patient's mood can be more variable within the interview, even labile, shallow, and blunted, or irritable without clear provocation. These patients may also appear to be totally unconcerned about the very symptoms that promoted a family member to bring the patient to the physician in the first place. In spite of this seeming aloofness from their symptoms, demented patients betray their concern about memory and concentration loss indirectly. The history may reveal elaborate efforts, such as note-taking and other methods, that the patient used to remind himself of everyday matters to be accomplished. The depressed patient has generally made no such efforts, so withdrawn is he or she from the world at large. This latter group demonstrates no sustained effort at these tasks; the demented patient can be seen to struggle at the simplest tasks of memory and concentration. In addition, the depressed patient, depending on the degree of withdrawal, may have lost many of the social graces by the time he or she sees the doctor. Dementia, in its early stages, does not tend to rob the patient of these interactive skills. It is only later in the course of the illness that the patient may show social improprieties.

Formal mental status examination reveals the depressed patient as seeming to neither know nor care about most current events. Demented patients, on the other hand, try to make a good showing and may contort an unusual event about which they are prompted into one that is more familiar, although usually temporally more distant. Demented patients may report a worsening of their symptoms during the evening and night. A pre-existing psychiatric history would not be unusual for the depressed patient, but is less common with the demented person.

History for substance use, although always important, is perhaps especially crucial among depressed and demented patients. In the case of depression, substance use often lessens the impulse control of the angry and hopeless patient, and can greatly increase suicide risk. Indeed, 25 percent of all suicide victims have alcohol in their body fluids at autopsy. The use of some drugs, such as alcohol or other central nervous system depressants, may directly worsen the affective state and aggravate the depressive affect. Resorting to the use of such drugs also reflects the efforts of some patients at self treatment or self-reproach. If the doctor uncovers such a history, it is often prudent to admit the patient for detoxification. This maneuver allows supervision of the patient and introduces a controlled environment. "Drying out" may unmask a clear depression or may reveal a picture more suggestive

of personality pathology. The latter finding suggests that the drug may have produced an organic mood disorder, rather than the existence of a true major depression. However, one must always be suspicious of the coexistence of all three—primary mood disorder, organic mood disorder, and personality disorder.

Substance use can also be an important factor in the etiology and maintenance of a dementia. Alcohol use is the paradigmatic example. Long-standing and heavy use damages the liver, stomach and upper gastrointestinal tract, pancreas, and brain. Coincident and chronic vitamin deficiencies, such as thiamine deficiency, markedly worsen cerebral functioning and can have catastrophic consequences, as in the example of Korsakoff's psychosis. This is the chronic, often irreversible, sequela of thiamine deficiency, sometimes unmasked after thiamine treatment of Wernicke's syndrome. However, apart from vitamin deficiency, alcohol alone can result in chronic, virtually irreversible dementia, often with characteristic cerebellar involvement. Patients demonstrate confabulation and poor short-term memory. Acute alcohol intoxication depresses affect and clouds memory and concentration. One should always repeat a thorough physical and mental status examination in such patients after the clearance of the acutely intoxicated state.

When the depressed patient is intoxicated, he is at greater risk for committing suicide. Any suicidal patient should be examined personally by the physician and should undergo psychiatric consultation. Transient suicidal ideation may respond to the careful and empathic taking of the history of the symptom. Such an interview may provide the opportunity to make sense of the symptom; the patient is often confused and embarrassed by his suicidal thinking, and a considerate physician can be of great assistance in helping to relieve these symptoms by the act of helpful listening. The physician must assess current risk, duration of the symptoms, and the origins and apparent purpose of the suicide. Chronic suicidal ideation or fantasies of dying are common in many patients with a chronic, severe medical illness. The fantasies may provide an avenue of escape or a sense of control that is not present in the patient's real life. One need not always hospitalize these patients to treat their suicidal ideation. Careful listening, an empathic approach to the fantasies, and the expression of understanding about their origins often help. This approach usually decompresses the symptom; acceptance of the symptom means that the patient need not hide it, and the impulse to act is often removed.

One should take a history of previous suicidal ideation, previous suicide attempts, and a family psychiatric history.[7, 8] The physician needs to uncover previous psychiatric history (including history for bipolar and depressive illness), suicide attempts, completed suicides, and substance use about the patient's family. A positive history for any of these factors increases the risk for suicide in the patient. Current lethality is assessed by looking for an elaborated plan of the suicidal act, specific and detailed fantasies about the reactions of family members and others close to the patient, and the possession of tools required for the act as planned (e.g., drugs, weapons, or easy access to windows or platforms at great height). Recent personal loss or other major psychosocial stressors, severe medical illness, advanced age, and interpersonal isolation also increase the risk for completed suicide in the patient with suicidal thoughts. These points should be explored in every depressed patient's history.

Treatment

Special management and knowledge are required for the successful treatment of depression in older patients.[2] The psychopharmacologic approach needs to be careful and judicious.[10, 11] Psychotherapy should be guided by an understanding of the life cycle and the resulting context of particular psychosocial stressors.[7] The nonsuicidal patient is discussed first.

Once a decision is made that the elderly patient is indeed significantly depressed, that is, has more than expectable reactive despondency, the physician should consider at least two treatment modes.[1-4] *Psychotherapy*, shunned for the elderly in previous years because of the alleged lack of "plasticity" in their personalities, is enjoying an appropriate revival for this age group. The psychiatrist tries to help the

patient make sense of the symptoms of depression, not only as an illness with biologic facets but also as a syndrome expressive of the person's inner state. Loss can be seen in the context of a life in its later stages. For the elderly patient, the content of the depression may include issues of creativity, stagnation, and sense of heritage. Damage to self-esteem can result. The addition of relative or significant helplessness secondary to debilitating disease should also be examined. Many elderly patients can benefit from such therapy. Indeed, their years of experience with themselves and with others often means that they bring to the therapy a degree of self-knowledge and a willingness for frank self-observation not often encountered to the same degree in younger, so-called ideal psychotherapy patients.

Pharmacologic agents also can be useful in the treatment of depression in the aged person. The psychiatrist can offer consultation regarding these drugs as well as help to exclude other medications that contribute to the depressive syndrome.[1, 5, 10, 11]

There are no antidepressants that have special efficacy in the elderly, contrary to some promotional assertions.[10] The major consideration when using these agents in the aged is that of side effects.[11] There are particular areas of vulnerability in the elderly, in addition to their altered pharmacokinetic functioning, that must be considered. Also, changes in the aging brain itself probably render the older person more susceptible to both the positive and the adverse effects of the cyclic antidepressants (CyAds) and other psychotropics. Efforts aimed at reducing adverse side effects must recognize all three factors: altered pharmacokinetics, altered brain, and knowledge of the agents themselves. Successful efforts allow the older patient greater tolerance of the drug, which is not a small element in the overall objective of regular dosing that usually lasts for at least several months.

Because of the well-known cardiac side effects of these drugs in the setting of the tricyclic overdose, many physicians inappropriately withhold antidepressants from depressed patients with heart disease.[14, 15] Cyclic antidepressants do cause powerful adverse cardiac effects in cases of overdose. However, prudent administration is safe in all but a few types of cardiac disease. For example, patients suffering myocardial infarction without symptomatic conduction problems or significant loss of cardiac output often can be carefully treated with CyAds 6 to 8 weeks after the infarction when cardiology consultation and electrocardiograms are available. Almost all patients with minor conduction delays can be treated with CyAds. In any patients for whom CyAds present a cardiac risk, examination of the EKG before and after starting the drug and after each dosage change, cardiac consultation, and even hospitalization are useful approaches.

Only in those patients who are symptomatic, that is, have low cardiac output, orthostatic hypotension, syncope, or severe angina as a result of their conduction problems or myocardial impairment, are CyAds contraindicated. In themselves, most dysrhythmias are not reason to avoid these drugs. Two conduction problems that warrant very close assessment before using these agents are Wolff-Parkinson-White syndrome and the syndrome of QT interval prolongation. The quinidine-like effects of the CyAds make persons with these two syndromes more susceptible to lethal ventricular arrhythmias. One should also be aware of the combined effect of the CyAds with other class I cardiac drugs (quinidine, disopyramide, and procainamide) on cardiac conduction. Drugs from two of these groups should be used in combination with great care and only after in-depth consultation with a cardiologist.

A guideline for the use of CyAds in the treatment of cardiac patients must include an abiding awareness of the potential lethality of depression in the elderly. By definition, this group of cardiac patients also has a severe medical illness. The decision to avoid CyAds should be accompanied by comprehensive planning for care of the patient's depression. Alternative treatments, including electroconvulsive therapy, are sometimes indicated and may offer lower overall risks than some CyAds. Psychotherapeutic treatment, involvement of the family, and attention to relief of cardiac symptoms play a critical role in the management of depressive affect and helplessness.[7] In some cases, the contraindicating conduction problem or issue of impaired low cardiac output may resolve, allowing use of the CyAd.

Cyclic antidepressants vary as to their proclivity for causing cardiotoxic effects. Past work with doxepin suggested that it may be more appropriate for this group of patients. More recent studies now suggest that this earlier work with doxepin was conducted at subtherapeutic levels.[10] Still, many authorities continue to recommend it as the preferred agent for cardiac patients. Nortriptyline has had fewer reported episodes of hypotension, which is of some consequence for the elderly, who are likely to sustain hip fractures after falls. Nortriptyline is also less sedating and less anticholinergic than other agents sometimes chosen by physicians, such as doxepin and amitriptyline. Among the traditional CyAds, desipramine is the least sedating and least anticholinergic. Desipramine also has a relatively low incidence of causing orthostatic hypotension. Compared with nortriptyline, desipramine has the possible disadvantage of being relatively more active in only one amine system—the noradrenergic system—as opposed to being more active in that *and* the serotonergic system, as occurs with nortriptyline.

Prostatism and other disorders adversely affected by anticholinergic drug activity occur with frequency in the elderly. Constipation, increased intraocular pressure associated with glaucoma, bladder outlet dysfunction, and dysmotility of the upper gastrointestinal tract may worsen when the patient is given drugs with strong anticholinergic effects. Cyclic antidepressants have anticholinergic activity that contraindicates their use in patients with untreated narrow angle glaucoma. In patients with the other aforementioned disorders, use of a CyAd with low anticholinergic activity may be possible without severe side effects. Trazodone and desipramine are examples that may be useful in these patients; however, trazodone is more sedating than desipramine and may cause priapism. A clinical trial for the patient involved, with close supervision and follow-up, is the wisest approach.

Changes in pharmacokinetics with aging can modify the clinician's approach to the prescribing of antidepressants to the elderly.[10, 11] Absorption of these drugs is usually not affected unless there has been major gastrointestinal surgery. Antacids may delay the speed, but usually not the efficacy, of absorption. Metabolism is somewhat slowed with aging because the activity of the liver enzymes that detoxify the drug is decreased. Drug interactions are of special interest here because the older patient with other medical illnesses is usually taking several medications. Of those commonly used, chronic alcohol, some steroids, and antiseizure medications will speed degradation of the CyAd and cause lowered serum levels for a given oral dose. Cimetidine, cigarette smoking, or acute alcohol intoxication will slow the rate of metabolism and result in higher blood levels.

In initiating administration of these medications in the depressed elderly patient, one should begin at a low dose, such as 10 to 25 mg per day of nortriptyline or its equivalent.[4, 12] Increases in dosage should be made gradually, such as 10 mg per day or every other day. Frequent follow-up visits, checks on orthostatic changes in vital signs, and performing EKGs when necessary, are important to the treatment.

Those changes in the brain that account for increased sensitivity to these drugs are not yet fully understood. Apart from the pharmacokinetic observations previously mentioned, these brain changes probably account for the increased incidence of side effects with psychoactive medications of all types for some elderly patients. The clinician can make a rough assessment of the cumulative sensitivity of the older patient by performing a mental status examination. Evidence of dementia and certainly of delirium suggest a greater likelihood of adverse side effects from psychotropic medications and argue for added caution in their use. In the case of the CyAds, the anticholinergic side effects are the major concern in the demented patient, who presumably has a greater sensitivity to any psychotropic agent. Anticholinergic delirium may result, producing disorganization, altered level of consciousness, impulsive and paranoid behavior, and visual or auditory illusions and hallucinations. There may be associated peripheral signs of anticholinergic toxicity, with tachycardia, dry and hot skin, and cutaneous vasodilatation. The risk for this toxic state is increased if the elderly patient is taking other medications that have anticholinergic activity. Examples include inhaled and oral anticholinergic agents used in certain pulmonary conditions, antihistamines, and most over-the-counter sedatives and hypnotics. In the latter group, the active ingredients are generally antihistaminic, with powerful anticholinergic effects. Labels of over-the-counter drugs often do not give separate prescribing recommendations for the elderly.

Some of the antidepressants, such as amitriptyline and doxepin, are quite sedating. For the elderly demented patient, the sedating effects of these CyAds can be enough to precipitate delirium. The risk is greater if the patient is already taking another sedating medication, such as an anxiolytic, a hypnotic, or alcohol.

If a particular antidepressant fails after an adequate trial, several points must be considered. The patient must take the medication daily, not as needed; at least 4 to 6 weeks are necessary to make a true assessment of the drug; the dose must be high enough—one may need to increase the daily dose until side effects begin to appear. This last point is often forgotten in treating the elderly, for whom caution is emphasized in an attempt to avoid inappropriately high doses. The psychiatrist should be involved to help evaluate the choice of the drug used. A review of the diagnosis is also helpful at this time. Bipolar illness, adjustment disorders, and undiagnosed organic mood disorders may account for the apparent failure of CyAds.

The psychiatrist may recommend switching to an antidepressant with activity in another biogenic amine system. In some patients, monoamine oxidase (MAO) inhibitors are a reasonable second choice to the CyAds.[4] With care to avoid drug interactions and adverse reactions to certain foods, this class of agents can provide relief to some patients with resistant depression. Electroconvulsive therapy (ECT) and stimulants are also alternatives when more conventional treatments fail or when urgency and severity of depressive symptoms dictate quick action.[4, 8] Although the risks of ECT are increased for the older patient, this form of treatment can still be safe, effective, and more rapidly acting than antidepressants.[16] Bipolar illnesses and some unipolar depressions continuing into later life may require lithium carbonate. Psychotic depressions often require a neuroleptic (i.e., major) tranquilizer in addition to the antidepressant.[9]

PARANOIA

Paranoia is a symptom of several psychiatric illnesses and syndromes.[8] The word is descriptive, not diagnostic, and its use should never imply the end of the search for etiology. Among the elderly, there are no truly unique causes of paranoia. Illnesses that produce paranoid thinking and behavior in younger persons can produce the same symptoms in older patients. Examples include schizophrenia and bipolar illness.[7] Dementia and delirium, more prevalent among the elderly, are associated with paranoid thinking in about 20 percent of cases.[17] The paranoid personality is rare, but it is seen in the aged. Poor vision or hearing may exacerbate mild paranoid thinking, and appropriate treatment of these sensory impairments may lessen paranoid symptoms.[2] Social isolation and deprivation can be so stressful as to worsen paranoid tendencies.[18]

Schizophrenia begins when the patient is young. A quick survey of the patient's history should reveal the long-standing psychiatric diagnosis of schizophrenia, with the commonly found record of hospitalizations and neuroleptic use. By old age, schizophrenia has often "burned out," leaving the so-called negative features, such as social withdrawal, suspiciousness, flat affect, and markedly decreased social functioning. After some questioning, the patient may give the history of at least occasional auditory hallucinations. Signs of disorientation, altered sensorium, or illusions are not characteristic, unless another diagnosis is also present. Paranoid thinking is usually mild and reflected in behavior rather than in overt complaints to others; the social withdrawal mandates little contact.

Appropriate management includes a careful medical history and physical examination for concurrent medical illness and contact with the patient's psychiatrist or mental health clinic. An effort should be made to ensure that an adequate supply of needed medications is available. Attempts to uncover adverse side effects, determine substance use, and document chronic movement disorders, such as tardive dyskinesia, are also indicated. Treatment almost always involves the use of appropriate antipsychotic agents.[2, 4] Hospitalization may be necessary, if the patient is suicidal or gravely disabled.

Drugs with marked anticholinergic effects and significant alpha adrenergic blockade (i.e., the lower potency neuroleptics) should be avoided in patients whose condition places them at risk for orthostatic faintness and anticholinergic delirium, as noted in the foregoing discussion of depression.[4] Although they generally do not cause these side effects, the higher potency agents may worsen an existing Parkinson's disease. With close observation, however, they are usually safe and effective in the elderly. An elderly patient with schizophrenia often has a history of treatment with several drugs. Many patients can tell the physician which one to choose if the chart or another source of data is not available. Initially, trying the drug used most successfully in the past is the best course for most patients. Paraphrenia, a condition of the elderly marked by a loosely constructed paranoid delusional system (perhaps related to the schizophrenias), often responds to neuroleptics.

Bipolar illness may begin after age 45, and a history of the illness is usually known by age 60.[9] Tricyclic antidepressants may precipitate a manic episode. Paranoia can be a manifestation of either depression or mania.[7] Paranoid thinking may escalate with the pace of the mania, especially in those prone to irritability rather than euphoria. Elderly manic patients often appear more confused and paranoid than do younger counterparts.[7] The disorder of mood, with racing thoughts and motor activity, and the decreased need for sleep are generally recognizable, and this syndrome usually precedes the onset of psychotic thinking. In the psychotic phase, the patient may be paranoid and suspicious, especially if one confronts or demeans the patient's grandiose ideas. Hallucinations, hypersexual behavior and seductiveness, and physical assaults may also appear in the severely manic person. In such instances, psychiatric consultation and hospitalization are necessary.

Management in earlier phases includes tests of serum lithium levels and, often, adding a neuroleptic to the regimen.[4] An elderly patient who had been taking lithium and a diuretic, and has stopped the diuretic without increasing the lithium dosage, may develop subtherapeutic blood levels of lithium. More commonly, the hypomanic patient stops taking lithium as part of a grandiose self-assessment of good health. Lithium toxicity can mimic severe mania; any manic patient new to the physician should undergo check of the blood lithium level. Adequate hydration should be advised for patients taking lithium, especially during warm weather and for those who exercise vigorously.

Up to 20 percent of demented patients may present with paranoia when they become delirious.[17] Clues to the likelihood of underlying dementia and delirium include an antecedent history of dementia, a drug recently added to the patient's regimen, fluctuation of sensorium and orientation over a period of hours, disturbed vital signs, and visual or auditory illusions, rather than hallucinations. The management should first involve a thorough diagnostic evaluation. The cause of the delirium or the exacerbation of the dementia should be vigorously sought. A contributing medical illness or drug, bacteremia, change in serum electrolytes, decreased arterial blood oxygenation, and deficiency of an important vitamin are all examples of possible triggers for delirium or worsening dementia and can result in symptoms that include paranoid thinking and behavior.[9]

Once the likely cause is found, specific corrective measures should be taken to treat the disturbance. At this point, it may be appropriate to administer neuroleptic agents in those paranoid, demented, or delirious patients who are agitated or potentially harmful to themselves or others.[4] The recommended treatment should begin with moderate doses of a high potency neuroleptic such as haloperidol to control agitation. Later, dosage is decreased to maintain control. An example of a beginning dose is 10 mg by mouth or 5 mg intravenously every 30 to 60 minutes until the patient is calm.

Paranoid personality is a rare, stable disorder characterized by generalized suspiciousness, social withdrawal, and hypervigilance in social situations. Because it is so uncommon and is seldom suspected, it may not appear in previous medical records. However, there is often reference to the patient's eccentricity, suspiciousness, or "strangeness." In contrast to paraphrenia, there is usually no specific delusional system, and hallucinations are absent. The patient is usually not in psychiatric care and is almost never on psychiatric medications. These patients come to the physician's attention when they refuse medications from a nurse or physician whom they do not know or balk at medical treatment that seems obviously necessary. Discussion with them reveals their suspiciousness about the physician's or nurse's motives. In contrast to schizophrenic patients, these persons do not have a classically deteriorating level of functioning, and may actually be employed. Management requires careful explanation of medical diagnoses and proposed treatments—including the patient in at least some aspects of decision making—and scrupulous respect for the patient's privacy and confidentiality. Psychiatric medications are usually refused and are often not necessary.

REFERENCES

1. Stoudemire GA: Selected organic mental disorders. In Hales RE, Yudofsky SC, eds: Textbook of Neuropsychiatry. Washington, American Psychiatric Press, 1987, p 125.
2. Reifler BV, Borson S: Geriatric psychiatry. In Michels R, Cooper AM, Guze S, et al, eds: Psychiatry, Vol 2. Philadelphia, JB Lippincott Co, 1987, p 1.
3. Thompson TL II: Psychosocial and psychiatric problems of the aged. In Schrier RW, ed: Clinical Internal Medicine in the Aged. Philadelphia, WB Saunders Co, 1982, p 29.
4. Salzman C: Management of psychiatric problems. In Rowe JW, Besdine RW, eds: Health and Disease in Old Age. Boston, Little, Brown & Co, 1982, p 115.
5. Cohen-Cole SA, Harpe C: Diagnostic assessment of depression in the medically ill. In Stoudemire A, Fogel BS, eds: Principles of Medical Psychiatry. Orlando, Grune and Stratton, 1987, p 23.
6. Linn L: Clinical manifestations of psychiatric disorders. In Kaplan HI, Sadock BJ, eds: Comprehensive Textbook of Psychiatry, 4th ed. Baltimore, Williams and Wilkins, 1985, p 579.
7. Liptzin B: Psychiatric Aspects of Aging. In Rowe JW, Besdine RW, eds: Health and Disease in Old Age. Boston, Little, Brown & Co, 1982, p 85.
8. Coni N, Davison W, Webster S: Ageing: the Facts. New York, Oxford, 1984, p 87.
9. Verwoerdt A: Clinical Geropsychiatry, 2nd ed. Baltimore, Williams and Wilkins, 1981, p 203.
10. Thompson TL II, Moran MG, Nies AS: Psychotropic drug use in the elderly. N Engl J Med 308:134; 194, 1983.
11. Vestal RE: Drug metabolism and therapeutics in

the elderly. In Steel K, ed: Geriatric Education. Lexington, Collamone Press, 1981, p 129.

12. Lehmann HE: Affective disorders: clinical features. In Kaplan HI, Sadock BJ, eds: Comprehensive Textbook of Psychiatry, 4th ed. Baltimore, Williams and Wilkins, 1985, p 801.

13. Butler RN: Geriatric psychiatry. In Kaplan HI, Sadock BJ, eds: Comprehensive Textbook of Psychiatry, 4th ed. Baltimore, Williams and Wilkins, 1985, p 1953.

14. Wendkos MH: Sudden Death and Psychiatric Illness. New York, SP Medical and Scientific, 1979, p 321.

15. Vieth RC, Raskin MA, Caldwell JH, et al: Cardiovascular effects of tricyclic antidepressants in depressed patients with cardiac disease. N Engl J Med 306:954, 1982.

16. Weiner RD, Coffey CE: Electroconvulsive therapy in the medically ill. In Stoudemire A, Fogel BS, eds: Principles of Medical Psychiatry. Orlando, Grune and Stratton, 1987, p 113.

17. Walker JI, Brodie HKH: Paranoid disorders. In Kaplan HI, Sadock BJ, eds: Comprehensive Textbook of Psychiatry, 4th ed. Baltimore, Williams and Wilkins, 1985, p 750.

18. Solomon P, Kleeman ST: Sensory deprivation. In Kaplan HI, Sadock BJ, eds: Comprehensive Textbook of Psychiatry, 4th ed. Baltimore, Williams and Wilkins, 1985, p 321.

CHAPTER 9

Alzheimer's Disease and Other Dementia States

Christopher M. Filley

Age steals away all things, even the mind. (Omnia fert ætas, animum quoque.)

VERGIL, Eclogues

Health depends as much on intellectual and emotional competence as on physical vigor. In older people, diseases of the nervous system often produce behavioral as well as physical impairments, and it has been estimated that neurologic illnesses account for 50 percent of the incapacitation in persons over the age of 65.[1] Alzheimer's disease (AD) and the other dementias comprise many of the diseases that affect behavior in the elderly and pose formidable challenges to the geriatric clinician.

In the 82 years since Alois Alzheimer published the first case of the disease that bears his name, AD has evolved from a rare neurologic illness to a major public health problem.[2, 3] As the population in industrialized countries ages, more people will be at risk for AD and most other dementias, and the prevalence of dementia will very likely increase over the next several decades.[4] Most of these illnesses are irreversible, and the emotional and financial burden for patients, family, and society is staggering. Alzheimer's disease, for example, causes a significant decrease in life expectancy and may be the fourth leading cause of death among adults in the United States.[5]

This chapter emphasizes clinically relevant descriptions of the dementias and practical guidelines for the physician's primary task, that is, the detection of reversible causes of dementia. Topics from the basic sciences that bear upon the care of demented patients are reviewed, and promising research directions are out-

lined. The first task is to deal with the difficult issues of definition and terminology, since the understanding of dementia depends on its recognition as an entity distinct from normal aging and from other neurobehavioral syndromes.

DEFINITION AND TERMINOLOGY

The definition of dementia has taken many forms, but common to all is the notion of intellectual impairment. A useful, recent attempt defines dementia as an acquired, persistent impairment in intellectual function, with deficits in three or more of the following five areas: memory, language, visuospatial function, cognition, and emotions or personality.[6] The term acquired distinguishes dementia from congenital mental retardation, and persistently characterizes dementia as a lasting syndrome that differs, for example, from the acute confusional state. The requirement for three or more areas of dysfunction highlights the widespread nature of impairment in dementia, differentiating it from a single impairment such as aphasia.[6] It is worth noting that no implications of progressive course or irreversibility are made, although many dementias are progressive and irreversible. Some, such as post-traumatic dementia, are usually static, and others, such as those associated with hypothyroidism, are often reversible. Dementia is simply a term used to describe a neurobehavioral syndrome; the diagnosis of dementia should serve to initiate a prompt and comprehensive search for a specific cause.

The term organic brain syndrome (OBS)

lingers on in clinical practice and in the literature. A patient with OBS is presumed to have a demonstrable pathophysiologic process in the brain and should be on a neurologic ward, whereas a patient with a functional illness belongs on a psychiatric service. Although such clinical decisions certainly need to be made, the term OBS lacks specificity; patients with dementia due to AD, acute confusion related to alcohol withdrawal, and nonfluent aphasia following a stroke are remarkably different clinically, yet all may be said to have OBS.[6] Furthermore, it is becoming increasingly accepted that *all* behavior, normal and otherwise, will be found to have a basis in brain activity, and that, as a result, all clinical presentations of abnormal behavior—from dementia to schizophrenia—are organic.[7] Neither our patients nor our understanding are well served by nonspecific designations such as OBS, and the use of this term is discouraged.

A final issue of terminology involves the subject of aging. Senescence is an appropriate designation for the process of normal aging. We avoid the word "senility" because it is imprecise and misleading. Alterations in mental status in the elderly are now recognized, and the clinician needs to appreciate these changes as normal phenomena of senescence.

MENTAL STATUS IN THE NORMAL ELDERLY

The nervous system, like other organ systems, is susceptible to age-related decrements in structure and function. In addition to changes in elemental neurologic function, such as stooped posture, slowed gait, impaired coordination, and hyporeflexia, there are also well-characterized changes in mentation, which are considered normal.[9, 10] The clinician examining an elderly patient must be aware of these changes, since often they raise the possibility of dementia. We will discuss two of the most common problems: "slowness" and forgetfulness.

It is common knowledge that elderly people slow down, not only physically but also mentally. Cognitive processes proceed at a slower pace, and obtaining a thorough history routinely takes longer than it does

with a younger patient. Formal neuropsychological research has confirmed these observations by demonstrating a difference between crystallized intelligence, the type required for manipulation of previously acquired knowledge, and fluid intelligence, that which is necessary for adapting to novel situations. The elderly consistently do worse on tests measuring fluid intelligence (the performance IQ of the Wechsler Adult Intelligence Scale) than on tests assessing crystallized intelligence (the verbal IQ).[11] This deficiency in ability to solve new problems may be caused by slower central processing of information.[10]

Forgetfulness is another frequent complaint in the elderly and is often noted by those who interact with them. This has been termed benign senescent forgetfulness, and involves the failure to recall relatively unimportant data, without significantly changing the life of the individual.[12] In true memory impairment, by contrast, important information is also lost, and the life of the individual may be substantially altered as a result. Persons with benign forgetfulness are aware of it and typically resort to circumlocution in an apologetic manner; those with malignant forgetfulness are usually unaware of the problem and may confabulate an erroneous response.[12] Age-related memory impairments are probably based on lowered efficiency of mental processes, a deficit suggesting a subtle impairment of neuroanatomic systems subserving arousal and attention.[10]

One should not conclude, however, that the elderly become incompetent as a result of these changes or that no special abilities are enhanced with age. Examples of very elderly persons who remain exceptionally productive are numerous, and the elderly in general may exceed the young in terms of wisdom, that is, the thoughtful consideration of events, which is informed by many years of experience.

MENTAL STATUS EXAMINATION

Administering an adequate mental status examination is crucial and requires considerable clinical skill. Despite the difficulties inherent in assessing behavior in patients with markedly different backgrounds and premorbid abilities, the mental status examination remains the best way to discover significant neurobehavioral impairment. A detailed mental status examination, as outlined in certain texts, appears to be an overwhelming task.[13] The following is a brief summary of areas assessed in the usual case of suspected dementia:

1. Arousal and attention—level of consciousness, concentration, vigilance
2. Memory—immediate, recent, remote
3. Language—fluency, auditory comprehension, repetition, naming, reading, writing
4. Visuospatial skills—drawing, copying, neglect, dressing
5. Cognition—abstraction, similarities, idioms, proverbs, multistep calculations
6. Emotion and personality—comportment, mood and affect, insight, thought content

Each of the six areas should be investigated because many dementias are distinguished by their unique combination of deficits, and more specific syndromes such as aphasia (language impairment) and amnesia (memory loss) will be uncovered. There is no single test or procedure that can provide an easy diagnosis; rather, the examiner's skill and perseverance are the keys to a proper neurobehavioral assessment.

Many standardized bedside tests of mental status have been developed. These have found most use in clinical research but may be helpful also to confirm or deny a clinical impression of dementia or to document the course of a patient's illness over time. Two short and useful tests are the Mini-Mental State Exam, and the Orientation Memory Concentration Test.[14, 15]

Finally, one may utilize formal neuropsychologic testing in cases of suspected dementia. Neuropsychologists are trained in the administration of a great variety of ingenious tests that assess many capabilities of an individual patient. In essence, they provide an extended, highly descriptive mental status examination. These tests are most helpful in the early stages of dementia, when deficits may be equivocal.

ALZHEIMER'S DISEASE

The first case of this important disease was described in a 55-year-old woman who died after a 4-year history of progressive dementia.[2] Later, cases involving older patients were described, and these had clinical and neuropathologic similarities to Alzheimer's case. A distinction then developed between those patients with onset before age 65 (presenile dementia) and those with onset at age 65 or older (senile dementia). In recent years, most authorities have viewed AD as a single disease, noting that no clinical or neuropathologic distinctions clearly separate early-onset from late-onset patients.[5] Younger patients may have a more rapidly progressive course or relatively more language impairment, but such differences need not imply a division of AD into two diseases, only a different vulnerability of the patient related to age at onset.[16, 17] In any case, use of the term AD, or "dementia of the Alzheimer type," is appropriate, given the present state of neurologic understanding.

Memory impairment is nearly always the initial manifestation of AD. Relatives, friends, or coworkers are often the first to note failing memory, and patients often remain unaware of their problem and may vehemently deny it. At this stage, neuroimaging and electrographic studies are likely to be normal, and differentiation from normal aging and depression may be difficult. As the disease progresses, impairments in language, visuospatial skills, and cognition become apparent. Personality and comportment are typically rather well preserved until later, but some apathy, indifference, and social inappropriateness may be apparent. Cerebral atrophy on computed tomographic (CT) or magnetic resonance imaging (MRI) scans is usually seen in later stages, and the electroencephalogram (EEG) shows diffuse slowing. Eventually, signs such as incontinence, myoclonus, or seizures may occur, and the terminal state is characterized by inanition, mutism, and a mercifully life-ending infection. Women have been affected more often than men, and the disease is most common after the 6th decade.[18] The average duration of survival after onset is 6 to 12 years.[18]

Autopsy studies show cerebral atrophy, with significant neuronal dropout in the hippocampus, neocortex, and elsewhere. Neuritic (senile) plaques, neurofibrillary tangles, and granulovacuolar degeneration are characteristic histologic changes that constitute the basis for definitive diagnosis. Recent interest has focused on the cholinergic system, which arises in the nucleus basalis of Meynert and ascends to the neocortex.[19] Careful studies have demonstrated correlations between degree of dementia and numbers of neocortical neuritic plaques and between degree of dementia and functional abnormalities of the cholinergic system.[20, 21] As enlightening as these findings are, however, attempts to treat memory and other deficits by enhancing cholinergic transmission have been disappointing.[22]

The cause of AD remains unknown. The disease is usually sporadic, although some families appear to transmit the disease in an autosomal dominant pattern.[23] The defective gene in such families has been found to be on chromosome 21, a finding that helps to explain the high incidence of AD in older patients with Down's syndrome (trisomy 21).[24] Other causes of AD are possible; viruses or prions and toxins such as aluminum and silicon have been studied, but AD must still be considered idiopathic.[25–27]

REVERSIBLE DEMENTIAS

The diseases that can cause reversible dementia comprise an important group. More than 60 causes of reversible or potentially reversible dementia are known, and some of these illnesses may be present in patients who appear to have AD.[28] An abbreviated list of more common causes is given in Table 9–1, and we will discuss each major category in some detail.

Perhaps most important are conditions caused by drugs and other toxins. Drug-induced dementias are often iatrogenic, and environmental toxins can be easily avoided or removed if detected. Medications such as anticholinergic compounds, benzodiazepines, antidepressants, lithium, antipsychotics, anticonvulsants, levodopa, many antihypertensive agents, steroids, and digitalis can cause cognitive impairment, and often a gratifying recovery follows simple withdrawal or reduction of such drugs. Among the nonprescription drugs, alcohol deserves special mention. In addition to the well known amnesic confabulatory state of Korsakoff's

psychosis, chronic alcoholism can produce a dementia in some patients.[29] Abstinence may improve patients with alcoholic dementia, and CT abnormalities may also improve after withdrawal of alcohol.[30, 31] Heavy metals (lead, arsenic, mercury) and many industrial and environmental agents may also cause dementia.

Mass lesions in or adjacent to the cerebrum are common and are easily detected by modern neuroimaging techniques. Neoplasms, hematomas, and abscesses can be found, and, depending on the number, size, location, and nature of the lesion(s), much recovery is often possible.

Normal pressure hydrocephalus (NPH) is another condition that causes dementia, in association with a gait disturbance and urinary incontinence.[32] Although the exact pathophysiology is not yet understood, many patients appear to improve after ventriculoperitoneal shunts are placed. Although criteria for shunt placement remain controversial, NPH should be considered a potentially reversible dementing illness.

A wide variety of systemic illnesses can cause dementia. Pulmonary failure, congestive heart failure, hypoxia, uremia, hepatic encephalopathy, electrolyte disturbances, and hypoglycemia all may be responsible and are routinely detected on initial examination or laboratory evaluation. Endocrinopathies can be responsible as well, particularly hypothyroidism. Deficiency states such as vitamin B_{12} or folate deficiency can cause dementia, and porphyria is a rare cause. Systemic malignancies may produce dementia through a variety of means, including paraneoplastic syndromes.

Inflammatory diseases, both infectious and noninfectious, are well known causes of dementia. General paresis, a form of neurosyphilis common in the preantibiotic era, is a dementia with prominent behavioral abnormalities such as grandiosity and disinhibition. Fungal meningitis, most often cryptococcal, and parasitic diseases, notably cysticercosis, should be considered, and herpes simplex encephalitis can cause severe dementia.[33] Noninfectious illnesses such as systemic lupus erythematosus, temporal arteritis, and sarcoidosis can also be beneficially treated.

Dementia resulting from trauma may show improvement over time, if compli-

TABLE 9–1. Reversible Causes of Dementia

Drugs and toxins
    anticholinergic compounds, benzodiazepines, antidepressants, lithium,
    antipsychotics, anticonvulsants, levodopa, antihypertensives, steroids,
    digitalis, alcohol, heavy metals, solvents, insecticides, carbon monoxide
Mass lesions
    neoplasms, hematomas, abscesses
Normal pressure hydrocephalus
Systemic illnesses
    pulmonary failure, congestive heart failure, hypoxia, uremia, hepatic
    encephalopathy, electrolyte disturbances, hypoglycemia, thyroid
    disturbances, parathyroid abnormalities, adrenal diseases, vitamin B_{12}
    deficiency, folate deficiency, porphyria, paraneoplastic syndromes
Inflammatory diseases
    Infections
        general paresis, fungal meningitis, cysticercosis, herpes simplex
        encephalitis
    Noninfectious conditions
        systemic lupus erythematosus, temporal arteritis, sarcoidosis
Traumatic brain injury
Depression

cations are avoided. Because its course is not progressive, this dementia has the potential for some spontaneous reversibility, although in severe cases residual deficits are common.

Finally, the subject of depression is discussed here because this entity can cause a reversible dementia as surely as can general paresis or drug toxicity. Cognitive impairment due to depression has been termed pseudodementia, as if there is no dementia at all, but, in fact, depressed patients show many similarities to individuals with reversible dementias.[34, 35] Depression is an example of a functional illness in which there is very likely a defect of central neurochemical systems; identification of biologically mediated disorders of mood and affect shows how the distinction between functional and organic diseases is becoming increasingly blurred. Because depression is usually completely reversible with antidepressant or other therapy, its clinical recognition is of great importance.

OTHER DEMENTING ILLNESSES

A large number of other illnesses may cause dementia, and their exact diagnosis often requires neurologic expertise. Although effective treatment for some aspects of these diseases exists—the motor disorder of Parkinson's disease, for example—the dementias are essentially ir-

reversible. A brief discussion of these entities will suffice to introduce their salient features; detailed descriptions may be found elsewhere.[36]

Multi-infarct dementia (MID) accounts for 10 to 20 percent of patients with dementia, and a common dilemma is the distinction between AD and MID. Often the two coexist, since both are common in the elderly. MID can be considered a progressive illness characterized by stepwise deterioration of cognitive function caused by the cumulative effects of repeated cerebral infarction. As can be expected, hypertension and diabetes mellitus are common in such patients; focal neurologic signs and multiple areas of infarction on CT or MRI scans are typical.[37] Multi-infarct dementia is *not* synonymous with arteriosclerotic dementia, a dated term implying dementia caused by progressive arteriosclerosis and reduced cerebral blood flow. Rather, it is a specific syndrome of dementia related to multifocal loss of brain tissue.[38] Binswanger's disease, a variant of MID in which subcortical infarction is prominent, has a similar presentation.[39] Treatment is directed at controlling the causes of infarction (e.g., hypertension, diabetes, cardiac valvular disease, and so on); reversal of symptoms and signs is not likely, but arrest of the disease progression can be achieved in some cases.

The acquired immunodeficiency syndrome (AIDS) has recently been added to the list of conditions that produce dementias. Experience with this alarming illness has led to the concept that dementia results from a progressive viral encephalitis that afflicts a significant number of AIDS patients.[40] Superimposed opportunistic infections and malignancies may also contribute to the AIDS-related dementia. At present, this disease is uncommon in the elderly. Creutzfeldt-Jakob disease (CJD) is another dementia caused by an infectious agent; patients typically have a 1 to 2-year course of dementia and prominent myoclonus. Although this is a rare disease, CJD has attracted much interest because it may be transmitted by a novel proteinaceous infectious agent known as a prion.[25]

Huntington's disease (HD) is a dementia that usually begins in young adulthood but can occur in the 6th to 8th decade.[41] Chorea is a diagnostic feature, and patients also develop atrophy of the caudate nuclei on CT or MRI scanning. Inheritance is autosomal dominant, and recent evidence has located the gene on the short arm of chromosome 4; a predictive test for some persons at risk for HD is now available.[41]

Parkinson's disease is a common disorder of movement in the elderly, and dementia has also been recognized in a substantial number of patients.[42] Progressive supranuclear palsy is a similar illness, characterized by supranuclear ophthalmoplegia, axial dystonia in extension, pseudobulbar palsy, and dementia.[43] A less common dementia is Pick's disease. Disorders of behavior and language typically precede deficits in memory, concomitant with atrophy of frontal and temporal lobes.[44] Patients with Pick's disease can be misdiagnosed as schizophrenic or manic because their behavioral disinhibition is often impressive.

Uncommon dementing illnesses in the elderly include spinocerebellar degenerations, amyotrophic lateral sclerosis/Parkinsonism/dementia complex, and idiopathic calcification of the basal ganglia. These are best referred for neurologic evaluation.

DIAGNOSIS

The first step in the evaluation of a demented patient is to be certain that a dementia is indeed present. Many syndromes can simulate dementia, and adequate history taking and examination, particularly of the mental status, should identify the correct syndrome in the majority of patients. Those with acute confusional state, for example, have a more abrupt onset and display a fluctuating level of consciousness and impaired attention. Aphasia, especially fluent aphasia, can also be difficult to recognize, but the onset is typically acute and related to a cerebral infarct, and the language disorder overshadows other neurobehavioral deficits. Amnesic patients may appear demented, but deficits other than memory loss are minimal. Psychiatric disorders such as schizophrenia, mania, and hysteria may present with syndromes akin to dementia, but these typically begin in younger age groups. Depression is a more difficult problem, since it often occurs in the elderly.

Once a determination is made that the patient is demented, specific clinical features can be useful. Systemic illnesses are often suggested by general physical findings, and neurologic abnormalities, such as multifocal motor deficits in MID or chorea in HD, can be helpful. There is no specific and sensitive test in laboratory evaluation that provides an exact diagnosis for most patients with dementia. Only cerebral biopsy or postmortem data gives definitive information, and biopsy is not indicated in the usual case. The clinician is left to identify those diseases that can be diagnosed confidently and to rule out reversible diseases in the remaining patients. A reliable diagnosis can be achieved using clinical means in most instances; using current methods, diagnostic accuracy in AD is now about 90 percent.[3]

The selection of laboratory tests is difficult, since performing all conceivable tests for dementia leads to unacceptable costs and risks to the patient. Rather, the clinician should select tests based on a reasonable expectation of the disease that may be present. It is our practice to conduct routine tests in all cases and reserve other tests for specific indications. In Table 9–2 are listed both categories of tests.

The single most important test is a CT or MRI scan. Computed tomography revolutionized neurologic diagnosis in the 1970s when it first appeared and continues to be used extensively as an effective means of viewing intracranial contents. Magnetic resonance imaging, first intro-

TABLE 9–2. Laboratory Tests for Dementia

Routine Tests

Biochemical survey (electrolytes, glucose, renal and
  hepatic function tests, calcium, phosphorus)
Complete blood count
Erythrocyte sedimentation rate
Serologic test for syphilis
Thyroid function tests
Vitamin B_{12} and folate levels
CT or MRI scan

Tests for Selected Cases

Lumbar puncture
Electroencephalogram
Isotope cisternogram
Arteriogram
Chest roentgenogram
Electrocardiogram
Toxicology screen
Heavy metal screen
Porphyrin screen

duced clinically in the early 1980s, offers even greater resolution of brain structure and is particularly useful for diseases of white matter.[45] Computed tomography presently has the advantage of greater availability, whereas MRI has the benefit of no risk of irradiation. Either scan is acceptable, and every patient with undiagnosed dementia should be evaluated using one of these tests.

Computed tomography initially gave much impetus to the goals of finding a diagnostic marker for AD and for predicting the degree of cognitive impairment. Unfortunately, normal aged individuals as well as demented patients can have cerebral atrophy, and some demented patients have normal CT scans.[46, 47] Furthermore, a relationship between CT measures and cognitive deficit in an individual patient may not be evident.[48] Work with MRI scanning has been only preliminary, and it remains to be seen whether brain atrophy on MRI will correlate with the degree of dementia.[49] In Figure 9–1 are shown CT scans of a normal elderly individual and of an AD patient; Figure 9–2 shows MRI scans of two similar individuals. Cerebral atrophy is certainly a common finding with both tests in AD, but neither test can give positive criteria for the disease. The diagnostic value of neuroimaging remains one of excluding other causes of dementia.

TREATMENT

The treatment of dementia may seem to be a distressingly brief topic, yet clinicians are faced daily with the need to care for afflicted individuals and their families, who bear a heavy burden as well. Caring for patients with chronic and incurable neurologic disease is indeed difficult, but it should be borne in mind that relatively few diseases in medicine are truly reversible. What follows is an outline of ways the physician can be helpful, because whereas many diseases are irreversible, none are untreatable.

Patients with reversible or potentially reversible dementias are a rather small, but very rewarding, group. Treatment may be simple, such as withdrawing psychoactive medications or administering penicillin for neurosyphilis, or complex, such as overcoming alcoholism or making the difficult decision to place a shunt in NPH. Specific treatment of the reversible dementias obviously depends on the cause; details of these treatments are found in standard neurologic textbooks.[36]

Treatment of AD and other irreversible dementias demands much more of the clinician. In these cases, great skill and sensitivity are required. We will review the attempts at pharmacologic treatment that have been made in AD and discuss some practical points of overall management.

A large number of drugs have been used to improve memory and other deficits in demented elderly patients. These include cholinomimetic drugs, neuropeptides, nootropics, vasodilators, and psychostimulants.[50] Among these drugs, the ergoloid mesylates have the most popularity, and many studies purport that they improve cognitive function.[50] These studies are flawed by methodologic problems, however, and most clinicians remain skeptical of their conclusions.[51] The most attractive drugs are the cholinomimetics, since a substantial body of evidence pointing to dysfunction of the cholinergic system in the brain has been assembled.[52] Choline, lecithin, and physostigmine have been studied rather thoroughly, and slight improvements in some cognitive tests have been documented with lecithin and physostigmine or with physostigmine alone.[53, 54] The most promising drug of this group is tetrahydroaminoacridine (THA), a centrally active cholinesterase inhibitor that showed good results in a recent preliminary study; a national multicenter trial of

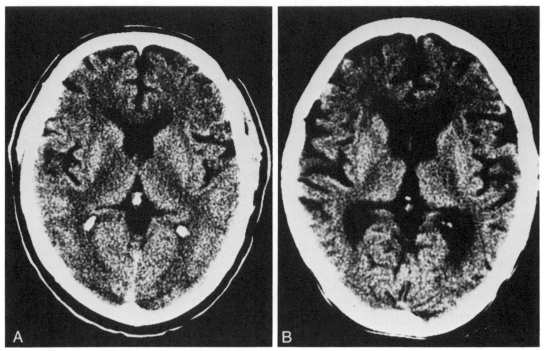

FIGURE 9–1. A, CT scans of a normal elderly individual and B, an AD patient. Cerebral atrophy is evident in B.

this agent has been initiated.[55] None of the pharmacologic treatments of AD are claimed to be a cure; all simply attempt to alleviate symptoms and signs. A curative drug must await advances in the understanding of etiology.

The most important role for the physician is the exclusion of reversible dementias. Specific diagnoses of irreversible diseases may be possible, but these remain of more academic interest. Once a diagnosis of AD or other irreversible process is made, prevention and treatment of medical problems can be helpful, if carried out appropriately. Specific behavioral problems can be effectively treated; we use

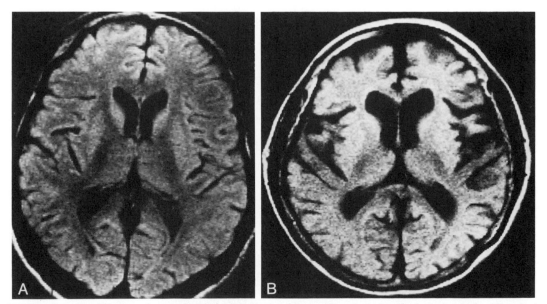

FIGURE 9–2. A, MRI scans of a normal elderly individual and B, an AD patient. Atrophy is present in the AD patient. Anatomy is better seen with this technique than with CT scans.

chloral hydrate for ensuring adequate sleep, haloperidol for agitation, and desipramine for superimposed depression. All medications must be closely monitored lest acute confusional states further exacerbate the behavioral decline. Patients should be provided with familiar and structured settings, and caregivers should have ample opportunity for respite from their demanding tasks. Finally, the physician can provide informed and sympathetic counseling to families as inevitable issues of competency, function (such as ability to drive a motor vehicle), and nursing home placement arise. Publications such as *The 36-Hour Day* (Johns Hopkins, 1987) and organizations such as the Alzheimer's Association can be extremely helpful with these and other issues.[56]

FUTURE DIRECTIONS

Although the threat of AD is a menacing one, much effort has been devoted to the detection of its cause or causes and to the discovery of effective treatments. Considerable excitement has been generated by the identification of cholinergic system deficiencies, but enthusiasm should be tempered by the recognition that other transmitter systems are also affected in AD and that replacing acetylcholine or any other neurotransmitter is not likely to produce a cure.[52, 57] Tetrahydroaminoacridine may be the best hope for effective treatment of AD at this point, and further data on this drug should soon be available.

Other areas of interest include detailed clinical, neuroradiologic, and neuropathologic studies aimed at establishing firm diagnostic criteria, information on the natural history of disease, and better understanding of brain/behavior relationships. Epidemiologic studies exploring risk factors and basic work on possible viral, toxic, and genetic factors in AD will be pursued. Another area with great potential significance is the study of nerve growth factor, a protein found in the central and peripheral nervous systems, that has the ability to enhance survival of damaged cholinergic neurons in experimental animal studies.[58] Neural implantation may also play a role in the treatment of AD.[59, 60] Finally, elegant imaging techniques such as positron emission tomography (PET) will doubtlessly shed further light on the basis of cognitive decline in dementia as well as on the foundations of thought and feeling in normal individuals.

Dementia in the elderly, particularly in AD patients, poses a challenge to all who work with the aged and care for them throughout senescence. The next few decades promise to yield important new information that will certainly aid in the difficult task of providing adequate care for this growing group of patients.

REFERENCES

1. Akhtar AJ, Broe GA, Crombie A, et al: Disability and dependence in the elderly at home. Age Ageing 2:102, 1973.
2. Alzheimer A: About a peculiar disease of the cerebral cortex. (Jarvik L, Greenson H, trans). Alzheimer Dis Assoc Dis 1:7, 1987.
3. Katzman R: Alzheimer's disease. N Engl J Med 314:964, 1986.
4. Besdine RW: Geriatric medicine: an overview. In Eisdorfer C, ed: Annual Review of Gerontology and Geriatrics, Vol 1. New York, Springer, 1980, p 135.
5. Katzman R: The prevalence and malignancy of Alzheimer disease. Arch Neurol 33:217, 1976.

DEFINITION AND TERMINOLOGY

6. Cummings JL, Benson DF: Dementia: A Clinical Approach. Boston, Butterworths, 1983, p 1.
7. Kandel ER: Brain and behavior. In Kandel ER, Schwartz JH, eds: Principles of Neural Science. New York, Elsevier Science Publishing Co Inc, 1985, p 3.
8. Cohen GD: Historical views and evolution of concepts. In Reisberg B, ed: Alzheimer's Disease: The Standard Reference. New York, The Free Press, 1983, p 29.

MENTAL STATUS IN THE NORMAL ELDERLY

9. Creasey H, Rapoport SI: The aging human brain. Ann Neurol 17:2, 1985.
10. Caine ED: Mental status changes with aging. Semin Neurol 1:36, 1981.
11. Hochanadel G, Kaplan E: Neuropsychology of normal aging. In Albert ML, ed: Clinical Neurology of Aging. New York, Oxford University Press Inc, 1984, p 231.
12. Kral VA: Senescent forgetfulness: benign and malignant. Can Med Assoc J 86:257, 1962.

MENTAL STATUS EXAMINATION

13. Strub RL, Black FW: The Mental Status Examination in Neurology. Philadelphia, FA Davis Co, 1977, pp 1–136.
14. Folstein MF, Folstein SE, McHugh PR: "Mini-mental state": a practical method for grading the

cognitive state of patients for the clinician. J Psychiatr Res 12:189, 1975.

15. Katzman R, Brown T, Fuld P, et al: Validation of a short orientation-memory-concentration test of cognitive impairment. Am J Psychiatry 140:734, 1983.

ALZHEIMER'S DISEASE

16. Seltzer B, Sherwin I: A comparison of clinical features in early- and late-onset primary degenerative dementia: one entity or two? Arch Neurol 40:143, 1983.
17. Filley CM, Kelly J, Heaton RK: Neuropsychologic features of early- and late-onset Alzheimer's disease. Arch Neurol 43:574, 1986.
18. Cummings JL, Benson DF: Dementia: A Clinical Approach. Boston, Butterworths, 1983, p 35.
19. Whitehouse PJ, Price DL, Clark AW, et al: Alzheimer disease: evidence for selective loss of cholinergic neurons in the nucleus basalis. Ann Neurol 10:122, 1981.
20. Blessed G, Tomlinson BE, Roth M: The association between quantitative measures of dementia and of senile changes in the cerebral grey matter of elderly subjects. Br J Psychiatry 114:797, 1968.
21. Perry EK, Tomlinson BE, Blessed G, et al: Correlation of cholinergic abnormalities with senile plaques and mental test scores in senile dementia. Br Med J 2:1457, 1978.
22. Bartus RT, Dean RL III, Beer B, et al: The cholinergic hypothesis of geriatric memory dysfunction. Science 217:408, 1982.
23. Matsuyama SS: Genetic factors in dementia of the Alzheimer type. In Reisberg B, ed: Alzheimer's Disease: The Standard Reference. New York, The Free Press, 1983, p 155.
24. St. George-Hyslop PH, Tarzi RE, Polinsky RJ, et al: The genetic defect causing familial Alzheimer's disease maps on chromosome 21. Science 235:885, 1987.
25. Prusiner SB: Novel proteinaceous infectious particles cause scrapie. Science 216:136, 1982.
26. Perl DP, Brody AR: Alzheimer's disease: x-ray spectrometric evidence of aluminum accumulation in neurofibrillary tanglebearing neurons. Science 208:297, 1980.
27. Nikaido T, Austin J, Treub L, et al: Studies in aging of the brain, II: microchemical analyses of the nervous system in Alzheimer's patients. Arch Neurol 27:549, 1972.

REVERSIBLE DEMENTIAS

28. Cummings JL, Benson DF, LoVerme S Jr: Reversible dementia: illustrative cases, definition, and review. JAMA 243:2434, 1980.
29. Lishman WA: Cerebral disorder in alcoholism: syndromes of impairment. Brain 104:1, 1981.
30. Ron MA: Brain damage in chronic alcoholism: a neuropathological, neuroradiological and psychological review. Psychol Med 7:103, 1977.
31. Ron MA, Acher W, Shaw GK, et al: Computerized tomography of the brain in chronic alcoholism: a survey and follow-up study. Brain 105:497, 1982.
32. Adams RD, Fisher CM, Hakim S, et al: Symptomatic occult hydrocephalus with "normal" cerebrospinal fluid pressure: a treatable syndrome. N Engl J Med 273:117, 1965.
33. Earnest MP, Reller LB, Filley CM, et al: Neurocysticercosis in the United States: 35 cases and review. Rev Infect Dis 9:961, 1987.
34. Wells CE: Pseudodementia. Am J Psychiatry 136:895, 1979.
35. Caine ED: Pseudodementia: current concepts and future directions. Arch Gen Psychiatry 38:1359, 1981.

OTHER DEMENTING ILLNESSES

36. Adams RD, Victor M: Principles of Neurology. New York, McGraw-Hill, 1985, p 311.
37. Hachinski VC, Iliff LD, Zilhka E, et al: Cerebral blood flow in dementia. Arch Neurol 32:632, 1975.
38. Fields WS: Multi-infarct dementia. Neurol Clin 4:405, 1986.
39. Babikian V, Ropper AH: Binswanger's disease: a review. Stroke 18:2, 1987.
40. Gabuzda DH, Hirsch MS: Neurologic manifestations of infection with human immunodeficiency virus: clinical features and pathogenesis. Ann Intern Med 107:383, 1987.
41. Martin JB, Gusella JF: Huntington's disease: pathogenesis and management. N Engl J Med 315:1267, 1986.
42. Lieberman A, Dziatolowski M, Kupersmith M, et al: Dementia in Parkinson disease. Ann Neurol 6:355, 1979.
43. Albert ML, Feldman RG, Willis AL: The "subcortical dementia" of progressive supranuclear palsy. J Neurol Neurosurg Psychiatry 37:121, 1974.
44. Lishman WA: Organic Psychiatry. Oxford, Blackwell Scientific Publications, 1978, p 527.

DIAGNOSIS

45. Doyle FH, Pennock JM, Orr JS, et al: Imaging of the brain by nuclear magnetic resonance. Lancet 1:53, 1981.
46. Earnest MP, Heaton RK, Williamson WE, et al: Cortical atrophy, ventricular enlargement and intellectual impairment in the aged. Neurology 29:1138, 1979.
47. Jacoby RJ, Levy R: Computed tomography in the elderly, 2. Senile dementia: diagnosis and functional impairment. Br J Psychiatry 136:256, 1980.
48. Freedman M, Knoefel J, Naeser M, et al: Computerized axial tomography in aging. In Albert ML, ed: Clinical Neurology of Aging. New York, Oxford University Press Inc, 1984, p 139.
49. Johnson KA, Davis KR, Buonanno FS, et al: Comparison of magnetic resonance and roentgen ray computed tomography in dementia. Arch Neurol 44:1075, 1987.

TREATMENT

50. Rosenberg GS, Greenwald B, Davis KL: Pharmacologic treatment of Alzheimer's disease: an overview. In Reisberg B, ed: Alzheimer's Disease: The Standard Reference. New York, The Free Press, 1983, p 329.
51. Yesavage JA, Tinklenberg JR, Hollister LE, et al: Vasodilators in senile dementias: a review of the literature. Arch Gen Psychiatry 36:220, 1979.

52. Drachman DA: The pharmacological basis for cholinergic investigations of Alzheimer's disease: evidence and implications. In Reisberg B, ed: Alzheimer's Disease: The Standard Reference. New York, The Free Press, 1983, p 340.
53. Thal LJ, Fuld PA, Masur DM, et al: Oral physostigmine and lecithin improve memory in Alzheimer disease. Ann Neurol 13:491, 1983.
54. Stern Y, Sano M, Mayeux R: Effects of oral physostigmine in Alzheimer's disease. Ann Neurol 22:306, 1987.
55. Summers WK, Mayovski LV, Marsh GM, et al: Oral tetrahydroaminoacridine in long-term treatment of senile dementia, Alzheimer type. N Engl J Med 315:1241, 1986.
56. Mace NL, Rabins PV: The 36-hour day: a family guide to caring for persons with Alzheimer's disease. Baltimore, Johns Hopkins University Press, 1981.

FUTURE DIRECTIONS

57. Mann DMA, Yates PO: Neurotransmitter deficits in Alzheimer's disease and in other dementing disorders. Hum Neurobiol 5:147, 1986.
58. Kromer LF: Nerve growth factor treatment after brain injury prevents neuronal death. Science 235:214, 1987.
59. Gash DM, Collier TJ, Sladek JR Jr: Neural transplantation: a review of recent developments and potential applications to the aged brain. Neurobiol Aging 6:131, 1985.
60. Katzman R: Commentary on review by Gash et al: potential usefulness and current limitations of neural transplantation in the aged brain. Neurobiol Aging 6:152, 1985.

CHAPTER 10

Drug Use

John G. Gerber
Eric P. Brass

The same medicine will both harm and cure me.
(Res eadem vulnus opemque feret.)

OVID, *Tristia*

The elderly population, defined arbitrarily as persons over age 65, is increasing in the United States, both in absolute numbers and as a fraction of the whole population. At the turn of the century, only 2 to 4 percent of the population was over 65 years of age, whereas in 1982, this fraction increased to 11.6 percent. It is estimated that by the early part of the next century, 20 percent of the population will be 65 years old or over. The dramatic increase in the number of elderly is no doubt due to increased life expectancy. Decreased infant mortality, improved nutrition, better health care delivery, and better compliance with preventive measures have served to keep the population healthy.

It is important to realize that there is no physiologic basis to define elderly as being over 65 years of age. This definition is societal in origin, associated with retirement programs and Social Security. Aging is a dynamic process and very much dependent on both genetic and environmental influences. Thus, a chronologic age of 65 years could mean a much younger or older individual on physiologic parameters.[19]

The elderly use more drugs per capita than the younger population. This represents both prescription and over-the-counter medications. Certainly, part of this greater drug use is related to the increased susceptibility of the elderly to both chronic and acute illnesses. In part because of the increased drug use, aged patients have 3 to 7 times as many adverse drug reactions as patients in the 20- to 29-year-old age group.[34] In addition, because aging is associated with declining physiologic processes, once adverse drug reactions occur, the elderly patient's ability to recover from them may be impaired as well. For these reasons, the practitioner must be aware of how to use drugs safely and efficaciously and, equally important, when to use drugs in the elderly. Because of altered physiologic functions that occur with aging, elderly patients will handle or respond to certain groups of drugs differently than will younger patients. In this chapter, the effect of aging on absorption, distribution, excretion, and end-organ responsiveness of drugs is reviewed. Specific examples will be provided when possible. In addition to the understanding of the effect of aging on pharmacokinetic parameters, the reader must realize that disease processes themselves may alter the way the body handles drugs. Overall, there is a large variability across a population group in the way a drug is processed by the body. Therefore, individualization of drug therapy remains the ideal method of approach.

DRUG ABSORPTION AND BIOAVAILABILITY IN THE ELDERLY

By far, the majority of drugs in clinical use are administered orally. Before these drugs reach the systemic circulation, they are in contact with the stomach, the small intestine (where most of the absorption takes place), and, via the portal circulation, the liver. Drugs that are rapidly and extensively metabolized by the liver will be extracted to a large extent during their first pass through the liver via the portal vein, thereby reducing the drug's systemic bioavailability. Once the drug reaches the systemic circulation, it can interact with key cellular components to exert a pharmacologic effect.

The gastrointestinal tract undergoes both physiologic and anatomic changes with aging that could potentially affect drug absorption. Nonetheless, studies have not demonstrated that these gastrointestinal changes affect drug absorption for the majority of the drugs used by the elderly.[30] However, not all drugs have been evaluated in this regard. Gastric acid production decreases with aging but gastric motility does not. With aging, there is about a 30 percent decrease in mucosal absorptive surface in the small bowel as well as a decrease in gastrointestinal motility. In addition, there is about a 40 percent reduction in small intestinal blood flow. Evidence suggests diminished absorption through the active transport systems involved with galactose, calcium, thiamine, and iron absorption in the elderly, but most drugs are passively absorbed, and for these drugs, the aging gut is not an obstacle.[24] Rather, diseases associated with aging or the concomitant administration of several drugs may contribute to abnormal drug absorption in the elderly patient. Antacids can decrease the absorption of chlorpromazine, tetracycline, cimetidine, isoniazid, and D-penicillamine, whereas cholestyramine can bind and decrease the absorption of phenobarbital, warfarin, thiazides, thyroxine, digitalis, glycosides, aspirin, acetaminophen, and penicillin. Drugs with anticholinergic effects can decrease motility and delay the absorption of many drugs.[41] Although these drug interactions can occur in patients of all ages, the likelihood of the use of multiple drugs is greater in the elderly.

The liver stands between drugs in the portal blood and the systemic circulation. Drugs that have high hepatic clearance (that is, the extraction ratio in each pass through the liver is greater than 30 to 40 percent) will be extensively metabolized by the liver during their first pass after absorption, thus reducing the drugs' systemic bioavailability. Aging has been reported to decrease the metabolic capacity of the liver. For orally administered high hepatic clearance drugs, the first pass elimination would therefore be reduced in the elderly, and consequently, the amount of drug reaching the systemic circulation would be expected to increase. Increased bioavailability has been described in the elderly for the β-adrenoceptor blocker, propranolol, a prototype high hepatic clearance drug. However, the variability in the hepatic extraction ratio for propranolol across a population group was of such magnitude that both the elderly and the young had overlapping values. This observation again stresses the importance of individualization of drug therapy because the genetic and environmental influences on hepatic metabolism of drugs produce a greater variation across a population than the effect of aging itself.

DRUG DISTRIBUTION IN THE ELDERLY

Once a drug reaches the systemic circulation, it is distributed throughout body fluids and tissues. Drug distribution is determined mainly by body composition and plasma protein binding. The body composition is altered by aging so that the total body water both in absolute terms and in percent of body weight is reduced by as much as 15 percent between the ages of 20 and 80. Lean body mass is decreased, but there is a marked increase in total body fat with age. This increase in total body fat is relatively greater in men than in women.[26]

In addition to alterations in body composition, plasma binding of drugs may be different in the young than in the elderly. Since it is the free drug concentration in the blood that determines the effect of the drug at its site of action, alterations in protein binding can significantly affect drug action for a given total drug concentration. Plasma concentration of albumin tends to decrease with aging, which is probably secondary to a decrease in albumin production by the liver.[40] The effect of this decrease in albumin concentration in the plasma has been suggested to result in a decrease in plasma protein binding capacity of acidic drugs like phenytoin, phenylbutazone, and warfarin. However, many of the basic drugs like lidocaine and propranolol bind mainly to α_1 acid glycoproteins, the concentration of which, if anything, increases with aging, and with acute or chronic inflammatory diseases.[36] Drugs like meperidine (Demerol) can also bind to erythrocytes with very high affinity. It appears that aging reduces the binding capacity to red blood cells, and Demerol binding has been demonstrated to decrease in elderly patients.

With known alterations in body composition as well as in protein binding, predictions can be made as to how the volume of distribution of drugs should be different in the elderly. The volume of distribution is simply the ratio of the mass of the drug in the body divided by its concentration in the blood. Thus, the higher the volume of distribution of the drug, a lower percentage of the total amount of the drug circulates in the intravascular compartment. The volume of distribution of any drug is determined by the relative affinity of the drug for the tissues versus for the blood. If a drug has a very high affinity for blood components but has a low affinity for tissue components, the volume of distribution will be small. Alternatively, if the drug has a very high affinity for tissue components but has a poor affinity for blood components, the volume of distribution would be greater because the drug would preferentially partition into tissue spaces. It is with this knowledge that predictions are made about the volume of distribution when the body composition is altered, as in the elderly.

Since total tissue water content is decreased in the aged, one would predict that the volume of distribution of drugs that distribute mainly into body water would be smaller in the elderly, if plasma binding is not altered. Antipyrine is a model drug that distributes into water spaces and remains essentially unbound in the plasma. Indeed, the volume of distribution of antipyrine has been reported to be reduced in the elderly.[37] Ethanol also distributes into water spaces, and the volume of distribution of ethanol is reduced in the elderly. For a drug such as diazepam, which is very lipophilic, the volume of distribution is increased in the elderly, presumably because of the increased total body fat content, as diazepam plasma protein binding is unaltered.[21] For a drug like digoxin, in which the large volume of distribution is secondary to the extensive tissue binding of the drug (primarily to muscle Na^+/K^+ ATPases), the decreased muscle mass in the elderly is associated with a decreased volume of distribution of digoxin.

How do changes in volume of distribution affect therapeutic use of drugs? Volume of distribution is one of the two determinants of the half-life of a drug. A greater volume of distribution produces a longer half-life, whereas a smaller distribution produces a shorter half-life. This relationship (Vd = volume of distribution; t½ = drug half-life) is given quantitatively as:

$$t\frac{1}{2} = \frac{.693 \times Vd}{plasma\ clearance}$$

Thus, alterations in the volume of distribution influence the dosage intervals of drugs used in chronic therapy. The larger the volume of distribution, the less frequently the drug has to be administered because the plasma concentration of the drug decays more slowly. However, since both the clearance and the effects of drugs are usually related to the free drug concentration, the steady-state effects of a maintenance dosage regimen should not be altered by the volume of distribution alone. Steady-state is defined as when the amount of drug taken in per unit of time equals the drug excreted per unit of time. At steady-state, only two variables determine the plasma level of the drug achieved: the amount of drug reaching the systemic circulation and the blood clearance of the drug. The volume of distribution, therefore, can be considered as a reservoir for drugs in the body. The blood concentration of the drug is in equilibrium with the tissue concentration of the drug. If the tissue reservoir for the drug is very large (large Vd), the rate of fall of the blood concentration of the drug will be slow, even if the clearance of the drug is high. In the absence of a loading dose, it may take a considerable period to reach a steady-state blood concentration if the drug's Vd is large, as a large reservoir for drug has to be filled. The partitioning of drug into this reservoir will delay the time it will take to reach steady-state. Since the drug that is partitioned into tissues and extravascular fluid spaces is not available for either metabolism or excretion, it will not play a role in determining the blood concentration at steady-state, but it will certainly determine the length of time it will take to reach that steady-state concentration.

This principle is very important to the understanding of pharmacokinetics in the elderly, in disease states, or in simple drug interactions. If the steady-state blood concentration of one drug at a fixed dosage is altered by a disease state or by another drug, this alteration must have occurred because of a change in either the bioavailability or the plasma clearance of the drug. An example is the effect of phenylbutazone on warfarin kinetics. It has been noticed that warfarin's effect on clotting factor synthesis is enhanced by the concurrent administration of the nonsteroidal anti-inflammatory drug, phenylbutazone. It was found that phenylbutazone interferes with warfarin metabolism, therefore decreasing the clearance of warfarin.[35]

Alterations in drug binding to plasma proteins may alter the drug's volume of distribution and/or the amount of free (unbound) drug in the plasma at any total plasma drug concentration. By decreasing the fractional protein binding (that is, drug bound as percentage of total drug in plasma) of a drug, the amount of free drug available to interact with its receptor is increased at an equivalent total drug concentration. Thus, interpretation of a total drug level under conditions of altered protein binding has to be reappraised. This concept is well understood in interpreting plasma phenytoin levels in uremia. Although the decrease in protein binding in the elderly for phenytoin is not as dramatic as in uremia, it could potentially result in excessive drug response at an apparent therapeutic total drug concentration.[14]

Since it is the free drug that interacts with a receptor and it is the free drug that is available for metabolism, alterations in protein binding per se will not change the drug dosage in the elderly, unless free drug clearance is affected as well. Thus, an important pharmacokinetic impact that changes in protein binding may have is the interpretation of total plasma concentrations during therapeutic drug monitoring. A total plasma phenytoin level of 20 μg/ml will not have the same implication when only 80 percent of the drug is bound to albumin, instead of the normal binding of 90 percent.

THE EFFECT OF AGING ON RENAL ELIMINATION OF DRUGS

There are numerous drugs in which the major mode of elimination is through the kidney. Some of the more important ones that are used frequently in the elderly population include digoxin, procainamide, the aminoglycoside antibiotics, penicillin, thiazide diuretics, clonidine, and the β-adrenergic blockers, atenolol and nadolol. Renal function deteriorates with age; the glomerular filtration rate at age 70 is about 60 percent of what it is at age 20. In addition, renal blood flow is decreased by 40 percent in the elderly, and maximal sodium and water conservation is impaired as well.[7] Because aging is associated with a decrease in muscle mass, the source of creatinine, using plasma creatinine alone as a measure of renal function can be very deceiving. A plasma creatinine of 1 mg per 100 ml in a 70-year-old person does not indicate the same glomerular filtration rate as a plasma creatinine of 1 mg per 100 ml in a 20-year-old person. Thus, one should never base the dosage of a renally excreted drug on plasma creatinine alone. Whenever possible, an endogenous creatinine clearance should be determined to estimate the glomerular filtration rate. If that is not practical, the practitioner should assume that in the elderly, there is a 40 percent reduction in renal function if the serum creatinine concentration is normal, and start a medication eliminated by renal excretion at a reduced dosage.

For drugs like digoxin, procainamide, and aminoglycosides, blood concentrations can be followed to assess the appropriateness of the dosing regimen. For the thiazide diuretics and clonidine, evaluating clinical response is the best way to follow the efficacy of these drugs. Interestingly, since the tubular transport system in the kidney is diminished with aging, drugs like furosemide that reach the active tubular site via the organic acid transport mechanism in the kidney require higher dosage in the elderly to achieve the same intratubular concentration and, therefore, an equivalent diuresis as in younger patients.

A number of dosage guidelines and nomograms have been developed on the basis of endogenous creatinine clearance. Since the variability of normal renal function independent of age is small and the effect of aging on this function is predictable, rational guidelines for therapy can be established for renally excreted drugs.

THE EFFECT OF AGE ON HEPATIC CLEARANCE OF DRUGS

Unfortunately, the variability of hepatic metabolism of drugs within a population is so large that simple predictions about alterations in dosage requirements with aging are impossible to make. Hepatic clearance of drugs is determined by both the intrinsic ability of the liver to metabolize a drug and the blood flow to the liver. The relative contributions of these two physiologic variables to the hepatic clearance of the drug is specific for each drug. For drugs that are extremely avidly metabolized by the liver (i.e., the liver has a large capacity to metabolize the drugs), the hepatic blood flow is the main determinant of the liver clearance. Propranolol, lidocaine, and many of the tricyclic antidepressant drugs belong to this class. These drugs have a high hepatic clearance and high hepatic extraction, and the extent of their metabolism is perfusion-limited. In the case of drugs for which the liver has a limited metabolizing capacity, it is the intrinsic enzymatic activity within the liver that determines the hepatic clearance. Warfarin, theophylline, and the barbiturates belong to this class. These drugs have a low hepatic clearance, and the extent of their metabolism is perfusion-independent. The majority of other drugs belong somewhere between these two extremes, in which both the enzymatic activity and the hepatic blood flow contribute to the determination of their hepatic clearance (Table 10–1).

Hepatic drug metabolism occurs primarily by two enzyme systems. Phase I reactions carried out by the microsomal mixed function oxidase system result in a more polar molecule from the parent compound that is frequently pharmacologically still active. Phase II metabolism results in conjugation of the molecule by glucuronidation, sulfation, or acetylation. Conjugated molecules are pharmacologically inactive and eliminated by the kidney or by the biliary system. It has been suggested that aging decreases phase I reactions. However, this effect is probably unrelated to any decrease in the enzymatic activity in the hepatocytes per se but, more likely, is secondary to the decrease in liver size associated with aging and, therefore, to a decrease in the total numbers of hepatocytes.[17] Phase II conjugation reactions have not been demonstrated to be affected by aging. However, in practical terms, the liver metabolism of a low clearance prototype drug, antipyrine (which is metabolized by the phase I reaction) was not different in the young or the old population. Although the mean hepatic clearance was lower in the elderly, there was such an overlap between the two population groups that meaningful population differences could not be demonstrated.[42]

The liver blood flow plays a critical role in determining the rate of metabolism of drugs with very high clearances. Liver blood flow is significantly reduced in the elderly as compared with the younger population. This would suggest that the hepatic clearance of high-clearance drugs is reduced in the elderly, and this difference has been demonstrated for intravenously administered propranolol.[39] In addition, the disposition of orally administered high-clearance drugs is complex. Since these drugs undergo significant first-pass liver metabolism, alterations in liver blood flow will affect the amount of drug reaching the systemic circulation. Thus, even though the systemic metabolism of these drugs is expected to be lower in the elderly because of the diminished hepatic blood flow, the systemic drug load would be expected to be lower as well. In addition, there is a large variability in the hepatic extraction of drugs via first pass caused by genetic and environmental factors, making age a relatively small component of any pharmacokinetic differences observed across a study population.

In summary, for drugs undergoing hepatic metabolism, individualization of drug therapy is of utmost importance. For drugs like β-adrenergic blocking agents that have high therapeutic indices, close clinical monitoring is not as important as

TABLE 10–1. Major Mode of Excretion of Commonly Used Drugs

Hepatic Excretion			Renal Excretion	
High Clearance *(> 500 ml/min)*	*Intermediate* *(100–500 ml/min)*	*Low Clearance* *(< 100 ml/min)*		
70 kg	*70 kg*	*70 kg*		
Amitriptyline	Acetaminophen	Carbamazepine	Acecainide	Hydrochlorothiazide
Chlorpromazine	Chloramphenicol	Chlordiazepoxide	Aminoglycosides	Lithium
Doxepin	Erythromycin	Diazepam	Amikacin	Methicillin
Hydralazine	Prazosin	Digitoxin	Amoxicillin	Methotrexate
Imipramine	Quinidine	Ibuprofen	Ampicillin	Nadolol
Lidocaine		Indomethacin	Atenolol	Penicillin
Meperidine		Phenobarbital	Captopril	Procainamide
Metoprolol		Phenylbutazone	Carbenicillin	Vancomycin
Nifedipine		Salicylic acid	Cefazolin	
Nortriptyline		(concentration	Cephalexin	
Propranolol		dependent)	Chlorothiazide	
Triazolam		Theophylline	Cimetidine	
Verapamil		Tolbutamide	Clonidine	
		Valproic acid	Digoxin	
		Warfarin	Disopyramide	
			Furosemide	

for drugs like lidocaine or warfarin, in which therapeutic monitoring is critical to avoid untoward side effects.

THE EFFECT OF AGING ON END-ORGAN RESPONSIVENESS TO DRUGS

Excessive drug response in the elderly can be a result either of pharmacokinetic alterations resulting in excessive blood levels of the drug or of increased sensitivity of the body to the drug. A change in end-organ responsiveness can result from alterations in receptor number or affinity, changes in the enzymes that eventually translate the effect of the drug, or structural changes in the end organ so that the organ cannot respond fully. Actual changes in the end-organ responses in the elderly have been described for only a few drugs. Elderly subjects have a quantitatively lower increase in heart rate to intravenous boluses of isoproterenol.[38] This effect does not seem to be secondary to alterations in the β-adrenergic receptor numbers or to affinity in the elderly, but it is likely caused by a post-receptor mechanism. The elderly also have an enhanced orthostatic response to antihypertensive agents. Aging is associated with an abnormal baroreceptor response to hypotension as well as with a reduction in peripheral venous tone. The enhanced orthostatic hy-

potension to sympatholytic drugs in the elderly is an example of excessive effect as a consequence of changes in tissue responsiveness associated with aging. Elderly patients have been described to have a reduced rate of synthesis of clotting factors when compared with a young population at an equivalent plasma concentration of free warfarin. Whether this increased sensitivity was secondary to altered vitamin K availability in the elderly or to a depressed ability to synthesize clotting factors was not elucidated. Nonetheless, investigators have reported that, in general, elderly patients require much less warfarin to achieve anticoagulation than the younger population.[27]

Elderly patients also seem to respond excessively to psychotropic drugs. One report examined psychomotor performance in elderly and younger subjects after receiving 10 mg of the benzodiazepine, nitrazepam. There were no pharmacokinetic differences between the two groups, but the elderly had significantly greater impairment of psychomotor performance as compared with the younger volunteers.[6] Elderly patients also frequently have paradoxical agitation to barbiturates. The etiology of this unusual response is unknown, but the routine use of barbiturates and sedative hypnotic agents is discouraged in the elderly.

These are some important examples of altered end-organ responsiveness in the elderly. This is a fertile, but still unexplored, territory in gerontology that urgently needs more work.

EFFECT OF AGING ON THE USE OF SPECIFIC DRUGS

The large number of drugs currently available for use and the explosion of interest in geriatric clinical pharmacology in recent years make an exhaustive review of all drugs used by the elderly far beyond the scope of this chapter. The following discussion attempts to briefly illustrate the aforementioned principles and to note the effects of some commonly used agents in elderly patients. The pharmacokinetic and pharmacodynamic changes observed during the use of these agents are summarized in Tables 10–2 and Table 10–3.

Anticoagulants

Coumarin anticoagulants such as warfarin are strongly protein-bound and metabolized by the liver. The dosage of anticoagulant must be individualized, using the prothrombin time to avoid complications from over-anticoagulation or under-anticoagulation. Most data suggest that the coumarin dose required for proper anticoagulation is lower in the elderly population as compared with young patients.[27] This appears to be related to an increased sensitivity of the liver to inhibition of clotting factor synthesis at any plasma total warfarin concentration in elderly patients. No dramatic pharmacokinetic changes with aging have been described for warfarin.

Drug interactions with warfarin are common and may have catastrophic effects.[35] These drug interactions may result from changes in warfarin absorption, protein binding, or metabolism. Additionally, pharmacodynamic interactions may result from administration of other drugs that alter hemostasis or by dietary changes in vitamin K availability. In the geriatric patient population, the frequent changes in medications (with or without notification of the physician) and the use of treatments such as influenza vaccine that may alter warfarin action or kinetics mandate great caution and frequent reassessment of the patient during the administration of warfarin.

Antihypertensive Drugs

Aging is associated with an abnormal baroreceptor response to hypotension as well as with a reduction in peripheral venous tone.[4, 12] Thus, it is not unusual to observe some orthostatic hypotension in the elderly on no medication. The use of drugs that further interfere with sympathetic function, such as clonidine and methyldopa, may result in severe orthostatic hypotension in this population. Prazosin, guanethidine, and reserpine may also cause significant orthostatic hypotension.

Alterations in the renin-angiotensin system also occur with aging; decreases in renin and aldosterone levels have been reported. The implications of this change on the pharmacologic control of blood pressure has not been completely defined. Elderly patients respond to angiotensin converting enzyme inhibitors with a decrease in blood pressure; however, the use of agents that work independent of the renin-angiotensin system has been recommended for treatment of hypertension in the elderly.[18]

Studies on pharmacokinetic alterations with aging in the handling of antihypertensive medications have been limited. Studies have suggested that the bioavailability of prazosin may be decreased in elderly patients. Also, the volume of distribution of prazosin is increased with aging, but the clearance is unchanged. The increased volume of distribution results in an increased half-life for prazosin in elderly patients.[23] As discussed below, the use of diuretics and β-adrenergic antagonists is complicated by both pharmacodynamic and pharmacokinetic changes related to aging.[32] The safest way to treat elderly hypertensive patients is to use drugs conservatively. The incidence of both cerebral and coronary arteriosclerosis is high in the elderly so that excessive hypotension can result in serious sequelae. The clinician needs to weigh the potential benefits of treatment of established hypertension in the elderly against the morbidity associated with the use of antihypertensive agents.

TABLE 10–2. Alterations in the Pharmacokinetics of Drugs with Aging

Drug	Vd	t½	Cl	Mechanism	Recommendation
Acetaminophen	D	U	D	?	No dose adjustment
Aminoglycosides	U	I	D	Reduced renal function	Reduce dose or increase dosing interval
Amitriptyline, Nortriptyline, Imipramine	?	I	D		
Atenolol	U	I	D	Reduced renal function	Assess efficacy clinically
Chlordiazepoxide	I	I	D	?	
Cimetidine	?	I	D	Reduced renal function	Reduce dose
Diazepam	I	I	U	?	Assess efficacy clinically
Digoxin	D	I	D	Reduced renal function	Reduce dose
Disopyramide	U	I	D	Reduced renal function	Reduce dose
Furosemide	I	I	D	Reduced renal function, decreased albumin	Not major factor in clinical use
Ibuprofen	?	?	D	?	
Lidocaine	I	I	D	Decreased hepatic blood flow	Reduce dose
Lithium	?	I	D	Reduced renal function	Reduce dose
Naproxen	?	?	D	?	Effect is small
Phenobarbital	?	I	?	?	Monitor levels
Phenylbutazone	I	U	?	Decreased albumin	
Phenytoin	I	?	I	Reduced albumin	Monitor levels, adjust dose with caution due to saturation kinetics
Prazosin	I	I	U		
Procainamide	U	I	D	Reduced renal function	Reduce dose
Propranolol	U	I	D	Decreased hepatic blood flow	Assess efficacy clinically
Quinidine	U	I	D	Decreased metabolism	Reduce dose
Raniditine	?	I	?	Reduced renal function; increase peak also seen	Reduced dose may be needed
Salicylate	I	I	D	Reduced renal function, decreased albumin	
Theophylline	U	I	D	?	Measure drug levels
Tocainide	U	I	D	Reduced renal function	Reduce dose
Trazadone	?	I	D	?	
Valproic acid	U	U	U	FREE drug clearance decreased, decreased protein binding	

? = Unknown; U = Unchanged; I = Increased; D = Decreased; Vd = Volume of distribution; t½ = Half-life; Cl = Clearance.

Antibiotics

Several antibiotics, including the penicillins, vancomycin, and the aminoglycosides are cleared primarily by the kidney, and hence their clearance will decrease with aging. This is particularly important with respect to the aminoglycosides, as their use is associated with a 5 to 10 percent incidence of nephrotoxicity.[25] The serum creatinine concentration may not be a reliable indicator of creatinine clearance in the elderly because creatinine production is also decreased as a result of the lower muscle mass in this population. Serum concentrations of the aminoglycosides can be measured to adjust the dosing regimen to minimize the cumulative aminoglycoside exposure, and, hopefully, to reduce the risk of toxicity. Fortunately, most antibiotics have a large margin of

TABLE 10–3. Alterations in Pharmacodynamics of Drugs with Aging

Drug	Alteration	Recommendation
Antihypertensive agents	Increased risk of orthostatic hypotension	Use agents cautiously
Benzodiazepines	Increased sensitivity	Use lower maintenance dose initially
β-adrenergic blockers	Decreased β-adrenergic responsiveness	Monitor efficacy/action clinically
Coumarin anticoagulants	Increased sensitivity	Use lower maintenance dose initially
Diuretics	Decreased intratubular concentration Increased sensitivity to complications	Monitor electrolytes and orthostatic blood pressure

safety, and any pharmacokinetic alterations with aging are not associated with clinically significant changes.

Antiepileptic Drugs

Phenytoin elimination is characterized by saturable kinetics. The drug is also extensively protein-bound, and only the free drug is available for metabolism and pharmacologic action. Age-related alterations in kinetics have been examined for phenytoin.[15] Protein binding of phenytoin decreases with aging, owing to the decrease in plasma albumin concentration. The total plasma clearance of phenytoin is increased in the elderly as compared with clearance in the younger population, but the free drug clearance may not be different in the two groups, reflecting the alteration in protein binding. The saturation kinetics of phenytoin limit the clinical utility of a detailed analysis of phenytoin clearance, as the elimination kinetics will alter in an individual patient as the dose is changed, regardless of the patient's age.[31] The plasma concentration at which phenytoin metabolism becomes saturated varies widely, and genetic factors probably overshadow any age-dependent alterations in phenytoin metabolism.

When treating a patient with phenytoin, the practitioner must understand that phenytoin metabolism may become saturated at plasma concentrations at or below therapeutic levels. Measurement of phenytoin levels may be useful in avoiding toxicity while maximizing efficacy, but alterations in protein binding may complicate the interpretation of total phenytoin levels in the elderly. If alterations in protein binding are suspected, a specific measurement of the free phenytoin concentration is available to clarify this clinical situation.

Phenobarbital is cleared primarily by hepatic metabolism. The data available suggest that the plasma half-life of phenobarbital is increased with aging. Either a change in plasma clearance or in the volume of distribution could be responsible for this change in half-life, and its clinical significance has not been defined. Limited data indicate that the pharmacokinetics of carbamazepine are not affected by aging.[16] Valproic acid's half-life, volume of distribution, and total drug clearance have not been reported to be different in young and elderly subjects.[29] However, valproic acid protein binding was shown to be decreased in the elderly subjects and the free drug clearance reduced.

Antiarrhythmic Drugs

A large number of antiarrhythmic agents are now in clinical use, including drugs eliminated by hepatic metabolism such as quinidine and lidocaine. Others are excreted to varying degrees by the kidney (procainamide, disopyramide, tocainide).[32] As would be expected, the decrease in creatinine clearance associated with aging results in decreased clearance of procainamide, tocainide, and presumably disopyramide.

Lidocaine elimination by the liver is flow-limited. Thus, it could be predicted that the decreased hepatic flow rates in the elderly would result in decreases in lidocaine clearance with aging, and this has been confirmed in some studies. Additionally, the volume of distribution of lidocaine increases with age. The result of both of these alterations is a prolonged half-life of lidocaine in elderly patients. The clearance of quinidine is approximately 35 percent lower in the elderly as compared with a younger population. Neither the volume of distribution nor the protein binding of quinidine is significantly affected by aging.

Digoxin

Digoxin is commonly used by the elderly population, and its use is associated with a high incidence of adverse reactions. Plasma digoxin levels are not uniformly predictive of toxicity and may be particularly misleading in patients over 65 years of age.[3] Digoxin is eliminated primarily through renal excretion. The decrease in creatinine clearance with aging correlates well with a decrease in digoxin clearance. Some investigators have reported a decrease in the volume of distribution of digoxin with aging, but the decrease in clearance is the dominant change with aging. Thus, the half-life of digoxin increases with aging, and the initial maintenance dose should be reduced in elderly patients. If further work confirms the reduction in the volume of distribution, the loading dose of digoxin used would also need to be reduced in the geriatric population.

β-Adrenergic Blockers

A large number of β-adrenergic blockers are now in clinical use, and complex pharmacokinetic and pharmacodynamic differences have been demonstrated for their use in elderly versus young patients. Propranolol has been the most studied in this respect. Propranolol is cleared by the liver in a flow-dependent manner. With aging, the clearance of propranolol is decreased, whereas its volume of distribution, protein binding, and bioavailability are unchanged. The half-life of propranolol is thus increased with aging.[39] However, there are also physiologic changes in the β-adrenergic system that occur with aging that may alter the action of β-adrenergic blockers. Some studies have demonstrated a decreased number of β-adrenergic receptors with aging and a decrease in the maximal cardiac response to isoproterenol, a β-adrenergic agonist.[32] How these changes in adrenergic function translate to the pharmacologic use of β-adrenergic blockers is complex and the subject of ongoing investigation, but may make the elderly patient either more or less susceptible to β-blockade with drugs like propranolol. Thus, clinical assessment is critical for balancing these varied pharmacokinetic and pharmacodynamic changes.

In general, the other β-adrenergic blockers available can be characterized as lipophilic compounds like propranolol, which are metabolized by the liver, or hydrophilic drugs like atenolol, which are eliminated by the kidney. Aging is associated with alterations in both hepatic blood flow and creatinine clearance, so that the clearance of both lipophilic and hydrophilic drugs is decreased in the elderly. No significant changes in the volume of distribution of these agents have been described, so the decrease in clearance leads to a prolongation of the half-life of these agents in the geriatric population.

Diuretics

As many as 45 percent of patients over 65 years of age admitted to an inpatient medical facility will be taking diuretics. Furosemide is commonly used in elderly patients. Its volume of distribution may increase slightly with age, but the dominant pharmacokinetic alteration is a decrease in clearance leading to a prolonged half-life.[1, 20] However, elderly patients are also relatively resistant to the diuretic action of furosemide. Furosemide needs to reach the intraluminal surface of the renal tubule to influence sodium chloride transport. Thus, the same decrease in renal function that results in lower furosemide clearance also decreases furosemide delivery to its site of action. These changes in the kinetics and action of furosemide need to be viewed in the context of frequent adverse reactions to diuretic therapy in geriatric populations.

Dehydration, prerenal azotemia, and hypotension are frequently associated with diuretic use in the elderly, whereas these complications are rarely observed in the younger population. The use of thiazide diuretics causes a greater potassium loss in the elderly as compared with younger patients.[9] There are no clear-cut explanations for these enhanced responses in the elderly, but altered dietary intake, less effective thirst recognition, and abnormal autonomic response to hypotension may contribute to these adverse effects. A practitioner, therefore, needs to be cautious when prescribing a diuretic for an elderly patient. Serum electrolyte determinations and measurement of orthostatic blood pressures will be helpful in avoiding serious complications. The combination of a diuretic and digoxin may be dangerous because hypokalemia and hypomagnesemia from the diuretic use can potentiate the cardiotoxicity of digoxin. Also, a decrease in renal function secondary to diuretic-induced dehydration can result in accumulation of digoxin to toxic levels.

Nonsteroidal Anti-inflammatory Drugs

Most nonsteroidal anti-inflammatory drugs (NSAID) are strongly protein-bound and are metabolized by the liver.[43] Aspirin is the mostly commonly used NSAID. It is rapidly converted to salicylate after absorption, and this conversion is unaffected by age. The volume of distribution for salicylate increases with age, whereas its clearance decreases. These changes result in a prolonged half-life for salicylate in the elderly. Pharmacokinetic studies have also been performed using some of the other NSAIDs. The volume of distribution of phenylbutazone is increased with age. As alternative drugs become available, phenylbutazone is used less frequently because of the risk of bone marrow toxicity. The clearances of ibuprofen and naproxen have been to shown to decrease with age, but for unclear reasons, the changes in ibuprofen clearance were seen in elderly men but not in elderly women. The pharmacokinetics of piroxicam and indomethacin have not been shown to change with age.

It should also be noted that while NSAIDs are useful drugs, they are associated with significant morbidity in the elderly.[43] Bleeding from peptic ulcers in patients over age 60 has been shown to be associated with NSAID use. Many of the recent reports of severe hepatic and renal toxicity secondary to NSAID use have occurred in elderly patients. As always, the clinician needs to assess carefully the risks and benefits of treatment with these agents in geriatric patients and to review periodically the need for their continued use.

Sedative, Antipsychotic, and Antidepressant Drugs

The consequences of aging on the proper use of psychoactive drugs are complex. Pharmacokinetic studies have been performed for only the minority of drugs. Many studies examining central nervous system (CNS) sensitivity to these drugs in the elderly do not take into account the possibility of altered clearances or protein binding. Aging may be associated with a decrease in mental agility, a decline in intellectual responsiveness and perception, and impaired learning ability and memory. Thus, it would not be surprising that the use of sedative hypnotic drugs would lead to adverse CNS reactions more commonly in the elderly. Unfortunately, this important interaction has not been explored in detail. It has been recognized for a long time that elderly patients frequently experience paradoxical agitation to barbiturates. The exact etiology of this reaction is unknown, but the routine use of barbiturates and sedative hypnotic agents should be minimized in the elderly.

The half-life of diazepam is increased approximately 4-fold in the elderly as compared with a young population.[21] This change in half-life is the result of an increased volume of distribution, without a change in clearance or protein binding. These kinetic changes would suggest on a pharmacokinetic basis alone that at steady-state, the total dose of diazepam should be unchanged in the elderly but that the dosing interval could be lengthened. The half-life of chlordiazepoxide is increased with aging caused by both an increase in the volume of distribution and a decrease in the clearance. Data also suggest that the elderly are more sensitive to the central depressant effect of benzodiazepines. Adverse CNS effects during flurazepam therapy are more common in the elderly than in younger patients.[11] Impairment of psychomotor performance after the administration of 10 mg of nitrazapam was greater in elderly subjects as compared with younger individuals, whereas no change in nitrazapam pharmacokinetics were observed.[6] Thus, it is prudent to begin elderly patients on a lower benzodiazepine dose than would be used in younger patients.

Limited data are available on alterations in the pharmacokinetics and pharmacodynamics of the antidepressants with aging. The clearances of amitriptyline, nortriptyline, and imipramine have been reported to be decreased in the elderly. The plasma half-life of trazadone is increased in the elderly, secondary to a decrease in clearance.

Analgesics

Early studies examining the effect of morphine sulfate and pentazocine hydrochloride on postoperative pain concluded that elderly patients were more sensitive to the analgesic effects of these narcotics.[2] Data indicate that neither the volume of distribution nor the elimination of morphine sulfate is different in young or elderly subjects.[28] However, the rate of distribution of morphine is faster in younger patients, which would result in higher plasma levels of the drug soon after administration in elderly patients. Higher Demerol levels have also been reported after administration of the drug to elderly patients as compared with young individuals. A detailed and complete analysis of pharmacodynamic and pharmacokinetic changes in narcotic analgesic handling in the elderly is not yet available.

Alterations in acetaminophen pharmacokinetics with aging are small. The volume of distribution for acetaminophen decreases, and there is also a trend towards decreased acetaminophen clearance as well. The combination of these changes results in little or no change in acetaminophen half-life with aging.[8]

Other Drugs

Lithium is excreted by the kidneys, and its clearance is decreased in the elderly. Cimetidine is eliminated by both renal and hepatic mechanisms, and its clearance is decreased with aging. Ranitidine, a histamine-2 antagonist similar to cimetidine, is also eliminated by both renal and hepatic mechanisms. The half-life of ranitidine is increased by approximately 40 percent in elderly patients as compared with a young population. Additionally, the peak ranitidine concentration after oral administration is higher in elderly patients, suggesting a decrease in the first-pass elimination of the drug with aging. Theophylline is cleared primarily via hepatic metabolism, and clearance has been reported to be decreased in elderly patients. For both lithium and theophylline, laboratory measurement of drug levels can be helpful in optimizing dosage regimens. The calcium channel blockers are being used with increasing frequency in elderly patients, but insufficient data are available concerning differences in their use in young versus older patients.

SUMMARY OF DRUG USE IN THE GERIATRIC POPULATION

The proper use of therapeutic agents in the elderly is important to optimal functioning. Yet data have repeatedly demonstrated that the incidence of adverse drug reactions in a geriatric population is 2 to 3 times that seen in young patients, reaching an incidence rate of above 20 percent in patients over 80 years old.[5, 22] The physician must be aware of this risk and its contributing factors as well as of techniques to minimize risk.

Physiologic changes that occur with aging result in predictable alterations in drug distribution and elimination, and an understanding of these alterations permit the clinician to use drugs in elderly patients rationally and safely. For drugs eliminated by renal excretion, the fall in glomerular filtration in the elderly will decrease drug clearance by as much as 50 percent. Hepatic drug metabolism is altered much less with aging, except for those drugs in which clearance is limited by the reduced hepatic blood flow in elderly patients. The use of measured drug levels to assist in clinical decision making (therapeutic drug monitoring) is one way to objectively assess whether the optimal dosing regimen has been chosen. Elderly patients often take a large number of medications (5 to 10 different drugs in most studies), which increases the risk of adverse drug interactions.[10, 33] Nonprescription medications should not be neglected in this regard. Additionally, elderly patients may be more sensitive to drug effects, both therapeutic and toxic, at any given drug concentration. The adverse effects of many drugs may be subtle, particularly when superimposed on the changes that occur with aging and the effects of underlying diseases. Thus, it is critical that the physician specifically question and examine the patient, keeping the potential for adverse drug effects in mind.

Optimal prescribing practices by the physician will not be sufficient if the patient does not take the medications properly. Several techniques can be employed to improve patient compliance.[13, 33] The obvious steps are to minimize the number of medications and to caution the patient about altering drug dosages. For some patients, it may be necessary to involve family members or visiting nurses in these discussions. Patients should also be informed of the potential hazards of over-the-counter drugs. The pharmacist can also work with the patient to reinforce the instructions of the physician, to provide special packaging that includes memory aids, and to keep accurate drug lists. Obviously, it is impossible to completely eliminate adverse drug reactions in the elderly; however, with care, these problems can be minimized and their consequences recognized and managed.

REFERENCES

1. Andreasen F, Hansen U, Husted JE, et al: The pharmacokinetics of frusemide are influenced by age. Br J Clin Pharmacol 16:391, 1983.
2. Belville JW, Forrest WH, Miller E, et al: Influence of age on pain relief from analgesics: a study of postoperative patients. JAMA 217:1835, 1971.
3. Boman K: Digitalis intoxication in geriatric inpatients. Acta Med Scand 214:345, 1983.
4. Caird FI, Andrew GR, Kennedy RD: Effect of posture on blood pressure in the elderly. Br Heart J 35:527, 1973.
5. Caird FI: Towards rational drug therapy in old age. J R College Physicians Lond 19:235, 1985.
6. Castelden CM, George CF, Marcer D, et al: Increased sensitivity to nitrazepam in old age. Br J Med 1:10, 1977.
7. Davies DF, Shock NW: Age changes in glomerular filtration rate, effective renal plasma flow, and tubular excretory capacity in adult males. J Clin Invest 29:496, 1950.
8. Divoll M, Abernethy DR, Ameer B, et al: Acetaminophen kinetics in the elderly. Clin Pharmacol Ther 31:151, 1982.
9. Friend DG: Drug therapy and the geriatric patient. Clin Pharmacol Ther 2:832, 1961.
10. Gosney M, Tallis R: Prescription of contraindicated and interacting drugs in elderly patients admitted to hospital. Lancet 2:564, 1984.
11. Greenblatt DJ, Allen MD, Shader RI: Toxicity of high-dose flurazepam in the elderly. Clin Pharmacol Ther 21:355, 1977.
12. Gribbon B, Pickering TG, Sleight P, et al: Effect of age and high blood pressure on baroreflex sensitivity in man. Circ Res 29:424, 1971.
13. Gryfe CI, Gryfe BM: Drug therapy of the aged: the problem of compliance and the roles of physicians and pharmacists. J Am Geriatr Soc 32:301, 1984.
14. Hayes MJ, Langmann MJS, Short AH: Changes in drug metabolism with age. Vol 1, Warfarin binding and plasma proteins. Br J Clin Pharmacol 2:69, 1975.
15. Hayes MJ, Langmann MJS, Short AH: Changes in drug metabolism with increasing age. Vol 2, Phenytoin clearance and protein binding. Br J Clin Pharmacol 2:73, 1975.
16. Hockings N, Pall A, Moody J, et al: The effect of age on carbamazepine pharmacokinetics and adverse effects. Br J Clin Pharmacol 22:725, 1986.
17. James OFW: Gastrointestinal and liver function in old age. Clin Gastroenterol 12:671, 1983.
18. Jenkins AC, Knoll JR, Dreslinski GR: Captopril in the treatment of the elderly hypertensive patient. Arch Intern Med 145:2029, 1985.
19. Jernigan JA: Update on drugs and the elderly. Am Fam Physician 29:238, 1984.
20. Kerremans ALM, Tan Y, van Baars H, et al: Furosemide kinetics and dynamics in aged patients. Clin Pharmacol Ther 34:181, 1983.
21. Klotz U, Avant GR, Hoyumpa A, et al: The effects of age and liver disease in the disposition and elimination of diazepam in adult man. J Clin Invest 55:347, 1975.
22. Leach S, Roy SS: Adverse drug reactions: an investigation on an acute geriatric ward. Age Ageing 15:241, 1986.
23. McNeil JJ, Drummer OH, Conway EL, et al: Effect of age on pharmacokinetics of and blood pressure responses to prazosin and terazosin. J Cardiovasc Pharmacol 10:168, 1987.
24. Montgomery RD, Haeney MR, Ross IN, et al: The ageing gut: a study of intestinal absorption in relation to nutrition in the elderly. Q J Med 47:197, 1978.
25. Moore RD, Smith CR, Lipsky JJ, et al: Risk factors for nephrotoxicity in patients treated with aminoglycosides. Ann Intern Med 100:352, 1984.
26. Novak LP: Aging, total body potassium, fat-free mass, and cell mass in males and females between ages 18 and 85 years. J Gerontol 27:438, 1972.
27. O'Malley K, Stevenson IH, Ward CA, et al: Determinants of anticoagulant control in patients receiving warfarin. Br J Clin Pharmacol 4:309, 1977.
28. Owen JA, Sitar DS, Berger L, et al: Age-related morphine kinetics. Clin Pharmacol Ther 34:364, 1983.
29. Perucca E, Grimaldi R, Gatti G, et al: Pharmacokinetics of valproic acid in the elderly. Br J Clin Pharmacol 17:665, 1984.
30. Plein JB, Plein EM: Ageing and drug therapy. Ann Rev Gerontol Geriatr 2:211, 1981.
31. Richens A: Clinical pharmacokinetics of phenytoin. Clin Pharmacokinet 4:153, 1979.
32. Rocci ML, Jr., Vlasses PH, Abrams WB: Geriatric clinical pharmacology. Cardiol Clin 4:213, 1986.
33. Royal College of Physicians: Medication for the elderly. J R College Physicians Lond 18:7, 1984.
34. Schmucker DL: Age-related changes in drug disposition. Pharmacol Rev 30:445, 1978.
35. Serlin MJ, Breckenridge AM: Drug interactions with warfarin. Drugs 25:610, 1983.
36. Sjoqvist F, Alvan G: Aging and drug disposition-metabolism. J Chronic Dis 36:31, 1983.
37. Vestal RE, Wood AJJ: Influence of age and smoking on drug kinetics in man: studies using model compounds. Clin Pharmacokinet 5:309, 1980.
38. Vestal RE, Wood AJJ, Shand DG: Reduced beta-adrenoceptor sensitivity in the elderly. Clin Pharmacol Ther 26:181, 1979.
39. Vestal RE, Wood AJJ, Branch RA, et al: Effect of age and cigarette smoking on propranolol disposition. Clin Pharmacokinet 1:135, 1976.
40. Wallace S, Whiting B, Runcie J: Factors affecting drug binding in plasma of elderly patients. Br J Clin Pharmacol 3:327, 1976.
41. Weiling PG: Interactions affecting drug absorption. Clin Pharmacokinet 9:404, 1984.
42. Wood AJJ, Vestal RE, Wilkinson GR, et al: Effect of aging and cigarette smoking on antipyrine and indocyanine green elimination. Clin Pharmacol Ther 26:16, 1979.
43. Woodhouse KW, Wynne H: The pharmacokinetics of non-steroidal anti-inflammatory drugs in the elderly. Clin Pharmacokinet 12:111, 1987.

CHAPTER 11

Parkinson's Disease and Other Movement Disorders

Earl W. Sutherland, III

Years steal
Fire from the mind as vigour from the limb,
And life's enchanted cup but sparkles near the brim.
BYRON, *Childe Harold*

PERSPECTIVE

The typical parkinsonian gait and tremor caricature old age, making this movement disorder one of the most dreaded afflictions of aging. Similarly, various tremors exact a disproportionate morbidity because of their visible signification of age. Thus, the clinician is confronted with a special responsibility to the elderly with disorders of movement both to treat the disease and to manage the patient.

The problem is compounded by the fact that many normally aging individuals move less, move more stiffly, and assume a stooped posture. In such a setting, the presence of the usually innocuous essential tremor may seem to be the ominous harbinger of parkinsonism. It has been estimated that one half of the elderly with tremorous conditions have essential tremor, one third have parkinsonism, and one sixth have one of a large variety of other conditions. Parkinson's disease itself occurs in 1 in 100 individuals over 60 years of age, and 50,000 new cases are identified annually. Currently, over a million individuals in the United States are afflicted. Essential tremor affects 1 in 25 individuals and begins at any age. The familial forms usually are expressed at the earliest ages. Thus, these are common disorders.

ESSENTIAL TREMOR

When tremor begins in older age, the main task is to distinguish essential tremor from parkinsonian tremor. Even before this distinction is made, however, physiologic tremor, familiar to all following a sustained posture, should be eliminated as a cause. Exaggeration of physiologic tremor may be seen in the older patient taking certain drugs. Among the most common offenders are bronchodilators (thcophylline and β-2 agonists such as albuterol, metaproterenol, and terbutaline); psychotropic agents (including tricyclic antidepressants, major neuroleptics, and lithium); thyroxine; valproic acid; and levodopa. The responses to cold, anxiety, and fatigue are also manifestations of enhanced physiologic tremor.

Whereas familial forms of essential tremor may begin in the young, sporadic forms begin later. In either case, amplitude increases with age, producing greater disability. Essential tremor typically worsens as affected individuals try to write, fasten buttons, tie shoes, or bring food or drink to their mouths. Often, modest amounts of alcohol may still the tremor. Of more practical value, β-adrenergic blockers, especially propranolol, are the first choice in therapy, with the use of primidone as an alternative therapy.[1]

The most reliable distinction of essential tremor from that of parkinsonism (in the absence of other typical signs of parkinsonism) is involvement of the head. This is rarely seen with the parkinsonian tremor but is typical in essential tremor. Usually, essential tremor is absent at rest, much unlike the parkinsonian tremor, but more severe cases may show a resting tremor. In an occasional individual, diagnosis is initially uncertain, which may explain why some patients with essential tremor develop typical parkinsonism.

DIAGNOSIS OF PARKINSON'S DISEASE

Parkinson's disease remains a clinically defined entity with little modification since James Parkinson's description of the disorder in 1817. The important contributions of Lewy (Lewy bodies in 1912), Tretiakoff (cellular loss in the substantia nigra in 1919), Carlsson (decreased cerebral dopamine in animal models in the late 1950s), and Hornykiewicz (decreased human striatal dopamine and improvement of parkinsonian symptoms with the dopamine precursor dl-dopa in 1961) have led to the possibility of diagnosis in the future through the use of a positron-emitting analog of levodopa such as 6-FD.[2] Computed tomography (CT) of the brain and conventional biochemical analyses add little to the diagnosis. Familial history does not seem to be relevant.[3] A syndrome discovered in some individuals (chiefly opioid abusers) exposed to the chemical MPTP (1-methyl-4-phenyl-1,2,3,6-tetrahydropyridine) closely resembles Parkinson's disease and strongly raises the possibility of an etiologic role of an environmental toxin. As yet, no clear such agents have emerged.[4, 5]

The clinical features of Parkinson's disease are excellently detailed in a book account by Sidney Dorros, a victim of the disorder. It is valuable to all clinicians treating this disease.[6] It is believed that individuals develop symptoms when about three fourths of their striatal dopamine has been lost.* This amount represents about fifty percent more loss than the maximum seen in normal aging. The four clinical features of parkinsonism are impoverishment of movement (bradykinesia), resting tremor, rigidity, and postural disorders that give rise to a stooped position and typical gait. In many individuals, it is the slowing down of movement that is the presenting complaint. A sensitive early sign is the loss of arm-swing when walking. Following the loss of spontaneous associated movements, facial expression diminishes ("masked facies"), and initiation of all voluntary movements becomes slow. Neurologic signs are usually asymmetric at first, but ultimately become bilateral. Tremor, which is at times the presenting feature, is typically lost during movement of the involved limb, the distal parts of which are most affected.

The "pill-rolling" appearance of the hands and the pronation-supination of the forearm are classic physical signs. Rigidity of the "cog-wheel" type and abnormal gait are usually not presenting features. The typical gait consists of short, shuffling steps, propelling a stooped body at an increasing rate (festination), as though to prevent a forward fall. With advanced disease, postural reflexes are impaired, greatly restricting mobility. Dementia is certainly not a feature of recently diagnosed Parkinson's disease, and its presence suggests an alternative diagnosis. Dementia may occur somewhat more commonly in patients with advanced disease than it does in the general population of the same age. More subtle cognitive defects may occur earlier. Depression seems more frequent in Parkinson's disease. Among those who don't succumb to the more common mortal events of age, death of the patient with Parkinson's disease is not caused by the disease per se, but rather by the many hazards of bedbound immobility.

Several disorders may resemble Parkinson's disease. They are generally much rarer, and all but exceptional cases display additional neurologic signs. The signs helpful in distinguishing these "Parkinson's plus" syndromes are outlined in Table 11–1. Most of these syndromes do not regularly respond to levodopa, which is another useful distinguishing criterion.

---

*The striatum, composed of the caudate and putamen, together with globus pallidus, the subthalamic nucleus (nucleus of Luys), and the substantia nigra are the major components of the basal ganglia. The basal ganglia are responsible for the initiation of movement and the smooth modulation of movement. Because much of the output of the basal ganglia is through the descending corticospinal (pyramidal) tracts, this regulator of movement is known as the extra-pyramidal system.

TABLE 11–1. Parkinson's Plus Syndromes

Syndrome	Usual Distinction From Parkinson's Disease
Progressive supranuclear palsy (Steele-Richardson-Olszewski)	Downward gaze disturbance Symmetric onset Presents with gait disturbance No rest tremor
Olivopontocerebellar atrophies	Cerebellar ataxia
Shy-Drager	Orthostatic hypotension Bladder disturbances
Post-encephalitic parkinsonism (Von Economo)	History Oculogyric crises Tics
Multiple small cerebral infarcts	Hyper-reflexia
Normal pressure hydrocephalus	Dementia early Gait disturbances without rest tremor
Carbon monoxide poisoning	Other signs of anoxic brain injury
Tardive dyskinesia	History of antipsychotic drug use
Wilson's disease	Patient is younger Kayser-Fleischer rings Decreased ceruloplasmin
Striatonigral degeneration	Neuropathologic only

Management

Efficacious therapy of Parkinson's disease exists, but as may be expected when the usual neuropathology is of progressive cellular loss, the disease ultimately becomes resistant to therapy.[7, 8] Thus, one direction of new therapy is to prevent progressive disease by treating the cause. The only good candidate for an etiologic agent presently is the toxic metabolite of MPTP, the formation of which is blocked by inhibiting monoamine oxidase-B. Although not approved for use in the United States, such an inhibitor, deprenyl, has been used for years in Europe and has proved useful in the management of the fluctuations of symptoms in Parkinson's disease. There is some potential evidence that deprenyl-treated patients may live longer.[9] These considerations have led to a major cooperative study of North Americans with early Parkinson's disease treated with deprenyl or with tocopherol (which acts as a chemical antioxidant), or with both.

The theory of present therapy is that symptoms are due to both a deficiency of dopamine and an unbalanced effect of acetylcholinergic neurons. The current four classes of drugs used to treat Parkinson's disease conform to this theoretical basis, namely, anticholinergics, amantadine, bromocriptine, and levodopa.

Nonpharmacologic therapy is, however, the cornerstone of management of Parkinson's disease. In early disease stages, exercise and the development of psychologic strategies for coping with a progressive disorder are important. In advanced disease, the use of mechanical devices for daily activities and association with support groups for victims and their caregivers help to maintain the quality of life. An extensive library of pamphlets and other resources for both professionals and patients is available through various local and national Parkinson's groups.

When should pharmacologic therapy begin? There is little or no support for the hopeful idea that worsening of the disease can be prevented by earlier drug treatment. Most clinicians avoid using medications until symptoms interfere with the individual's lifestyle, a threshold best decided upon with the patient.

Anticholinergic drugs (Table 11–2) have often been considered as the first line of pharmacotherapy. This is because of their efficacy in reducing tremor and rigidity and their low cost compared with other agents. However, anticholinergics provide little benefit for bradykinesia or postural disturbances. Moreover, they may induce serious side effects such as constipation, urinary retention, and increased intraocular pressure. Cognitive and behavioral effects may be severe, and some clinicians minimize the use of this category of drugs primarily for these reasons.

Amantadine is also especially useful in early disease. This drug, a product used for influenza A prophylaxis, augments dopaminergic function, probably mainly at

TABLE 11–2. Drugs Used to Treat Parkinson's Disease

Drug	Dosage Forms	Usual Range of Daily Dose
Anticholinergics		
Benztropine mesylate (Cogentin; generic)	0.5, 1, and 2 mg tablets 1 mg/ml injectable	0.5–6 mg
Biperiden (Akineton)	2 mg tablet 5 mg/ml injectable	2–16 mg
Diphenhydramine HCl (Benadryl; generic)	25 and 50 mg capsules 12.5 mg/ml elixir 10 and 50 mg/ml injectable	50–200 mg
Ethopropazine HCl (Parsidol)	10 and 50 mg tablets	50–800 mg
Procyclidine HCl (Kemadrin)	5 mg tablet	7.5–20 mg
Trihexyphenidyl (Artane; generic)	2 and 5 mg tablets 2 mg/5 ml elixir 5 mg sustained release capsule	1–15 mg
Amantadine (Symmetrel; generic)	100 mg tablet 50 mg/5 ml syrup	100–300 mg
Bromocriptine (Parlodel)	2.5 and 5 mg tablets	5–100 mg
Levodopa/carbidopa (Sinemet)	100/10, 100/25, and 250/25 mg tablets	400–1500/25–150 mg

postsynaptic sites. Benefits may be seen in all symptoms, but the effects are not sustained although often, relief of symptoms may be achieved again after several weeks without use of the drug. Adverse effects of amantadine are the least severe among antiparkinsonian drugs, although confusion may be noted and dependent edema can be annoying.

Among the dopamine agonists, bromocriptine is the only drug widely used. It may be taken as a single agent, but its greatest utility appears as an adjunct to therapy with levodopa.[10, 11] Although less potent than levodopa, bromocriptine usually produces a more even effect and may extend the duration of relatively symptom-free disease.

The most important drug in treating Parkinson's disease is levodopa. In the United States, levodopa is mostly administered in combination with carbidopa, an inhibitor of dopa decarboxylase that does not cross the blood-brain barrier. Early use of levodopa, without carbidopa, was marked by cardiac stimulation and nausea and vomiting, mainly caused by the peripheral formation of dopamine, catalyzed by systemic dopa decarboxylase. Both of these side effects are uncommon when adequate doses of carbidopa are used, i.e., 70 to 100 mg daily.

The pharmacokinetics of levodopa are complicated. The desired product, dopamine, fails to cross the blood-brain barrier, thus, its immediate precursor, levodopa, is used. Levodopa is partially broken down within the stomach so that drugs that delay gastric emptying, such as the anticholinergic drugs used to treat Parkinson's disease, could impair efficacy. Antacids or H_2-blockers (cimetidine, ranitidine, famotidine) could speed gastric emptying. Levodopa, an amino acid, is absorbed by means of a saturable carrier transport system that is highly specific for neutral amino acids. A very similar system of transport is present at the blood-brain barrier with kinetics so that levodopa must always compete with the normal array of amino acids in the blood for transport into the central nervous system (CNS).

A decrease of levodopa's beneficial actions after a meal high in protein, secondary to competitive effects at either the enteric or CNS site, has been elegantly demonstrated.[12] An unpredictable response to levodopa is often related to the extracerebral pharmacokinetic variables; the patient should be educated by the physician about these matters. In chronic disease, a wearing-off phenomenon occurs, in which the duration of action of levodopa is shortened. As there is no known change in peripheral metabolism of the drug, it has been hypothesized that the progressive loss of nigrostriatal cells results in both less formation and more rapid destruction of dopamine, since there is less neuronal capacity for storage. Unfortunately, the obvious solution of administering more levodopa is not always successful because excessive levels produce a variety of dyskinesias. At times, baclofen is required to control these side effects. Maintenance of more constant levodopa blood levels may be obtained by frequent smaller doses. The addition of bromocriptine may also help the wearing-off syndrome.

With chronic Parkinson's disease, about half of patients experience abrupt swings from nearly normal function to akinesia or severe tremor. At times symptoms are relieved by more levodopa and at times, they clear spontaneously in minutes to hours. The cause of this on-off phenomenon is uncertain, and therapy has been disappointing. Lithium has been tried, and a new class of drugs, which are partial agonists of dopamine receptors, may prove useful; both of these therapeutic approaches, however, remain experimental.[13, 14]

In advanced disease, independence is lost and side effects of the drugs become limiting. Conceivably, an extension of the neurosurgical engraftment techniques reported by Madrazo can offer new hope in advanced stages.[15]

Four national organizations for victims of Parkinson's disease and their caregivers are:

American Parkinson Disease Association, Inc.
116 John Street
New York, NY 10034
(212) 732-9550

National Parkinson Foundation, Inc.
1501 NW Ninth Avenue
Miami, FL 33136
(305) 547-6666 or (800) 327-4545

Parkinson's Disease Foundation
640 W. 168th Street
New York, NY 10032
(212) 923-4700

United Parkinson Foundation
360 W. Superior Street
Chicago, IL 60610
(312) 644-2344

REFERENCES

1. Findley LS: The pharmacological management of essential tremor. Clin Neuropharmacol 9 (Suppl 2):S61, 1986.
2. Martin WRW, Calne DB: Imaging techniques and movement disorders. In Marsden CD, Fahn S, eds: Movement Disorders 2. London, Butterworths, 1987, p 4.
3. Ward CD, Davoisin RC, Ince SE, et al: Parkinson's disease in 65 pairs of twins and a set of quadruplets. Neurology 33:815, 1983.
4. Snyder SH, D'Amato RJ: MPTP: a neurotoxin relevant to the pathophysiology of Parkinson's disease. Neurology 36:250, 1986.
5. Langston JW: MPTP: the promise of a new neurotoxin. In Marsden CD, Fahn S, eds: Movement Disorders 2. London, Butterworths, 1987, p 73.
6. Dorros S: Parkinson's: A Patient's View. New York, Warner Books, 1981.
7. Markham CH, Diamond SG: Long-term follow-up of early dopa treatment in Parkinson's disease. Ann Neurol 19:365, 1986.
8. Goetz CG, Tanner CM, Shannon KM: Progression of Parkinson's disease without levodopa. Neurology 37:695, 1987.
9. Birkmayer W, Reiderer P: Deprenyl prolongs the therapeutic efficacy of combined L-DOPA in Parkinson's disease. Adv Neurol 40:475, 1981.
10. Helm MMM, Elton RL: Low dosages of bromocriptine added to levodopa in Parkinson's disease. Neurology 35:206, 1985.
11. Rinne UK: Early combination of bromocriptine and levodopa in the treatment of Parkinson's disease: a 5 year follow-up. Neurology 37:826, 1987.
12. Nutt JG, Woodward WR, Hammerstad JP, et al: The "on off" phenomenon in Parkinson's disease: relation to levodopa absorption and transport. N Engl J Med 310:483, 1984.
13. Coffey CE, Ross DR, Ferren EL, et al: Treatment of the "on-off" phenomenon in Parkinson's with lithium carbonate. Ann Neurol 12:375, 1982.
14. Lieberman A, Gopinathan G, Neophytides A, et al: Advanced Parkinson's disease: use of a partial dopamine agonist, ciladopa. Neurology 37:863, 1987.
15. Madrazo I, Drucker-Colin R, Diaz V, et al: Open microsurgical autograft of adrenal medulla to the right caudate nucleus in two patients with intractable Parkinson's disease. N Engl J Med 316:831, 1987.

CHAPTER 12

Cerebrovascular Disease

Michael P. Earnest
Jeffrey A. Cohen

I'm growing fonder of my staff;
I'm growing dimmer in the eyes;
I'm growing fainter in my laugh;
I'm growing deeper in my sighs;
I'm growing careless of my dress;
I'm growing frugal of my gold;
I'm growing wise; I'm growing—yes—
I'm growing old.

J. G. SAXE, *I'm Growing Old*

Cerebrovascular disease is a major cause of morbidity and mortality in the elderly. It is the third leading cause of death (after heart disease and cancer) among persons 65 years of age and older in the United States. Annually, about 140,000 persons over age 65 die of stroke, but, more commonly, cerebrovascular disease produces chronic neurologic disability. The American Heart Association estimated that there were 1,830,000 survivors of stroke in the United States in 1984.[6, 7]

Fortunately, both the incidence and mortality rate associated with cerebrovascular disease have declined in recent decades (Fig. 12–1).[7, 8] Improved treatment of medical conditions predisposing to stroke (risk factors), especially hypertension, has resulted in the decreased incidence.[8, 9] Reduced mortality probably is related both to the decreasing incidence of stroke and to lower case fatality rates because of improved acute medical care for stroke patients.

Epidemiologic studies have identified multiple risk factors for stroke, including aging, heart disease, diabetes mellitus, hypertension, smoking, use of birth control pills, hyperlipidemia, excessive alcohol use, and transient ischemic attacks.[7, 9] Treatment of risk factors reduces the individual's risk of having a stroke and also may reduce the recurrence rate in patients who already have had a stroke.

DEFINITIONS

Stroke is a generic term denoting an acute focal neurologic deficit due to cerebrovascular disease that persists longer than 24 hours. Equivalent but less useful terms are cerebral thrombosis, cerebrovascular accident (CVA), and cerebral apoplexy. A clinical stroke syndrome generally is associated with a demonstrable focal lesion in the brain or spinal cord.

Transient ischemic attack (TIA) refers to a stroke-like event that lasts less than 24 hours. A TIA generally has no associated structural lesion of the central nervous system (CNS) but is thought to be caused by temporary dysfunction of a portion of the brain caused by transient ischemia.

CEREBROVASCULAR PATHOLOGY

Many different types of vascular lesions cause stroke and TIAs (Table 12–1).[5, 10, 11] The most common lesion is atherosclerosis, often located in the carotid or vertebral arteries in the neck. A less frequent but still common process is hypertensive vascular disease, affecting the small penetrating arteries within the brain. These vessels develop thick, hyalinized walls (lipohyalinosis) and microscopic dilatations (microaneurysms) that may lead to either occlusion or to rupture of the vessel. Even less common vascular processes underlying stroke are arteritis (e.g., temporal arteritis), fibromuscular dysplasia, arterial dissection, venous occlusion, and amyloid angiopathy. The last is a rare but distinct vasculopathy of the elderly in which the walls of small- and medium-sized vessels of the brain have amyloid deposition,

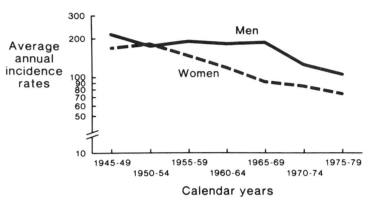

FIGURE 12–1. Five-year average annual incidence rates per 100,000 population for all first episodes of stroke in Rochester, Minnesota. (From Whisnant JP: The decline of stroke. Stroke 15:160, 1984. By permission.)

which eventually leads to occlusion or rupture.[14] Temporal arteritis is another rare, but treatable, cause of stroke in the elderly.[15]

PATHOPHYSIOLOGIC MECHANISMS OF STROKE

There are two distinct types of brain lesions that cause clinical stroke syndromes: brain infarction (BI) and intracranial hemorrhage (ICH) (see Table 12–1). Brain infarction can occur by several mechanisms, including:

1. Thrombotic occlusion of a large artery (e.g., carotid or middle cerebral) or small artery (e.g., lenticulostriate) superimposed on atherosclerotic or hypertensive vascular lesions

2. Embolic occlusion, often caused by a blood clot or platelet clump embolus traveling from a cardiac or proximal carotid artery lesion

3. Hypoperfusion, usually due to profound systemic hypotension, which causes inadequate perfusion of brain tissue distal to a severely stenotic artery

4. Rarely, spasm of an intracranial vessel following subarachnoid hemorrhage.[2–5, 10, 11]

Intracranial hemorrhage can occur as a hemorrhage into the parenchyma of the brain (IPH), a hemorrhage into the intracranial cerebrospinal fluid cisterns, a subarachnoid hemorrhage (SAH), or a combined IPH and SAH.[1–5] Parenchymal hemorrhages usually are caused by rupture of a small vessel within the brain, commonly a vessel weakened by hypertensive vascular disease. However, a con-

genital arteriovenous malformation (AVM) or a vessel weakened by amyloid angiopathy also may rupture to cause IPH. Therapeutic anticoagulation is a notorious cause of IPH in the elderly over age 70. Liver disease, thrombocytopenia, other bleeding disorders, and occult metastatic tumors are less common precipitants. An SAH usually is caused by rupture of a congenital (berry) aneurysm of the circle of Willis but also may be caused by rupture of an AVM.

CLINICAL SYNDROMES

Brain Infarction

Brain infarction characteristically presents when a patient awakens with or has the acute onset of a focal neurologic deficit.[1–5] The patient has no headache and is fully alert. The typical neurologic signs of large vessel (e.g., carotid or middle cerebral artery) occlusion are hemiparesis, often with sensory loss and abnormal reflexes in the same distribution. If the infarction is in the dominant hemisphere, the patient has language dysfunction (dysphasia or aphasia). Thrombotic occlusion cannot be reliably distinguished from embolic occlusion based on neurologic history and signs alone.

Three varieties of BI are less common but are important to recognize. Progressing infarction (stroke-in-evolution, stroke-in-progression) occurs as a typical BI at its onset, but over the next 24 to 36 hours, the deficit worsens, often intermittently improving and then deteriorating.[12] This course usually is caused by severe stenosis

TABLE 12–1. Vascular Lesions and Pathophysiologic Mechanisms Causing Stroke

Brain Infarction (BI)
  Large vessel occlusion—carotid, middle, anterior, posterior cerebral, and vertebrobasilar arteries—atherosclerosis in the artery causing thrombosis large embolus, usually from cardiac source
  Branch vessel occlusions on surface of brain—atherosclerosis
    small emboli, usually from heart or from ulcerated atherosclerotic plaque at carotid origin
    vasculitis
  Penetrating vessel occlusions causing lacunar infarctions—
    hypertensive vascular disease
    atherosclerosis in large vessel at the origin of the penetrating artery
    vasculitis
    amyloid angiopathy
  Hypoperfusion—
    systemic hypotension superimposed on a focal cerebrovascular stenosis
  Vascular spasm—
    following subarachnoid hemorrhage
    associated with migraine
Intracranial Hemorrhage (ICH)
  Intraparenchymal hemorrhage (IPH)—
    rupture of penetrating artery due to hypertensive vascular disease
    arteriovenous malformation (AVM)
    amyloid angiopathy
    tumor (glioma or metastasis)
    secondary IPH following large infarction
  Subarachnoid hemorrhage (SAH)—
    rupture of congenital arterial (berry) aneurysm
    AVM
  Medical causes of ICH
    therapeutic anticoagulants
    occult bleeding disorder, liver disease, thrombocytopenia, etc.

of a large artery, producing slow failure of brain perfusion.

The second unusual syndrome is multi-infarct dementia (MID).[13] The most common case is the patient who has several major BIs, which result in dementia. However, some patients with severe hypertensive or atherosclerotic cerebrovascular disease have a course of progressive dementia, often punctuated by the occurrence of minor strokes. The underlying pathology is usually multiple small deep gray and white matter cerebral infarctions.[13] Amyloid angiopathy commonly produces an MID syndrome.[14]

In the third type, occlusion of small penetrating vessels within the brain, usually resulting from hypertensive vascular disease, may cause several distinct clinical syndromes (lacunar stroke syndromes).[16]

The most common is pure motor hemiplegia, a syndrome in which the weakness has no associated sensory, language, or other signs of cortical dysfunction.

Intracranial Hemorrhage

This syndrome usually presents quite differently than BI. The patient has a sudden, severe headache, often with nausea and vomiting, plus neurologic signs and depression of consciousness.[1–5] The pulse and blood pressure usually are severely elevated, and the patient has tachypnea. An intraparenchymal hemorrhage usually causes profound hemiparesis, but clinical signs alone do not reliably distinguish parenchymal hemorrhage from SAH.

One distinctive location of IPH (i.e., cerebellum) must be recognized because immediate therapy may be lifesaving. Cerebellar hemorrhage causes an acute, severe occipital headache and ataxia, often with vertigo and vomiting.[17] The patient usually has severe hypertension.

CLINICAL LABORATORY EVALUATION

Patients with BI require an extensive evaluation for underlying medical conditions commonly associated with stroke in the elderly.[18] Basic laboratory tests include complete blood count, urinalysis, electrolytes and serum chemistry and lipid profiles. A serologic test for syphilis and erythrocyte sedimentation rate (ESR) will disclose two important causes of vasculitis, meningovascular syphilis and temporal arteritis.[15] Platelet count, prothrombin time, and partial thromboplastin time will determine the coagulation status.

Electrocardiography (ECG) is important to exclude acute myocardial infarction, arrhythmia, or other cardiac abnormality. A routine chest x-ray probably is indicated for general medical purposes. An echocardiogram may show valvular lesions, intracardiac thrombi, or a hypokinetic ventricular wall, which may be a source of emboli.

Noninvasive vascular tests, including ultrasound imaging and flow studies, may be performed to demonstrate atherosclerotic lesions in the cervical carotid artery that cause stenosis or act as a source for emboli to the brain.

Lumbar puncture (LP) is reserved for patients in whom the cerebrospinal fluid (CSF) chemistry or cytologic tests will establish a cause for the stroke. Patients with suspected CNS infection or vasculitis and those with clinical symptoms of an SAH but nondiagnostic computed tomography (CT) brain scan require an LP.

NEURORADIOLOGIC EVALUATION

The first, and usually immediate, test done in an elderly stroke patient is a CT scan of the head. This will demonstrate a nonvascular lesion (e.g., tumor, subdural hematoma, or brain abscess) that may present as an apparent stroke. It also will disclose the pathophysiologic mechanism of the vascular injury to the brain (Fig. 12–2). Intracranial hemorrhage appears as a high-density abnormality, either in the parenchyma or in the subarachnoid space, whereas ischemic infarction shows little if any abnormality within the first 12 hours after onset of symptoms. Brain infarction appears later on CT scan as a focal low-density region.

A magnetic resonance image (MRI) scan may be helpful when the CT scan is not diagnostic. The MRI scan more reliably demonstrates lacunar infarctions, infarctions in the vertebrobasilar arterial system, and cerebral infarctions early in their course (i.e., within the first 12 hours).

Arteriography (angiography) usually is reserved for patients with the following conditions:

1. Cerebral infarction of the large vessel type in patients who have made a good recovery and who, by general medical criteria, are low-risk candidates for carotid endarterectomy

2. Progressing cerebral infarction not responding to anticoagulation

3. Suspected vasculitis

4. SAH in patients who are awake and are neurologically and medically good risks for surgical ablation of a berry aneurysm or AVM.

For patients with progressing infarction or SAH, arteriography is performed as early as possible to expedite decisions about possible surgical intervention. Ar-

teriography for patients in the first category is done several weeks after the acute stroke.

CLINICAL MANAGEMENT OF STROKE

Early Management of All Stroke Patients

All patients with an acute stroke require immediate steps to ensure an optimal oxygen supply to the brain and adequate glucose and blood perfusion.[1–5] Administration of nasal oxygen probably is indicated. If there is clinical evidence of hypoglycemia, a serum glucose determination is made, and intravenous glucose is given. Because hyperglycemia may exacerbate ischemic brain injury by increasing the acidosis within the ischemic tissue, however, glucose administration is not routinely indicated. The patient's blood pressure and cardiac rate and rhythm should be controlled to ensure optimal cardiac output. An ECG is done to exclude cardiac disease.

As soon as the physician is confident that the patient is medically stable, a CT scan of the head is obtained. This will exclude nonvascular lesions, define the mechanism of the cerebrovascular event (see Figure 12–2), and guide further management.

Management of Large Vessel Infarction

After a CT scan demonstrates that no hemorrhage and no nonvascular lesion are present, management is focused on several distinct goals (Table 12–2): (1) preserving ischemic but noninfarcted brain; (2) closely observing the patient's neurologic signs for evidence of progressive infarction; (3) searching for occult medical disorders precipitating the BI; (4) preventing and treating medical complications of stroke; (5) rehabilitating the patient; and (6) preventing future strokes.

Around the acutely infarcted brain tissue lies a zone of ischemic but viable tissue. That zone may recover to function again, or it may undergo infarction. Treat-

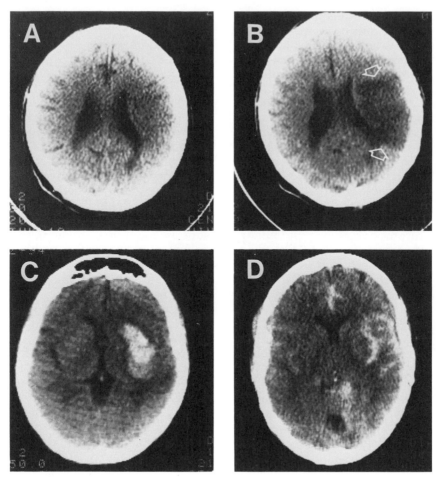

FIGURE 12–2. Head CT scan sections. A, Right cerebral brain infarction at 12 hours. B, The same infarction (arrows) at 11 days. C, Hypertensive intraparenchymal hemorrhage. D, Subarachnoid hemorrhage in both sylvian fissures, the interhemispheric fissure, and under right occipital lobe. (From Schrier RW, ed: Medicine: Diagnosis and Treatment. Boston, Little, Brown & Company, 1988, p 447. By permission.)

ment to reverse the ischemia and to preserve neurophysiologic function requires careful maintenance of optimal oxygenation, blood glucose, and brain perfusion during the first 48 to 72 hours following the onset of stroke symptoms. Brain perfusion depends on adequate rehydration of the dehydrated patient—a condition frequently present in the elderly stroke victim—and management of blood pressure

TABLE 12–2. Management Steps for Large Vessel Brain Infarction

Exclude a nonvascular lesion
Preserve the brain
Observe for and halt progressive ischemia
Determine if occult medical disorders are present
Treat complications of stroke
Rehabilitate the patient
Prevent future strokes

and cardiac rate and rhythm to ensure optimal cardiac output. Many medical and physical therapies have been advocated as effective measures to reverse brain ischemia, including hyperbaric oxygen, corticosteroids, blood volume expansion, hemodilution, prostacyclin, fibrinolysins, and so forth.[3] Unfortunately, none has proved effective when rigorously tested in clinical trials. Currently, there is no "magic bullet" to treat BI; good general medical care is the best care.

Progressing infarction initially is recognized by worsening neurologic signs without medical explanation (i.e., there is no hypoxia, hypoglycemia, hypertension, cardiac arrhythmia, or other medical cause). If a CT scan does not show secondary hemorrhage into the BI, the diagnosis of progressing infarction is established. Once ICH has been excluded by the CT scan, full anticoagulation therapy with intravenous heparin is instituted.[12]

The evaluation for occult medical disorders includes all of the aforementioned appropriate laboratory tests. If an infectious or a vasculitic process is suspected, an LP is indicated to search for elevated protein, decreased glucose, or excessive white blood cells in the CSF. An echocardiogram is valuable for patients who may have had an embolic BI.

Medical complications that commonly occur in stroke patients are pneumonia, congestive heart failure, urinary tract infections, thrombophlebitis, pulmonary emboli, and decubitus ulcers. Other frequent complications include depression, spasticity with contractures of the paralyzed limbs, and subluxation of the shoulder caused by the dependent weight of a flaccid arm. Daily physical examinations for early signs of complications are required so that treatment can be instituted before serious damage occurs.

Hypertension is commonly present in patients with acute BI, in some because of chronic hypertension, although it also may be a response to the stroke. The mechanisms of hypertension secondary to BI are not known but probably reflect increased tone of the sympathetic nervous system. Treatment of hypertension in the acute phase of a BI is advisable only if there is significant elevated diastolic pressure (e.g., to 105 mmHg). Lesser degrees of hypertension often resolve within a few weeks without treatment. Overzealous antihypertensive therapy can cause hypotension in the elderly stroke patient, especially when sitting or standing, and can exacerbate the ischemic brain injury.

Depression is common among stroke patients, in part as a normal response to a disabling illness and in part caused by brain lesion impairment of the individual's affect. Early psychological counseling is valuable to minimize the distress of the depression and lessen its impact on the patient's recovery.

Rehabilitation begins as soon as the patient's medical and neurologic conditions are stable. Emotional support by the medical and nursing staff as well as getting the patient out of bed as soon as possible are important early steps. Physical, speech, and occupational therapy consultations initiate the formal physical rehabilitation. If major neurologic deficits are present, admission to a rehabilitation unit is indicated. Details of long-term rehabilitation are presented in a subsequent section.

Future strokes are prevented by treating the underlying medical conditions that precipitated the current BI. Control of hypertension and treatment of cardiac disease are the most effective preventive measures. Treatment of hypertension usually is instituted several weeks after the stroke. Antihypertensive drugs are administered in low doses, and the blood pressure is monitored frequently, with the patient at rest as well as while sitting or standing.

Patients with a cardiac lesion that produced an embolus causing the BI usually are treated with intravenous heparin while in the hospital and with oral anticoagulants after discharge. The duration of oral anticoagulation therapy depends on the specific nature of the cardiac process. However, caution is necessary when anticoagulation is used to treat elderly patients; age over 60 and duration of therapy beyond 1 year are both associated with a high risk of morbidity or mortality from hemorrhagic complications of anticoagulation.[19] Such therapy should be as brief as possible, and appropriate blood tests should be performed frequently to monitor the level of anticoagulation. Chronic anticoagulation is not indicated for patients with a completed thrombotic BI.

The rare patient with stroke caused by vasculitis should be given high-dose corticosteroids or immunosuppressants.[15] Treatment should continue for several months and then be reduced gradually and discontinued if symptoms do not recur.

Patients who have had a probable thrombotic BI and have made a good recovery should be considered for noninvasive cerebrovascular studies and possible angiography. If a lesion of the cervical carotid artery is discovered, surgical consultation is appropriate.

The patient's later outpatient care requires regular medical evaluations to monitor for both recurrence of stroke symptoms and development of medical or neuropsychological complications. The role of medications to reduce platelet activity (antiplatelet agents), such as aspirin, sulfinpyrazone, and dipyridamole, is not established. Daily long-term aspirin intake may reduce the risk of future strokes, but the efficacy, proper dose, and duration of its effect have not been established.

Management of Lacunar Infarction

Recognition of a lacunar infarction syndrome is important because this type of BI is almost always caused by occlusion of intraparenchymal arterioles resulting from hypertensive vascular disease. A CT scan is necessary to exclude the possibility of a small parenchymal hemorrhage, an event that on rare occasion can mimic a lacunar infarction. Once the diagnosis is established, anticoagulation, arteriography, noninvasive vascular studies, and echocardiography usually are not done. Management is guided by the aforementioned steps concerning good general medical and nursing care, preventing complications, rehabilitating the patient, and preventing future strokes. Control of hypertension is the critical medical therapy.

Management of ICH

The presence of ICH is suspected by the characteristic clinical presentation and is proven by an immediate CT scan. This procedure discloses the type of ICH present, its location, size, and any secondary hydrocephalus caused by obstruction of CSF flow. If the clinical history suggests ICH, but the CT shows no blood, a lumbar puncture is required to diagnose an SAH. About 10 percent of patients with SAH will have a nondiagnostic CT.

Intracranial hemorrhage causes brain injury by focal ischemic, toxic effects of extravascular blood and mass effect. Mass effect includes both local pressure by the hemorrhage, causing injury to nearby brain tissue, and also diffusely increased intracranial pressure (ICP), affecting function of the entire brain. Management of ICH is similar to that for BI but also includes treatment to reduce the mass effect of the hemorrhage (Fig. 12–3). Once an ICH has been identified, dexamethasone is given to reduce inflammatory reaction to the blood and to reduce elevated ICP. If clinical signs of transtentorial brain herniation are present, an event frequently caused by a large parenchymal hemorrhage, endotracheal intubation and hyperventilation are required, and an osmotic diuretic (usually mannitol) and sometimes a loop diuretic (usually furosemide) are given to reduce brain edema and ICP.

Hypertension, often to a severe degree, is present in almost every patient with an ICH. It is a response to ICP and to the direct toxic effects of blood on the brain and meninges. Blood pressure should be maintained near the upper limits of normal for patients with parenchymal hemorrhages. The goal is to maintain adequate cerebral perfusion in spite of the increased ICP. However, for patients with SAH, blood pressure should be maintained near the lower limits of normal or even slightly hypotensive (e.g., 90/60 mmHg). The low blood pressure theoretically reduces the risk of a second rupture of the aneurysm that caused the SAH.

Early consultation with a neurologist or neurosurgeon will provide guidance concerning management of hypertension, treatment of ICP, and decisions about arteriography and surgery.

Surgery is done for SAH patients with an aneurysm documented by an arteriogram and who are awake and in acceptable medical and neurologic condition. The surgery often is performed as soon as possible to prevent a second rupture of the aneurysm, an event that commonly occurs 5 to 10 days after the initial SAH. Surgery generally is not indicated for comatose or severely brain-injured patients with SAH or for patients who have an IPH. A very important exception is the patient with a cerebellar parenchymal hemorrhage. The patient presents with a sudden, severe occipital headache, vomiting, and ataxia, followed by depression of consciousness. The blood pressure is severely elevated. An emergency CT scan demonstrates hemorrhage in the cerebellum, with secondary hydrocephalus. Immediate surgery to drain the hemorrhage may save the patient's life by preventing lethal compression of the brainstem from the mass effect of the hematoma.[16]

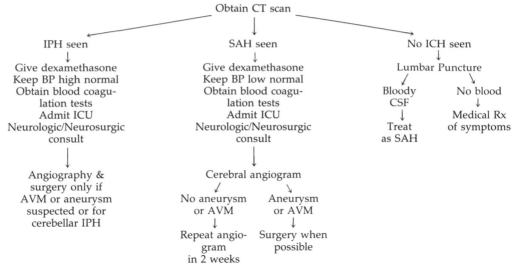

FIGURE 12–3. Management of the patient with suspected intracranial hemorrhage.

REHABILITATION OF THE STROKE SURVIVOR

Approximately 85 percent of patients with BI and 60 percent of those with ICH survive the acute illness. Most survivors have some degree of long-term neurologic disability. Elderly patients who survive stroke live an average of over 4 years, so maximum therapy must be given to restore independent status as fully as possible. With proper therapy and support services, over 80 percent of survivors can return to their prior residence, and 70 percent will be independent in daily self-care activities.[20, 21] The best setting for accomplishing these goals is a dedicated rehabilitation unit that provides comprehensive services including physical, occupational, and speech therapies, social services, psychologic counseling, and support services for returning to the home. The patient's spouse, children, and other support persons are encouraged to participate in the rehabilitation program and discharge planning. Therapy may be continued on an outpatient basis for several months.

After discharge from the rehabilitation program, the physician should periodically reassess the patient's level of function. The patient and family are questioned about any problems that the patient may have with climbing stairs, dressing, bathing, cooking, and other activities of daily living or with recurring falls. If such problems occur, further rehabilitation therapies may be helpful, even years after the stroke.

TRANSIENT ISCHEMIC ATTACKS

These attacks cause no persisting neurologic deficit. Most are thought to be caused by small emboli entering into the intracranial circulation that are quickly fragmented or resorbed, leaving no permanent tissue damage. Transient ischemic attacks are an important risk factor and warning symptom of future stroke. Approximately 20 to 30 percent of patients having a first TIA will have a completed stroke within 3 years.[22]

The clinical symptoms of TIAs are divided into two patterns: those with symptoms that indicate a carotid–middle cerebral artery distribution event and those that indicate vertebrobasilar ischemia (Table 12–3). Carotid distribution TIAs produce hemiparesis, hemisensory abnormality, and, if the dominant hemisphere is involved, dysphasia or aphasia. Although not originating from cerebral ischemia, transient monocular blindness (TMB or amaurosis fugax) is an important symptom

TABLE 12–3. Transient Ischemic Attack Symptoms by Vascular Supply

Carotid Artery Territory	Vertebrobasilar Territory
Hemiparesis	Vertigo
Hemisensory deficit	Auditory symptoms
Aphasia	Ataxia
Monocular blindness	Diplopia
	Dysarthria
	Dysphagia
	Bilateral facial or limb sensory symptoms
	Bilateral weakness
	Hemianopsia or total blindness
	Drop attacks
	Syncope

of carotid territory ischemia. Transient monocular blindness is sudden loss of vision in one eye only that usually resolves completely in a few (less than 30) minutes. It is due to retinal ischemia because of inadequate perfusion through the ophthalmic artery, the first major intracranial branch of the internal carotid artery. The occurrence of TMB and cerebral ischemic symptoms together indicates a greater than 80 percent probability of an atherosclerotic lesion at the origin of the internal carotid artery.

Vertebrobasilar TIAs or the vertebrobasilar insufficiency (VBI) syndrome is manifested by some combination of motor, sensory, cranial nerve, visual, or cerebellar symptoms and signs. The symptoms can include vertigo, nausea, vomiting, ataxia, diplopia, hemianopsia, total loss of vision, dysarthria, dysphagia, facial numbness, bilateral limb weakness or sensory symptoms, faintness, syncope, and, rarely, sudden falling without loss of consciousness (drop attacks). Vertebrobasilar insufficiency symptoms are difficult to distinguish from those of inner ear disease, orthostatic hypotension, and anxiety, so the diagnosis of a vertebrobasilar TIA often is problematic.

Patients with TIAs require a full evaluation for occult medical diseases (as described for the patient with a stroke), including blood and urine tests, cardiac evaluation, and a CT scan, to exclude a nonvascular lesion (brain tumor, subdural hematoma) masquerading as a TIA. Patients with carotid distribution symptoms require either noninvasive vascular studies

or an arteriogram of the appropriate carotid artery to determine whether a surgically treatable stenosis or a source of emboli (i.e., ulcerated atherosclerotic plaque) at the origin of the internal carotid artery is present. Those with VBI usually do not require vascular studies, because surgery of that vascular system is associated with excessive morbidity and mortality.

Medical management includes treatment of any stroke risk factors that are identified by the physical examination or laboratory tests. Antiplatelet agents have been demonstrated to reduce future incidence of stroke following TIAs.[23, 24] The most effective drug is probably aspirin. Anticoagulation with heparin or oral anticoagulants is probably best reserved for patients in whom the TIAs cannot be controlled by antiplatelet agents. However, some authors recommend first prescribing anticoagulation therapy for a few months and then changing to antiplatelet therapy.

Surgical treatment of severe carotid artery stenosis or an ulcerated plaque involves a carotid endarterectomy. In the elderly, this procedure carries significant risk of morbidity and mortality.[25] It should be performed only after careful evaluation of the general medical condition to ensure that the patient is a low-risk candidate for surgery and after consideration of alternative medical therapies.

ASYMPTOMATIC BRUITS

About 4 percent of a population over age 60 has a bruit of a cervical carotid artery. Such bruits usually indicate underlying atherosclerotic disease and are associated with an increased risk of future stroke.[26, 27] However, there is no convincing evidence that arteriography followed by carotid endarterectomy reduces future stroke morbidity or mortality. Such an aggressive course probably should be undertaken only if noninvasive vascular studies demonstrate a stenosis of the internal carotid artery that is impeding blood flow significantly *and* if the combined, documented morbidity and mortality for these procedures in the physician's specific hospital are less than 2 percent.

REFERENCES

CEREBROVASCULAR DISEASE—TEXTS AND REVIEWS

1. Barnett HJM, Stein BH, Mohr JP, et al: Stroke: Pathophysiology, Diagnosis and Management. New York, Churchill Livingstone, 1986.
2. Adams RD, Victor M: Cerebrovascular diseases. In Adams RD, Victor M: Principles of Neurology, 3rd ed. New York, McGraw-Hill, 1985, p 569.
3. Grotta JC: Current medical and surgical therapy for cerebrovascular disease. N Engl J Med 317:1505, 1987.
4. Hachinski V, Norris JW: The Acute Stroke. Philadelphia, FA Davis, 1985.
5. Kistler JP, Ropper AH, Martin JB: Cerebrovascular diseases. In Braunwald E, Isselbacher KJ, Petersdorf RG, et al, eds: Harrison's Principles of Internal Medicine, 11th ed. New York, McGraw-Hill, 1987, p 1930.

EPIDEMIOLOGY OF CEREBROVASCULAR DISEASE

6. Posner JD, Gorman KM, Woldow A: Stroke in the elderly: I. Epidemiology. J Am Geriatr Soc 32:95, 1984.
7. Whisnant JP: The decline of stroke. Stroke 15:160, 1984.
8. Garraway WM, Whisnant JP: The changing pattern of hypertension and the declining incidence of stroke. JAMA 258:214, 1987.
9. Davis PH, Dambrosia JM, Schoenberg BS, et al: Risk factors for ischemic stroke: a prospective study in Rochester, Minnesota. Ann Neurol 22:319, 1987.

PATHOLOGY AND PATHOPHYSIOLOGY OF STROKE

10. Meyer FB, Sundt TM Jr, Yanagihara T, et al: Focal cerebral ischemia: pathophysiologic mechanisms and rationale for future avenues of treatment. Mayo Clin Proc 62:35, 1987.
11. Kurtzke JF: Epidemiology. Pathophysiology of strokes, Unit I. In Barnett HJM, Stein BH, Mohr JP, et al, eds: Stroke: Pathophysiology, Diagnosis and Management, Vol I. New York, Churchill Livingstone, 1986, p 3.

SPECIAL CEREBROVASCULAR SYNDROMES

12. Millikan CH, McDowell FH: Treatment of progressing stroke. Stroke 12:397, 1987.
13. Rosen WG, Terry RD, Fuld PA, et al: Pathological verification of ischemic score in differentiation of dementias. Ann Neurol 7:486, 1980.
14. Okazaki H, Reagan TJ, Campbell RJ: Clinicopathological studies of primary cerebral amyloid angiopathy. Mayo Clin Proc 54:22, 1979.
15. Caselli RJ, Hunder GG, Whisnant JP: Neurologic disease in biopsy-proven giant cell (temporal) arteritis. Neurology 38:352, 1988.
16. Fisher CM: Lacunes: small, deep cerebral infarcts. Neurology 15:774, 1965.
17. Heros RC: Cerebellar hemorrhage and infarction. Stroke 13:106, 1982.

LABORATORY AND RADIOLOGIC EVALUATION OF CEREBROVASCULAR LESIONS

18. Mohr JP: Overview of laboratory studies. Diagnostic studies for stroke, Unit II. In Barnett HJM, Stein BH, Mohr JP, et al, eds: Stroke: Pathophysiology, Diagnosis and Management, Vol I. New York, Churchill Livingstone, 1986, pp 183–278.

HEPARIN ANTICOAGULATION FOR BRAIN INFARCTION

19. Ramirez-Lassepas M, Quinones MR: Heparin therapy for stroke: hemorrhagic complications and risk factors for intracerebral hemorrhage. Neurology 34:114, 1984.

REHABILITATION OF STROKE SURVIVORS

20. Gresham GE: The rehabilitation of the stroke survivor. In Barnett HJM, Stein BH, Mohr JP, et al, eds: Stroke: Pathophysiology, Diagnosis and Management, Vol II. New York, Churchill Livingstone, 1986, p 1259.
21. King PS, Yang RCZ: Rehabilitation medicine. In Cassel CK, Walsh JR, eds: Geriatric Medicine, Vol 2. New York, Springer-Verlag, 1984, p 303.

TRANSIENT ISCHEMIC ATTACKS

22. Mohr JP, Pessin MS: Extracranial carotid artery disease. In Barnett HJM, Stein BH, Mohr JP, et al, eds: Stroke: Pathophysiology, Diagnosis and Management, Vol I. New York, Churchill Livingstone, 1986, p 313.
23. The Canadian Cooperative Study Group: A randomized trial of aspirin and sulfinpyrazone in threatened stroke. N Engl J Med 299:53, 1978.
24. The American-Canadian Co-operative Study Group: Persantine aspirin trial in cerebral ischemia, Part II: endpoint results. Stroke 16:406, 1985.
25. Committee on Health Care Issues, American Neurological Association: Does carotid endarterectomy decrease stroke and death in patients with transient ischemic attacks? Ann Neurol 22:72, 1987.

ASYMPTOMATIC CAROTID BRUITS

26. Chambers BR, Norris JW: Outcome in patients with asymptomatic neck bruits. N Engl J Med 315:860, 1986.
27. Meissner I, Wiebers DO, Whisnant JP, et al: The natural history of asymptomatic carotid artery occlusive lesions. JAMA 258:2704, 1987.

SENSORY AND SKIN PROBLEMS

CHAPTER 13

The Aging Eye

Roger H.S. Langston

He that is strucken blind can not forget
The precious treasure of his eyesight lost.
                    SHAKESPEARE, *Romeo and Juliet*

Aging brings a number of changes to the eye and to the life of the elderly patient. Some are natural annoyances that must be tolerated, and some represent significant diseases. A large portion of the geriatrician's work, whether or not he is an ophthalmologist, is to interpret and explain these changes to patients. Blindness is a problem clearly associated with increasing age, and many elderly patients naturally fear this potentiality when they develop any new ocular symptoms. This chapter outlines some of the more common "normal" aging changes, as well as some of the common diseases of the aging eye, as a background in understanding the elderly patient's ocular problems.

COMMON OPHTHALMIC SYMPTOMS

Diminished vision is by its nature a potentially serious symptom. It is usually caused by changes that occur in the eye, although it can be caused by problems in the visual pathways or occipital cortex. In evaluating decreased vision, consider that sudden change is always an indication of significant disease. Slowly progressive loss may result from a fairly benign problem, such as the need for a change in glasses or the development of cataract, or from more serious conditions. If the patient maintains good vision under some circumstances (for example, maintaining good near vision while losing distance vision) the problem is much less likely to be serious than if vision is decreased under all circumstances.

Fluctuations in vision associated with lighting are fairly common with aging and are generally caused by some cataract or other opacity in the ocular media. With age, the pupil tends to become smaller and the iris less reactive to changes in lighting. In addition, the lens of the eye darkens and may develop some opacities. The retina also becomes less sensitive. All of these changes cause the elderly patient to have problems in adapting to either very bright or dim illumination. Fluctuations in vision, especially darkening of vision, which occurs independent of lighting conditions, are more sinister and often are due to carotid or vertebral transient ischemic attacks (TIA) or, occasionally, to elevated intraocular or intracranial pressure.

When a patient complains of poor vision, it is important to ascertain if this is present in one or both eyes, at near or far distance, and with or without glasses, for reasons that are obvious to a physician, but not necessarily to the patient. A description of how the patient noticed the visual change can be helpful. For example, a patient may think he has sustained a sudden loss of vision when he covers one eye and discovers that the vision is poor in the other eye, although the vision loss in fact may have been slowly progressive but suddenly noticed. Similarly, most patients are not conscious of their visual fields, and if they have a transient loss of the left visual field resulting from a TIA, for example, they may interpret this as a loss of vision in the left eye, unless they checked the vision in each eye separately. In this example, the distinction, of course, is significant in differentiating between ocular or carotid artery disease versus cerebrocortical or vertebral artery disease. Patients who notice difficulty with reading may have poor near vision, but the complaint also can be caused by a scotoma from ocular or cerebral disease, by dyslexia from a stroke or by diminished mental faculties from Alzheimer's disease or other dementia states.

A scotoma, or loss of part of the visual field, always represents serious disease and warrants prompt evaluation. Uniocular scotomas are commonly caused by glaucoma or retinal disease. Binocular scotomas are commonly due to stroke or cerebral tumors.

Photopsia (flashing lights in the visual field) can be caused by migraine, but in the elderly, this symptom is commonly due to vitreous traction, which may be associated with developing retinal detachment. Photopsia requires ophthalmic evaluation.

Metamorphopsia, or distorted vision, is usually related to retinal disease, especially macular disease, although it can be caused by a cataract or by corneal disease. In the elderly patient, metamorphopsia should be cause for a prompt ophthalmologic examination, as it may indicate retinal pathology that is treatable only if detected early.

Diplopia (double vision) is pathologic. Binocular diplopia implies a misalignment of the eyes. Its onset in the elderly most frequently results from an extraocular muscle palsy caused by diabetes or vas-cular occlusion, although it has a wide variety of causes ranging from tumor to myasthenia gravis. Monocular diplopia is almost always caused by cataract or other opacity in the eye.

Burning, stinging, itching, and dryness are common ocular symptoms associated with irritation of the conjunctiva and cornea. In the absence of any visual symptoms and ocular inflammation or discharge, tear substitutes may be used for temporary relief. Itching, which is worsened by rubbing the eyes, is suggestive of an allergy.

Foreign-body sensation in the eye may be associated with corneal disease and warrants an evaluation with a slit lamp because this tissue is delicate, and damage to it can easily lead to loss of vision.

Deep pain in the eye itself is a serious symptom. It usually represents significant intraocular inflammation, which is potentially vision-threatening. Ocular inflammation usually also causes photophobia, that is, pain in the eye when exposed to light. Nonophthalmic problems in the distribution of the trigeminal nerve, caused by dental or sinus disease, for example, occasionally lead to referred pain in the eye.

Headache, even headache behind the eyes, is rarely related to ocular disease, unless it is associated with a concurrent decrease in vision. It is possible to develop a brow ache or headache from fatigue caused by prolonged use of the eyes when driving, reading, and so on. In this case, however, there will be a clear relationship between the headache and these activities. Often, this symptom is easily relieved by a change in eyeglass prescription or even by reassurance that the headache does not represent ocular disease.

In any elderly patient with headache, especially if there are associated symptoms of scalp tenderness, painful chewing, proximal myalgias, or weight loss, the diagnosis of temporal arteritis should be considered. This condition can lead to sudden, permanent visual loss if it is not treated with oral corticosteroids.

PRESBYOPIA

The shape of the lens of the eye can be altered by the action of the ciliary muscles, which allows a change in focus from distance to closeness. This is called accommodation. In a young child, the near point of accommodation is almost at the nose. With age, however, the lens becomes progressively harder and denser, and its shape is less able to change. This leads to a progressive inability to focus on near objects and, for the average person, leads to a need for reading glasses at about age 45. The process is progressive, and stronger reading glasses become necessary over time, requiring that the reading material be held closer to the eyes. Stronger reading glasses also have a narrower working range. For this reason, most persons are happiest when they do not change eyeglass prescriptions until they clearly need to because of fatigue with near work or because their "arms are too short."

CATARACT

In addition to becoming harder and denser with age, the lens of the eye also tends to become somewhat opaque. This is called cataract. Although some cataracts are associated with diseases, such as diabetes, or with drug toxicity (e.g., oral corticosteroids), the vast majority of cataracts are age-related or "senile" cataracts. Cataracts are very common with aging; the incidence of vision decrease caused by cataracts in the United States has been found to be 18 percent between ages 65 and 74 and 46 percent between ages 75 and 85.[1]

Generally, the only symptom caused by cataracts is blurred vision; however, depending on the type of cataract, the blurring may be worse at distance or at closeness. In all cases, cataract leads to increasing problems with glare, so that vision is ordinarily best in a moderately lit room and is worse in bright sunlight, when looking at someone in a doorway or against a window with light behind them, or when trying to see a traffic light against a bright sky. These examples suggest why patients with developing cataracts may function perfectly well in their own homes but still find their lifestyles substantially compromised. A cataract is best seen through a dilated pupil with a slit lamp microscope, but it can also be visualized

with an ophthalmoscope as a dark opacity in the red reflex from the retina.

Patients are often concerned about when the cataract should be removed. In rare cases, a cataract may need to be removed for medical reasons, but in more than 99 percent of cases, the only reason to remove a cataract is to permit the patient to see better. Because the results of cataract surgery are the same regardless of when it is performed, the patient can decide when to have surgery based on how he or she is functioning. Surgery is appropriate when the patient's lifestyle is affected. Clearly, this will be different for the active, driving, working patient than for the bedridden, nursing home resident.

Modern cataract surgery with intraocular lens implantation is ordinarily successful. Over 95 percent of patients with otherwise normal eyes achieve reading- and driving-quality vision. The surgery is usually performed in an outpatient setting and requires minimal postoperative restrictions. A description of this modern procedure is sometimes useful for an apprehensive patient who remembers a grandparent in bed for a week with sandbags around the head following cataract surgery.

TEAR DEFICIENCY

The cornea is not a naturally wettable surface. Although the tear film contains wetting agents and stabilizers (chiefly mucin and lipids), there is a definite tendency for the tear film to break up and for the cornea to dry. Continuous production of tears by the ocular adnexa and spreading of the tears over the cornea by blinking of the eyelids is necessary to keep the cornea comfortable and healthy.

Aging generally causes diminished tear secretion, that is, a decrease in the quality and quantity of the tears produced in a resting, nonirritated state. Although this is rarely severe enough to cause vision loss from corneal scarring, it commonly leads to a chronic feeling of dryness and burning in the eyes. The symptoms tend to be worse in artificial heat and when the humidity is low and are often exacerbated by reading, watching TV, or driving, caused by the decreased blinking rate during these activities. Dust, smoke, and fumes also increase irritation caused by tear deficiency.

Most patients with a tear deficiency find treatment less than satisfactory. Controlling the environment is difficult, and tear substitutes have a transient effect. Although ointments give more relief, they blur the vision. Often, the most a physician can do is to reassure the patient that the problem is not vision-threatening, although this advice may not be possible for patients with a severe tear deficiency associated with ocular pemphigoid and certain other pathologic states. A decrease in vision in a patient with tear deficiency is cause for prompt referral to an ophthalmologist because the tear deficient eye is particularly susceptible to infection.

EYELID PTOSIS

With age, the skin of the lids becomes thinner and wrinkled, and the subcutaneous tissues and ligaments become more lax. This leads to drooping lids. In the upper lid, the ptosis is usually a cosmetic concern, but occasionally, the lid will droop enough to cover part of the pupil and interfere with the upper visual field. (In such cases, third-party medical insurance payers may cover the cost of correction). In the lower lid, the laxity may lead to senile ectropion, in which the lid tends to fall away from the eye, leading to chronic tearing. This often causes the patient to wipe constantly at the eyes, exacerbating the problem. The patient with lid laxity should blot tears gently, pushing the lid up and in rather than wiping laterally, which tends to increase the problem. Although senile ectropion is unlikely to be vision-threatening, the chronic tearing and irritation of the exposed conjunctiva can be very annoying to the patient. The definitive treatment is lid surgery. Both ptosis of the upper lid and ectropion of the lower lid can result from pathologic processes such as third- or fifth-nerve palsies or tumors of the skin or meibomian glands.

VITREOUS FLOATERS AND RETINAL DETACHMENT

The major cavity of the eye, behind the lens and in front of the retina, contains a gel formed largely of collagen fibrils and hyaluronic acid. This is the vitreous humor. (The modern term is the vitreous body.) With advancing years, the gel normally separates into a watery component and clumps and strands of collagen. These are seen by patients as black specks and strands, often initially interpreted as being a fly or something else in the external environment. The floaters tend to come and go, but eventually move forward in the eye and settle out of the axis of vision and thus become less noticeable to the patient. They are innocuous, but annoying. As part of the same aging process, the collagen fibrils shrink and pull away from the retina. As they do so, they stimulate the retina and produce photopsia, usually in the periphery of the vision. Rarely, the retina will tear when the vitreous pulls on it, and a retinal detachment can occur as fluid leaks through the tear. In this case, the patient will have the sensation of a curtain or shade coming in from the periphery and obscuring his vision.

A retinal detachment is unlikely to be seen with the ordinary handheld ophthalmoscope because detachments usually start in the peripheral retina beyond the area that can be visualized with this instrument.

Any patient with a dramatic increase in floaters or photopsia in the vision should be warned about retinal detachment. An ophthalmologic examination should be performed promptly, since retinal detachment surgery is more successful when treated in its early stages.

MACULAR DEGENERATION

Only one portion of the retina is capable of high-grade, fine, discriminatory vision such as that needed for reading and driving. This is the macula. It subserves the central few degrees of the visual field. The remaining retina is capable only of perceiving relatively large objects. Unfortunately, the macula is prone to degenerative changes with aging. In the United States, age-related macular degeneration is the leading cause of new cases of legal blindness (i.e., vision of 20/200 or less) in patients over age 65. Its prevalence in the Framingham study was 9 percent.[2]

The visual result of macular degeneration is a central scotoma, a small spot in the center of the vision where objects are not well seen. Ordinarily, this is slowly progressive. At first, patients may have trouble only when reading; they may miss or confuse some letters in the words. Progressively, the scotoma enlarges, so that all of the central vision is gone, and activities such as reading and driving are quite impossible to perform. Patients will not be able to see the face of the person talking to them and will have to recognize people by their voices. This is, of course, devastating to the elderly patient especially because it is almost never treatable and is never reversible. Although the rate of change in macular degeneration is usually slow, it is always progressive. It may be asymmetric but is generally bilateral.

The only positive factor in this condition is that it is never completely blinding. The process is largely confined to the macular region, and the rest of the retina remains normal. Experience shows that most patients with macular degeneration maintain the ability to dress and groom themselves and generally function fairly well in a controlled, familiar environment such as their own homes. They usually do need assistance when away from familiar areas.

The diagnosis of macular degeneration is made with the ophthalmoscope. The earliest changes are drusen, yellowish spots in the macula, and clumping and dispersion of the retinal pigment epithelium. Later, the entire macula may be atrophic and scarred.

The vast majority of patients with age-related macular degeneration have a so-called dry form of the condition, which is untreatable. A few patients will develop vascular nets underneath the neurosensory retina, which can be treated with a laser to retard the progress of the disease. Because this possibility exists, all patients with macular degeneration should be examined by an ophthalmologist at least once.

Although magnifying lenses have limited value in macular degeneration, a low-vision clinic or sight center is often useful to the patient by offering various low-vision aids as well as counseling and support.

There is growing evidence that visible and ultraviolet radiation (UVR) can damage the retina over the years. It may be particularly sensible for patients with macular degeneration to avoid direct exposure to bright sunlight and to wear tinted sunglasses to exclude blue and ultraviolet light when they are outdoors.[3]

GLAUCOMA

Glaucoma is primarily a disease associated with aging; it is unusual in persons under the age of 40 and occurs with increasing frequency with increasing years. Approximately 11.5 million people in the United States have glaucoma.[4]

By definition, glaucoma is a disease manifest by increased pressure in the eye, leading to damage to the optic nerve and to loss of vision. If untreated, it leads to progressive and irreversible loss, first of peripheral vision and, finally, of central vision. With treatment, the damage and visual loss can ordinarily be arrested; however, an optic nerve that has been damaged by glaucoma is more susceptible to further damage. Therefore, it is important to detect glaucoma in its early stages.

Because patients are not aware of intraocular pressure, and self-monitoring devices do not exist, it is advisable that all adults have an annual intraocular pressure check as part of a complete eye examination. This is especially important for blacks, diabetic patients, and persons with a family history of glaucoma, all of whom are more likely to develop glaucoma as they become older.

The diagnosis of glaucoma is made on the basis of increased cupping of the optic nerve head associated with characteristic visual-field defects. If the disease is treated early, the only manifestation may be an elevated intraocular pressure, although elevated pressure alone usually is not diagnostic, as the general population shows a wide variation in intraocular pressure. If the patient falls into a high-risk group (for example, a patient with diabetes), the ophthalmologist may elect to treat on the basis of a suspiciously high pressure only.

Advanced glaucoma leads to a loss of the peripheral visual field. Some patients may maintain a small central field that allows them to read or watch TV quite well. However, they remain disabled by the peripheral field loss because it limits their ability to ambulate or, for example, to notice someone enter a room, unless they happen to be looking directly at the doorway. An impression of the effect of this deficit can be achieved by looking through a tube of cardboard or rolled paper and attempting to walk about, even in a familiar room.

Glaucoma is ordinarily treated with topical medications. Beta-blockers such as timolol are the first line of treatment, and miotics such as pilocarpine are used if further treatment is needed. The latter is less satisfactory because its use leads to problems with pupil adaptation to changing lighting conditions, especially in patients with some cataract. Epinephrine compounds have been found useful. Oral carbonic anhydrase inhibitors, laser treatment, or surgery may be necessary if topical medications do not control the pressure.

Regular use of medication is critical to prevent further eye damage in patients with glaucoma. Elderly, forgetful, and confused patients often require some help and support to remember to take medications. This is especially true when the medication is prophylactic, and there is no obvious, visual benefit noticed by the patient.

SOCIAL ASPECTS OF VISION LOSS

The major effect of diminishing vision in elderly patients is loss of independence. Sight-impaired patients need help with many activities, such as driving, reading, hobbies, and work, that gave them pleasure and reinforced feelings of competence and personal value. They may even have to give up some of these activities entirely and must learn to rely on others more than they have in the past. Consequently, they need to maintain, and even improve, their social skills. For some patients, this comes easily; for others, it is difficult, either because of ingrained personality traits or because of concomitant disabilities, especially deafness. In all cases, however, patients need a network of support to keep from withdrawing and becoming despondent.

Many sight-impaired patients are reluctant to ask for help for fear of being a burden or of being taken advantage of. It is important, therefore, that they be in an environment that is automatically supportive. This may be a nursing home or retirement facility, but support can often be effectively arranged at home if services are scheduled and reliable, and if communication is regular. The arrangement of these supports is generally beyond the responsibility of the physician, but he should be aware of the facilities available in the community so that he can refer patients and their families to the local sight center and social service agencies. In addition to the practical benefits (free phone directory assistance, Meals-on-Wheels, and so on), these efforts help patients to understand that they are not alone and that the community continues to care about them.

REFERENCES

1. Kahn HA, Leibowitz HM, Ganley JP, et al: The Framingham eye study: outline and major prevalence findings. Am J Epidemiol 106:17, 1977.
2. Framingham Monograph: Surv Ophthalmol (Suppl) 24:335, 1980.
3. Marshall J: Radiation and the aging eye. Ophthalmic Physiol Opt 51:241, 1985.
4. National Advisory Eye Council (US): Vision Research: a national plan, 1983–1987, Vol 1. Bethesda, National Institutes of Health, 1983.

CHAPTER 14

Hearing Problems

Richard H. Nodar

Old age doth in sharp pains abound;
We are belabored by the gout,
Our blindness is a dark profound,
Our deafness each one laughs about.
Then reason's light with falling ray
Doth but a trembling flicker cast.
Honor to age, ye children pay!
Alas! my fifty years are past!
                BÉRANGER, *Cinquante Ans.*

One of the most common responses from senior citizens when asked if they have hearing loss is, "I can hear, but I can't understand." There are many other retorts that usually suggest that people "mumble." These responses are understandable when one considers the effects of aging on the hearing mechanism.

Hearing loss associated with advancing age is labeled presbycusis (also presbyacusis and presbyacousis). It is usually bilateral, symmetric, and sensorineural. Auditory sensitivity is normal or near-normal in the low frequencies, with increasingly poorer sensitivity at frequencies above 1000 Hz (Fig. 14–1). If the hearing loss is not compounded by acoustic trauma, noise exposure, or previous pathologic conditions, its onset is gradual, almost insidious. This renders detection and acknowledgment difficult and resisted. Often, it is the patient's loved ones or coworkers who first notice the problem and recommend remediation.

Presbycusis usually begins to interfere with communication after 60 years of age. Because the individual can still detect low frequencies and certain consonants within normal tolerances, understanding in quiet is good or, at least, possible. However, two barriers to communication for the elderly are (1) background noise, and (2) distance. Either of these barriers is enough to frustrate attempts to communicate by two or more persons, although only one has the hearing loss. Consequently, the presbycusic person may tend to withdraw from participating in social situations, i.e., they become quiet at restaurants, wedding receptions, family gatherings, and so on.

CLINICAL PICTURE

A hearing test should be a part of the routine examination for patients over age 60. If a hearing test cannot be given, at least the following three questions should be asked when obtaining the patient's history: (1) "Do you have any history of hearing loss, noise exposure, or ear surgery?" (2) "Do you feel you have a hearing problem?," and (3) "Does your spouse think you have a hearing problem?" The most common answer to the third question is "Yes, but . . .", followed by an excuse blaming others for mumbling or an explanation of their own "concentration" on other things. Clinical experience indicates that if the mate believes a patient has a hearing loss, the mate is usually correct. In his work, Nodar lists typical responses to questions asked during the history taking.[3]

A complete audiologic evaluation will include *tympanometry*—a measure of middle-ear function; *pure-tone audiometry*—a test of auditory sensitivity across a range of frequencies from 125 Hz to 8000 Hz, including air-conduction and bone-conduction thresholds; *speech reception thresholds* (SRT)—a measure of the weakest level of understanding during continuous discourse; and *word discrimination scores* (WDS)—an assessment of the individual's ability to make fine speech discriminations when speech is loud enough for him to hear clearly.

The presbycusic patient will usually present with the following test results:

1. Normal tympanometric pressure peaks

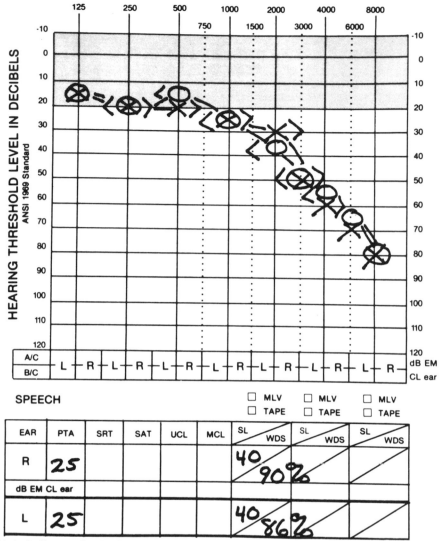

FIGURE 14–1. Audiogram showing binaural, symmetric high-frequency sensorineural hearing loss with bone conduction and air conduction thresholds interweaving. Also shown are the pure-tone averages and the word discrimination scores.

2. Acoustic reflexes at low and mid-frequencies and elevated or absent reflexes at high frequencies

3. Pure-tone thresholds within tolerance or at near-normal tolerance, with a loss of sensitivity in the high frequencies (see Fig. 14–1)

4. Interweaving air conduction and bone conduction scores (see Fig. 14–1)

5. Good agreement between the SRT and their respective pure-tone averages (three-frequency [.5,1,2 kHz] average for each ear)

6. Good to fair WDS for each ear (± 86 to 96 percent)

Naturally, abnormalities in any of the above tests merit an otolaryngologic con-sultation. Furthermore, if the diagnosis given by the otolaryngologist is presbycusis, and medical and surgical intervention is not recommended, rehabilitation in the form of hearing aids should be considered.

HEARING AIDS

Any device that assists the hearing-impaired individual to communicate with others is included in the broad classification of a hearing aid. However, the common notion suggests that a hearing aid is an electroacoustic device that amplifies sound. It is generally not true that a hearing aid cannot help an individual with a sensorineural hearing loss; this belief is, for most cases, erroneous and antiquated. Today, hearing aids have been developed to a degree that most senior citizens could benefit from them. However, it is important that they are properly fit by an audiologist and, in most cases, that patients wear two hearing aids. It should be noted that the three symptoms of a person with deafness in one ear are that (1) the patient cannot hear on the off side, (2) the patient cannot understand in a noise field, and (3) the patient cannot localize sound. If hearing-impaired persons are fitted with only one hearing aid, they will experience the same problems as persons with unilateral hearing loss. Ideally, the elderly patient should be fitted as soon as the hearing loss is detected. Hearing aids do not produce natural sounds; however, a gradual introduction to amplification is far easier for several reasons:

1. Hearing aids are complex and quite small. Manipulation of the controls, the battery, and the earmold (if necessary) will be easier at age 60 than at age 80.

2. As hearing sensitivity decreases, individuals "lose touch" with their acoustic environment. Once aided, a common complaint is, "This thing is noisy." Actually, our society is noisy, with air conditioners, background music, typing, and so on, and patients simply have not heard the background noise for a number of years.

3. Because low-frequency sensitivity is at or near normal, those frequencies are allowed to pass through a vent, permitting the patient to hear a combination of natural and amplified sounds, which is more pleasant than listening only to amplified sounds.

4. Acknowledgment of a hearing problem by patients is much easier on their families, coworkers, and others such as physicians and waitresses.

I tell my patients when everyone (including professionals) tells you that you have a hearing loss, and you deny it, you're only fooling one person. Today, hearing aids seem to carry a stigma akin to what spectacles suffered 50 years ago. I believe that professionals must help the hearing-impaired person to accept his hearing loss and to explore the benefits of amplification.

Phonemic Regression

This term was coined by Carhart to describe behavior in the elderly that appeared related to hearing but could not be explained on the basis of hearing loss.[1] Elderly individuals with normal thresholds up to 2 kHz did not do well in certain speech tests if tests were recorded and hurried. Given time, the elderly patient may respond correctly. Furthermore, if instructions were given in short, uncomplicated, unhurried sentences, understanding was clearer. Davis felt that generalized cerebral arteriosclerosis is probably the most common cause of misinterpreted responses.[1] If an elderly person appears confused, slow down and speak clearly in shorter sentences. In addition, give the individual a little more time to reply than you would give a 20-year-old.

Tinnitus

Tinnitus, or ringing in one or both ears, often accompanies presbycusis. The single term, tinnitus, is used to describe a multiplicity of auditory experiences, such as ringing, buzzing, hissing, and cricket-type sounds. It is not unusual for a presbycusic patient to present with a primary complaint of tinnitus, although a hearing loss is present as well. In most cases, hearing aids will be very beneficial in the relief from tinnitus because they raise the "noise floor," obscuring the tinnitus as well as facilitate communication.

CONCLUSION

The auditory system is our primary vehicle for communication. Hearing permits us to constantly scan our environment for danger or for any novel change within a circumscribed area—even when we are asleep. We tend to take hearing for granted because we cannot close our ears and experience deafness as we can close our eyes and experience blindness. In addition to interaction with others, hearing permits us to interact and react to events nearby. Our ears can "see" behind us, around corners, through walls, ceilings, and floors. Detection of malfunctioning machinery (e.g., automobiles and printers) is often a result of detecting an unusual sound.

The hearing-impaired individual is hampered not only by face-to-face communication but also by telephone, radio, and television use, an inability to hear digital watch alarms, tea kettles, doorbells, emergency vehicle sirens, and many other signals. Therefore, understanding, sympathy, and appropriate referral are indicated whenever hearing loss is present. Unfortunately, most physicians know very little about hearing loss and hearing aids and when to recommend them. Referrals to audiologists for assessment, otologists to exclude active pathology, and audiologists for rehabilitation are most appropriate.

REFERENCES

1. Nodar RH: The effects of aging and loud music on hearing. Cleve Clin Q 53:49, 1986.
2. Lichtenstein MJ, Bess FH, Logan FA, et al: Validation of screening tools for identifying hearing-impaired elderly in primary care. JAMA 259:2875, 1988.
3. Nodar RH: Hearing loss and hearing aids. Generations XII, 1:39–40, Fall 1987.
4. Davis H, Silverman SR: Hearing and Deafness. New York, Holt, Rinehart and Winston, 1947.

CHAPTER 15

Oral and Dental Problems

Steven R. Gordon

Last scene of all,
That ends this strange, eventful history,
Is second childishness, and mere oblivion,
Sans teeth, sans eyes, sans taste, sans everything.
SHAKESPEARE, *As You Like It*

TOOTH LOSS

Historically, the elderly have been characterized as being edentulous. Paintings, photographs, and even quotations from Shakespeare have promoted this image of aging. Whereas in years past this may have been accurate, the picture is changing to one of an increasingly dentulous older population. This dramatic shift results, in large part, from advances in public dental health including education of the public, availability of dental care, and fluoridation of water supplies. From 1957 to 1971, the percentage of edentulous persons in the United States over 65 years old decreased from more than 60 percent to approximately 51 percent.[1, 2] The most recent national data available indicate that this downward trend had continued to 41 percent in the 1985–1986 period, although the latter study evaluated only the elderly who were employed or who had visited community senior citizens centers.[3] The older and poorer elderly have higher rates of edentulism, so 41 percent is probably an underestimate of the current level of edentulousness.[2, 3] As further evidence of the continuing decline in toothlessness, only 32 percent of the elderly aged 65 to 69 years old were found to be edentulous, compared with 49 percent of those age 80 and over. Similar trends were found in two recent statewide oral health surveys in Iowa and North Carolina.[4, 5]

As the percentage and number of elderly with remaining natural teeth increase, it follows that the prevalence of dental diseases associated with natural teeth, such as dental caries and periodontal disease, will also increase.

DENTAL CARIES

Dental caries is a process of progressive tooth surface destruction associated with the presence of bacterial plaque on the tooth surface. Demineralization occurs in response to acid produced by the bacteria after exposure to sucrose and other sugars. Conditions that facilitate this scenario contribute to the formation of dental caries, and include poor oral hygiene, which allows bacterial plaque to build up on tooth surfaces, and diets with significant amounts of refined carbohydrates, which cause production of acids by these bacteria.

There are two general types of caries. *Coronal caries* initiates in the enamel-covered crown of the tooth, and *root caries* initiates in the cementum covering the root (Fig. 15–1). In addition, caries is described as being primary when a previously unblemished surface develops dental decay and as secondary, or recurrent, when decay starts adjacent to a previously placed dental restoration.

Caries has traditionally been viewed as of only minor significance in the elderly. This belief was supported by data from national surveys (1960–1962 and 1971–1974). Both surveys reported prevalence rates of only 0.5 to 0.7 carious teeth per dentate individual between 65 and 69 years of age.[6, 7] The 1985–1986 National Institute of Dental Research (NIDR) survey also found only 0.66 decayed teeth per person in the population aged 65 and older.[3] Despite these low numbers, there is evidence that caries continues to be a significant problem in this age group. If the incidence of caries is considered per number of remaining teeth rather than per

129

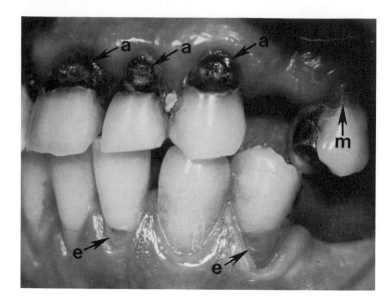

FIGURE 15–1. *Root surface caries: e (early), m (moderate), a (advanced).*

person, the prevalence in the elderly is actually higher than that in younger adults.[3, 8]

By any measure, root surface caries is far more prevalent in the elderly than in younger age groups. The rate per person is 3.75 times greater, whereas the rate per tooth is more than 5 times greater in the older population.[3] Although problems with poor oral hygiene and cariogenic diets can occur in patients of all ages, some predisposing factors are more commonly found among the elderly.

Gingival recession is one such predisposing factor. Root surfaces normally covered and protected by bone and gingiva in the healthy mouth are exposed to the oral environment as a result of gingival recession. Cementum, which forms the surface layer of the root, is more vulnerable to dental caries than enamel, which covers the crown of the tooth.[9] That surface vulnerability, combined with the more difficult problems of oral hygiene around exposed roots, helps to explain the high prevalence of root surface caries in older individuals. Banting and coworkers found that 83 percent of a group of institutionalized older persons with gingival recession had some root surface caries. Ninety percent of the group had gingival recession.[10]

Decreased salivary flow is another predisposing factor for root surface caries.[11] Although research is still being done on the relationship between salivation and advanced age, current knowledge indicates that parotid gland flow does not decrease.[12, 13] Recent evidence has shown that salivation of the submandibular gland and the minor salivary gland may diminish with age.[14, 15] Factors other than normal aging appear to be far more important causes of xerostomia in the elderly. Many medications, including antidepressants, antipsychotics, tranquilizers, antihistamines, decongestants, antihypertensives, diuretics, antineoplastics, and antispasmodics, cause diminished salivation as a side effect.[16] Radiation therapy to the salivary glands or adjacent structures, sicca syndrome, and general dehydration can also cause diminished salivation.

This major change in the oral environment can potentially decrease the diluting and cleansing effects of saliva. Some artificial saliva substitutes are commercially available to help alleviate the symptoms associated with xerostomia, but successful use of these agents requires extremely motivated patients willing to reapply the solution orally approximately every 30 minutes. Pilocarpine HCl (5 mg tid) has been suggested to systemically treat xerostomia from Sjögren's syndrome, head and neck radiation therapy, and idiopathic xerostomia.[17a] In the absence of meticulous oral hygiene, patients suffering from diminished salivation are at risk for dental caries.

PERIODONTAL DISEASE

Periodontal disease causes progressive inflammatory destruction of the anatomic structures surrounding the roots of teeth and is thought to result from bacteria on the teeth adjacent to the sites of destruction. Red, edematous gingiva that bleeds easily around the teeth is thought to be a sign of gingival and periodontal disease. Periodontitis is commonly associated with poor oral hygiene and leads to gingival recession, increased tooth mobility, and, ultimately, tooth loss (Fig. 15–2). Although symptomatic abscesses or acute infection can accompany periodontitis, like caries, it generally is asymptomatic until well advanced.

The early stages of periodontal disease are extremely common in older persons. In the 1985–1986 national survey of dental health, 88 percent of the dentate elderly had some gingival recession, and almost 50 percent had some area of bleeding gingiva. Advanced disease is also not uncommon. Approximately one third of the patients in the survey had suffered 6 mm or more of vertical bone loss in at least one of the dental test sites examined.[3] A number of authors have suggested that periodontal disease is responsible for more tooth extractions during middle and late adulthood than any other cause.[17, 18]

The earlier the signs and symptoms of periodontal disease are noted and evaluated and preventive therapy begun, the better the prognosis is for retaining the tooth. Possible treatments for periodontal disease range from thorough cleaning of the teeth and root surfaces with or without minor gum surgery to extraction of roots and teeth. For elderly patients, conservative therapies are more commonly advocated.

COMPLETE DENTURES

Although the percentage of elderly who are edentulous has dropped, the total number of persons in the United States over the age of 65 has risen by an even greater rate during the same period. Thus, there are actually more older people using dentures today than in the past. At best, dentures are a poor substitute for natural teeth. The continuous process of resorption of the alveolar ridges underlying the dentures causes a progressive loss of stability and retention after the dentures are made. This loss of bone height, combined with normal wear of the chewing surfaces of the teeth, eventually causes a loss in apparent facial height (i.e., vertical dimension of occlusion) when the upper and lower teeth are closed together. The consequent exaggerated creasing at the corners of the mouth, compression of the lips, and protrusion of the chin can make long-time denture users appear considerably older than their chronologic age (Fig. 15–3).

Use of poorly fitting dentures can cause both reversible and irreversible damage to

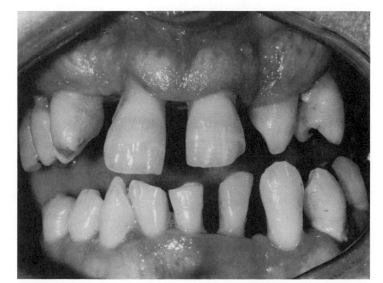

FIGURE 15–2. Periodontal disease associated with gingival recession and increased tooth mobility.

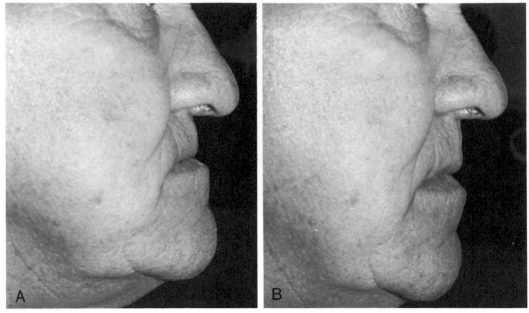

FIGURE 15–3. A, *Dentures with inadequate vertical dimension of occlusion result in exaggerated creasing at corners of mouth, compression of lips, and protrusion of chin, making patient appear older.* B, *New dentures for same patient create more youthful appearance.*

the supporting mucosa and bone.[19] Often asymptomatic, these physical changes generally go unnoticed by the denture user. Denture adhesives can accelerate this process both by masking the real problem of poor fit and by overfilling the potential space between denture and underlying mucosa, causing pressure that speeds resorption of soft tissue and bone.

Steps can be taken to prevent and correct some of these degenerative changes. As a general rule, individuals using dentures should see a dentist at least once a year. Dentures that are becoming loose but still have adequate appearance and chewing (occlusal) surfaces in contact can be relined to improve the fit. Relief of some localized areas of irritation can be achieved by making minor adjustments to the dentures; however, dentures with multiple problems generally should be remade.

Denture users should develop the following daily habits to optimize oral health:[19]

1. All edentulous individuals should thoroughly clean their mouths at least once a day. This can be done most conveniently with a soft toothbrush or facecloth used on all intraoral surfaces that come in contact with the dentures.

2. Dentures should be removed and rinsed after each meal and cleaned thoroughly with a brush at least once a day.

3. Dentures should be removed from the mouth for at least several hours each day; while sleeping at night is probably most convenient. The dentures should soak in clean water or in a standard denture cleanser when not in the mouth.[19]

USE OF DENTAL SERVICES

Despite the high levels of dental service needed by all categories of elderly individuals, use of services has historically remained low. National data from 1957 to 1975 indicate that the elderly made fewer dental visits on average than any other adult age group.[20] This was confirmed most recently by the 1985–1986 NIDR survey, which found that 37.5 percent of the elderly had seen a dentist within the previous 12 months, compared with 58.5 percent of 18- to 64-year-olds.[3] More revealing is a comparison of dentulous and edentulous elderly. Whereas 54.5 percent of older dentate individuals had dental service during the same period, the utilization rate was only 13.0 percent for the edentulous elderly. In fact, 49.1 percent of this edentulous group had not had a dental visit in more than 5 years. As may be expected, the older and poorer elderly saw a dentist even less frequently than the younger or wealthier elderly.[1] Close to 51 percent of the highest income group of elderly reported a dental visit in 1975, compared with 16.5 percent of the lowest income group.

Wealthier, younger, and more dentulous elderly do not have more dental problems than the poorer, older, edentulous elderly, so it is clear that the need for dental care is not a good predictor of demand for care. Because early and middle stages of dental caries, periodontal disease, and even oral cancer are often asymptomatic (as are many denture problems) oral discomfort is a relatively infrequent motivator to seek dental care. Most public dental health investigators now feel that lack of perceived need for care is the best explanation for the low use of dental services by the elderly.[21]

ORAL PATHOLOGY

The incidence of oral pathology increases with age (Fig. 15–4).[22, 23] In the United States, it represents 5 percent of all malignancies in men and 2 percent in

women; it is even more common in other parts of the world, representing as much as 70 percent of all malignancies in some areas of the Far East.[22, 24] In general, 75 percent of patients with oral cancer survive 5 years, if lesions are small and localized, but this decreases to only 25 percent if regional lymph node involvement has occurred.[24] The prognosis for older individuals is worse (Fig. 15–4).[23] Similar to skin cancer, early detection allows the best chance for a positive outcome. Over 90 percent of oral malignancies are squamous cell carcinoma, and they can appear on any oral mucosal surface (Fig. 15–5).[22] Age, tobacco use, and alcohol consumption have been associated with the incidence of oral cancer, and other factors such as poor dentition have also been suggested.[25, 26]

ORAL EXAMINATIONS

Changing or eliminating risk factors such as tobacco use and alcohol consumption is difficult, and changing the risk factor of advanced age is impossible. The best hope for minimizing the significant morbidity and mortality associated with oral cancer is frequent, regular oral examinations. Unfortunately, as noted, the ma-

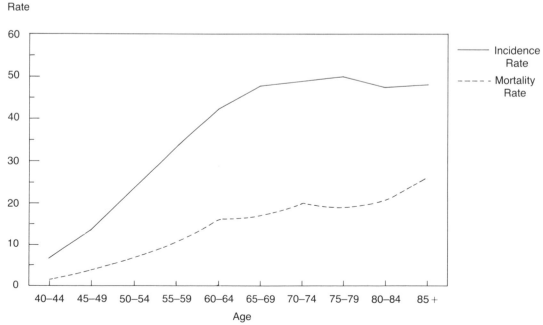

FIGURE 15–4. Incidence and mortality rates/100,000 population for cancer of the buccal cavity and pharynx.

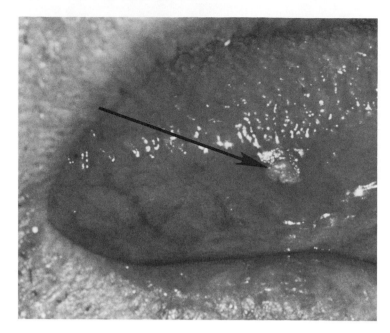

FIGURE 15–5. Squamous cell carcinoma on lateral border of tongue.

jority of elderly persons, especially those who are edentulous, fail to seek dental care regularly. They do continue to seek physician care, however. A national study from 1974 to 1976 found that whereas 78.7 percent of elderly persons visited a physician during a 12-month period, only 29.5 percent saw a dentist.[27] To encourage oral examinations, it would be beneficial for physicians to simply recommend to their patients that they see a dentist every 2 to 3 months for individuals at greatest risk for disease to every 12 months for others. Unfortunately, many barriers, such as cost, fear, and lack of transportation, prevent some elderly from seeking dental care. For the benefit of these patients, it is important that the physician be able to perform oral screening examinations; techniques for accomplishing this have been described for both edentulous and dentulous patients.[19, 28]

QUALITY OF LIFE

In addition to oral pathology that is life-threatening, oral disease has several important consequences that can potentially affect quality of life. These include chewing ability, appearance, phonetics, and subsequent need for dental treatment.

There is general agreement that decreased quality of natural dentition is associated with decreased chewing ability, despite high individual variation.[29, 30] Previous research has stongly suggested that the number of teeth with contact of occlusal surfaces when the jaws meet is correlated with masticatory efficiency, especially in the posterior segments.[31] Thus, as teeth are lost and not replaced, the ability to chew efficiently is diminished. Fortunately, fixed bridges that are cemented in place act much like intact natural teeth for masticatory efficiency. Removable partial dentures effect only a partial improvement in masticatory performance, which is still inferior to that produced with intact natural dentition.[32, 33] Masticatory efficiency with complete dentures is inferior to that with intact natural dentition; dentures are reported to be one sixth as efficient.[34, 35]

Despite these documented decreases in masticatory performance associated with tooth loss, the effect on diet is unclear. Masticatory efficiency has been studied exhaustively with test foods, but the reports on the relationship between performance and dietary selection and nutritional status are conflicting. Research from the Veterans' Administration Longitudinal Study on Normative Aging has shown that subjective estimates of food preference are associated with perceived ease of chewing.[33, 34] This suggests that diet may change as a result of self-perceived chewing problems, and evidence was found to support this among a group of very elderly, independently living persons.[36]

Unreplaced missing teeth can present aesthetic and phonetic problems. Even when restored, only the most carefully made prostheses, either fixed or removable, do not look like artificial replacements. Problems with aesthetics and phonetics are tolerated or go unnoticed by some denture users; however, these problems can consciously or unconsciously affect image and dignity of users in the eyes of others. Family, friends, and health caregivers may react negatively to these problems.

RECENT DEVELOPMENTS

Although dental implants have been in use since the 16th century (with varying degrees of success), progress in this area during the past 20 years has attracted much recent public attention. There are currently three types of dental implants: endosteal, subperiosteal, and transosteal, which have in common the function of supporting or stabilizing dental prostheses such as bridges or dentures. All require surgery to place them into or on the mandible or maxilla, sometimes necessitating general anesthesia. Several techniques require more than one surgical procedure before the dental prostheses can be started. The implant substructures in contact with the bone are made with a variety of materials, ranging from ceramics and hydroxyapatite to pure titanium. Only one of these techniques, involving endosseous titanium posts, has been classified as "provisionally acceptable" by the American Dental Association Council on Dental Materials, Instruments, and Equipment. By carefully selecting implant recipients, the developers of this technique have demonstrated a success rate of more than 90 percent over 5 years.[37] No one technique is appropriate for all situations, and there are some osseous sites that cannot be restored with any of the techniques currently in use. Many older individuals with missing teeth could be helped by dental implants, but the high cost and surgical risk greatly limit their application, even where the oral anatomy would be favorable. In addition, individuals who have lost teeth through dental neglect must become sufficiently motivated to maintain these implants with immaculate oral hygiene. However, it appears that the rapid developments in implant dentistry will eventually yield clinically useful techniques for many older patients.

Progress in preventive dentistry, although less dramatic than progress with implants, is of much greater use and has far wider public health care implications. For older adults, most attention has focused on topical rinses and gels containing fluoride or chlorhexidine gluconate.

Fluorides for topical use come in many formulations. Those designed for home use are less concentrated than the fluoride solutions applied professionally by the dentist or dental hygienist. When used at least once a day, these home rinses are extremely effective in preventing new caries and in arresting and remineralizing early carious lesions (Fig. 15–6).[38] Because the salivation rate is considerably lower during sleep, the most effective time to apply the fluoride solutions is at bedtime.

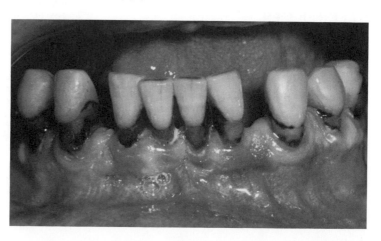

FIGURE 15–6. Brown areas on roots of teeth are early carious lesions, which remineralized following aggressive home use of fluoride gel.

After approximately 2 weeks, an equilibrium level of intraoral fluoride is established that remains consistent between daily fluoride applications.[39] Wescott and coworkers reported that by using a 0.4 percent stannous fluoride gel self-applied daily at bedtime, a 100 percent reduction in teeth "amputated" at the gingival margin because of deep caries and a 99 percent reduction in additional carious surfaces among patients who have had orofacial irradiation occurred.[40] This group of patients ordinarily demonstrates an extremely high caries rate because of the severe xerostomia resulting from radiation to the salivary glands. There is evidence that fluorides are effective even in the presence of dental microbial plaque.[41, 42] The use of topical fluoride rinses and gels is widely accepted as an effective means for preventing dental caries in adults. They hold great promise for populations of the elderly at particular risk for dental caries associated with orofacial irradiation and for institutionalized individuals.

Chlorhexidine, another effective adjunct to regular daily oral hygiene, has recently received USFDA approval as a mouthrinse to treat and prevent gingivitis. In a 6-month trial using 0.12 percent chlorhexidine gluconate mouthrinse in adults, Grossman and colleagues found reductions of 37 percent in the occurrence of gingivitis, 39 percent in the severity of gingivitis, 44 percent in bleeding owing to gingivitis, and 61 percent in amount of dental microbial plaque.[43] Chlorhexidine and some of the more concentrated fluoride solutions for home use are available by prescription only.

REFERENCES

1. Bureau of Economic Research and Statistics: Utilization of dental services by the elderly population. Chicago, American Dental Association, 1979.
2. National Center for Health Statistics: Edentulous Persons, United States, 1971. Vital and Health Statistics Series 10, No 89. US DHEW Pub No (HRA) 74–1516, June 1974.
3. National Institute for Dental Research: Oral health of United States adults. The national survey of oral health in the US: employed adults and seniors: 1985–1986. US DHHS, NIH Pub No 87–2868, August 1987.
4. Ettinger RL, Beck JD, and Jacobsen J: Removable prosthodontic treatment needs: a survey. J Prosthet Dent 51:419, 1984.
5. Schonfeld WH, Warren-Hicks D: Estimating the need for dental care and dental health manpower in North Carolina. In Bawden JW, DeFriese GH, eds: Planning for Dental Care on a Statewide Basis. Chapel Hill, Dental Foundation of North Carolina, 1981, p 122.
6. National Center for Health Statistics: Decayed, missing, and filled teeth in adults, United States, 1960–62. Series 11, No 23. DHEW Pub No 1000. Washington, 1967.
7. National Center for Health Statistics: Decayed, missing, and filled teeth among persons 1–74 years, United States. Series 11, No 223, US DHHS Pub No 81–1673. Hyattsville, MD, 1981.
8. Glass RL, Alman JE, Chauncey HH: A ten year longitudinal study of caries incidence rates in a sample of US male adults. Caries Res 21:360, 1987.
9. Hoppenbrouwers PMM, Driessens FCM, Borggreven JMPM, et al: The vulnerability of unexposed human dental roots to demineralization. J Dent Res 65:955, 1986.
10. Banting DW, Ellen RP, Fillery ED: Prevalence of root surface caries among institutionalized older persons. Community Dent Oral Epidemiol 8:84, 1980.
11. Ravald N, Hamp SE: Prediction of root surface caries in patients treated for advanced periodontal disease. J Clin Periodontol 8:400, 1981.
12. Baum BJ: Evaluation of stimulated parotid saliva flow rate in different age groups. J Dent Res 60:1292, 1981.
13. Chauncey HH, Borkan G, Wayler A, et al: Parotid fluid composition in healthy aging males. Adv Physiol Sci 28:323, 1981.
14. Pedersen W, Shubert M, Izutsu K, et al: Age dependent decreases in human submandibular gland flow rates as measured under resting and post-stimulation conditions. J Dent Res 64:822, 1985.
15. Gandara B, Izutsu K, Truelove E, et al: Salivary characteristics in patients with oral lichen planus. J Dent Res (Spec Iss) 64:378, 1985.
16. Handelman SL, Baric JM, Espeland MA, et al: Prevalence of drugs causing hyposalivation in an institutionalized geriatric population. Oral Surg 62:26, 1986.
17. Spolsky VW: The epidemiology of gingival and periodontal disease. In Carranza FA, ed: Glickman's Clinical Periodontology, 5th ed. Philadelphia, WB Saunders Co, 1979, p 346.
17a. Fox PC, Atkinson JC, Macynski A, et al: Pilocarpine for treatment of salivary hypofunction: A six-month trial. J Dent Res (Spec Iss) 68:315, 1989.
18. Amsterdam M, Abrams L: Periodontal prosthesis. In Goldman HM, Cohen DE, eds: Periodontal Therapy, 5th ed. St Louis, CV Mosby Co, 1973, p 977.
19. Gordon SR, Jahnigen DW: Oral assessment of the edentulous elderly patient. J Amer Geriatr Soc 31:797, 1983.
20. National Center for Health Statistics, National Health Survey Series B; Vital and Health Statistics Series 10. In Bureau of Economic Research and Statistics: Utilization of dental services by the elderly population. Chicago, American Dental Association, 1979.
21. Bailit HL, Wilson AA: Dental services in the elderly population. In Holm-Pedersen P, Loe H,

eds: Geriatric Dentistry. Copenhagen, Munksgaard Int Pubs Ltd, 1986, p 386.

22. Bhaskar SN: Synopsis of Oral Pathology, 5th ed. St Louis, CV Mosby Co, 1977.

23. National Institutes of Health: Surveillance, epidemiology, and end results: incidence and mortality data, 1973–77. NIH Pub No 81–2330. Washington, US GPO 1981, p 66.

24. Shklar, G: Oral pathology in the aging individual. In Toga CJ, Nandy K, and Chauncey HH, eds: Geriatric Dentistry. Lexington, Massachusetts, Lexington Books, DC Heath & Co, 1979, p 127.

25. Katz RV, Meskin LH: The epidemiology of oral diseases in older adults. In Holm-Pedersen P, Loe H, eds: Geriatric Dentistry. Copenhagen, Munksgaard Int Pubs Ltd, 1986, p 221.

26. Graham S, Dayal H, Rohrer T, et al: Dentition, diet, tobacco, and alcohol in the epidemiology of oral cancer. J Natl Cancer Inst 59:1611, 1977.

27. National Center for Health Statistics: State estimates of disability and utilization of medical services. Hyattsville, Maryland, DHEW Pub No 78–1241 (PHS), 1978.

28. Gordon SR, Jahnigen DW: Oral assessment of the dentulous elderly patient. J Amer Geriatr Soc 34:276, 1986.

29. Manly RS, Braley LC: Masticatory performance and efficiency. J Dent Res 29:448, 1950.

30. Yurkstas AA: The effect of missing teeth on masticatory performance and efficiency. J Prosthet Dent 4:120, 1954.

31. Manly RS, Shiere F: The effect of dental deficiency on mastication and food preference. Oral Surg 3:674, 1950.

32. Abel LF, Manly RS: Masticatory function of partial denture patients among Navy personnel. J Prosthet Dent 3:382, 1953.

33. Wayler AH, Muench ME, Kapur KK, et al: Masticatory performance and food acceptability in persons with removable partial dentures, full dentures, and intact natural dentition. J Gerontol 39:284, 1984.

34. Chauncey HH, Muench M, Kapur K, et al: The effect of the loss of teeth on diet and nutrition. Int Dent J 34:98, 1984.

35. Kapur KK, Soman S: Masticatory performance and efficiency in denture wearers. J Prosthet Dent 14:687, 1964.

36. Gordon SR, Kelley SL, Sybyl JR, et al: Relationship in very elderly veterans of nutritional status, self-perceived chewing ability, dental status and social isolation. J Amer Geriatr Soc 33:334, 1985.

37. Adell R, Lekholm U, Rockler B, et al: A 15 year study of osseointegrated implants in the treatment of the edentulous jaw. Int J Oral Surg 6:387, 1981.

38. Billings RJ, Brown LR, Kaster AG, et al: Clinical and microbiologic evaluation of contemporary treatment strategies for root surface dental caries. Gerodontics 1:20, 1985.

39. Duckworth RM, Morgan SN, Murray AM: Fluoride in saliva and plaque following use of fluoride-containing mouthwashes. J Dent Res 66:1730, 1987.

40. Wescott WB, Starcke EN, Shannon IL: Chemical protection against post-irradiation dental caries. Oral Surg 40:709, 1975.

41. Yankell SL, Stoller NH, Green PA, et al: Clinical effects of using stannous fluoride mouthrinses during a five-day study in the absence of oral hygiene. J Periodont Res 17:374, 1982.

42. Tinanoff N, Klock B, Camosci DA, et al: Microbiologic effects of SnF_2 and NaF mouthrinse in subjects with high caries activity: results after one year. J Dent Res 62:907, 1983.

43. Grossman E, Reiter G, Sturzenberger OP, et al: Six-month study of the effects of chlorhexidine mouthrinse on gingivitis in adults. J Periodont Res 16:33, 1986.

CHAPTER 16

Geriatric Dermatology

James E. Fitzpatrick
J. Ramsey Mellette, Jr.

As a white candle
In a holy place,
So is the beauty
Of an aged face.
JOSEPH CAMPBELL, The Old Woman

The study of dermatologic diseases in the elderly requires a basic knowledge of structural changes that occur in aging skin and their impact on function. It is important to discriminate between intrinsic changes caused by aging and secondary changes caused by internal influences (i.e., hormonal changes) or external influences (e.g., sun exposure).

Intrinsic changes of the epidermis include a slight decrease in thickness associated with a decrease in corneocyte adhesion and an increase in cytoarchitectural disarray of keratinocytes. Functionally, these alterations result in impaired barrier function, which makes geriatric skin more prone to dryness and irritant contact dermatitis. Important appendageal changes include a decrease in the total number of eccrine glands, resulting in impaired thermoregulation, and an androgen-mediated decrease in the total number of hair follicles. This is not functionally important, but cosmetically, it often has a negative impact on both self-image and society's perception of the individual.

Melanocytes are also often lost from the hair bulb, resulting in graying of the hair. The dermis becomes relatively thinner, acellular, and avascular. It has been calculated that the total amount of collagen in the dermis decreases at a rate of 1 percent per year throughout adult life.

These changes result in susceptibility to injury and impaired injury response. Subcutaneous fat tends to atrophy in acral areas, subjecting underlying tissues to injury and hypertrophy in selected truncal areas such as the waist in men and the thighs in women. These are changes that our society regards as cosmetically undesirable.[1]

The most important *extrinsic changes* result from cumulative exposure of the skin to ultraviolet radiation (UVR) from the sun. Darker skin, which produces more melanin, is less likely to demonstrate severe changes because of melanin's protective effect. Chronic solar damage has a profound effect on both the epidermis and dermis. Epidermal changes include atrophy, dyspigmentation, and epithelial dysplasia; the last change may result in the development of malignancies. In the dermis, chronic sun exposure damages fibroblasts, which respond with the production of an abnormal elastotic material known as solar elastosis. The presence of this material, combined with epidermal changes, produces most of the age-related skin changes including dyspigmentation and a leathery texture with overlying wrinkles (Fig. 16–1).[2, 3]

Survey studies have demonstrated that skin diseases are more common in the elderly than in the general population. Results have varied, depending on the population surveyed, but in general, the most common complaint is pruritus (29 percent), and the most common dermatoses are solar elastosis, xerosis, dermatophytoses, senile purpura, contact dermatitis, and seborrheic dermatitis. The most common benign skin tumors are seborrheic keratoses, cherry hemangiomas, nevi, acrochordons, and sebaceous hyperplasia. The most common premalignant

The opinions or assertions contained herein are the views of the authors and are not to be considered as reflecting the views of the Department of the Army or the Department of Defense.

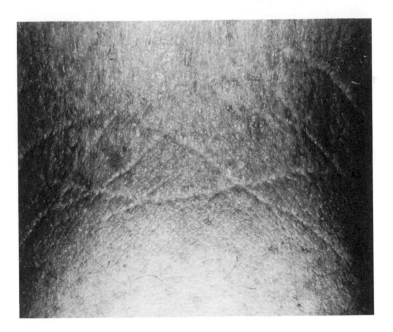

FIGURE 16–1. *Cutis rhomboidalis nuchae. Leathery skin, wrinkles, and dyspigmentation on sun-exposed skin on the back of the neck. Note the more normal appearing skin at the base of the neck.*

tumor is actinic keratoses, and the most common malignant tumors are basal cell carcinomas, followed by squamous cell carcinomas and malignant melanomas.[4, 5]

COMMON INFLAMMATORY SKIN CONDITIONS

Xerosis

Xerosis or dry skin is perhaps the most common dermatosis and a frequent cause of pruritus in the elderly population.[5] Loss of sebaceous and eccrine function probably plays an important role, but other factors including diminished corneocyte adhesion are also important. Xerosis is more prevalent during the winter and is characterized by dry white scale that is usually more severe on the extremities. Fissure formation is variable, but in severe cases they may become widened and inflamed, producing a condition called erythema craquelé. Xerosis is best treated by avoiding irritants such as highly alkaline soaps and by hydrating the skin followed by applying an emollient. Severe cases may require the application of emollients containing lactic acid or one of its salts.

Seborrheic Dermatitis

Seborrheic dermatitis is named for its tendency to occur in areas of high seba-

ceous activity. The most common locations are the scalp, ears, eyebrows, sides of the nose, and the sternal area. Occasional cases may be more extensive. The primary lesion is erythema, associated with variable white scale, but in some cases, the scale may have a yellow, greasy appearance. The etiology has not been established, but recent studies have suggested that seborrheic dermatitis may be a host response to *Malassezia ovalis*, a yeast normally found in large numbers in the scale. Glabrous, or non-hairy, skin is usually treated with 1 percent hydrocortisone cream, but broad-spectrum topical antifungal agents (ketoconazole and miconazole) have also been used.[6] If stronger corticosteroid creams are required, the diagnosis should be reassessed. Hair-bearing areas are usually managed with topical keratolytics, tar preparations, and cytostatic shampoos (zinc pyrithione and selenium sulfide).

Acne Rosacea

Acne rosacea is a common condition (up to 12 percent incidence in some studies) often seen in patients with seborrheic dermatitis.[4] It is a chronic inflammatory acneiform eruption that typically involves the mid-face, with the forehead and chin also affected at times. In milder forms of the disease, there is slight flushing in

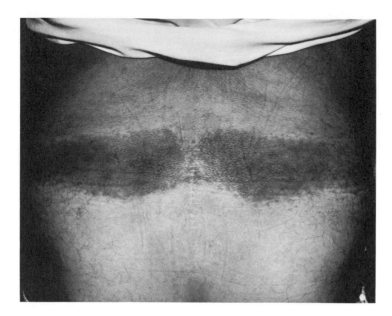

FIGURE 16–2. *Allergic contact dermatitis. Erythema secondary to allergy to chemical compounds in elastic waistband of underwear.*

affected areas associated with variable hyperplasia of the sebaceous glands. In some cases, the sebaceous hyperplasia tends to affect the distal half of the nose and may change the contour, producing a condition called rhinophyma. In more severe cases, acneiform papules and pustules may be present. The inflammation is usually treated with topical agents (erythromycin or clindamycin) or oral antibiotics (tetracycline), but occasionally, topical sulfur medications or mild corticosteroids are used. Rhinophyma is best treated by surgical ablation.[7]

Contact Dermatitis

Contact dermatitis may develop secondary to either an irritant or an allergic contact mechanism. Structural changes in the aged skin, with resultant impairment of the barrier function, make the elderly more prone to this condition. The most common irritants are alkaline soaps and over-the-counter astringents. Irritant dermatitis usually occurs rapidly following application and often burns or stings, but it may also be pruritic. It rarely blisters and typically does not extend past the site of application.

Allergic contact dermatitis is often indistinguishable from irritant contact dermatitis. Allergic contact dermatitis is usually more intensely pruritic, may extend past the point of application, is more commonly vesiculobullous, and new lesions may continue to develop for up to 2 or 3 weeks following exposure (Fig. 16–2). Although immune function diminishes with age, allergic contact dermatitis actually appears to be more common in the elderly.

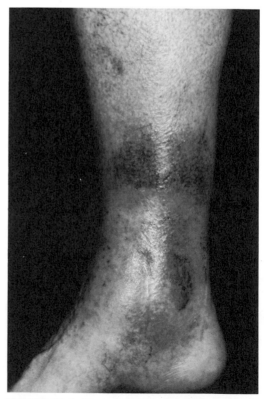

FIGURE 16–3. *Stasis dermatitis. Classic location with edema, superficial varicosities, erythema, and brownish puncta secondary to hemosiderin deposition.*

In many cases, the cause can be determined by physical examination and history, but other cases may require patch testing with suspected offending agents. The treatment in both cases requires removal of the offending agent and the topical application of a corticosteroid cream. Irritant dermatitis can usually be treated with a low- to medium-potency corticosteroid cream, whereas true allergic contact dermatitis often requires more potent topical corticosteroids. Occasional extensive cases may require oral antihistamines or corticosteroids.

Stasis Dermatitis

Stasis dermatitis is a relatively common condition that usually affects middle-aged or elderly individuals.[5] The underlying cause appears to be valvular incompetence that results in inadequate venous circulation. The single most common anatomic location is the medial paramalleolar region, but more extensive involvement of the lower half of the leg is common. Clinically, stasis dermatitis is characterized by variable edema, varicosities, erythema, scale, and characteristic reddish brown puncta caused by hemosiderin deposition. Secondary excoriations, ulceration, and infection may also develop (Fig. 16–3).

Stasis dermatitis is treated with elevation and supportive stockings to reduce edema. The dermatitis usually responds to mild- to moderate-potency corticosteroid creams. Superficial secondary infections should be treated with oral antibiotics, whereas cellulitis should usually be treated with intravenous antibiotics. The optimal topical management of stasis ulcers is controversial, but occlusive dressings are useful to promote re-epithelialization.

Bullous Pemphigoid

Bullous pemphigoid is a blistering disorder usually seen in patients over age 60. It is an autoimmune condition in which antibodies are directed against the basement membrane zone at the epidermal/dermal junction. Clinically, it is characterized by a pruritic eruption that usually involves the trunk and extremities.

In 20 percent of cases, the mucosa may also be involved. The lesions are typically tense, fluid-filled blisters that do not break easily, but erythematous urticarial plaques may also be present.

The diagnosis can be established by biopsy and direct immunofluorescent studies, which usually demonstrate a linear deposition of IgG (gamma G immunoglobin) and C_3 at the basement membrane zone. The treatment of choice is oral corticosteroids, although other forms of immunosuppressive therapy have also been used successfully. Mild cases may respond to topical application of a potent corticosteroid cream. In approximately half of all patients, the disease will spontaneously remit and medication may be discontinued.[8]

Pemphigus Vulgaris

Pemphigus vulgaris most commonly occurs between the ages of 40 and 60, but a significant incidence occurs in the elderly. Like bullous pemphigoid, it is an autoimmune disease, but in this case antibodies are directed against the intercellular substance between keratinocytes and indirectly results in loss of cohesion between cells. Clinically, it is characterized by large flaccid blisters of the skin that rupture quickly, leaving raw erythematous ulcerations. The oral mucosa is more frequently involved than in bullous pemphigoid and is often the presenting manifestation. Differentiation from bullous pemphigoid is based on clinical appearance, biopsy results, and direct immunofluorescent studies. The treatment of choice is high-dose oral corticosteroids in severe cases, but other forms of immunosuppressive therapy have been used successfully. Unlike bullous pemphigoid, the disease is not benign, and even with proper therapy the mortality rate may reach 30 percent of all cases.[8]

COMMON INFECTIONS OF THE SKIN

Dermatophytosis

Fungal infections of the skin are relatively common in the elderly population.

In one study done on patients over the age of 64, 79 percent had evidence of dermatophytic infections.[4] The most common sites are the feet (tinea pedis), followed by the nails (onychomycosis) and hands (tinea manuum). Infection of the scalp (tinea capitis) is very rare in the elderly. On the palms and soles, the infection usually presents as diffuse scaling that is exaggerated in the skin creases (Fig. 16–4). The presence of erythema is variable. In occasional cases, bullous lesions may develop. Onychomycosis is frequently present and clinically appears as distal subungual hyperkeratosis that may ultimately involve the entire nail. The diagnosis is best established by scraping the affected skin or subungual hyperkeratotic debris with a no. 15 blade. The scrapings are placed on a slide, and a drop of 10 percent potassium hydroxide (KOH) is added. Gentle heating is applied to enhance clearing of the specimen. The slide is then examined under a light microscope for the presence of hyphae. Fungal cultures are considerably less sensitive in establishing the diagnosis.

Dermatophyte infections can be treated with topical antifungals (spectazole, clotrimazole, miconazole, or ciclopirox olamine creams) in mild cases or with oral griseofulvin in resistant or extensive infections. Onychomycosis (particularly in toe nails) is very resistant to eradication, and not all cases should be treated. Oral griseofulvin is the treatment of choice but carries only a 10 to 20 percent cure rate, even after 6 to 12 months of therapy. Severely dystrophic or thickened nails may become painful or cosmetically unacceptable and may require surgical removal.[9]

Candidiasis (Moniliasis)

Candidiasis is caused by the yeast *Candida albicans.* Unfortunately, different clinical terms including thrush (oral candidiasis), intertrigo (infections of body folds), perlèche (angle of the mouth), and erosio interdigitalis blastomycetica (infection of the finger webs) are used to describe candidiasis. Other common sites of infection include the genitoanal area and periungual tissues.

Candidiasis is more commonly seen in the diabetic, obese, or immunocompromised patient. Clinical lesions vary, depending on the site, but generally consist of erythematous papules with occasional pustules. In moist areas, maceration is often present. The diagnosis is established by KOH examination, which demonstrates both yeast and hyphal structures, and by culture. Mild cases are best treated by topical preparations (nystatin, clotrimazole, miconazole, spectazole, ciclopirox olamine), whereas severe or extensive cases may require oral ketoconazole.

Herpes Zoster (Shingles)

Herpes zoster is a recrudescence of an infection caused by the varicella-zoster virus that has been dormant in a nerve root ganglion. It is increasingly common with advancing age. Clinically, it is characterized by a prodrome of variable neuralgic pain, followed by the appearance of grouped vesicles on an erythematous base

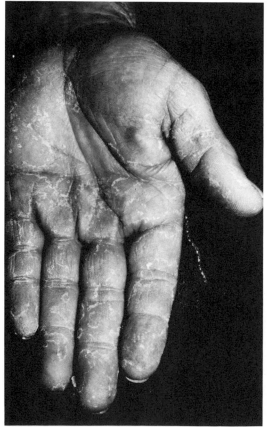

FIGURE 16–4. *Tinea manuum. Scaling secondary to chronic dermatophyte infection.*

in a dermatomal distribution. The most commonly affected dermatomes are C2, L2, and the fifth cranial nerve. Dissemination more commonly occurs in immunocompromised patients (Fig. 16–5).

The lesions usually begin to crust in the second week but may become gangrenous or demonstrate progressive enlargement in immunocompromised patients. The diagnosis can usually be made on clinical grounds but can be confirmed by Tzanck preparation findings of multinucleated giant cells or by culture. Oral acyclovir is the treatment of choice for herpes zoster. In the younger patient, the infection resolves without sequelae, but in older patients, post-herpetic neuralgia may persist for months.[10]

BENIGN TUMORS

The development of skin tumors is commonly associated with aging. Virtually all adults over age 65 have at least one, and usually several, benign tumors.

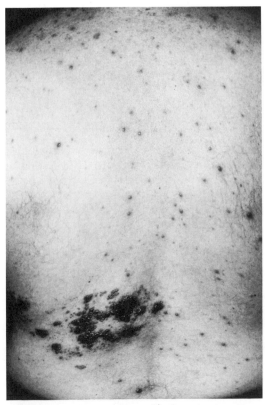

FIGURE 16–5. Herpes zoster with dissemination. Hemorrhagic vesicles in a dermatomal distribution and numerous individual vesicles secondary to dissemination. The patient had an underlying lymphoma.

Acrochordons (Skin Tags)

Acrochordons are very common tumors in the aged and often begin in middle age. They are pedunculated, flesh-colored to brown, and have a predilection for areas subject to friction such as the neck, axillae, and groin (Fig. 16–6). Obesity is commonly present in affected individuals. Recently, an association with colonic polyps has been proposed.[11] Because such polyps may be the source of colonic adenocarcinoma, an appropriate gastrointestinal work-up may be considered if deemed clinically relevant. Treatment is usually by scissor excision or electrocautery, both procedures that can be performed without anesthesia.

Seborrheic Keratosis

Sometimes referred to as a delayed birthmark, seborrheic keratosis is probably dominantly inherited but is not commonly seen before the fifth decade. It is uncommon in black individuals. Clinically, seborrheic keratosis has a verrucous or pebbly surface, ranges in color from light tan to dark brown, and is sharply demarcated and appear to be "stuck on" the skin surface. It is most commonly seen on the trunk but may occur on the face and extremities.

The sudden appearance of numerous seborrheic keratoses on clear skin with rapid increase in size and number is known as Leser-Trélat sign.[12] Although rare, it is probable that this sign is a marker of internal malignancy, usually adenocarcinoma, in the elderly.

Seborrheic keratosis is easily treated either by freezing with skin refrigerant followed by curettage or by freezing with liquid nitrogen. Rarely, malignant melanoma may resemble seborrheic keratosis, so accuracy of diagnosis is imperative before treatment is initiated.

Stucco Keratosis

Stucco keratosis is a small, papillomatous, whitish lesion that also has a "stuck on" appearance and is characteristically seen on the lower extremities of the el-

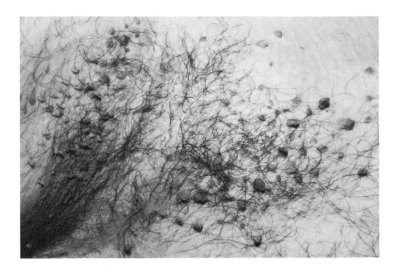

FIGURE 16–6. Acrochordons. Multiple flesh-colored to tan pedunculated papules in the axilla of an obese person.

derly. It is similar to seborrheic keratosis and has no medical significance.

Keratoacanthoma

Keratoacanthoma is a rapidly growing tumor usually found on sun-exposed surfaces of the middle-aged and elderly.[13] It begins as an erythematous, dome-shaped papule that enlarges to 1 to 2 cm in diameter over several weeks and develops a keratin-filled central crater (Fig. 16–7). After several months, the lesions usually involute spontaneously, often leaving a scar. Rarely, multiple keratoacanthomas may be present, either with the classic morphology and clinical course or as small, persistent lesions, which may be dominantly inherited.

Keratoacanthomas may resemble several other lesions including actinic keratosis, verruca vulgaris, and squamous cell carcinoma. The diagnosis is best made by obtaining an incisional biopsy through the center of the lesion, encompassing the entire diameter. With an established diagnosis, any remaining tumor may be excised or treated with intralesional 5-fluorouracil.

Cherry Hemangioma

These are typically 1 to 5 mm diameter vascular neoplasms commonly seen on the trunk of the middle-aged and elderly. They are deep red in color and may regress with extreme age. They have no potential for malignant transformation, are not subject to bleeding, and treatment is usually not attempted.

Sebaceous Hyperplasia

The face is the usual site of this benign skin tumor associated with both the middle-aged and elderly. Ranging in size from 1 to 3 mm, sebaceous hyperplasia tumors contain mature sebaceous glands and on close observation can be seen to have a central pore. They have a yellowish color, and large ones can sometimes be mistaken for basal cell carcinomas. Treatment is usu-

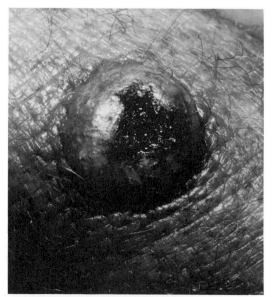

FIGURE 16–7. Keratoacanthoma. Crateriform lesion with central keratin plug and a history of rapid growth.

ally not necessary, but when requested, freezing with liquid nitrogen is sometimes helpful.

Venous Lakes

These are collections of dilated venules that occur on the lips, ears, and faces of the elderly. They are usually deep purple or blue in color and rarely exceed 5 mm in diameter. They may mimic melanotic lesions and are occasionally excised to exclude malignant melanoma. Removal, when desired, is usually accomplished under local anesthesia with a shave excision and gentle electrocautery of the base.

Melanocytic Nevi

The common benign pigmented lesions of melanocytic origin include junctional, compound, and intradermal nevi and lentigines.

Most nevi are acquired during the first 2 decades of life, so that the young adult will average in excess of twenty. The junctional nevus is typically flat, is darkly pigmented, and contains melanocytes at the dermal/epidermal junction. With maturation, the melanocytes will migrate downward into the dermis, producing a combined dermal and junctional component (compound nevus) and, finally, may be situated only in the dermis (intradermal nevus). Older nevi may lose pigment and regress altogether; therefore, the elderly frequently have only a few nevi.

Lentigo

Lentigines may arise in any age group but when acquired in the elderly, they are referred to as lentigo senilis or solar lentigo ("liver spots"). They are brown macules caused by localized areas of mild epidermal hyperplasia, associated with increased numbers of melanocytes and increased melanin pigment production. They are common on sun-exposed surfaces, with a predilection for the dorsum of the hands. Lentigines may be indistinguishable from freckles that are induced entirely by ultraviolet light. Freckles contain a normal number of melanocytes, which produce an abnormally large amount of melanin. A particular type of lentigo—lentigo maligna—is discussed under precancerous tumors.

PREMALIGNANT AND MALIGNANT TUMORS

Solar irradiation, especially in the 290 nm to 320 nm range, is responsible for much of what is recognized as sunburn and contributes significantly to the development of many age-related changes in the skin. These include wrinkling, atrophy, irregular pigmentation, lentigines, freckles, and precancerous keratoses.[14] Additionally, the vast majority of squamous cell carcinomas, most basal cell carcinomas, and, very probably, many malignant melanomas are induced in some way by solar irradiation.[15] All three cancers occurred more often in fair-skinned people with light eyes (grey, blue, green) who burn easily and rarely tan. Skin cancer is much less prevalent in darker-skinned individuals. Much of the sequelae of solar irradiation can be prevented by the judicious use of sun screens and by the avoidance of exposure to the sun. Overzealous programs of sun avoidance, however, may conflict with a healthy outdoor lifestyle, so care should be taken to not make "sun cripples" of the geriatric population.

Actinic Keratosis

Actinic keratoses are seen predominantly after middle age in fair-skinned people.[16] They are particularly common on the dorsum of the hands and arms, on the face, and on the scalp of bald men. They are erythematous and covered with a scale and may range in size from a few millimeters to over 4 cm (Fig. 16–8). These lesions are considered precursors of squamous cell carcinomas of the slow-growing type and rarely metastasize.

Application of liquid nitrogen to a solitary lesion or treatment with topical 5-fluorouracil for extensive lesions is usually effective therapy. Avoidance of excessive sun exposure and use of protective sun screens with a sun protective factor (SPF) of 15 or higher will help prevent recurrences.

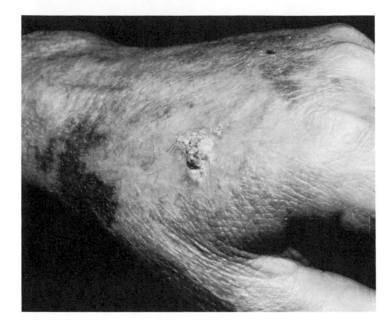

FIGURE 16–8. Actinic keratosis. Hyperkeratotic papule on a background of severe solar damage. Note presence of senile purpura.

Bowen's Disease (Squamous Cell Carcinoma In Situ)

Bowen's disease represents squamous cell carcinoma in situ. It may occur on sun-exposed, covered skin and mucosal surfaces. In the skin, there is an irregular erythematous plaque with an overlying scale. The lesion is usually sharply demarcated, a feature that clinically helps differentiate it from actinic keratosis (Fig. 16–9). On mucosal surfaces, where it is known

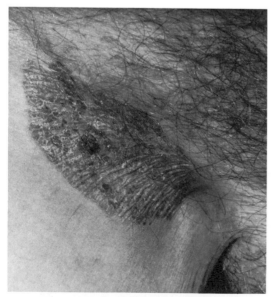

FIGURE 16–9. Bowen's disease. Erythematous, scaly plaque of groin initially treated as a dermatosis.

as Queyrat's erythroplasia, the lesions are erythematous and sharply demarcated, with a velvety surface.

A history of arsenic exposure can sometimes be implicated in the development of Bowen's disease, and it is possible that in these cases, there is an increased incidence of visceral malignancy, especially carcinoma of the lung. Arsenical keratosis of the palms and soles, which are histologic correlates of Bowen's disease, may also be seen with arsenic ingestion.

If the lesions are small, surgical excision is the treatment of choice, since the atypical cells may extend downward around follicular structures. Destruction of lesions by freezing and electrodesiccation may also be effective. On mucosal surfaces, especially the genitalia, topical 5-fluorouracil will often effect cures without the need for potentially mutilating surgery.

Lentigo Maligna (Hutchinson's Freckle)

Lentigo maligna is usually a large hyperpigmented macule with an irregular border situated most commonly on the sun-damaged skin of the face of the elderly, but it may also occur at other sites. It is very slow growing and may attain a diameter of several centimeters. Approximately one third of all lentigo malignas will develop into a malignant melanoma.[17]

Treatment is usually by surgical excision, but it must be tailored to the individual patient and lesion.

Basal Cell Carcinoma

Basal cell carcinoma is the most common skin cancer.[18] It occurs predominantly in fair-skinned people on sun-exposed surfaces, especially the face, but it may also be seen in scars, in irradiated skin, and after chronic arsenic exposure. Basal cell carcinomas usually begin as small, pearly, translucent nodules with prominent telangiectasias; however, they may be quite subtle, presenting as small areas of induration, atrophy, or superficial ulcers with crust formation (Fig. 16–10). They typically enlarge by peripheral extension and may reach several centimeters in diameter. Basal cell carcinomas rarely metastasize but are commonly invasive and locally destructive, if not treated early and adequately.

Treatment modalities include curettage and electrodesiccation, scalpel excision, irradiation, cryosurgery, and Mohs' micrographic surgery. Cure rates over 95 percent can be expected for most primary basal cell carcinomas, when appropriately treated.

Squamous Cell Carcinoma

Squamous cell carcinoma is the second most common skin cancer. It occurs most often in fair-skinned people past middle age. Squamous cell carcinomas usually arise on sun-exposed skin, often from a pre-existing actinic keratosis. With the exception of those occurring on the lips, in which a 12 to 15 percent metastatic rate may be encountered, actinically induced squamous cell carcinomas rarely metastasize. Metastases are much more likely to occur in areas of late radiation dermatitis, scars, and chronic ulcers.

Early squamous cell carcinomas are ill-defined erythematous areas of induration and scaling. The surface is often friable and may bleed easily. Ulceration may develop early or late. With continued growth, the surface may appear granular, and there may be considerable necrosis.

Treatment is determined by the size, location, and type of skin from which the tumor arises. For small cancers (under 1 cm) on sun-damaged skin, simple excision with some form of histopathologic margin control will often suffice. For larger tumors and tumors arising on the lips, in scars, and in ulcers in irradiated skin, more radical therapy may be necessary.

Malignant Melanoma

Malignant melanomas are seen most commonly in fair-skinned individuals with light hair and eyes. As with basal cell

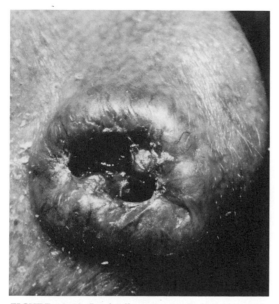

FIGURE 16–10. Basal cell carcinoma. Rodent ulcer with rolled, pearly border on the back of an ear.

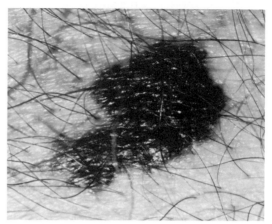

FIGURE 16–11. Superficial spreading malignant melanoma. Black lesion with occasional areas of brown with an irregular (notched) border and irregular surface.

carcinomas and squamous cell carcinomas, exposure to ultraviolet light is considered to be an important etiologic factor. Data have recently been reported showing that malignant melanoma is one of the most rapidly increasing cancers in the world, with an 83 percent increase in incidence over the last 7 years.[19] From an incidence of 1 in 1500 in 1930, it has increased to 1 in 135 in 1987, and it is expected to reach an incidence of 1 in 90 by the year 2000.

There are four major types of malignant melanoma arising in the skin: (1) lentigo maligna melanoma, arising in a lentigo maligna; (2) superficial spreading melanoma; (3) nodular melanoma; and (4) acral-lentiginous melanoma (Fig. 16–11). Acral-lentiginous melanoma occurs on the palms, soles, nail beds, mucocutaneous junctions, and some mucosal surfaces. All but nodular melanoma are usually slow growing, with a superficial growth phase before deep invasion. The nodular melanoma invades early, but it may still exhibit radial growth prior to invasion.

Early malignant melanomas typically demonstrate asymmetry; irregular borders; irregular pigment with shades of tan, brown, and black; and large size, usually larger than 7 mm. These features are exaggerated with continued growth, and the lesions may exhibit areas of regression so that some areas may appear depigmented. Nodular melanomas especially may be amelanotic from inception.

Because virtually all malignant melanomas have a preinvasive phase in which they are confined to the epidermis and are not subject to metastases, the key to survival is early detection and removal. Valuable prognostic information can be obtained by histopathologic determination of thickness (Breslow level) and depth (Clark's levels), so that whenever possible, the entire lesion should be excised for diagnosis.

Treatment of primary malignant melanoma is by surgical excision. There is a growing body of evidence suggesting that wide surgical margins do not improve survival; therefore, many surgeons are opting for conservative excisions that result in reduced morbidity and improved cosmesis.[20, 21]

REFERENCES

1. Fenske NA, Lober CW: Structural and functional changes of normal aging skin. J Am Acad Dermatol 15:571, 1986.
2. Fenske NA, Sekula S: Solar-induced skin changes. Am Fam Physician 26:109, 1982.
3. Goldberg LH, Altman A: Benign skin changes associated with chronic sunlight exposure. Cutis 34:33, 1984.
4. Tindall JP: Skin changes and lesions in our senior citizens. Cutis 18:359, 1976.
5. Beauregard S, Gilchrest BA: A survey of skin problems and skin care regimens in the elderly. Arch Dermatol 123:1638, 1987.
6. Skinner RB, Jr, Noah PW, Taylor RM, et al: Double-blind treatment of seborrheic dermatitis with 2% ketoconazole cream. J Am Acad Dermatol 12:852, 1985.
7. Wilkin JK: Rosacea. Int J Dermatol 22:393, 1983.
8. Lever WF: Pemphigus and pemphigoid: a review of advances made since 1964. J Am Acad Dermatol 1:2, 1979.
9. Hernandez AD: An approach to the diagnosis and therapy of dermatophytosis. Int J Dermatol 19:540, 1980.
10. Reuler JB, Chang MK: Herpes zoster: epidemiology, clinical features, and management. South Med J 77:1149, 1984.
11. Beitler M, Eng A, Kilgour M, et al: Association between acrochordons and colonic polyps. J Am Acad Dermatol 14:1042, 1986.
12. Veneicie PY, Perry HO: Sign of Leser-Trelat: report of two cases and review of the literature. J Am Acad Dermatol 10:83, 1984.
13. Rook A, Whimster I: Keratoacanthoma: A thirty year retrospect. Br J Dermatol 100:41, 1979.
14. Forbes PD, Davies RE, Urbach F: Aging, environmental influences, and photocarcinogenesis. J Invest Dermatol 73:131, 1979.
15. Urbach F, Forbes PD: Photocarcinogenesis. In Fitzpatrick TB, Eisen AZ, Wolff K, Freedberg IM, Austen FK, eds: Dermatology in General Medicine, 3rd ed. New York, McGraw-Hill, 1987, p 1475.
16. Gilchrest BA: Age associated changes in the skin: overview and clinical relevance. J Am Geriatr Soc 30:129, 1982.
17. Wayte DM, Helwig EB: Melanotic freckle of Hutchinson. Cancer 21:893, 1968.
18. Mackie RM: Tumors of the skin. In Rook A, Wilkinson DS, Ebling FJG, Champion RH, Burton JL, eds: Textbook of Dermatology. Oxford, Blackwell, 1986, p 2375.
19. Rigel DS: What's new in malignant melanoma? Presented in symposium on cutaneous tumors, Annual Meeting of the American Academy of Dermatology, San Antonio, December 7, 1987.
20. Day CL, Mihm MG, Jr, Sober AJ, et al: Correspondence on width of excision for melanoma. N Engl J Med 307:440, 1982.
21. Lang NP, Stair JM, Degges RD, et al: Melanoma today does not require radical surgery. Am J Surg 184:723, 1984.

CHAPTER 17

Skin Problems Associated with Pressure

Gerit D. Mulder
Stephen F. Albert

Youth is the time for the adventures of the body, but age for the triumphs of the mind.
LOGAN PEARSALL SMITH,
On Reading Shakespeare

This chapter discusses the treatment of pressure ulcers through the use of new technology. Although the prevention of lesions is important, reducing associated morbidity and mortality can only be accomplished through appropriate care, once lesions are present.

Pressure sores are commonly encountered clinical problems among patients with chronic disease, particularly those in an institutionalized setting. Between 25 and 85 percent of patients with spinal cord injuries develop pressure ulcers, resulting in a 7 to 8 percent mortality incidence.[1, 2] During hospitalization, 3 to 4.5 percent of patients develop pressure sores, especially those who are comatose, dehydrated, elderly, incontinent, nutritionally depleted, neurologically debilitated, or immobile.[3]

CLASSIFICATION AND LOCATION

Ninety-six percent of pressure sores are located on the lower half of the body, 67 percent are in the pelvic area, and 29 percent are on the lower extremities.[4] The more commonly involved sites include the sacrum, ischial tuberositates, trochanters, heels, and lateral malleoli. The differential diagnoses of pressure sores must include local abscess, fungal/bacterial infection, vasculitis, and necrotic malignancy.

The clinical staging of pressure sores, the most widely used of which was established by Shea, may serve as a guide to the selection of therapy.[5] They are grade I—soft tissue inflammation with loss of epidermis; grade II—full-thickness skin ulcer extending to subcutaneous fat; grade III—ulceration extending into subcutaneous fat with extensive undermining of skin; and grade IV—ulceration extending to muscle, bone, and joints.

ETIOLOGY AND PREDISPOSITION

Of the many factors that contribute to the development of pressure sores, the four most critical are pressure, shearing force, friction, and moisture. *Pressure* (the force exerted on a unit area) over a bony prominence is of particular importance.[6]

Studies by Guyton, Granger, and Taylor have demonstrated that with the application of external pressure, interstitial fluid pressure increases when venous limb pressure (12 mmHg)[7] is exceeded, there is a marked increase in total tissue pressure. The final results are increased capillary arteriolar pressure, filtration of fluid from capillaries, edema, autolysis, and ischemia. Furthermore, lymphatic vessels may occlude, leading to accumulation of anaerobic metabolic waste products and, ultimately, to tissue necrosis.[8]

Experimental studies have indicated that a constant pressure of 70 mmHg applied for over 2 hours produces irreversible tissue damage. With intermittent pressure relief, minimal tissue damage was noted.[2, 9] These results suggest that the critical period of pressure application is within the 1- to 2-hour range, with irreversible changes occurring after this time.[6] Thus, an inverse relationship exists between pressure and time in the formation of an ulcer.

Shearing force is created by the sliding of adjacent surfaces of laminar elements, providing a progressive relative displacement.[10] Reichel reported that shear is generated when the head of the bed is raised, causing the torso to slide down and transmit pressure to the sacrum and deep fascia.[11] Whereas the skin remains fixed secondary to friction with the bed, the loosely attached superficial fascia slides over the more firmly attached deep fascia. Tension then develops in the tissue, placing stretch and angulation on the blood vessels, which leads to thrombosis, ischemia, and undermining of the dermis. The vessels particularly affected are the posterior branches of the lateral sacral arteries and the superficial branches of the superior gluteal artery. Additionally, subcutaneous fat, which lacks tensile strength and is particularly vulnerable to mechanical forces, accentuates the shearing phenomenon.

Friction is the force created when two surfaces in contact move across each other. This may occur when a patient is pulled across the bedsheets or when spasticity causes an extremity to rub against an adjacent surface. Friction accelerates the onset of ulceration by removing the outer protective stratum corneum. In addition, when friction and shear forces are applied to pigskin, which is similar to human skin, the minimal pressure needed to produce skin damage dropped from 70 mmHg to 45 mmHg.[2] These pressures are easily produced in humans.

Moisture caused by fecal or urinary incontinence or by perspiration increases the risk of pressure ulcer formation by 4 to 5 times. This is primarily due to maceration of the epidermis, which allows tissue necrosis to occur more readily.

Predisposing factors to pressure sore formation include any variable that alters the metabolism of normal cells, leading to a subsequent alteration in their response to the ischemic effect of pressure. Anemia, blood dyscrasia, and blood vessel fragility decrease the amount of oxygen available to tissues. Cardiovascular disease may result in poor perfusion of the capillary beds. Edema increases capillary pressure while widening the distance between skin cells and their blood supply, which results in both a compromised blood supply to the skin and a reduction in the efficiency of oxygen delivery. Poor nutrition, with subsequent loss of subcutaneous tissue, emphasizes bony prominences. Inadequate protein reserves decrease tissue vitality and hinder wound healing.[12]

The elderly are especially prone to develop pressure ulcers secondary to increased susceptibility to trauma because of diminished epidermal thickness, dermal collagen, and tissue elasticity. Immobilization and neurologic impairment paralysis as well as decreased sensation all contribute to ulcer formation.

Exton-Smith and Sherwin studied the correlation between impaired mobility and the risk of pressure ulceration.[13] They concluded that a key factor in the development of pressure sores was decreased movement. They noted the importance of identifying patients at high risk for developing these lesions. An assessment scale was developed, based on clinical parameters such as physical condition, mental condition, activity, mobility, and incontinence.[14, 15]

COMPLICATIONS

The multiple complications resulting from pressure ulcers can be life-threatening.[16] In a septic patient, pressure ulcers should be considered a cause of infection when no other obvious sources of infection are present. Surgical consultation is recommended, and antibiotic therapy should include coverage for gram-negative and anaerobic organisms.[17] Commonly, there is invasion into bone leading to pyarthroses, osteomyelitis, and joint disarticulation.[18] Although pressure ulcers frequently appear to be superficial, a deep sinus tract extending to the joint space may exist. Sinography is particularly useful as a differential technique.[19, 20] Standard radiography and bone scans should also be performed.

Pressure sores may communicate with deeper soft tissue structures, including the bowel and bladder. The formation of heterotopic calcifications may occur, providing foci for new pressure sores and increased susceptibility to tetanus.[21] Newman reported that systemic amyloidosis, a frequently reported complication of spinal cord injury in older literature, may be a consequence of these chronic suppurative ulcers.[22]

PREVENTION

Pressure ulcer prevention must include skin care, pressure relief, positioning, and evaluation of nutritional and metabolic status of the patient. A clinical assessment of risk must first be made. High-risk patients should be given aggressive nursing care. The skin needs to be carefully monitored every 2 hours for early signs of tissue breakdown and should be free of stool, urine, and moisture. The patient should be lifted, not dragged, across a surface to avoid abrading the epidermis. Sheets should be kept loose on the patient. Genuine sheepskin boots, mats, and elbow protectors help reduce friction.

The most important aspect of prevention is pressure relief. The most simple and frequently used mechanism of pressure relief—rotation of the patient—should be performed at least every 2 hours. An inexpensive and useful technique for pressure relief is the strategic placement of soft pillows (usually six or more) to create a bridging effect. Pressure-relieving products and devices are intended to alter or diminish pressure over bony prominences at regular intervals or to disperse pressure through a molding effect.[12] Examples include the waterbed the air mattress, the air-fluidized bed, the silicone gel pad, and the polyurethane foam mattress. These products may be useful adjuncts to quality nursing. The literature on each device must be carefully analyzed because variations exist among devices.

Positioning of bedridden patients is important for pressure redistribution and ulcer prevention. The supine and 30° oblique positions are the most favorable. The prone and 90° positions should be avoided in the elderly.

The occurrence of pressure ulcers in wheelchair-bound patients continues to be a source of frustration. None of the available cushions adequately reduce capillary pressure to a level sufficient enough to eliminate the need for pressure relief at regular intervals.[23] Risk of ulcer occurrence is reduced by doing a push-up from the seat or by moving in the wheelchair, causing a shift in pressure and allowing blood to flow to tissues. Donuts are to be avoided because of both the undesirable distribution of stress and the potential for vessel occlusion.

Correction of nutritional and metabolic deficiencies is important in the prevention of pressure ulcers. In some cases, dietary supplements, anabolic steroids, parenteral vitamins, small doses of insulin before meals for diabetic patients, and intravenous hyperalimentation may improve these deficiencies. Tissue oxygen should be maintained in the normal range. Control of diabetes and edema will decrease the susceptibility of the skin to mechanical destruction.

MANAGEMENT

General wound care principles, including both local and systemic therapies, apply in the treatment of pressure sores. Systemically, the most important treatment is optimal nutrition. Recently, hypoalbuminemia, which is commonly caused by malnutrition, has been identified as a risk factor for pressure sore development.[24] Protein and carbohydrate deficiencies and deficiencies in a number of vitamins and minerals, such as zinc, magnesium, calcium, copper, and vitamin C, can slow wound healing.[25] The oxygen level in the blood must be sufficient to maintain Po_2 in the normal range, assuming that normal cardiac output and normovolemia are present. Improved oxygenation through the use of hyperbaric oxygen, which increases the supply of oxygen within plasma, and ultrasonography, which increases local circulation, are believed to expedite wound healing, although more studies are needed to justify their use.

Underlying medical conditions such as anemia, spasticity, congestive heart failure, and diabetes mellitus should be corrected or controlled. Systemic infections need treatment. If bacteremia occurs, systemic antibiotics are indicated.[26]

Local treatment for pressure sores incorporates four basic principles based on the ulcer's classification. In addition, excellent nursing care is required for any management plan. Because 70 to 90 percent of pressure sores are superficial, most can be managed with conservative therapy.[6] Table 17–1 outlines currently available treatment modalities.

The first principle of treatment is *elimination of local pressure from the ulcer site.* The same principles as for prevention apply; however, once an ulcer has developed, it is important not to allow the patient to lie on the ulcer for even a short period of time.

Debridement (i.e., removal of necrotic tissue) is the second principle of treatment. There are two forms of debridement: selective and nonselective. Selective debridement, in which only necrotic tissue is removed, can be accomplished through use of enzymes, through synthetic membrane dressings, or by surgery (although surgical debridement in patients with peripheral vascular disease is to be avoided). Synthetic membrane dressings may aid in the process of debridement. Enzymes dissolve the necrotic tissue and are quite safe and easy to use, although results are seen only after long-term therapy. Surgical debridement is the most efficient form of therapy and gives a rapid result.

Nonselective debridement, the indiscriminate removal of tissue from the wound, includes wet-to-dry dressings and vigorous wound irrigation. The use of wet-to-dry dressings is a simple method for rapid removal of small amounts of necrotic tissue. Neither method of nonselective debridement should ever be used on nonnecrotic wounds because they will remove delicate epithelium and granulation tissue. A grossly contaminated or necrotic ulcer, however, often benefits from vigorous wound irrigation.

Disinfection of the ulcer site is the third principle of treatment. Bendy and associates found that pressure ulcers with a count of less than 1×10^5 bacteria per ml of exudate spontaneously healed.[27] A study by Krizek and Robson suggested that skin grafting and delayed closure procedures are more likely to be successful if the bacterial counts have been reduced to less than 1×10^5 bacteria per gm of wound tissue.[28] Systemic antibiotics do not appear to be effective in eradicating bacterial colonization of the wound itself.[26]

There are numerous topical antibiotics for pressure sores; however, their effectiveness in healing is uncertain. They may also contribute to the development of resistant organisms. Benefits are questionable when compared with saline-saturated gauze dressings that are changed every 4 hours.[29] A preliminary study by Gomolin and Brandt showed favorable results in treating foul-smelling and purulent ulcers with topical metronidazole.[30] Ulcers of this type, which are grossly contaminated, should be irrigated with an antiseptic. An experimental study by Lineaweaver and coworkers indicated the optimal antibacterial, yet not cytotoxic, concentrations of povidone-iodine and sodium hypochlorite to be 0.001 percent and 0.005 percent, respectively.[31] Various topical agents may interact and inactivate one another and, therefore, should not be used together.[29] Shrosbree and Engel reported that dextranomer is beneficial to the repair of deep penetrating sores.[32]

Once granulation tissue appears, all disinfectants should be discontinued. Continued use will irritate the wound and diminish host defenses, resulting in increased bacterial numbers.

The fourth principle of treatment addresses the use of *dressings.* The purpose of a dressing is to protect the lesion from external contamination and to assist in creating an optimal environment for wound-healing. The seven types of dressings used to treat pressure ulcers are dry, nonadherent, nonocclusive, occlusive, periodic wet, wet, and wet-to-dry. It has been shown that occlusion plays an important role in the healing of wounds. Of the numerous materials available to physicians, the recent addition of synthetic membranes has been of great benefit. Three basic types of membranes exist, which are hydrocolloid, polyurethane film, and gel bio-dressings.[33] Each type of dressing has its own distinct advantages, disadvantages, and considerations. (A complete listing, however, is beyond the scope of this chapter.)

Surgical intervention is generally required with deeper (grades III and IV) pressure ulcers and ulcers associated with sepsis. Surgery includes excision of ulcerated areas, split-thickness or full-thickness skin grafting, resection of bony prominences, formation of large rotational flaps,

TABLE 17–1. Current Treatment Modalities for Pressure Ulcers

Modality	Indication	Consideration
Systemic antibiotics	Systemic infections	Useful in reducing bacterial tissue counts
Antiseptics (e.g., Povidone iodine; hydrogen peroxide; sodium hypochlorite; acetic acid)	Grossly contaminated wounds	Appropriate concentrations necessary; possible inactivation with other topical agents
Enzymes (e.g., collagenase; fibrinolysin; desoxyribonuclease)	Necrotic wounds	BID or TID applications; results within 3 to 14 days generally Discontinue when granulation tissue appears
Synthetic membranes; (Synthetic dressings)	Open draining lesions	Numerous contraindications including osteomyelitis; bone or tendon exposure; infection; ischemic ulcers; excessive drainage; extensive sinus tracts; friable periwound tissue; wounds of a pathologic nature
Hydrocolloids	Excellent for low to moderate exudate wounds	Often leak and are messy; poor retention; possible maceration; on high exudate wounds may damage and tear friable periwound tissue (especially in geriatric patients)
Polyurethane films	Superficial wounds with little to no exudate	Generally difficult to apply; poor exudate retention or absorption; easily disrupted and removed from wound site; not recommended on deeper lesions
Hydrogels	Superficial wounds	QD applications; nonadhesive, difficult to maintain on wound
Pressure-relieving devices Static (e.g., foam, overlap water, gel, and air-filled devices)	Patient must be able to move independently	Simply provide cushioning and more even weight distribution
Dynamic (e.g., alternating pressure pads; air support therapy, electrical stimulation	For immobile patients	Useful in prevention as well as therapy; electricity required; more expensive than static devices

and creation of additional padding, using muscle flaps. Limb amputation at various levels and even hemicorporectomy may be necessary.[32, 34]

After a pressure sore has healed, the patient must build up tolerance to pressure on the affected area. This is a gradual process that requires the patient to increase the time of lying on the previous ulcer site in increments from 5 to 20 minutes. The indicator of tolerance is the disappearance of erythema and/or induration after 20 minutes of pressure relief. When this does not occur, the time increments must be shortened.

INNOVATIONS IN TREATMENT

New technology during the last decade has focused on the development of improved dressings and pressure-relieving devices. Present research is directed towards materials and devices that will have an effect on cellular and wound-repair activity.

Growth factors are presently being studied in great depth.[35] Collagen matrices that may facilitate wound re-epithelialization are also being investigated.[36, 37] Recent studies have shown injected glutaraldehyde cross-linked collagen to be a useful treatment for the prevention of pressure-related ulcers in diabetic patients.[38]

Electrical stimulation may serve as a useful adjunct in the treatment of more severe pressure ulcers.

In summary, prevention, although not always possible, is the best treatment. Once an ulcer occurs, the appropriate choice of an effective modality and use of newly available treatment may reduce mortality and morbidity associated with the occurrence of the common pressure ulcer.

REFERENCES

1. El-Toraei I, Chung B: The management of pressure sores. J Dermatol Surg Oncol 3:507, 1977.
2. Dinsdale S: Decubitus ulcers: role of pressure and friction in causation. Arch Phys Med Rehabil 55:147, 1974.
3. Petersen NC, Bittman S: The epidemiology of pressure sores. Scand J Plast Reconstr Surg 5:62, 1971.
4. Vasconey LO, Schneider WJ, Jurkiewicz MJ: Pressure sores. Curr Probl Surg 14(4):1, 1977.
5. Shea DJ: Pressure sores: classification and management. Clin Orthop 112:89, 1975.
6. Reuler HB, Cooney TG: The pressure sore: pathophysiology and principles of management. Ann Intern Med 94:661, 1981.
7. Guyton AC, Granger HJ, Taylor AE: Interstitial fluid pressure. Physiol Rev 51:527–63, 1971.
8. Krovskop TA, Reddy NP, Spencer WA, et al: Mechanisms of decubitus ulcer formation: a hypothesis. Med Hypotheses 4:37, 1978.
9. Kosiak M: Etiology of decubitus ulcers. Arch Phys Med Rehabil 42:19, 1961.
10. Tepperman PS, DeSwirek CS, Chiarcossi AL, et al: Pressure sores: prevention and step-up management. Postgrad Med 62:83, 1977.
11. Reichel SM: Shearing force as a factor in decubitus ulcers in paraplegics. JAMA 166:762, 1958.
12. Delisa JA, Mikulic MA: Pressure ulcers: what to do if preventive management fails. Postgrad Med 77:209, 1985.
13. Exton-Smith AN, Sherwin RW: The prevention of pressure sores: significance of spontaneous bodily movements. Lancet 2(7212):1124, 1961.
14. Norton D, McLaren R, Exton-Smith AN: An investigation of geriatric nursing problems in hospitals. London, National Corporation for the Care of Old People, 1962.
15. Exton-Smith AN: Prevention of pressure sores: monitoring mobility and assessment of clinical condition. In Kenedi RM, Cowden JM, eds: Bedsore Biomechanics. Baltimore, University Park Press, 1976, p 133.
16. Conway H, Stark RB, Weeter JC, et al: Complications of decubitus ulcers in patients with paraplegia. Plast Reconstr Surg 7:117, 1975.
17. Bryan CS, Dew CE, Reynolds KL: Bacteremia associated with decubitus ulcers. Arch Intern Med 143:2093, 1983.
18. Waldvogel FA, Vasey H: Osteomyelitis: the past decade. N Engl J Med 303:360, 1980.
19. Lopez EM, Aranha GV: The value of sinography in the management of decubitis ulcers. Plast Reconstr Surg 53:208, 1974.
20. Putnam T, Calenoff L, Betts HB, et al: Sinography in the management of decubitis ulcers. Arch Phys Med Rehabil 59:243, 1978.
21. LaForce FM, Young LS, Bennett JV: Tetany in the United States (1965–1966): epidemiologic and clinical features. N Engl J Med 280:569, 1969.
22. Newman W, Jacobson AS: Paraplegia and secondary amyloidosis. Am J Med 15:216, 1953.
23. Kosiak M: An effective method of preventing decubital ulcers. Arch Phys Med Rehabil 47:742, 1966.
24. Allman RM, Laprade CA, Noel LB, et al: Pressure sores among hospitalized patients. Ann Intern Med 105:337, 1986.
25. Pollack SV: Systemic drugs and nutritional aspects of wound healing. Clin Dermatol 2(3):68, 1984.
26. Galpin JE, Chow AW, Bayer AS, et al: Sepsis associated with decubitus ulcers. Am J Med 61:346, 1976.
27. Bendy RH, Nuccio PA, Wolfe E: Relationship of quantitative wound bacterial count to healing of decubiti: effect of topical gentamicin. Antimicrob Agents Chemother 4:147, 1964.
28. Krizek TJ, Robson MC: Evolution of quantitative bacteriology in wound management. Am J Surg 130:579, 1975.

29. Xakallis GC, Garzone P: Pressure ulcers. Am Fam Physician 35:159, 1987.
30. Gomolin IH, Brandt JL: Topical metronidazole therapy for pressure sores of geriatric patients. J Am Geriatr Soc 31:710, 1983.
31. Lineaweaver W, Howard R, Soucy D, et al: Topical antimicrobial toxicity. Arch Surg 120:267, 1985.
32. Shrosbree RD, Engel P: The treatment of decubitus ulcers with dextranomer. S Afr Med J 59:902, 1981.
33. Mulder GD: Synthetic membranes: use in diabetic ulcers. Clin Podiatr Med Surg 4:419, 1987.
34. Campbell RM, Delgado JP: The pressure sore. In Converse JM, ed: Reconstructive Plastic Surgery, 2nd ed. Philadelphia, WB Saunders Co, 1977, p 3763.
35. Knighton D, Fiegel VD, Austin LL, et al: Classification and treatment of chronic nonhealing wounds. Ann Surg 204:322, 1986.
36. McPherson J, et al: Effect of a fibrillar collagen and fibrillar collagen-heparin complex on wound healing. Palo Alto, Collagen Corp Res Rep W-84-276, 1985.
37. McPherson J, et al: Effect of several collagen-based implant preparations in the guinea pig dermal wound healing model. Palo Alto, Collagen Corp Res Rep W-84-226, 1984.
38. Mulder GD, Jahnigen D, Vandepol CJ: The role of injectable collagen in the prevention of recurrent diabetic ulcers. J Am Podiatr Med Assoc 78:238–242, 1988.

SECTION V

GENITOURINARY PROBLEMS

CHAPTER 18

Urinary Incontinence and Catheters in the Elderly Male and Female

Richard R. Augspurger

All sorts of allowances are made for the illusions of youth; and none, or almost none, for the disenchantments of age.
    R. L. STEVENSON, *Virginibus Puerisque: Crabbed Age and Youth*

As the proportion of Americans over the age of 65 increases over the last decade of this century, one of the greatest challenges to face the U.S. health care system will be the management of urinary incontinence. Urinary incontinence can be defined as the involuntary loss of urine of sufficient amounts to cause psychologic, economic, or health problems. Urinary incontinence is a common major medical problem in the elderly.

It is estimated that between 15 and 30 per cent of community-dwelling elderly experience urinary incontinence. In 5 to 10 per cent of these individuals, the incontinence is of sufficient quantity to soak their clothes and thus require pads.[1, 2] The institutionalized elderly have a much higher incidence (40 to 60 per cent) of urinary incontinence.[3]

The cost of management of the incontinent patient is significant. In 1984, the estimated expense to the economy of caring for the incontinent elderly was $8.1 billion for both the direct costs (diagnosis, treatment care, and rehabilitation) and indirect costs (lost productivity and time).[4] This translates into $1.8 billion incurred by nursing homes to manage incontinence, or $2.90 to $11.90 a day more than the cost of treatment of continent nursing home patients. The community-dwelling elderly incurred $4.8 billion in direct costs and $1.5 billion in indirect costs. The total figure exceeds the combined amount spent annually for coronary artery bypass surgery and renal dialysis.[1]

The psychosocial impact is great, not only on the patient, but also on the families and caregivers. Urinary incontinence produces social isolation through the avoidance of social contacts with family and friends. It contributes to depression, decreases self-esteem, and is yet another area in which the elderly experience loss of control over their lives. Significant stress is often placed on the caregivers. Finally, it is a major factor contributing to the admission of the elderly to nursing homes.

The medical consequences of urinary incontinence are also important. Urinary incontinence can result in decubitus ulcers, skin breakdown, and the necessity of placing urethral catheters. Infection and stones associated with catheters and balanitis associated with external collecting devices all lead to increased morbidity and mortality in the elderly. The lowest nursing home cost for indwelling catheter management is $2.90 per day; however, there is a three-fold increase in mortality and significant rise in morbidity that increase the cost to $2888 per year, which is not much different from the cost of $2072 to $4532 of noncatheter management.[3]

Urinary incontinence should *not* be accepted as a normal part of aging. Too often, this has been a neglected area of medical care in the United States. Until now, urologists have not shown much interest or participated in the evaluation and care of this segment of the population.[5] The elderly tend to minimize or deny their urinary incontinence, and less than one in five elderly individuals seek medical care. Those who seek help find that only one of three physicians will institute even the most rudimentary evaluation.[3] The minimal workup for urinary incontinence is estimated at $500 to $1000.

Two thirds of the incontinent population can be cured with appropriate treatment, and the other one third can benefit from palliative measures.[1] It appears to be cost efficient to evaluate all incontinent elderly so that appropriate treatment can be instituted. Thus, better education of the elderly and the medical community that urinary incontinence is not a normal process of aging is needed. This chapter attempts to address the pathophysiology, diagnosis, and management of urinary incontinence in the elderly as one step in the educational process.

ANATOMY AND NEUROUROLOGY

To understand the pathophysiology of urinary incontinence and thus its treatment, a basic discussion of the normal anatomy, neurology, and physiology of the bladder is presented below.

The bladder is a smooth muscle storage organ of the urinary tract. Urine produced in the kidneys passes down the ureters to enter the bladder. As urine enters the bladder, the bladder muscle relaxes to accommodate between 450 and 500 ml of urine. The urine does not leak out of the urethra because of the sphincter mechanisms. There are two sphincters: the internal sphincter, which is smooth muscle, and the external sphincter, which is skeletal and smooth muscle (Fig. 18–1). At capacity, voiding occurs voluntarily. The detrusor contracts, the proximal sphincter funnels open, and the distal sphincter relaxes, allowing urine to pass from the bladder.

The normal processes of urine storage and voiding are under the control of the central nervous system (CNS). Several theories of neurologic control have been proposed.[6] The main reflex center for the bladder (Fig. 18–2) appears to be located in the mesencephalic-reticular formation, that is, the brain stem micturition center (BSMC). A less dominant center, the spinal cord micturition center (SCMC), also plays a role.

Sensory, proprioceptive fibers arising in the bladder pass by way of the pelvic nerves and the posterior columns to the BSMC. Motor fibers originating in the BSMC travel via the reticulospinal tracts to the detrusor motor nucleus in the intermediolateral grey cell column of the sacral spinal cord (S2–S4). From the detrusor motor nucleus, parasympathetic fibers traverse the pelvic nerves, synapse in the pelvic ganglia, and innervate the detrusor muscle. The neurotransmitter is the cholinergic agent acetylcholine (Fig. 18–3). Suprasacral interruption of the pathway releases the SCMC from inhibition. Thus, a low-capacity bladder with unsustained, uninhibited contractions of the detrusor muscle develops.

Supraspinal areas modulate the detrusor reflex through inputs on the BSMC (see Fig. 18–2). The detrusor motor area is located in the prefrontal portion. Fibers pass via the internal capsule to synapse at BSMC. Other CNS areas, that is, the thalmus, basal ganglia, and cerebellum, have inputs into the BSMC. The overall effect is one of inhibition of the detrusor reflex;

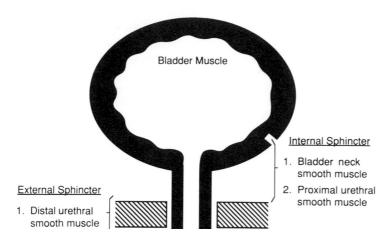

Bladder Muscle

Internal Sphincter

1. Bladder neck smooth muscle
2. Proximal urethral smooth muscle

External Sphincter

1. Distal urethral smooth muscle
2. Skeletal muscle

FIGURE 18–1. Schematic diagram of the bladder and urinary sphincter. The internal sphincter consists of bladder neck smooth muscle and the proximal urethral smooth muscle. The external sphincter consists of the distal urethral smooth muscle and skeletal, striate, external sphincter.

therefore, interruption of these pathways results in loss of voluntary control over the detrusor reflex. This is characterized by a sustained uninhibited detrusor contraction.

Sympathetic innervation (see Fig. 18–3) originates in the thoracolumbar spinal cord (T-10–L-2). The efferent fibers pass via the hypogastric nerve and synapse in the inferior mesenteric, hypogastric, and pelvic ganglia. The dome of the bladder is innervated primarily by beta-adrenergic fibers, with the bladder neck innervated by alpha-adrenergic fibers. Stimulation of the beta-adrenergic fiber results in detrusor muscle relaxation, whereas stimulation of alpha-adrenergic fibers causes contraction and tightening of the bladder neck.

In summary, storage of urine is a sympathetic response that occurs with tightening of the bladder neck and relaxation of the dome during adrenergic stimulation. Voiding is under parasympathetic control, with contraction of the detrusor and relaxation of the sphincters. An understanding of these neuropharmacologic principles aids in both the understanding of the side effects of medicines and the selection of the appropriate medicines employed in the treatment of urinary incontinence.

The striate (skeletal) external sphincter is under voluntary control. It is more highly developed in males than in females. Motor fibers arise in the pudendal motor area in the medial aspect of the central sulcus. Fibers pass through the internal capsule and corticospinal tract to synapse on the pudendal motor nucleus in the ventral grey of the sacral cord (see Fig. 18–3). Motor fibers pass by way of the pudendal nerve to the external striate sphincter. Suprasacral interruption of this pathway produces spasticity in the striate external sphincter.

There is a reciprocal innervation be-

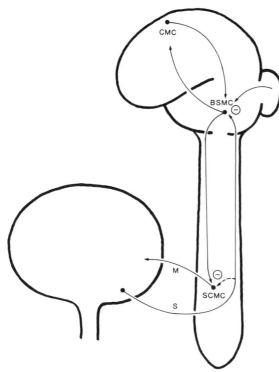

CMC

BSMC

M

S

SCMC

FIGURE 18–2. The reflex arcs associated with micturition: motor neuron (M); sensory neuron (S); cortical micturition center (CMC); brain stem micturition center (BSMC); sacral cord micturition center (SCMC).

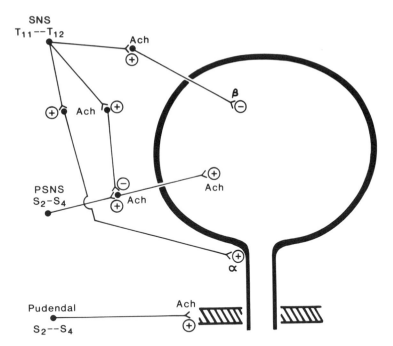

FIGURE 18–3. Diagram of the dual innervation of the bladder by the sympathetic nervous system (SNS) and the parasympathetic nervous system (PSNS). The neurotransmitters, acetycholine (Ach), norephinephrine (alpha, beta) are indicated. − = inhibitory effect; + = stimulating effect.

tween the striate external sphincter and the detrusor muscle. Thus, a detrusor contraction produces reflex relaxation of the striate external sphincter and vice versa. To maintain a sustained coordinated detrusor contraction and relaxation of the external sphincter, an intact spinal cord to level of the BSMC is required. Any lesion below the BSMC can produce dyscoordination between the bladder and sphincter, resulting in detrusor-sphincter dyssynergia.

PATHOPHYSIOLOGY

With the normal aging process, changes occur in the lower urinary tract. Although there is a lack of definitive data, it appears that with aging, the capacity of the bladder, the ability to postpone voiding, compliance of the urethra and bladder, and the length and closing pressure of the urethra all decrease. In contrast, uninhibited detrusor contractions and residual urine increase. The elderly—unlike younger individuals—excrete two thirds of daily ingested fluid after 8 or 9 PM. This fact, along with the higher incidence of sleep disorders, leads to nocturia, even in the normal elderly.[1]

In themselves, these age-related changes do not cause urinary incontinence; they are also present in normal, continent elderly patients. They do, however, reduce the ability of the lower urinary tract to withstand further insults. From these changes, two important principles arise: (1) incontinence in the elderly is more likely to be due to a precipitant outside the lower urinary tract; and (2) reversal of the precipitant frequently is sufficient to restore continence, even if any underlying urologic abnormality is not corrected.[1]

Urinary incontinence occurs when the intravesical pressure exceeds the bladder outlet resistance. Any condition in which the bladder, bladder outlet, or both fail to function will result in incontinence. Urinary incontinence in the elderly can be divided into two categories—transient and established.

The causes of *transient incontinence* can be recalled by the mnemonic DIAPPERS (Table 18–1).[1] Because transient incontinence occurs commonly and correcting the underlying condition will, in most cases, restore continence, transient causes of incontinence need to be addressed in the evaluation of all incontinent elderly patients.

One major area of transient incontinence is the iatrogenic-induced incontinence secondary to pharmacotherapy. Many elderly patients are taking one or more medications, many of which have

TABLE 18–1. Common Causes of Transient Incontinence

Mnemonic Designation	Cause
D	Delirium or confusional state
I	Infection, urinary (symptomatic)
A	Atrophic urethritis or vaginitis
P	Pharmaceuticals
	Sedative Hypnotics, especially long-acting agents
	Loop diuretics
	Anticholinergic agents
	Antipsychotics
	Antidepressants
	Antihistamines
	Antiparkinsonian medications
	Antiarrhythmics
	Opiates
	Alpha-adrenergic agonist and antagonists
	Calcium channel blockers
P	Psychologic disorders, especially depression
E	Endocrine disorders (e.g., hypercalcemia, hyperglycemia)
R	Restricted mobility
S	Stool impaction

(From Resnick NM, Yalla SV: Aging and its effect on the bladder. Semin Urol 5:82, 1987; by permission.)

significant side effects on the bladder (Table 18–2).[7] A drug history needs to be carefully sought. Many elderly also take over-the-counter cold preparations, which contain alpha-adrenergic agents. The drugs may, therefore, cause neck contraction and failure to empty the bladder. Often, the elderly do not volunteer a history of over-the-counter drug use because these medicines have not been prescribed by their physicians.

Established incontinence, as well as transient incontinence, can result from either a failure to empty the bladder or a failure to store urine. Failure to empty the bladder can be a result of decreased bladder contractility, increased bladder outlet resistance (obstruction), or both. This combination results in urinary retention and overflow incontinence and accounts for 7 to 11 per cent of total cause. In the male patient, this most commonly results from prostate hypertrophy (see Chapter 19) or urethral strictures. In the female, diabetes, with resultant diabetic neuropathy and flaccid neurogenic bladder, is the more common cause. The diagnosis is made by the findings of an elevated residual urine, large bladder capacity (> 900 cc), and decreased sensation of bladder filling.

Failure to store urine can have various etiologies. Functionally, it results from increased bladder pressure, decreased bladder outlet resistance, or a combination of these. The two main areas are stress incontinence and detrusor instability.

Stress urinary incontinence accounts for 3 to 10 per cent of cause in females, but it is rare in males. Stress incontinence is characterized by leakage of urine associated with the sudden increase in intra-abdominal pressure, as with coughing, sneezing, or laughing. Diagnosis is made by objective demonstration of distention of the bladder neck and urethra, associated leakage of urine, and stoppage of the incontinence with elevation of the bladder neck.

TABLE 18–2. Drugs and Their Effects on the Bladder

Drug Class	Effect
Diuretics	Increased urinary output
Anticholinergics	Decreased bladder contractility; urinary retention
Sedatives/hypnotics	Some decreased attention to bladder clues
Antipsychotics	
Antidepressants	
Antiarrhythmics	
Alpha-adrenergic agents	
Agonists	
Antiallergy medications	Bladder neck closure; urinary retention
Cold medications	
Antagonists	Relaxation of bladder neck; incontinence
Antihypertensives	
Beta-blockers	Bladder neck closure; urinary retention
Calcium channel blockers	Decreased bladder contractility; urinary retention
Narcotics	Decrease bladder contractility; urinary retention
Nonsteroidal antiinflammatory agents	Decreased bladder contractility; urinary retention

Detrusor instability is the most common cause of urinary incontinence and accounts for 40 to 60 per cent of total cause. The etiology of the abnormal bladder contractions is often unclear. They can occur with normal aging, in the presence of bladder outlet obstruction, or with loss of cortical inhibition of the voiding reflex commonly associated with parkinsonism, cardiovascular accident (CVA), and dementia. Diagnosis is made by demonstrating an involuntary rise in bladder pressure greater than 15 cm of water on cystometry. This is often associated with a smaller than normal bladder capacity. A subset of this group is an uninhibited detrusor contraction but with impaired contractility (DHIC).[1] The condition is defined as uncontrolled detrusor contraction with impaired bladder emptying, leaving over one third of bladder contents as residual urine. This diagnosis is likely, provided bladder outlet obstruction, spinal cord lesion, detrusor-sphincter dyssynergia, fecal impaction, bladder suppressants, and volitional inhibition of the detrusor have been excluded. DHIC can be difficult to diagnose, but it is felt to be the most common cause of incontinence in the institutionalized elderly.[1]

EVALUATION

The elderly incontinent patient is not often provided the same thorough evaluation given younger individuals. This occurs not only because the patient minimizes his or her symptoms but also because there appears to be a lack of awareness in the medical community of the significance of incontinence in the elderly. Both because incontinence is not a consequence of aging and because many causes are readily treatable, a large percentage of the incontinent elderly would benefit from a basic urologic evaluation. An extensive, costly urodynamic assessment is not necessary in most cases, but the evaluation needs to be comprehensive enough to determine whether readily reversible causes of incontinence exist. Several authors have proposed screening protocol that will allow identification of 70 to 90 per cent of the treatable causes of incontinence.[5, 7, 8] In general, this can be accomplished by using the approach outlined in Table 18–3.

TABLE 18–3. Evaluation of Urinary Incontinence

Screening Protocol
Take thorough medical history
Perform physical examination
Evaluate urine analysis, including culture and sensitivity
Determine post-void residual urine
Perform cystometric studies using water or CO_2
Observe for stress incontinence

The key elements in the history are related to potentially reversible conditions. Irritative symptoms of dysuria, frequency, and urgency suggest possible urinary tract infection or atrophic vaginitis or urethritis. Leakage with cough, sneezing, or activity has a high correlation with the findings of stress incontinence on physical examination. Urinary frequency must be evaluated with regard to both volume and time. A voiding diary, in which time and volume voided are recorded for 24 to 48 hours, is often helpful. High-volume frequency can be caused by diuretics or diabetic glucosuria, whereas low-volume frequency, especially when associated with urgency, is often related to an unstable bladder. It must be kept in mind, however, that one third of the elderly with detrusor instability give no history of urgency.

Nocturia without daytime frequency relates to the inability of elderly to excrete urine during the day. Bed wetting, voiding frequent small amounts, and incontinence may suggest overflow incontinence or urinary retention. Decreased flow rate, which is a complaint primarily of males, can be caused by bladder outlet obstruction or poor bladder contractility and must be differentiated.

Other important aspects of the history include (1) identifying all prescription and over-the-counter medicines that the patient has at home; (2) assessing surgical history, including all gynecologic, urologic, colorectal, and neurosurgical procedures; (3) determining if neurologic disease exists, such as CVA, parkinsonism, or spinal stenosis; and (4) assessing changes in mobility and limitations in activities. In the cognitively impaired patient, much information will need to be provided by the caregiver.

During the physical examination, attention should be directed to the patient's mental capacity, psychologic and behavioral disturbances, and mobility and manual dexterity. The lower abdomen should be palpated for bladder distention. Pelvic and rectal examinations are needed to evaluate for fecal impaction, pelvic masses, presence of pelvic prolapse, and size and consistency of the prostate. A limited urologic-neurologic examination should evaluate sensation in the perineal area (S2–S4 distribution), anal sphincter tone, and presence of the bulbocavernosus and anal reflexes.

The minimal laboratory test performed should be a urine analysis and urine culture and sensitivity. At times, plasma electrolytes, blood urea nitrogen (BUN), and serum creatinine, along with a fasting blood sugar evaluation, can be helpful. An intravenous pyelogram (IVP) and voiding cystogram should be done only when indicated by the initial evaluation.

The final steps in the evaluation are catheterization for measurement of residual urine, and a simple cystometrogram, using water or CO_2. It is felt by Castleden and colleagues that the treatment of elderly incontinent patients without cystometry is analogous to treating a patient with cardiac arrhythmia without an electrocardiogram (ECG).[9] The cystometrogram gives the volume-pressure status of the bladder. At the bedside, this can be easily performed with a catheter tip syringe and sterile water for irrigation. The plunger is removed from the syringe, and the syringe is connected to the catheter. With the syringe held 15 cm above the pubis, water is instilled in 50-ml increments and the pressure is recorded. (The patient is instructed not to urinate.) The first sensations of bladder filling and fullness are noted. Any sudden rise in bladder pressure or leakage around the catheter that the patient cannot inhibit confirms the diagnosis of detrusor instability (Fig. 18–4). The cystometrogram not only documents uninhibited detrusor contractions but also gives information about bladder compliance, sensation, and, in some settings, capacity.

At the end of the test, the bladder is filled and the catheter is removed. Observation for leakage during coughing and sneezing in both the supine and upright positions tests for stress incontinence. Finally, the patient is asked to urinate so that the force and caliber of the stream can be observed, flow rates can be determined, and voided volume can be recorded.

The above tests can identify 70 to 90 per cent of the causes of incontinence so that the appropriate therapy can be instituted. Cystoscopy should be done when indicated for hematuria, suspected bladder tumor, interstitial cystitis, or persistent urinary tract infections. Sophisticated urodynamic evaluations (e.g., urethral pressure profiles, multichannel studies with fluoroscopy) should be reserved for patients who fail to respond to therapy or for those who require surgical intervention.

TREATMENT

Therapy for urinary incontinence depends on the cause of the condition. First, the causes of transient incontinence should be identified because they are often easily reversed. Delirium and underlying medical causes, such as congestive heart failure or urinary tract infection, should be recognized and treated. Urinary tract infections should be treated with antibiotics, although the relationship between asymptomatic bacteriuria and incontinence has not been clearly established. Atrophic vaginitis and urethritis are treated with topical or oral estrogens. Drug-induced incontinence is modified by stopping or changing drug therapy. Re-

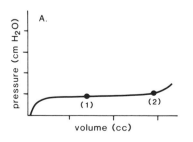

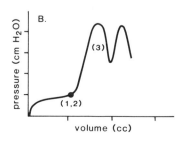

FIGURE 18–4. A, A normal cystometrogram. First sensation to urinate (1); sensation of bladder fullness (2). B, Abnormal cystometrogram demonstrating detrusor instability with uninhibited detrusor contraction and a low-volume bladder (3) with leakage around the catheter.

stricted mobility can be helped by changes in environment, such as the use of a bed pan or bedside commode, and clothing that allows easier access with elastic bands, in place of buttons for easier access. Treatment for fecal impactions should be instituted.

General methods are available, such as behavior therapy, timed voiding, bladder retraining, prompted voiding, and biofeedback. These methods are discussed under the treatment of detrusor instability, but they can have applications in treating other types of incontinence. The use of an indwelling catheter (discussed below) should be avoided, if possible.

The elderly are particularly susceptible to the side effects of uropharmacologic therapy, thus limiting its usefulness. Therefore, the initial doses should be about one half of the recommended dosage. In the elderly, the effectiveness of some treatment regimens has not been proved through controlled clinical trials.

As noted, failure to empty the bladder can result from poor bladder contractility or from the presence of bladder outlet obstruction. By far the most common cause of urinary retention in males is bladder outlet obstruction secondary to prostate hypertrophy. (A discussion of treatment is included in Chapter 19.)

In those patients who have a noncontractible bladder without outlet obstruction, pharmacotherapy can be directed at attempting to increase detrusor contractility or decreasing the bladder outlet resistance. The lack of clinical efficacy of the oral cholinergic agonist bethanechol (urecholine, Duvoid) has been demonstrated in several clinical studies that have measured such objective data as changes in cystometrics and decrease in residual urines.[10] It is agreed that an oral dose of 200 mg is required in a denervated bladder to produce the same effect as a subcutaneous dose of 5 mg.[10]

Bladder outlet resistance can be decreased through alpha-adrenergic blockade. The two drugs most commonly used are phenoxybenzamine (Dibenzyline) 10 mg/day, which can be increased to maximum dose of 60 mg/day, and prazosin (Minipress) 2 to 3 mg/day, which can be increased to a maximum dose of 20 mg/day in divided doses. Several side effects of these drugs may occur in the elderly, es-

pecially orthostatic hypotension, reflex tachycardia, nasal congestion, and sedation. Therefore, caution should be used with these drugs.

The mainstay of treatment of urinary retention is clean, intermittent self-catheterization. If patients have good use of their hands, they can usually perform intermittent self-catheterization. This can be tested by the patient's ability to write his or her name. The technique of clean, intermittent self-catheterization is well known (Table 18–4). A minimum schedule of three to four times a day must be maintained, and catheterized volume of 350 to 500 ml is the maximum acceptable amount. If larger volumes are obtained, the frequency of the catheterizations needs to be increased. For the cognitively impaired, the caregiver should be trained to assist, and a schedule that will provide continence, prevent infection, and avoid taxing the caregiver should be developed.

Other forms of therapy are available (Table 18–5) but are reserved for special situations. These therapies are not discussed in detail here.

Stress urinary incontinence is the failure to store bladder urine, which can be treated in several ways. If atrophic vaginitis is present, oral or local estrogens will help restore the normal urethral mucosa and enhance the alpha-adrenergic effect. For mild stress incontinence, alpha-adrenergic stimulants, such as ephedrine 25 to 50 mg four times a day, phenylpropanolamine 50 mg three times a day, or imipramine (Tofranil) 25 mg three to four times a day, are effective in some cases. However, most patients with moderate or severe stress incontinence will not show a complete response, and incontinence will persist.

TABLE 18–4. Technique of Clean Intermittent Catheterization

Procedure
Wash catheter and hands with soap and water
Clean meatus with soap and water
Apply water-soluble lubricant to catheter tip
Insert catheter until urine returns
Empty bladder completely
Remove catheter and wash and rinse with water; dry
Store catheter until next use

TABLE 18–5. Treatment of Failure to Empty

Increase Intravesical Pressure/Bladder Contractility
    External compression—Credé/Valsalva maneuver
    Pharmacotherapy
        Increase contractility
            Cholinergic medications (e.g., Bethanechol)
            Prostaglandins
        Block inhibition
            Alpha-adrenergic antagonists
    Electrical stimulation
        Direct—bladder pacemaker
        Spinal cord—nerve roots
    Reduction cystoplasty

Decrease Bladder Outlet Resistance
    Surgical treatment of anatomic obstruction
        (TURP, repair of urethral sphincter)
    Smooth muscle sphincter
        Pharmacotherapy
            Alpha-adrenergic antagonists
            Beta-adrenergic agonists
        Surgery
            Incision of bladder neck
            Y-V plasty of bladder neck
    Striate sphincter
        Pharmacotherapy
            Skeletal muscle relaxants
            Alpha-adrenergic antagonists
        Biofeedback
        Surgery
            Urethral dilation
            External sphincterotomy
            Pudendal nerve interruption

Circumvention
    Intermittent self-catheterization
    Continuous catheterization
    Urinary diversion

The mainstay of treatment is a bladder neck suspension procedure. This can be performed as an open surgical procedure, such as with the Marshall-Marchetti-Krantz operation, or endoscopically with minimal invasion, such as with the Raz procedure. If the patient is not a surgical candidate, pessaries—donut-shaped devices that are inserted into the vagina to elevate the bladder neck and compress the urethra against the pubis—can be employed with moderate success.

Detrusor instability, which accounts for 40 to 60 per cent of cases of incontinence, can be approached on a multimodality basis. One of the cornerstones of treatment is behavioral therapy, which includes bladder retraining, biofeedback, habit training, timed voidings, and prompted voidings.

For the cognitively impaired patient, good success can be achieved with timed and prompted voiding. With timed voiding, a diary is kept to document the time interval between voidings and incontinence episodes. Once this interval is established, a toileting schedule is developed. The patient is taken to the toilet on a fixed voiding schedule. With habit training, the time interval is initially fixed and adjusted during treatment. With prompted voiding, the patient is asked about the need to urinate at fixed time intervals. When he or she gives a positive response, the patient is then taken to the bathroom. The group of cognitively impaired patients will show a response to treatment; however, once treatment is stopped, the majority of patients revert to pretreatment levels of incontinence.[11]

The ambulatory individual with higher cognitive levels can be treated through bladder retraining (bladder drill) and biofeedback, with or without the use of pharmacotherapy. The success rates approach 75 to 90 per cent.[12, 13] In bladder retraining, the patient urinates on a mandatory predetermined schedule at the risk of incontinence. The intervals between voiding are then gradually increased. In a second option, the patient can urinate on a self-determined schedule. Initially, a voiding diary is kept and is analyzed both for volume voided and for time interval. The patient then tries to extend the interval by 30 minutes or by a volume of 30 to 60 ml. At the end of 1 month, the voiding diary is rechecked to determine what progress has been made.

During biofeedback, certain parameters are monitored, such as changes in cystometry or sphincter electromyography (EMG) recordings. The patient then attempts to inhibit the abnormal detrusor contraction or relax the external sphincter with visual or auditory stimuli as a guide to success.

Pharmacotherapy for bladder instability has been the mainstay of treatment.[14] Drugs that inhibit the detrusor contraction have been used most frequently. Anticholinergic medicines, including propantheline bromide (Probanthine and others) in doses of 15 to 30 mg four times a day; oxybutynin chloride (Ditropan), which also has a direct smooth muscle relaxant effect, in doses of 5 mg three to four times a day; and atropine in doses of 0.4 mg four times a day, exert their effect by blocking the acetylcholine-induced stimulation of the postganglionic, parasympathetic cholinergic receptors sites on the bladder smooth muscles. Other agents that act directly on bladder smooth muscle by producing relaxation include dicyclomine hydrocholoride (Bentyl) 20 mg three to four times a day and flavoxate hydrochloride (Urispas) 100 to 200 mg three to four times a day. They have been employed with some success. Tricyclic antidepressants such as imipramine (Tofranil) and nortriptyline (Pamelar) act through both a weak antimuscarinic effect and a strong, direct inhibiting effect on bladder smooth muscle. The initial dose is 25 mg at bedtime, which can be increased to a maximum of 150 mg. They also may be given in divided doses. The author has found this to be the most useful drug category for treatment of detrusor instability in the elderly.

Once incontinence is controlled and maintained, the use of behavioral modification, along with pharmacotherapy, may allow slow tapering off of medications. Most bladder regimens take 6 to 12 months to achieve long-lasting results. If detrusor contractions persist, other more invasive procedures can be employed (Table 18–6).

When sphincter incompetence is present (e.g., post-prostatectomy incontinence in men, neurologic lesions affecting the urethra and periurethral muscles, or nonfunctional fibrotic urethra in females), alpha-adrenergic medicines in doses described in the section on the treatment of stress incontinence can be used. Limited success is usually achieved. Another option is the implantation of an artificial urinary sphincter. This device is made up of three components: an occlusive cuff that can be placed around the urethra, a pressure balloon reservoir that controls the pressure in the cuff, and a pump that is placed in the labia or scrotum that controls the device (Fig. 18–5). The artificial urinary sphincter has a success rate of between 75 and 90 per cent in selected elderly patients. Its reliability is much improved over that of earlier models. Other surgical procedures can also be employed to increase bladder outlet resistance.

Despite the many modalities available, many elderly individuals remain incontinent. Palliative procedures can be very helpful to prevent scalding of the skin and skin breakdown, protect clothing and bedding, and prevent odor. Such procedures include the use of absorbent pads, pants, and undergarments and, for male patients, external collecting devices. As a last resort, an indwelling Foley catheter can be employed. The use of indwelling Foley catheters should be discouraged, even though this is the "simple solution." Lower urinary tract infections are common in the chronically ill elderly who are maintained on catheter drainage. The elderly also experience the more severe catheter-associated complications.[15] Late complications include stones, sepsis, and, in males, epididymitis, periurethral abscess and fistula formation, and stricture formation.

With catheterization, bacteriuria will develop in 50 per cent of patients within 2 weeks and in 100 per cent within 6 weeks. Trauma to the bladder mucosa then allows access to the bacteria into the bladder wall, thus establishing infection. Any agent that increases trauma to the bladder mucosa, such as changes of the catheter, detrusor spasms, catheter blockage with overdistention of the bladder, irrigations, and stones, will promote infection.[16]

Management of the indwelling catheter should be aimed at minimizing infection. The use of prophylactic antibiotics, bladder irrigations, and bladder instillations

TABLE 18–6. Treatment of the Failure to Store Bladder Urine

Decrease Bladder Contractility
Pharmacotherapy
  Anticholinergic medications
  Smooth muscle relaxants
Surgery
  Hydrodilatation
  Nerve interruption
    Subarachnoid block
    Selective sacral rhizotomy
    Peripheral bladder denervation; cystolysis
  Augmentation cystoplasty
Reflex inhibition—electrical stimulation of anal
  sphincter

Increase Sphincter Resistance
Pharmacotherapy
  Alpha-adrenergic agonist
  Antihistamines
  Beta-adrenergic antagonists
Surgery
  Urethral or urethrovesical suspension
  Reconstruction of proximal urethra
  Urethral plication
  Periurethral Teflon injection
  Urethral compression
  Artificial urinary sphincter

Circumvention
Urinary diversion

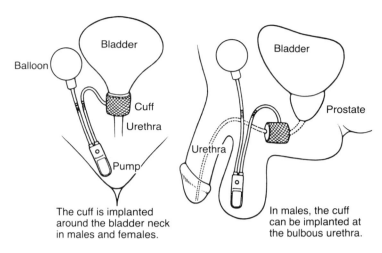

Balloon

Bladder

Cuff

Urethra

Pump

The cuff is implanted around the bladder neck in males and females.

Bladder

Prostate

Urethra

In males, the cuff can be implanted at the bulbous urethra.

FIGURE 18–5. *The American Medical Systems artificial urinary sphincter.*

and frequent catheter changes all have been unsuccessful in eliminating bacteriuria, encrustation, and obstruction. These measures are worth abandoning, since they lead to increased trauma to the mucosa and a potentially higher incidence of infection. More effective measures include taking in adequate fluid, avoiding catheter manipulation, and exchanging the catheter either when urine flow is decreased or when infection is suspected.[16]

Finally, the physician, caregiver, and patients are often in need of information and resource aids. Several organizations have been established to promote the treatment of urinary incontinence.

HIP (Help for Incontinent People),
Inc.
P.O. Box 544
Union, SC 29379

The Simon Foundation
P.O. Box 815
Wilmette, IL 60091

Continence Restored, Inc.
785 Park Ave.
New York, NY 10021

CONCLUSIONS

Through better education, both the elderly population and the medical community should accept that incontinence is not an inevitable consequence of aging. More incontinent elderly patients should be encouraged to seek evaluations so that appropriate treatment can be instituted. The physician must keep in mind that incontinence in the elderly is often caused by precipitants outside of the urinary tract and that by correcting the precipitant, incontinence can be reduced.[1] With appropriate treatment, urinary incontinence can be controlled, the quality of life of the elderly can be improved, and health care expenditures for this condition can be controlled.

REFERENCES

1. Resnick NM, Yalla SV: Aging and its effect on the bladder. Semin Urol, 5:82, 1987.
2. Diokno AC, Brock BM, Herzogar AR, et al: Prevalence of urologic symptoms of the noninstitutionalized elderly (abstr). J Urol 133:179A, 1985.
3. Ouslander JG, Kane RL: The costs of urinary incontinence in nursing homes. Med Care 22:69, 1984.
4. Hu TW: The economic impact of urinary incontinence. Clin Geriatr Med 2:673, 1986.
5. Rohner TJ, Iqou JF: Urinary incontinence in the elderly. AUA update series, Vol V, Lesson 26, 1, 1986.
6. Wein AJ, Raezer DM: Physiology of micturition. In RJ Krane, MB Siroky, eds: Clinical Neuro-Urology. Boston, Little, Brown & Co, 1979, p 1.
7. Badlani GH, Smith AD: Pharmacotherapy of voiding dysfunction in the elderly. Semin Urol 5:120, 1987.
8. Ouslander JG, Staskin S, Orzeck S, et al: Diagnostic tests for geriatric incontinence. World J Urol 4:16, 1986.
9. Castleden CM, Duffin HM, Aswen NH: Clinical and urodynamic studies in 100 elderly incontinent patients. Br Med J 282:1103, 1981.
10. Wein AJ: Drug treatment of voiding dysfunction, Part I: evaluation of drugs: treatment of emptying

failure. AUA update series, Vol 7, Lesson 14, 106, 1988.

11. Schnelle JF: Management of geriatric incontinence in nursing homes. J Appl Behav Anal 16:235, 1983.

12. Jarvis GJ: A controlled trial of bladder drill and drug therapy in the management of detrusor instability. Br J Urol 53:565, 1981.

13. Cardozo L, Stanton SL, Hafner S, et al: Biofeedback in the treatment of detrusor instability. Br J Urol 50:250, 1978.

14. Wein AJ: Drug treatment of voiding dysfunction, Part II: drug treatment of storage failure. AUA update series, Vol 7, Lesson 15, 114, 1988.

15. Warren JW, Muncie HL Jr, Bergquist EJ, et al: Sequelae and management of urinary infections in the patient requiring chronic catheterization. J Urol 125:1, 1981.

16. Seiler WO, Stahelin HB: Practical management of catheter associated UTI's. Geriatrics 43:43, 1988.

CHAPTER 19

Diseases of the Prostate

Robert E. Donohue

Marilyn A. Davis

E. David Crawford

Old age isn't so bad when you consider the alternative.

MAURICE CHEVALIER,
New York Times, quoted

The prostate gland is a musculoglandular structure—conical in shape and located in the pelvis—that bridges the bladder neck and membranous urethra. The normal post pubertal prostate measures approximately 3.5 cm transversely at its base and about 2.5 cm in its vertical and anteroposterior dimensions. It weighs about 18 gms.

Disease of the prostate occurs more often than disease of any other internal organ in men. It accounts for the most common urologic cancer as well as the most common benign, proliferative abnormality of any internal organ, i.e., benign prostatic hypertrophy. The incidence of these two disease entities increases with age, and yet a high proportion of prostatic lesions remain clinically insignificant. Autopsy studies have documented that 30 per cent of men age 50 and older will be found to have evidence of carcinoma of the prostate.

PROSTATITIS

Prostatitis is a perplexing disease that requires very specific clinical and laboratory investigations in order to establish the diagnosis and to properly categorize the type of prostatitis present. The majority of cases are not due to bacterial infection, but are secondary to pathogenic processes, which cause inflammation of the prostate. In an elderly patient population, the diagnosis and treatment require persever-

ance and precision. The classification system is based on a set of urine and prostatic cultures and the microscopic examination, known as the segmented urine culture technique, described by Meares and Stamey.[1]

There are two types of infectious prostatitis: acute bacterial prostatitis and chronic bacterial prostatitis.[2] A patient with acute bacterial prostatitis is generally quite ill, experiencing systemic toxicity with fever, chills, lower back and sacral pain, perineal pain, and varying degrees of urinary obstruction. Rectal examination reveals an enlarged, tender, boggy prostate. It is unwise to perform a vigorous prostatic massage because this may induce bacteremia. Acute bacterial prostatitis is relatively rare in young men; however, the elderly population has an increased incidence caused by the frequent use of indwelling, urethral catheters.

Chronic prostatitis can be of either bacterial or nonbacterial etiology and presents with varying degrees of dysuria, frequency, nocturia, or sharp, diffusely radiating perineal or lower back pain. The disease is characterized by periods of exacerbation and remission. Chronic bacterial prostatitis is the most common cause of recurrent urinary tract infections in men with a normal intravenous pyelogram (IVP). Prostatodynia is the fourth type of prostatitis recognized and is, basically, pain in the prostate with no abnormal findings in the prostatic secretions or cultures.

Microorganisms most commonly gain access to the prostate gland in a retrograde fashion by ascending the urethral route. Theoretical seeding of the prostate with bacteria-laden urine is supported by the fact that prostatic calculi can contain extraneous constituents originating in the urine. Rarely, hematogenous or lymphogenous routes are implicated in bacterial prostatic infection. There is some evidence that prostatitis may be sexually transmitted, in that partners of patients who have the disease will often have positive vaginal introitus cultures for the same organism.

Nonbacterial prostatitis is felt to be inflammatory in nature, produced by irritants such as caffeine, alcohol, dietary factors, pharmacologic agents, and even physical activity. Increased intravesical pressure generated by heavy lifting or exercise against a closed external urethral sphincter can force urine into the prostatic ducts, creating a chemical prostatitis. Psychogenic factors such as stress and anxiety play an unquantifiable but demonstrable role in the promotion of prostatitis. Iatrogenic factors can also predispose the patients to bacterial prostatitis, including, as noted, indwelling urethral catheters, surgical manipulation of the lower urinary tract, and transurethral resection of the prostate.

The most common organisms involved in bacterial prostatitis parallel those seen with urinary tract infections, including the enteric organisms *Escherichia coli*, *Pseudomonas*, *Enterobacter*, *Klebsiella*, and *Proteus*. Gram-positive pathogens are rarely cultured. Mixed cultures involving multiple organisms have been reported but are rare in the absence of indwelling, foreign bodies such as a urethral catheter. Nonbacterial prostatitis is a common disease entity and may be precipitated by agents such as *Trichomonas*, *Ureaplasma*, and *Chlamydia*.

Diagnosis

The sine qua non for the diagnosis is the segmented urine culture technique. With this method, it is possible to localize the infection to the prostatic substance. In order to perform these cultures, the patient reports to the clinic with a full bladder, and his external meatus is cleansed with soap and water. Antiseptic solutions should be avoided, since one drop in a collected specimen can inhibit growth. The patient is asked to void 5 to 10 ml of urine in a container, which is then labeled (VB_1); this is followed by the classic, midstream

collection, labeled (VB_2). At this point, a prostatic massage is carried out and these secretions are collected in a container labeled expressed prostatic secretion (EPS). The patient voids 10 more ml in another container labeled (VB_3). It is helpful to have these containers prelabeled and available at the time of the collection of the specimens, and to inform patients, especially the elderly, in advance, of exactly what the procedure entails. The technique takes no longer than 5 minutes and is a cost-effective measure, considering that many patients are needlessly placed on antimicrobial regimens when, in fact, they do not have a bacterial prostatitis. These cultures and sensitivities, if performed in the hospital laboratory, can be quite expensive, exceeding $170. To reduce the cost of separate processing for cultures, a culture plate containing eosin-methylene blue (EMB) or MacConkey's agar can be divided into four quadrants and each sample swabbed on a separate quadrant. The technique is not as precise as that performed in a commercial laboratory, but it is easy to visualize positive culture results and to make a determination of whether there is a differential growth between the EPS or VB_3 and VB_1 or VB_2.

To make a diagnosis of a chronic bacterial prostatitis, there should be at least a 1 log difference in the growth between the EPS or VB_3 and VB_1 and VB_2. However, any colony count is significant. For example, 1000 organisms in the EPS with 100 or less in VB_1 and VB_2 would indicate prostatitis. The next step is to examine the expressed prostatic secretions for white blood cells, oval fat bodies, and lecithin granules. Table 19–1 outlines the microscopic evaluation of the EPS, showing that in both chronic bacterial and nonbacterial prostatitis, there are increased numbers of white cells and oval fat bodies and decreased lecithin granules. The culture serves to establish the presence of bacteria. Prostatodynia rarely produces any abnormalities of the EPS, and cultures are always negative.

Other urological abnormalities, including carcinoma in situ, stones, urethral diverticula and strictures, may mimic the symptoms of prostatitis. Additionally, subtle urologic voiding dysfunctions, including detrusor sphincter dyssynergia,

TABLE 19–1. Microscopic Evaluation of Expressed Prostatic Secretions in the Diagnosis of Prostatitis*

	Chronic Bacterial Prostatitis	Nonbacterial Prostatitis	Prostatodynia
WBC	Increased	Increased	Normal
Oval fat bodies	Increased	Increased	Rare
Lecithin granules	Decreased	Decreased	Normal

*Prostatic massage is generally deferred in an acute bacterial presentation.

are known to precipitate nonbacterial prostatitis.

Treatment

Once the diagnosis of a bacterial prostatitis is made, the proper antibiotic must be chosen. The ideal antibiotic does not become ionized in the blood and is lipid soluble in its nonionized form; however, it ionizes at the pH of prostatic fluids. These characteristics cause the drug to diffuse into the gland, become ionized, and thus accumulate in prostatic tissue by a process known as ion-trapping. The prostate possesses a barrier, analogous to the blood-brain barrier, which is breached in acute infection, allowing bacteria, as well as antibiotics, to diffuse freely into the gland. However, after resolution of the acute process, penetration of antimicrobial agents into the prostate becomes dependent on their lipid solubility and ionization potential.

In the patient acutely ill with prostatitis, therapy should be started with an aminogycoside and ampicillin. These antibiotics are continued until the septic process abates, and the patient is then given oral antimicrobial agents, based on the sensitivity of the offending organism. In general, the antibiotic chosen has properties that allow it to penetrate into the prostate, including carbenicillin and trimethoprim-sulfamethoxazole.

Data from clinical trials evaluating the efficacy of various antibiotics in chronic prostatitis are limited. It would appear that the ideal theoretical drug would be lipid soluble, thus promoting its passage into the prostate, and have a spectrum covering most common organisms associated with prostatitis. The first drug of choice is carbenicillin indanyl sodium (2 382-mg tablets taken four times a day for 1 month). Patients allergic to penicillin should be given trimethoprim-sulfamethoxazole (1 tablet taken twice a day for one month). Alternative drugs include the quinolones and tetracyclines.

Patients failing to respond to these regimens should be re-evaluated, and consideration given to a nonbacterial prostatitis. Urodynamic disorders may be effectively managed with short courses of anticholinergic agents such as oxybutynin. Those patients with symptoms precipitated by infrequent voiding may benefit from timed voiding, such as q.2h trials. Approaches such as sitz baths and administration of antiinflammatory agents and low-dose diazepam may be beneficial. In patients with prostatodynia, work and lifestyle patterns contributing to perineal, musculoskeletal dysfunction should be evaluated.

The diagnosis and treatment of prostatitis are clinically challenging. With our current understanding of the pathogenesis of the disease, it can now be more precisely defined and comprehensively managed. The segmented urine culture technique and microscopic examination of the expressed prostatic secretions are of paramount importance in classifying the disease. The discovery of effective antibiotics that penetrate into the prostate now leads to cure of the disease in a substantial number of patients. In nonbacterial prostatitis and prostatodynia, a careful, meticulous screening and diagnostic work-up is indicated, followed by appropriate management strategies to alleviate the numerous etiological causes.

BENIGN PROSTATIC HYPERPLASIA

The prostate gland, an accessory sexual gland, is responsible for 30 per cent of the ejaculate in the male. In the elderly male, growth of this gland causes elongation, tortuosity, and compression of the posterior urethra and leads to significant bladder outlet obstruction often requiring surgical correction.

From birth until puberty, the prostate undergoes slow growth, but with puberty it undergoes a rapid increase in size until approximately age 20.[3] It remains constant at a weight of about 20 gm until about age 45, when the onset of benign prostatic hyperplasia (BPH) commences, and the volume increases.

In the fifth decade, the incidence of BPH in men is approximately 23 per cent, whereas in the ninth decade, it increases to 88 per cent. Twenty years ago, it was predicted that 10 per cent of men age 40 who lived to age 80 would require surgical correction for significant prostate obstruction. A current reappraisal states that a 50-year-old man has a 25 per cent chance of requiring prostatectomy during his lifetime.[4]

The pathogenesis of BPH remains unclear and the etiology debatable.[5] The role of the testis, intracellular dihydrotestosterone, and androgen/estrogen synergism are all being researched.

Symptoms of prostatic disease can be obstructive or irritative. The obstructive manifestations of prostatic disease are hesitancy in initiating urination, weakened urinary stream, the inability to terminate urination abruptly without dribbling, incomplete emptying of the bladder at the time of voiding, the inability to void at all, acute urinary retention, and overflow incontinence (continuous leakage of a small volume of urine without bladder emptying). The irritative symptoms are dysuria, urgency, and frequency.

As the obstruction of the posterior urethra by elongation, tortuosity, and compression from prostatic tissue progresses, 50 to 80 per cent of males develop an unstable bladder with frequency, urgency, and some urge incontinence.[6] Their residual urine increases and nocturia and daytime frequency occur. Often, a mass may appear in the lower abdomen, i.e., distended bladder, and overflow incontinence ensues.

At times, the patient may suffer from silent prostatism. The patient's symptoms do not represent the primary effects of urethral compression and tortuosity but the secondary systemic effects of bladder neck obstruction. These symptoms are (1) acute urinary retention, (2) overflow incontinence, (3) renal failure with blood urea nitrogen (BUN) and serum creatinine elevation, and (4) uremia. Acute retention, the final result of the progression of obstructive symptoms or silent prostatism, can be precipitated also by delay in voiding, alcohol, or the use of anticholinergics, antidepressants, tranquilizers, and decongestants.

Diagnosis

The physical examination of the patient with BPH includes monitoring of the vital signs and a generalized examination. Evaluation of the abdomen should include suprapubic percussion for a distended bladder and evaluation for the presence of inguinal hernia. Rectal examination is most easily and effectively completed with the patient on his knees and elbows on the examining table. The examiner does not assume any uncomfortable position during the performance of this examination, and the examination is facilitated in the obese male.

Inspection of the perineum and lower back is carried out, noting scars from previous laminectomies, detecting pilonidal sinus, and assessing fissures, fistulas, and hemorrhoids.

Rectal examination should include an evaluation of the anal sphincter tone and determination of the presence or absence of a narrowing just proximal to the anal sphincter muscle, suggestive of either a previous aggressive hemorrhoidectomy or assessment of adenocarcinoma of the rectum.

The prostatic examination should include an evaluation for size, symmetry, nodularity, and hardness. The prostate should be considered normal in size or enlarged and symmetric or asymmetric. The presence of nodules should be detected using two techniques. In the initial technique, the examining finger should traverse the median sulcus and then run superficially across the surface of each lateral lobe from the median sulcus to the lateral border of the gland to detect gross nodularity. In the second technique, each area of each lobe should be compressed individually and the prostatic tissue evaluated beneath the rectal wall for nodules that are not obvious. Any abnormality on either assessment should be diagrammed, highlighting its position for future comparison examination. The consistency of the prostate should be assessed and described as normal or hard and hard areas diagrammed. Just above the prostate, the distal portion of the vas deferens may be palpated superiorly toward the midline and the seminal vesicles detected laterally. The rectal lumen should be palpated as far as possible to determine patency, the rectal wall palpated for abnormalities or growths, and a guaiac test completed for occult blood in a stool specimen removed with the gloved hand.

Laboratory evaluation should consist of urinalysis, culture and sensitivity, if appropriate, and assessment of residual urine. The patient should then be instructed to collect 5-second urine flow rates at the first morning void for 7 days. Less than 10 ml per second or 50 ml per 5 seconds suggests obstruction. A peak flow, usually more than 15 ml per second, also offers functional information.

Cystoscopy is the study of choice for the evaluation of outlet obstruction. By direct vision, the lumen and lining of the entire urethra are studied, and the anatomic relationship of the obstructing lobes (subtrigonal, subcervical, and lateral) of the prostate is visualized. The presence of bladder calculi, tumors, cystitis, and vesical hemorrhage can be easily detected. The changes in the bladder musculature (trabeculations, cellules, and diverticula) caused by the outlet obstruction can be seen directly. The sites in the trigone for the openings of the ureters can be seen, renal and ureteral hematuria diagnosed, and ureteral emptying recorded. The presence of a urethral stricture, a bladder neck contracture, and/or significant residual adenomatous prostatic tissue can be confirmed in patients with recurrent outlet obstructive symptoms after previous transurethral prostatectomy.

The differential diagnoses of symptomatic BPH are (1) benign prostatic hypertrophy; (2) uncontrolled diabetes mellitus; (3) transitional cell carcinoma of the bladder; (4) carcinoma in situ of the bladder (CIS); (5) uninhibited neurogenic bladder; (6) flaccid neurogenic bladder; (7) adenocarcinoma of the prostate; (8) bladder calculus; (9) prostatitis; (10) meatal stenosis; (11)

urethral stricture disease; and (12) bladder neck contracture.

Excretory urography yields excellent information about the anatomy of the urinary tract, renal anomalies, excretory capability of the kidneys, presence of renal masses, and filling defects of the collecting system. The anatomy, course, and caliber of the ureters are delineated; the presence of bladder wall trabeculations, cellules and diverticula, and effects of prostatic obstruction determined; and bladder filling evaluated. A post-void film yields information about the degree of bladder emptying.

In the patient experiencing urgency and frequency, bladder pressure studies and cystometrography (either with water or with carbon dioxide) can be performed. Urgency and frequency also mandate a voided urine cytology to exclude transitional cell carcinoma in situ (CIS) in patients without obvious neurogenic disease. The direct observation of the urinary stream by the examining physician, a study that has fallen into disfavor recently, deserves to be used in selected cases.

Treatment

Table 19–2 lists the current and experimental methodologies for treatment of BPH. Therapy for this disorder remains mostly surgical. Historically, castration and antiandrogens have been tried without much success.[7, 8] Intermittent self-catheterization is a nonsurgical therapy that has been employed successfully for generations. The patient catheterizes himself frequently enough in the day so that he never accumulates a volume of 500 ml at the time of any one catheterization. However, the risk of infection persists.

Alpha adrenergic blockers, dibenzylene, and prasozin have been most effective in relaxing the bladder neck to allow a better stream, greater force of stream, higher flow rates, and more complete emptying.[9–11] Dibenzylene has significant side effects and is poorly tolerated by the elderly patient. Prasozin seems to work as well and has fewer side effects. 5-alpha-reductase inhibitors have also been studied. The use of the first generation 5-alpha-reductase inhibitor, which blocks the conversion of testosterone into dihydrotestosterone, had

TABLE 19–2. History of Treatment of Benign Prostatic Hyperplasia (BPH)

Treatment/Procedure	Date First Performed
Intermittent catheterization	?
Suprapubic transvesical prostatectomy	1880
Perineal prostatectomy	1894
Castration	1898
Transurethral prostatectomy (TUR)	1929
Retropubic prostatectomy	1945
Transurethral incision of the prostate	1965
Alpha adrenergic blockers	1980
Anticholesteremic agents (Candicidin)	1980
Antiandrogens	1980s
Luteinizing hormone–releasing hormone analogues	1980s
Flutamide	1980s
Balloon dilatation	1987

? = Unknown

to be discontinued because of toxicity. A new 5-alpha-reductase agent with less toxicity, which must be given prior to the onset of BPH at approximately age 40, is now being studied.

Successful surgery for prostatic hyperplasia dates back to the 1880s, when the suprapubic prostatectomy was introduced. Other successful surgical procedures were perineal prostatectomy in the 1890s, transurethral resection of the prostate (TURP) in the 1920s, and simple retropubic enucleation of the prostate for benign disease in the 1940s. With better optics, better instrumentation, and more sophisticated application of electronic technology in the practice of urology, TURP has become the most popular method of prostatectomy, even for significantly enlarged glands.

Spinal or continuous epidural anesthesia is the preferred method of anesthesia for the surgical procedure. The conscious patient allows the anesthesiologist to closely monitor mental status and alert the surgeon to hypervolemic problems early.

The intraoperative complications of TURP include bleeding, capsular perforation, bladder perforation, and urinary extravasation. Excessive absorption of irrigating fluid may result in hypovolemia, restlessness, confusion, nausea, or vomit-

ing. If undetected, convulsions, coma, and death may occur.

The postoperative complications include secondary hemorrhage, acute urinary retention, urinary retention caused by clot formation from secondary hemorrhage, bladder neck contracture, and urethral stricture. Total urinary incontinence due to sphincteric injury occurs in about 1 per cent of patients. More commonly, patients with preoperative urgency continue to have urgency and urgency incontinence that will respond to anticholinergics.

Sexual function is affected as well. The removal of the prostate gland and occlusion of the ejaculatory ducts draining the seminal vesicles can eliminate ejaculation at orgasm. The seminal vesicles contribute 70 per cent to the volume of ejaculate. If the ejaculatory ducts empty into the urethra with orgasm, the loss of the bladder neck may lead to retrograde passage of this ejaculation into the bladder.

Impotence also occurs after TURP. The exact incidence remains to be determined. Not enough attention has been given to the objective preoperative assessment of erectile function, and therefore postoperative impotence is difficult to evaluate and interpret. Excessive periprostatic extravasation of irrigating fluid during TURP may contribute to impotence.

Recent studies show that in patients whose prostates weigh under 30 to 35 gm as estimated by rectal examination, unilateral or bilateral surgical incisions of the prostate and bladder neck beginning at the posterior trigone and ending near the apex of the prostate, allow for adequate voiding and complete emptying and have been accompanied by a significant reduction in morbidity and mortality as compared with TURP.[12, 13] The incision is made deeply through the prostatic tissue from the posterior wall of the trigone, just medial to the ureteral orifice, down to and alongside the verumontanum in the distal prostatic urethra. With this incision, the bladder neck and prostatic urethra are widely opened. When this is accomplished unilaterally, approximately 40 per cent of the patients experience retrograde ejaculation. When it is performed bilaterally, approximately 70 per cent of the patients experience this ejaculation phenomenon. Whether or not the transurethral incision of the prostate will stand the test of time remains to be seen. Effective voiding can be restored, however, and except for retrograde ejaculation, sexual function remains unaffected.

In summary, benign prostatic hypertrophy affects males 40 years of age and older. It may be associated with significant alteration in lifestyle and the preferred therapy continues to be surgery for correction of bladder outlet obstruction. The role of 5-alpha-reductase inhibitors in the prevention of the disease and the role of the transurethral incision of the prostate in its treatment both need to be evaluated further.

CANCER OF THE PROSTATE

Cancer originating in the prostate gland is the most commonly occurring tumor in males in the United States, exceeding lung cancer for the first time in 1988.[14] Considered a rare phenomenon in the 19th century, presently prostate cancer is viewed as a disease process with an extremely morbid and mortal potential, with over 26,000 attributable deaths annually.[14] A relatively uncommon disease in men under age 40, the mean age at presentation is 72 years. No specific etiologic factors are known.[15] Endogenous hormonal influences are implied because dihydrotestosterone, the intracellularly active metabolite of testosterone, is essential to prostatic growth and metabolism. Geographic patterns show higher incidences of prostate cancer in northern and western European countries and apparent lower incidences in eastern Europe and Japan.[16] Incidence rates in black males are roughly twice that of white males in the United States, with corresponding mortality statistics.[16] Rising disease rates in immigrants from countries considered low risk for prostate cancer suggest environmental initiating or promoting factors. Genetic factors are suggested, with familial distributions observed.

With increasing life expectancy, a corresponding increase in prostatic cancer can also be anticipated. Incidence data identifying latent (clinically unsuspected) carcinomas range from 0.85 per cent in Alexejew and Dunajewski's large random series to 66.7 per cent per 100 males over age 80 as reported by Rullis and colleagues.[17, 18]

Diagnosis

Prostate cancer is curable if diagnosed while localized to the prostate gland; however, detection while the cancer is confined within the prostatic capsule is accomplished in only 10 to 15 per cent of presentations. Prior to 1936, rectal examination was the only test for the detection of a suspicious prostatic lesion. With the description of serum acid phosphatase by Gutman in 1936, the field of biologic markers as potential indicators of the presence of tumors was introduced.[19] Since that time, numerous biologically active substances, including prostatic acid phosphatase (PAP) and prostate specific antigen (PSA), have been examined. Radioimmunoassay of PAP is not entirely specific for prostate cancer; approximately 6 per cent of patients with elevated PAP have exclusively benign hypertrophy of the prostate.

Prostate specific antigen, as identified by Wang and associates in 1979, is antigenically distinct from PAP; however, because PSA is also present in men with benign prostatic hypertrophy, differentiation between cancer and BPH at low concentrations of PSA is almost impossible. The findings of Chu and coworkers suggest that simultaneous PSA and PAP measurements may enhance the clinician's ability to assess the likelihood of the presence of prostate cancer and monitor activity of the disease and its response to therapy.[21] The level of other markers such as carcinoembryonic antigen, lactic dehydrogenase (LDH), and urinary hydroxyproline may tend to rise with disease progression and fall with disease response, but the low percentage of efficiency does not justify their use as prostate cancer markers.

Newer modalities, specifically aspiration cytology and transrectal ultrasonography, have been promoted in the detection of prostate cancer. The technique of fine needle aspiration of sheets of cells for cytologic review, first reported by Esposti in 1956 and popularized in European centers, is now being applied in the United States.[22] However, the bioptic gun technique with the ability to yield cores of tissue has been demonstrated to be a high-yield, cost-effective procedure with low morbidity. Transrectal ultrasonography, although not a cost effective, sensitive, or specific screening test, provides computerized images for viewing the entire prostatic structure and enhances the clinician's accuracy in guiding biopsy or aspiration needles to suspicious sites.

The digital rectal examination of the prostate gland is the most cost-efficient test, with no compromise of diagnostic accuracy.[23] As suggested by Guinan and associates, adherence to American Cancer Society guidelines for annual digital examination of the prostate gland for men over 40 years of age is recommended.[23]

The differential diagnosis of a prostatic nodule includes carcinoma (50 per cent), BPH, granulomatous prostatitis, tuberculosis, prostatic calculi, and phlebolith of the rectal wall. Histologic evaluation is needed to establish a definitive diagnosis; therefore, once the clinical suspicion of a prostatic cancer has arisen, the next step is prostatic biopsy. The common method used to confirm the diagnosis is needle biopsy of the prostate, performed either transperineally or transrectally. Needle biopsy may be done on an outpatient basis. It is simple to perform, relatively safe, and reliable. Needle tract tumor seeding is rarely reported. Other more invasive methods of prostatic biopsy include transurethral resection of the prostate and open perineal biopsy. Papanicolaou (PAP) stains of prostatic fluid, obtained by prostatic massage, are positive in approximately 80 per cent of patients with an established diagnosis of advanced (stage C and D) prostatic cancer.

The interpretation of prostatic biopsies by pathologists is often frought with difficulty due to the similarity of a number of benign and malignant processes that can coexist.[24] The majority of prostatic carcinomas are adenocarcinomas, which are believed to arise from the epithelium lining the peripheral acini. In addition to these conventional carcinomas, a number of rare, unconventional ones also exist. Ductal carcinomas are often papillary or cribriform. Those arising at the junction of large ducts with the prostatic urethra are known as periurethral prostatic duct carcinomas. Central, ductal tumors tend to be locally aggressive and metastasize later in their natural history. Endometrioid carcinomas, once thought to arise from the prostatic utricle, produce both PSA and PAP. They are, therefore, believed to be a variant of ductal carcinoma. Mucinous carcinomas are uncommon (0.4 to 3.0 per cent); however, as many as 10 to 20 per cent of acinar carcinomas contain areas of mucin production. The possibility of invasive colorectal carcinoma should always be excluded in these cases. Other rare tumors such as pure transitional cell carcinomas, small cell (neuroendocrine) carcinomas, adenoid cystic carcinomas and carcinosarcomas have been reported.

Once the diagnosis of prostatic carcinoma has been established, a histologic grade is assigned in an attempt to predict the patient's prognosis. To date, over 40 prostatic cancer grading systems have been described. This is because prostatic carcinomas are often composed of a variety of histologic patterns admixed even in small biopsy fragments. Although a number of criteria have been examined for their prognostic significance, only two—glandular architectural and nuclear anaplasia—have consistently proved to be of value. The Gleason system is one of the most widely used and depends entirely on glandular architecture. In this approach, the two most predominant patterns of carcinoma are assigned scores ranging from 1 to 5. The scores are then added to obtain a pattern sum for that patient. These sums have been shown to be predictive of stage and survival in large series of patients when used alone or in combination with clinical staging.

The system developed for use by the National Prostatic Cancer Project (NPCP) uses both the glandular architecture and the nuclear detail approaches.[25] A number of other workers have presented modifications of these techniques. Although at present, no single system has been universally adopted, it has been recommended that the Gleason system serve as a standard against which other systems be compared.

Recently, the definition of premalignant states, such as atypical hyperplasia and dysplasia, has raised a possibility of identifying patients at an earlier stage. These two lesions occur in both the presence and absence of BPH and seem, therefore, to be independent. In series of patients, both of these lesions have been shown to be present in association with small volume, early tumors and with more advanced disease. With continued evaluation, atypical hyperplasia or dysplasia may provide a means to improve our ability to detect patients at risk for developing clinically significant disease before it has invaded or metastasized.

Staging of Prostatic Carcinoma

After histologic confirmation, a staging work-up is done to evaluate localized extent and metastatic status with awareness of the tumor's propensity to spread via blood vessels and lymphatics. Radiologic examinations include excretory urography, chest x-ray, bone scan, and bone survey or spot films of suspicious areas. Hepatomegaly or abnormal liver function requires further hepatic evaluations. Pelvic and periaortic nodes are evaluated by pelvic computed tomography (CT). Because microscopic lymphatic metastases are not imaged, however, pelvic lymphadenectomy remains the most accurate method for assessment of lymph node status. Transrectal ultrasonography may suggest size, shape, consistency, and delineate the prostatic capsule. Magnetic resonance imaging (MRI) may prove to be of value in distinguishing between benign prostatic hypertrophy and cancer because it illustrates the seminal vesicles and prostate capsule and delineates the interface between the prostate gland and contiguous structure.

Prostate cancer is clinically staged A through D, with stage A disease unsuspected at digital rectal examination and incidentally found on pathologic examination of resected prostate tissue. Subdivided into A_1 and A_2 disease, A_1 is pathologically graded as well-differentiated or moderately well-differentiated tumor, with foci of tumor representing less than 5 per cent of resected tissue. A_2 disease is moderately or poorly differentiated tumor involving over 5 per cent of the resection. Presently, with conservative medical management being considered a cost-effective alternative to surgical resection for mild or moderate degrees of obstructive uropathy, the percentage of stage A disease identification may fall.

Stage B disease is palpable tumor confined to the prostate; B_1 disease is a unilobar nodule less than 2 cm, B_2 is a unilobar nodule over 2 cm, and B_3 is bilobar nodule or diffuse disease confined to the gland. Stage C disease is clinically determined to involve seminal vesicles or adjacent structures. Stage D represents metastatic disease, with D_1 suggesting regional involvement and D_2 documenting tumor metastatic to bone, other organs, or nodes above the aortic bifurcation.

Management of Disease

Stage A_1 disease is managed by follow-up needle biopsies of the prostate gland 6 to 8 weeks after the initial prostatectomy. If no residual tumor is detected, routine prostate screening recommendations are followed. Documentation of residual tumor results in reclassification of the patient into clinical stage A_2.

Complete surgical removal of the prostate gland, including the seminal vesicles, remains the treatment of choice for stage A_2, B_1, and B_2 lesions. Significantly higher overall survival rates have been obtained with radical prostatectomy than with external-beam radiotherapy or interstitial radiation implantation techniques. A retropubic approach is preferred because the limited pelvic lymphadenectomy can be followed by radical prostatectomy if the nodal frozen sections are negative for tumor. Although the perineal approach facilitates vesicourethral anastomosis and decreases blood loss, the pelvic lymphatics are not accessible and another surgical approach for adequate evaluation must be performed.

Rectal injuries and severe hemorrhage are infrequent complications of radical prostatectomy. Postoperative complications include a 6 per cent risk of partial to complete urinary incontinence and lesser risks of bladder neck contracture and urethral stricture. Impotence, which had been an inevitable sequela of complete surgical removal of the prostate, can be avoided in most cases by use of the Walsh technique, which spares the pelvic nerve plexuses involved in penile erection. Pharmacologic induction of erection with intracorporeal injection of papaverine is widely used.

The role of radiotherapy as a curative modality in prostate cancer has generated considerable controversy. External-beam megavoltage radiotherapy has controlled disease limited to the prostate in an impressive number of patients. New implantation techniques for delivering radiation directly to target prostate tissue, used alone or with external-beam therapy, offer local control without loss of potency.

More than 50 per cent of all prostate cancer lesions initially judged to be clinical stage C are actually stage D_1, with local lymphatic disease, or even D_2 disease, with micrometastatic foci of tumor to bone. The curative potential for either radiotherapy or surgical intervention in advanced-stage lesions is slight. Although 5-year survival figures comparing radiotherapy with radical prostatectomy are similar, at 10 and 15 years, the survival figures favor radical prostatectomy as the therapy of choice. Radiotherapy is, however, clearly indicated in patients who are not good surgical candidates.

Advanced prostate cancer (stages C, D_1, and D_2 disease) can be viewed as a chronic condition that patients can live with comfortably for a long time. The myth that advanced malignancies are not amenable to therapeutic intervention should be dispelled.

Since the demonstration of the androgen-dependent nature of prostate cancer by Huggins and Hodges in 1941, hormonal manipulation has been the cornerstone of therapy for advanced malignancy. Initially, Huggins thought that androgen deprivation had the potential to cure metastatic disease; however, continued evaluation demonstrated recurrence in most patients between 12 and 24 months after orchiectomy. Manifestations vary in severity from indolent to aggressive.

The adult testes produce 95 per cent of serum testosterone; the adrenal glands produce the remaining 5 per cent. An intact hypothalamic-pituitary-gonadal axis is required to maintain physiologic levels of testosterone. Interruption at any point in this axis will circumvent the prostate supply of androgens, depriving the gland of testosterone and producing subjective or objective improvement in disease activity and symptom control. A number of pharmacologic agents and surgical interventions are designed to disrupt the axis.

Bilateral orchiectomy is the time-honored and most cost-effective method for permanent disruption of the axis. It is a simple surgical procedure with minimal morbidity and continues to be effective as initial therapy for symptomatic advanced-stage disease. Serum testosterone is permanently reduced to castrate levels, and impotence results. Patients who refuse orchiectomy may be treated with daily oral diethylstilbestrol (DES) at an adequate suppression dosage (1 mg three times a day). DES blocks the axis at the hypothalamic level, with remission rates approximating those of orchiectomy. Complications include salt and water retention, embolic and thromboembolic episodes, cardiovascular compromise, testicular atrophy, and decreased libido. DES-associated gynecomastia can be prevented by delivery of 400 rad to each breast before administration of the drug. DES continues to be widely used and is an effective, cost-efficient therapy.

Hypophysectomy for control of symptomatic advanced prostate cancer has had disappointing results. Investigators have successfully synthesized a luteinizing hormone–releasing hormone (LHRH) that is far more powerful than the naturally occurring hormone. Long-term supraphysiologic doses of synthetic LHRH paradoxically cause androgen depletion, perhaps as a result of pituitary depletion or desensitization to the abundance of circulating LHRH. Luteinizing hormone–releasing hormone analogues appear to be effective, although expensive, agents with acceptable side effects (primarily, hot flashes). It is suggested that LHRH analogues work more effectively in combination with antiandrogens, which compete with dihydrotestosterone for binding sites on prostate cells.

Tumor cell heterogeneity, a major cause of development of resistance to a formerly effective therapeutic maneuver, is demonstrated by prostate cancer cell lines that can be grown synthetically in the absence of androgens.

In the continuing search for long-term control of the heterogeneous prostate cancer cell lines, a number of chemotherapeutic agents have been evaluated in clinical trials as single agents, combination therapy, or adjuvant therapy. Complete responses to chemotherapy in stage D_2 prostate cancer have not been documented. Partial responses have not been sustained. Subjective responses or disease stabilization have been commonly observed, with the most effective chemotherapeutic agents being cyclophosphamide, 5-fluorouracil, cisplatin, doxorubicin, and methotrexate.[27]

SUMMARY

Early-stage diagnosis of prostate cancer when a cure is a likely outcome is clearly within the realm of current clinical realities. Advances in tumor markers, scanning, imaging, and cytologic and tissue specimen evaluations greatly enhance the clinician's ability to localize tumor, define scope of activity, and predict and monitor response to therapy. New strategies in hormonal manipulation offer promise in contributing to enhancement of quality of life for patients with advanced prostate cancer. Finally, the elucidation of combined therapeutic regimens to control androgen-sensitive and androgen-independent prostatic cancer cells encourages a multidisciplinary approach to this major disease entity.

REFERENCES

1. Meares EM Jr, Stamey TA: Bacteriologic localization patterns in bacterial prostatitis and urethritis. Invest Urol 5:492, 1968.
2. Crawford ED: Diagnosis and treatment of prostatitis. Hosp Pract 20:77, 1985.
3. Berry SJ, Coffey DS, Walsh PC, et al: The development of human benign prostatic hyperplasia with age. J Urol 132:474, 1984.
4. Lytton B, Emery JM, Harvard BM: The incidence of benign prostatic hyperplasia. J Urol 99:639, 1968.
5. Wilson JD: The pathogenesis of benign prostatic hyperplasia. Am J Med 68:745, 1980.
6. Turner-Warwick R: Clinical urodynamics. Urol Clin North Am 6:171, 1979.
7. Deming CL: The effect of castration on benign hypertrophy of the prostate in man. J Urol 33:388, 1935.
8. Caine M, Perlberg S, Gordon R: The treatment of benign prostatic hypertrophy with flutamide (SCH 13521): a placebo-controlled study. J Urol 114:564, 1975a.
9. Caine M, Perlberg S, Shapiro A: Phenoxybenzamine for benign prostatic obstruction: review of 200 cases. Urology 17:542, 1981.
10. Paulson DF, Kane RD: A prospective study in the pharmaceutical management of benign prostatic hyperplasia. J Urol 113:811, 1975.
11. Caine M, Pfau A, Perlberg S: The use of alpha adrenergic blockers in benign prostatic hypertrophy. Urology 48:255, 1976.
12. Orandi H: Transurethral incision of the prostate. Urology 12:187, 1978.
13. Edwards L, Powell C: An objective comparison of transurethral resection and bladder neck incision in the treatment of prostatic hypertrophy. J Urol 128:325, 1982.
14. American Cancer Society: 1986 Cancer facts and figures. Ca 39:3, 1989.
15. Murphy GP, et al: Prostate Cancer Part A: Research, Endocrine Treatment, and Histopathology. New York, Alan R Liss, 1987.
16. Jacobi GH, Hohenfellner RF. Prostate Cancer. Baltimore, Williams & Wilkins, 1982, p 15.
17. Alexejew M, Dunajewski L: Prostatakarzinom im kindesalter. Urol Chir 1:64, 1930.
18. Rullis I, Shaeffer IA, Lilien OM: Incidence of prostatic carcinoma in the elderly. Urology 4:295, 1975.
19. Gutman EB, Sproul EE, Autman AB: Significance of increased phosphatase activity of bone at the site of osteoblastic metastases secondary to carcinoma of the prostate gland. Am J Cancer 28:485, 1946.
20. Wang MC, Valenzuela LA, Murphy GP, et al: Purification of a human prostate-specific antigen. Invest Urol 17:159, 1979.
21. Chu TM, Murphy AP: What's new in tumor markers for prostate cancer? Urology 27:487, 1986.
22. Esposti PL: Cytologic diagnosis of prostatic tumors with the aid of transrectal aspiration biopsy: a critical review of 1,110 cases and a report of morphologic and cytochemical studies. Acta Cytol 10:182, 1966.
23. Guinan P, Bush I, Ray V, et al: The accuracy of the rectal examination in the diagnosis of prostate cancer. N Engl J Med 303(9):499, 1980.
24. Miller GJ: An atlas of prostatic biopsies: dilemmas of morphologic variance. In Fenoglio-Preiser CM, Wolff M, Rilke F, eds: Progress in surgical pathology, Vol VIII. Philadelphia, Field and Wood, 1988, p 81.
25. Mostofi FK: Grading of prostatic carcinoma. Cancer Chemother Rep 59:111, 1975.
26. Fowler JE, Mills SE: Operable prostatic carcinoma: correlations among clinical stage, pathological stage, Gleason histologic score and early disease-free survival. J Urol 133:49, 1985.
27. Scher HI, Sternberg CN: Chemotherapy of urologic malignancies. Semin Urol 3(4):239, 1985.

CHAPTER 21

Renal Disease

Moshe Levi
Robert W. Schrier

Youth is a gift of nature; age is a work of art.
ANON.

The aging process has well recognized effects on renal function and anatomy. This process has been systematically studied in humans and experimental animals and has been the subject of several recent review articles, textbook chapters, and monographs.[1-9] This chapter provides a practical and updated overview of the well documented, age-related changes that occur in renal function, which will be very useful for the medical student and house officer providing medical care to elderly patients.

RENAL ANATOMY

Advancing age is associated with progressive loss of renal mass in humans, with renal weight decreasing from 250 to 270 gm in young adulthood to 180 to 200 gm by the eighth decade. The loss of renal mass is primarily cortical, with relative sparing of the renal medulla. The total number of identifiable glomeruli falls with age, in accordance with the changes of renal weight. The number of hyalinized or sclerotic glomeruli identified on light microscopy increases from 1 to 2 percent during the third to fifth decade to as high as 30 percent in some apparently healthy 80 year olds, with a mean prevalence after age 70 of approximately 10 to 12 percent.[10] Changes also occur in the intrarenal vasculature with age, independent of hypertension or other renal disease. Normal aging is associated with variable sclerotic changes in the wall of the larger renal vessels, which are augmented in the presence of hypertension. Smaller vessels are spared, with fewer than 20 percent of senescent kidneys from nonhypertensive subjects displaying arteriolar changes.[10] Microangiographic and histologic studies have identified two very distinctive patterns of change in arteriolar-glomerular units with senescence.[11, 12] In one type, hyalinization and collapse of the glomerular tuft are associated with obliteration of the lumen of the preglomerular arteriole and a resultant loss in blood flow. This type of change is seen primarily in the cortical area. The second pattern, seen primarily in the juxtamedullary area, is characterized by the development of anatomic continuity between the afferent and efferent arterioles during glomerular sclerosis. The end point is thus loss of glomerulus and shunting of blood flow from afferent to efferent arterioles. Blood flow is maintained to the arteriolar rectae verae, the primary vascular supply of the medulla, which do not decrease in number with age.

RENAL PHYSIOLOGY AND PATHOPHYSIOLOGY

Renal Blood Flow

A progressive reduction in renal plasma flow (paraminohippuric acid [PAH] clearance) of approximately 10 percent per decade from 600 ml/min/1.73 m² in the 20- to 29-year-old age group to 300/ml/min/1.73 m² in the 80-to 89-year-old age group is known to occur.[13] The decrease in renal blood flow is associated with significant increases in both the afferent and efferent arteriolar resistance.[14] The increase in the efferent arteriolar resistance may explain the age-related increase in filtration fraction.[13, 14] The exact relationship between renal plasma flow and cardiac output as a function of aging is not well established. Some studies have shown an age-related decrease in cardiac output, whereas others have shown no decrease in cardiac output with age. Furthermore, there is a small but definite decrease in the renal fraction of the cardiac output (RBF/CO).[15]

These later studies suggest that the major determinant of reduced renal blood flow with age is associated with functional or anatomic changes in the renal vasculature. A study using the xenon washout technique to measure renal blood flow in 207 healthy potential renal donors ranging from 17 to 76 years of age also showed an age-related linear reduction in mean blood flow per gm of kidney weight.[16] There was a parallel reduction in the rapid component flow rate as well as in the percent of flow entering the rapid component (Fig. 21–1). Since the rapid component is thought to provide an index of cortical flow, the finding of a preferential decrease in cortical blood flow as a function of aging is consistent with the histologic studies showing a selective loss of cortical vasculature and preservation of medullary flow. This histologic and functional demonstration of selective decrease in cortical flow may also explain the observation that filtration fraction actually increases with ad-

vancing age because outer cortical nephrons have a lower filtration fraction than do juxtamedullary nephrons.

Whether the age-related decrease in renal blood flow results from anatomic or functional changes in the renal vasculature has been studied by two groups of investigators. In one study, renal hemodynamics following intravenous administration of pyrogen was measured; the other measured renal hemodynamics following intra-arterial administration of acetylcholine and angiotensin.[14, 16] During both pyrogen and acetylcholine administration, the vasodilator response was greater in the younger subjects compared with the older subjects. On the other hand, the vasoconstrictive response to angiotensin was identical in young and old subjects. These studies suggest that although the aging renal vasculature does respond to vasoconstriction and vasodilatation, the response to vasodilatation is markedly blunted and anatomic changes, rather than functional vasoconstriction, may be largely responsible for the age-related decrease in renal blood flow.

The relationship of the age-related increase in filtration fraction to the increased prevalence of glomerulosclerosis in the aging kidney has not been definitely established. In view of recent interest in the possible role of hyperfiltration in the even-

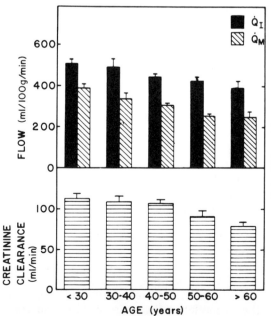

FIGURE 21–1. Relationship between age, renal perfusion rates, and creatinine clearance. There is a significant reduction in mean renal blood flow (Q_M) with age (p<0.001); a parallel reduction in the rapid-component flow rate (Q_1) occurs also with age (p<0.001). (From NK Hollenberg, DF Adams, HS Solomon, et al: Senescence and the renal vasculature in normal man. Circ Res 34:309, 1974.)

tual glomerulosclerosis in insulin-dependent diabetes mellitus, essential hypertension, and other forms of chronic renal disease, a similar role for hyperfiltration propagating glomerulosclerosis in the aging kidney has also been suggested.[5, 17] This phenomenon may be responsible for the acceleration of renal functional impairment in elderly patients with hypertension.[18] Studies in the aging rat reveal that long-term dietary sodium or protein restriction, which would decrease the filtration fraction, results in significant decreases in the incidence and severity of age-related renal lesions, renal functional impairments, and proteinuria.[19–21] These animal studies have definite implications for the prevention or attenuation of renal disease in the elderly.

Glomerular Filtration Rate (GFR)

A progressive, age-related decline in the GFR is well known to occur in men and women.[13–16, 22–24] In a cross-sectional study of 548 healthy volunteers who participated in the Baltimore Longitudinal Study of Aging, creatinine clearance was found to show a progressive linear decline from 140 ml/min/1.73 m^2 at age 30 to 97 ml/min/1.73 m^2 at age 80, at an approximate rate of 0.8 ml/min/1.73 m^2 per year (Fig. 21–2).[22] In another study of 446 normal subjects, the age-related decline in creatinine clearance was found to be much steeper in blacks than in whites.[23] This may reflect an increased propensity for glomerulosclerosis in blacks.[25]

Follow-up studies of 254 normal subjects in the Baltimore Longitudinal Study on Aging with 5 to 14 serial creatinine clearance determinations obtained between 1958 and 1981 also reveal a mean decrease in creatinine clearance of 0.75 ml/min/year and an increase in the rate of loss of creatinine clearance with age.[24] Of interest is the fact that 29 (36 percent) of the 254 subjects followed had no absolute decrease in creatinine clearance, and seven of these subjects actually had a statistically significant increase in creatinine clearance over time.[24] These observations may have important implications in understanding of the age-related decline in the GFR. Furthermore, they also provide impetus to identify potential metabolic, hemodynamic, and hormonal factors that may modulate the age-related alterations in renal function.

The highly significant decrease in GFR that occurs with age is not usually accompanied by an elevation in serum creatinine concentration (Table 21–1).[22] Since muscle mass, from which creatinine is derived, falls with age at approximately the same rate as GFR, the rather striking age-related loss of renal function is not reflected by an increase in the serum creatinine. Thus, serum creatinine usually underestimates the decline in GFR in the elderly. Creatinine clearance needs to be obtained or estimated by one of the commonly used formulas in clinical situations in which the absolute value of the GFR needs to be known (e.g., when adjusting the dosage of drugs in which clearance is accomplished by renal excretion). The following are the most commonly used formulas.[26, 27]

$$\text{Creatinine clearance (ml/min/1.73 m}^2\text{)} = (133 - 0.64) \times \text{age}$$

$$\text{Creatinine clearance (ml/min)} = \frac{(140 - \text{age}) \times \text{weight (kg)}}{72 \times \text{serum creatinine (mg/dl)}}$$
(15 percent less in females)

Either of these two formulas yields a quite reasonable estimation of the GFR. In fact, there is a very close correlation ($r = 0.85$) between calculated creatinine clearance (using formula 2) versus measured creatinine clearance.[26]

An important consequence of the age-related decrease in renal blood flow, GFR, or both is the potential predisposition to enhanced ischemic or toxic renal injury. In addition to the absolute decrease in renal blood flow, the autoregulatory capacity of the renal vasculature is also impaired. Thus, the risk of hemodynamically induced acute renal failure following severe volume depletion, septic shock, and major vascular surgery is increased. Failure to properly adjust the dosage of renally excreted drugs including aminoglycoside antibiotics, nonsteroidal anti-inflammatory drugs, and radiocontrast agents may also increase the incidence of toxin-induced renal failure.

The most important clinical implication for the age-related decrease in GFR is the need for adjustment of the dosage of medications that are either directly excreted by

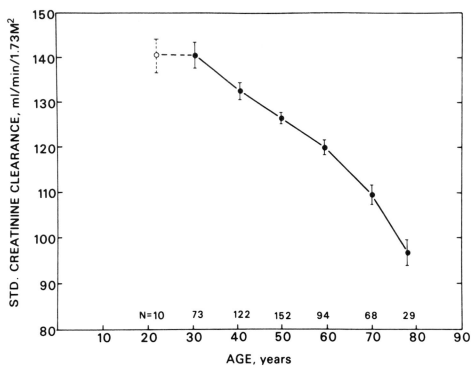

FIGURE 21–2. *Cross-sectional differences in standard creatinine clearance with age. The number of subjects in each age group is indicated above the abscissa. Values plotted indicate mean ± SEM. (From Rowe JW, Andres J, Tobin D, et al: The effect of age on creatinine clearance in men: a cross-sectional and longitudinal study. J Gerontol 31:155, 1976.)*

the kidney via glomerular filtration or tubular secretion and medications of which activate metabolites, formed in the liver, are eliminated by the kidney.[29] When adjusting the dosage of such medications, it is therefore very important to measure or estimate GFR, not only according to serum creatinine but also according to one of the aforementioned formulas. In Figure 21–3 and Table 21–2 are provided useful and practical guidelines for dose modification of commonly used drugs requiring adjust-

TABLE 21–1. Cross-Sectional Age Differences in Creatinine Clearance, Serum Creatinine, and 24-Hour Creatinine Excretion

Age (yr)	Number of Subjects	Creatinine Clearance* (ml/min/1.73m²)	Serum Creatinine Concentration (mg/100 ml)	Creatinine Excretion (mg/24 hr)
17–24	10	140.2*	0.808	1790.0
		3.7	0.026	52.0
25–34	73	140.1	0.808	1862.0
		2.5	0.010	31.0
35–44	122	132.6	0.813	1746.0
		1.8	0.009	24.0
45–54	152	126.98	0.829	1689.0
		1.4	0.008	18.0
55–64	94	119.9	0.837	1580.0
		1.7	0.012	22.0
65–74	68	109.5	0.825	1409.0
		2.0	0.012	25.0
75–84	29	96.9	0.843	1259.0
		2.9	0.019	45.0

(From Rowe JW, Andres R, Tobin JD, et al: The effect of age on creatinine clearance in men: a cross-sectional and longitudinal study. J Gerontol 31:155, 1976.)
*Values indicate standard error of the mean (SEM).

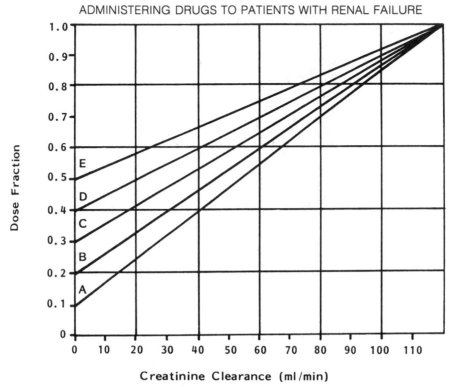

ADMINISTERING DRUGS TO PATIENTS WITH RENAL FAILURE

Creatinine Clearance (ml/min)

FIGURE 21–3. Dose fraction as a function of creatinine clearance. Lines A through E are "dosing lines" appropriate for different drugs based on the dose fraction of anephric patients. (From Aronoff GA, Abel SR: Principles of administering drugs to patients with renal failure. In Bennett WM, McCarron DA, guest eds: Renal Disease and Hypertension; Brenner BM, Stein JH, eds: Contemporary Issues in Nephrology, Vol 17. New York, Churchill Livingstone, 1987.)

ment in patients with a decrease in the GFR. In addition, it is also useful to monitor the serum levels of drugs that have a narrow therapeutic-to-toxic ratio.

Fluid and Electrolyte Balance

Under normal circumstances, age has no effect on plasma sodium or potassium concentrations, blood pH, or ability to maintain normal extracellular fluid volume. The adaptive reserve mechanisms responsible for maintaining constancy of the extracellular fluid volume and composition in response to stress are, however, impaired in the elderly.

Sodium-Conserving Ability

The ability of the aged kidney to conserve sodium in response to sodium deprivation is impaired.[57] Clearance studies in young and elderly subjects have shown a decreased distal tubular capacity for so-

dium reabsorption in the elderly.[31] The distal tubular dysfunction could be caused by anatomic changes in the aging kidney, such as interstitial fibrosis. Additionally, functional and hormonal changes, such as increased medullary blood flow or decreased renin-aldosterone activity, could also impair distal tubular reabsorption of sodium.

Renin Aldosterone System

There are important age-related alterations in the renin-aldosterone system. Basal plasma renin concentration or activity is decreased by 30 to 50 percent in elderly subjects in spite of normal levels of renin substrate.[32] During maneuvers designed to stimulate renin secretion (e.g., upright posture, 10 meq/day sodium intake, and furosemide administration), the differences in plasma renin activity are further amplified (Fig. 21–4).[33, 34] There is a similar 30 to 50 percent decrease in plasma aldosterone levels in elderly sub-

TABLE 21–2. Dose Fraction Regression Lines and Preferred Method of Dosage Modification of Commonly Used Drugs that Require Dose Adjustment in Patients with Decreased Renal Function

Drug	Method	Regression Line*
Aminoglycosides	I	A
Amikacin	I	A
Gentamicin	I	A
Kanamycin	I	A
Netilmicin	I	A
Streptomycin	I	A
Tobramycin	I	A
Antifungals		
Flucytosine	I	C
Antituberculous drugs		
Ethambutol	I	E
Antiviral agents		
Acyclovir	I	B
Amantadine	I	A
Aztreonam	I	C
Cephalosporins		
Cefaclor	I	D
Cefadroxil	I	C
Cefamandole	I	B
Cefazolin	I	C
Cefonicid†	I and D	D
Ceforanide	I	B
Cefotaxime	I	E
Cefoxitin	I	C
Cefsulodin	I	A
Ceftazidime	I	B
Ceftizoxime	I	A
Cefuroxime	I	B
Cephalexin	I	E
Cephalothin	I	E
Cephapirin	I	E
Cephradine	I	B
Moxalactam	I	C
Imepenem/Cilastin	I	E
Metronidazole	I	E
Penicillins		
Amdinocillin	I	C
Amoxicillin	I	E
Amoxicillin/clavulanate potassium	I	E
Ampicillin	I	E
Azlocillin	I	E
Carbenicillin	I	B
Methicillin	I	D
Mezlocillin	I	E
Penicillin G	I	E
Piperacillin	I	E
Ticarcillin	I	B
Ticarcillin/clavulanate potassium	I	C
Sulfonamides		
Co-trimoxazole	I	C
Sulfamethoxazole	I	C
Sulfisoxazole	I	E
Trimethoprim	I	E
Vancomycin	I	A
Analgesics		
Acetaminophen	I	E
Propoxyphene	D	C
Sedatives, Psychotherapeutics		
Lithium carbonate	D	D
Lorazepam	D	E
Antiarrhythmic agents		
Disopyramide	I	B
Procainamide	I	C
Tocainide	D	E

TABLE 21–2. Dose Fraction Regression Lines and Preferred Method of Dosage Modification of
Commonly Used Drugs that Require Dose Adjustment in Patients with
Decreased Renal Function *Continued*

Drug	Method	Regression Line*
Cardiac glycosides		
Digoxin	D	E
Diuretics		
Acetazolamide	I	D
Agents for gout		
Allopurinol	D	C
Colchicine	D	E
Miscellaneous		
Cimetidine	I	E
Metoclopramide	D	E
Ranitidine	I	E

(From Aronoff GA and Abel SR: Principles of administering drugs to patients with renal failure. In Bennett WM and McCarron DA, guest eds: Pharmacotherapy of Renal Disease and Hypertension, Contemp Issues Nephrol, Vol 17. Brenner BM and Stein JH, eds, NY, Churchill Livingstone, 1987, p 1.)

*See Figure 21–3. Lines A through E are dosing lines; D indicates dose change, I indicates interval change.

†Requires both altered dose (D) and dose interval (I).

jects during recumbency and normal sodium intake that becomes more pronounced during upright posture, sodium restriction, and furosemide administration.[32–35] The aldosterone deficiency appears to be related to the renin deficiency and not to intrinsic adrenal gland defects, since both plasma aldosterone and cortisol responses to corticotropin (adrenocorticotropic hormone [ACTH]) infusion are normal in the elderly.[33]

Thus, during sodium restriction, impaired renin-aldosterone response may result in decreased renal tubular reabsorption in the elderly. In fact, clearance studies in young and elderly subjects have

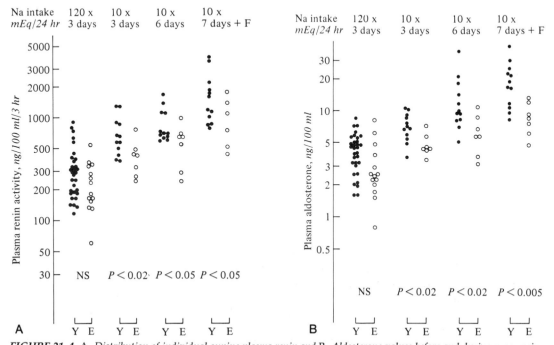

FIGURE 21–4. A, *Distribution of individual supine plasma renin and B, Aldosterone values before and during progressive sodium depletion in young and elderly healthy subjects. Y = young subjects; E = elderly subjects. Values indicating statistical significance refer to difference between young and elderly subjects. Plasma renin activity values are those obtained at incubation pH 5.7. (From Weidmann P, DeMytteraere-Bursztein S, Maxwell MH, et al: Effect of aging on plasma renin and aldosterone in normal man. Kidney Int 8:325, 1975.)*

shown marked improvement in distal tu-bular sodium reabsorption in the elderly following treatment with aldosterone.[36]

Decreased activity of the renin-angiotensin system also has implications for the diagnosis of renin-dependent hypertension, especially renovascular hypertension. High furosemide-stimulated plasma renin activity or a positive saralasin test is more likely to indicate the presence of renal vascular hypertension in the elderly than in the young.[37] On the other hand, because of the low renin profile in the aged, renal vascular hypertension may be underdiagnosed in elderly patients, especially with the use of routine screening tests. The decreased activity of the renin-angiotensin system in the elderly may also have implications for the treatment of hypertension, although controlled studies in this area are lacking.

Renal Concentrating Ability

Renal concentrating ability is well known to decline with age in humans.[38–42] The concentrating ability of the kidneys, as measured by the urinary-specific gravity in 38 healthy men, declined from 1.030 at age 40 years to 1.023 at age 89 years.[38] The maximal urine osmolality, measured following 12 to 24 hours of dehydration, is inversely related to age (Fig. 21–5).[39] The maximal urine osmolality was 1,109 mOsm/kg in 31 subjects age 20 to 39 years, compared with 1,051 mOsm/kg in 48 subjects age 40 to 59 years, and 882 mOsm/kg in 18 subjects age 60 to 79 years.[39] The age-related decline in the concentrating defect does not correlate to the age-related decline in the GFR.

Studies in humans suggest that the concentrating defect is due to an intrarenal defect rather than to a failure in the osmotic release of arginine vasopressin (AVP).[40–44] Following intravenous infusion of hypertonic saline (3 percent sodium chloride [NaCl]) in 9 younger subjects (21 to 49 years of age) and 3 older subjects (54 to 92 years of age), plasma AVP levels rose 4.5 times the baseline in the older subjects compared with 2.5 times the baseline in the younger subjects, despite similar free water clearances.[78] The slope of the plasma AVP concentration (% baseline) versus serum osmolality as an index of the sen-

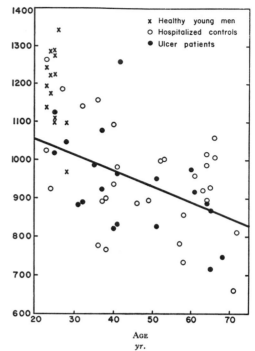

FIGURE 21–5. *Maximum urine osmolality in healthy young men, hospitalized controls, and patients with ulcer, showing a decrease with age. The solid line represents the regression slope for hospitalized patients. (From Lindeman RD, Van Buren HC, Raisz LG: Osmolar renal concentrating ability in healthy young men and hospitalized patients without renal disease. N Engl J Med 262:1306, 1960.)*

sitivity of the osmoreceptor was significantly increased in the older subjects. In addition, in the same study, intravenous infusion of ethanol caused a progressive decline in plasma AVP levels in the younger subjects, as would be expected, but failed to have a similar effect in the older subjects. In contrast, the volume-pressure-mediated AVP release decreases with age.[45]

Recent studies in humans reveal an age-related increase in solute excretion and osmolar clearance during dehydration.[42] This phenomenon, which may be a reflection of an impaired solute transport by the ascending Henle's loop, may be responsible for the impairment in the urine concentrating ability in elderly subjects. This possibility is supported by clearance studies in water-diuresing subjects that demonstrate a decrease in the sodium chloride transport in the ascending Henle's loop in elderly subjects.[31, 36] This defect in solute transport by the thick ascending limb of Henle's loop could diminish inner medullary hypertonicity and thereby impair urinary concentrating ability. Relative to cortical blood flow, an increase in medullary blood flow (as suggested by the xenon washout studies) could also cause an increase in the removal of solutes from the medullary interstitium and thereby contribute to the decreased maximal urinary osmolality.

The age-related impairments in renal concentrating and sodium-conserving abilities are associated with an increased incidence of volume depletion and hypernatremia in the elderly. Under normal physiologic conditions, increased thirst and fluid intake are natural defense mechanisms in response to volume depletion and hypernatremia. The apparent deficit in thirst and regulation of fluid intake in the elderly, however, may further contribute to the increased incidence of dehydration and hypernatremia.[46, 47] In practice, drugs that inhibit the thirst mechanism and the synthesis and release of AVP and drugs that inhibit the renal tubular action of AVP (especially lithium and demeclocycline) are therefore best avoided (Table 21–3). The use of osmotic diuretics, enteral feeding containing high protein and glucose, and bowel cathartics should also be carefully monitored in the elderly.

The incidence of severe hypernatremia in the elderly exceeds one case per hospital per month.[48, 49] Hypernatremia in the elderly may present with primary neurologic or psychiatric symptoms, which could delay the diagnosis. If not promptly diagnosed and treated, hypernatremia leads to coma, seizures, and death. In fact, in adults, acute elevation of serum sodium above 160 meq/l is associated with a 75 percent mortality rate. Even in the absence of death, the neurologic sequelae can be severe in the elderly.

Renal Diluting Ability

Renal diluting ability is also impaired as a function of aging.[40, 41] In water-diuresing subjects, minimal urine osmolality was significantly higher, 92 mOsm/kg in the older subjects (age 77 to 88) compared with 52 mOsm/kg in the younger subjects (age 17 to 40). Mechanisms of the impaired diluting ability in the elderly have not been well studied; in addition to the role of impaired GFR, inadequate suppression of

TABLE 21–3. Recommended Drug Modifications

Drugs that Inhibit Vasopressin Synthesis and/or Release
Norepinephrine
Fluphenazine
Haloperidol
Promethazine
Oxilorphan
Butorphanol
Morphine (low doses)
Alcohol
Carbamazepine
Glucocorticoids
? Phenytoin
Clonidine
Muscimol
Cisplatinum

Drugs that Inhibit Peripheral Action of Vasopressin
Lithium
Demeclocycline
Colchicine
Vinblastine
Methoxyflurane
Glyburide, acetohexamide, and tolazamide
Amphotericin B
Methicillin
Gentamicin
Isophosphamide
Propoxyphene
Furosemide and ethacrynic acid
Angiographic dyes
Osmotic diuretics
Cisplatinum
Lomustine (CCNU)

(From Levi M, Berl T: Water Metabolism. In Gonick HC, ed: Water Metabolism, Vol 9. Chicago, Yearbook Medical Publishers, 1986, p 410.)

AVP release or impaired solute transport in the ascending Henle's loop may also play a role.

The age-related impairment in maximal diluting ability and the enhanced osmotic release of AVP are associated with a high incidence of hyponatremia in the elderly. A random sampling of 160 patients in a chronic illness facility showed that 36 patients had hyponatremia, with a mean serum sodium of 120 meq/l, and 27 of these patients were symptomatic.[51] In another study, a survey of hospitalized patients in a geriatric unit during a 10-month period revealed that 77 patients, or 11 percent, had plasma sodium concentrations below 130 meq/l.[52] Diuretics, especially the combination of hydrochlorothiazide and amiloride, and hypotonic intravenous fluid administration were determined to cause the hyponatremia in 56 of these patients. Forty-seven were symptomatic, and the mortality rate for the hyponatremic patients was twice the overall rate for the geriatric unit.

Other reports also confirm that thiazide diuretics are a major cause of hyponatremia in the elderly.[53] The well-known effect of thiazide diuretics to impair the renal diluting ability under normal physiologic conditions seems to be compounded in elderly patients with a pre-existing renal diluting defect. In addition, thiazide diuretics, when used in combination with chlorpropamide, which is known to potentiate the peripheral action of vasopressin, have synergistic effects in impairing the renal diluting ability.[54] In practice, drugs or agents that stimulate the nonosmotic release of AVP and drugs that potentiate the renal tubular action of AVP must be used with extreme caution in the elderly (Table 21–4).

The signs and symptoms of hyponatremia are most likely related to cellular swelling and cerebral edema caused by the water movement as a result of the lowering of extracellular fluid (ECF) osmolality. Patients may present with symptoms of lethargy, apathy, disorientation, muscle

TABLE 21–4. Recommended Drug Modifications

Drugs that Potentiate Vasopressin Synthesis and/or Release

Acetycholine
Nicotine
Apomorphine
Morphine (high doses)
Epinephrine
Isoproterenol
Histamine
Bradykinin
Prostaglandins
β-Endorphin
Cyclophosphatmide IV
Vincristine
Insulin
2-deoxyglucose
Angiotensin
Lithium

Drugs that Potentiate Peripheral Action of Vasopressin

Nonsteroidal anti-inflammatory agents (short-term)
Acetaminophen
Chlorpropamide
Tolbutamide

(From Levi M, Berl T: Water Metabolism. In Gonick HC, ed: Current Nephrology, Vol 9. Chicago, Year-book Medical Publishers, 1986, p. 434.)

cramps, anorexia, nausea, or agitation and with signs ranging from depressed deep tendon reflexes to pseudobulbar palsy and seizures. Differentiation of these symptoms from primary neurologic or psychiatric disease is important so that one can promptly institute appropriate therapy and avoid severe neurologic sequelae.

Acid Base Balance

Elderly subjects can maintain the pH and bicarbonate of blood within the normal range, and their basal acid excretion is not different from that in healthy, younger volunteers. When senescent kidneys are challenged with an acute acid load, however, they do not increase their acid excretion to the same degree as kidneys in young volunteers.[55, 56] In an earlier study following a standard oral ammonium chloride acid load, the older subjects (age 72 to 93) excreted only 19 percent of the acid load compared with 35 percent excreted by the younger subjects (age 17 to 35) over an 8-hour period.[55] Urinary ammonia accounted for less of the total acid excretion in the older subjects—59 percent in the older subjects compared with 72 percent in the younger subjects. In this study, the decrease in both of these parameters was paralleled by a nearly equal drop in inulin clearance, so that acid excretion per unit GFR was almost identical in both younger and older subjects. This finding suggests that the decrease in acid excretion in the elderly results from a decreased renal tubular mass rather than from a specific tubular defect.

A more recent study of elderly subjects with less impaired GFR, however, has reached a different conclusion. In this study, the minimal urinary pH and net acid excretion, even when factored for GFR, were significantly decreased in the older subjects.[56] There were no differences in the titratable acid excretion, but the older subjects showed a significant reduction in ammonium excretion, even when factored for GFR—34 mol/min in the elderly compared with 51 mol/min in the younger subjects. This study, therefore, suggests an intrinsic tubular defect in ammonium excretion as a function of aging. It is not known whether this defect is due to anatomic changes or to functional defects, including the hypoaldosteronism that is frequently encountered in the aged.

Potassium Balance

Studies of the effects of aging on renal and extrarenal adaptation to high potassium loads or dietary potassium deprivation in humans are lacking. Two different studies conducted in the 1950s suggest that both total body potassium and total exchangeable potassium decrease with age in both genders and that these decreases are more marked in women than in men.[57, 58] They may relate to the decrease in muscle mass with advancing age.

The effects of aging on potassium adaptation has been studied in the aged rat.[59] In this study, the efficiency of the kaliuretic response to intravenous infusion of potassium chloride and the rise in plasma potassium were identical in both the young and aged rat. Following a period of dietary high potassium intake, however, the efficiency of kaliuretic response to intravenous potassium chloride was impaired in the aged rat, and also the rise in plasma potassium was significantly higher. Following bilateral nephrectomy, the rise in plasma potassium concentration was also higher in the aged rats when they were on a high potassium, but not normal potassium intake. This renal and extrarenal impairment in potassium adaptation was thought to be caused by a decrease in renal and colon Na,K-ATPase activity. Whether these findings also apply to human aging remains to be determined.

The presence of a renal acidification defect and decreased activity of the renin-angiotensin-aldosterone system may be the cause of the increased incidence of type 4 renal tubular acidosis (RTA), or the syndrome of hyporeninemic hypoaldosteronism in the elderly.[60] In fact, in a recent large clinical series, the mean age of the patients was 65 years.[60] In addition, the elderly are at increased risk for developing hyperkalemia with potassium-sparing diuretics, including spironolactone and amiloride, and drugs that inhibit the renin-angiotensin system, especially indomethacin, beta-blockers, and converting enzyme inhibitors (Table 21–5).[19, 61, 62]

TABLE 21–5. Recommended Drug Modification

Drugs that May Predispose to Hyperkalemia

Potassium-sparing diuretics
  Spironolactone
  Triamterene
  Amiloride

Beta-blockers
Prostaglandin synthesis inhibitors
Converting enzyme inhibitors

CLINICAL RENAL DISEASE

Acute Renal Failure

The age-related decreases in renal blood flow, GFR, and tubular transport of sodium and water make the elderly more susceptible to acute renal failure.

A major cause of acute renal failure in the elderly is prerenal failure, i.e., decreased perfusion of the kidney leading to a functional and potentially reversible type of acute renal failure. A decrease in cardiac output; gastrointestinal losses caused by vomiting, diarrhea, or bleeding; renal losses due to glycosuria; and use of diuretics may all result in prerenal failure (Fig. 21–6).

The elderly are also predisposed to intrinsic acute renal failure (i.e., acute tubular necrosis). In an earlier study, major surgery accounted for about 30 percent of cases of acute renal failure in the elderly.[64] Hypotension during or after surgery, postoperative fluid loss due to gastrointestinal or fistulous drainage, anesthetic toxicity, arrhythmias, and myocardial infarction (MI) are common postsurgical complications in the elderly that may result in acute renal failure. Infection accounts for another 30 percent of cases of acute renal failure in the elderly.[64] Gram-negative infections are associated with endotoxin-induced vasoconstriction, which, in the susceptible individual, may result in acute tubular necrosis. In addition, most of the antibiotics used to treat serious in-hospital infections are associated with a high incidence of acute tubular necrosis or acute interstitial nephritis. Age is a well-known risk factor for developing aminoglycoside nephrotoxicity.[65] The reasons may include overdosage as a result of inaccurate esti-

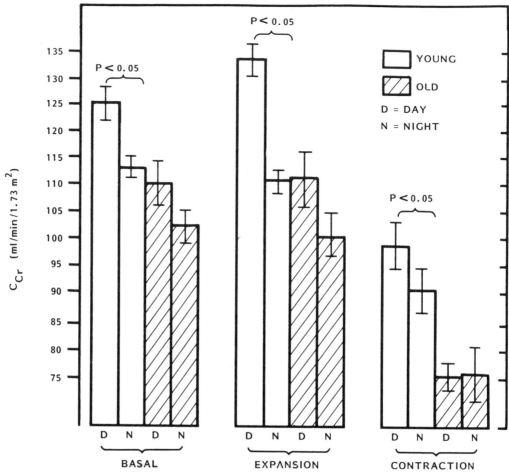

FIGURE 21–6. *Day and night C_{Cr} values compared between whites <40 years and whites >40 years (mean SEM) during basal, volume expansion, and volume contraction. (From Luft FC, Fineberg NS, Miller JZ, et al: The effects of age, race and heredity on glomerular filtration rate following volume expansion and contraction in normal man. Am J Med Sci 279:15–24, 1980.)*

mation of the GFR, and pre-existent age-related decrease in renal blood flow and tubular damage, which may enhance the hemodynamic and tubular toxic effects of aminoglycoside antibiotics. The elderly are also at increased risk for radiocontrast-induced renal failure.[66] The mechanisms of radiocontrast-induced renal injury are not completely understood but include hemodynamic effects and direct tubular toxic effects, which, because of pre-existent renal defects, predispose the elderly to enhanced renal toxicity. In a recent study of mainly medical patients, nephrotoxic antibiotics and contrast media in fact accounted for 25 percent of the cases of acute renal failure.[67] Another major cause of intrinsic renal failure in the elderly are

the nonsteroidal anti-inflammatory drugs (NSAID).[68] This is of special concern because ibuprofen, a NSAID, is available as an over-the-counter medication. Inhibition of renal vasodilatory prostaglandin biosynthesis caused by NSAIDs potentiates the renal vasoconstrictive effects of endogenous alpha adrenergic system, angiotensin II, and vasopressin. In the presence of an already reduced renal blood flow, this may result in acute renal failure.

One of the most significant causes of renal failure in the elderly is urinary obstruction. A deficiency of bladder sensation plays a major role in the renal consequences of prostatic hypertrophy in the elderly.[69] The symptoms of prostatism such as urinary frequency, difficulty in starting or stopping micturition, and nocturia may not be apparent to the patient. A significant number of patients may thus present with symptoms of end-stage renal disease rather than with prostatism. In addition, in clinically significant prostatism, the residual urine is often infected, which may potentiate impairments in tubular function and reduction in renal blood flow and the GFR caused by the obstruction. Prompt diagnosis and treatment of obstruction are therefore necessary to prevent significant renal damage.

Most elderly patients respond well to treatment of acute renal failure with dialysis, but the mortality remains high at 50 to 55 percent.[67] As in the adult population, prompt initiation of hemodialysis or peritoneal dialysis may alleviate the uremic symptoms and may prevent uremic complications such as infection, gastrointestinal bleeding, and cardiac failure, which are the major causes of increased mortality in the elderly patient with acute renal failure. Although the chances for recovery of renal function in the elderly patient with acute renal failure would be predicted to be markedly decreased, in a recent British study, more than 50 percent of patients age 65 years and over who were treated with hemodialysis or peritoneal dialysis for acute renal failure eventually recovered sufficient renal function to end the need for further dialysis.[70]

Chronic Renal Failure

Many forms of chronic renal failure are more commonly seen late in life because the renal disease is secondary to other age-dependent medical diseases. Atherosclerotic disease of the renal vasculature causing renovascular hypertension and renal ischemia; diabetes, hypertension, or chronic glomerulonephritis causing glomerulosclerosis; and prostatic hypertrophy causing hydronephrosis most commonly lead to chronic renal failure in the elderly. The clinical presentation of chronic renal failure in the elderly is often quite different than in the adult patient population. The elderly often present with decompensation of pre-existent medical conditions, such as congestive heart failure, hypertension, peptic ulcer disease, or

dementia, rather than with specific symptoms of uremia. In addition, the level of serum creatinine may underestimate the actual renal reserve, since in the presence of decreased muscle mass, serum creatinine does not rise in direct proportion to the reduction in the GFR. If the renal failure is advanced and no reversible causes can be identified, including renal artery stenosis and urinary tract obstruction, early dialysis is advisable to prevent the disabling symptoms of uremia and organ dysfunction that may become irreversible. Age itself should not be the sole criteria for selection for dialytic therapy. In the absence of major extrarenal organ dysfunction, the elderly adjust to dialysis quite well, and their longevity rate, although not as favorable as that in younger patients, is not markedly reduced as a result of end-stage renal disease.[71]

Renal Vascular Disorders

A major cause of vascular disease of the kidney in the elderly is atheroembolism. It occurs when cholesterol crystals and other forms of atheromatous debris are dislodged from eroded aortic atherosclerotic plaques occluding the arcuate and intralobular arteries of the kidney.[72] Renal cholesterol embolization has been reported to occur after abdominal trauma; aortic catheterization; surgery for aortic aneurysm; and abdominal, coronary, or carotid angiography. The patient may present with a combination of symptoms including lower extremity focal digital necrosis, gastrointestinal bleeding, pancreatitis, MI, retinal ischemia, cerebral infarction, hypertension, and uremia. It may be associated with fever, increased erythrocyte sedimentation rate, eosinophilia, and hematuria without casts. Episodic and labile hypertension due to renal artery emboli is a common finding.

Renal cholesterol embolization results in a major reduction in the GFR within 1 to 4 weeks.[72] This helps to differentiate it from radiocontrast-induced acute renal failure, which usually occurs within 1 to 4 days after the angiographic procedure. The renal insufficiency usually progresses to end-stage renal disease, but in a recent report of five patients, only two of them developed end-stage renal disease. Because renal cholesterol embolization occurs most commonly in men over 60 years of age with severe atherosclerotic disease, angiographic procedures should be replaced with noninvasive radionuclear studies in elderly patients, unless the clinical condition warrants otherwise. Cholesterol embolization should be considered in the differential diagnosis of acute renal failure in elderly patients, especially when it occurs after major vessel surgery or angiography.

Another major cause of renovascular disease in the elderly is renal artery thrombosis, which also occurs in patients with severe and generalized atherosclerotic disease. It may present as unilateral disease causing renovascular hypertension, as bilateral disease causing de novo acute renal failure, or as acute worsening of chronic renal failure.

Glomerulonephritis

Acute glomerulonephritis is receiving increased attention as a disease in which the presentation and prognosis are clearly age related. Acute glomerulonephritis in the elderly usually presents as congestive heart failure rather than hypertension, hematuria, and proteinuria.[73] Often, the presenting symptoms of acute glomerulonephritis in the elderly are ascribed to coexistent disease, and unless one maintains a high index of suspicion, the diagnosis can be overlooked.

A disease that appears to be more prevalent in the elderly is rapidly progressive or idiopathic crescentic glomerulonephritis. In an autopsy series of 44 elderly patients who died of renal disease and in an analysis of 115 patients over age 60 who underwent renal biopsy, 28 and 19 patients, respectively, had the diagnosis of idiopathic crescentic glomerulonephritis.[74, 75] The elderly patient with idiopathic crescentic glomerulonephritis appears to have a different disease from that seen in younger patients. Hemoptysis is rare, and circulating antiglomerular basement membrane antibodies are not often detected. Glomerular immunofluorescence studies reveal either granular deposits of IgG or are negative. The disease usually progresses to end-stage renal disease, and it is not clear whether the elderly respond to treatment with steroids, immunosuppressive agents, anticoagulants, and plasmapheresis.

Another important cause of acute glomerulonephritis in the elderly is diffuse proliferative glomerulonephritis, which usually occurs in association with a major infection, especially post-streptococcal glomerulonephritis (PSGN), resulting from pyodermal infections.[74] In elderly patients, oliguria and volume overload are the most common features of PSGN and, hence, it is easily confused with congestive heart failure. The outcome of the disease is similar to that in the younger age groups in that most patients recover renal function.

When compared with patients younger than age 60 (Table 21–6), the elderly also have a higher incidence of vasculitis and Wegener's granulomatosis, whereas the incidence of systemic lupus erythematosus is significantly lower.[75]

Nephrotic Syndrome

Nephrotic syndrome is a commonly diagnosed renal disease in the elderly, and membranous glomerulonephritis is its most commonly diagnosed cause (see Table 21–6). There is also a surprisingly high incidence of minimal change disease in the elderly. In one series of 25 patients over age 60 with nephrotic syndrome, six had minimal change disease and five had membranous glomerulonephritis. This incidence is similar to that seen in 75 patients between the ages of 15 and 59 with nephrotic syndrome.[76] In another series, membranous glomerulonephritis was diagnosed in 15 patients, and minimal change disease was diagnosed in nine patients.[75] Thus, renal biopsy seems to be essential to establishing the correct histologic diagnosis in the elderly patient with nephrotic syndrome. This is especially true because of the high frequency of minimal change disease in the elderly, who respond equally as well to steroids and immunosuppressive agents as the younger patients.[75, 76] A certain subset of the elderly patients with membranous glomerulonephritis may also respond to steroid therapy, although the effectiveness of steroids in the treatment of membranous glomerulonephritis is becoming less clear.

Another cause of the nephrotic syn-

TABLE 21–6. Comparative Incidence of the Different Renal Diseases in 115 Elderly Patients and 455 Patients Younger Than 60 Years

Diagnosis	Percentage of Elderly Adults (> age 60)	Percentage of Other Patients (< age 60)
Idiopathic crescentic glomerulonephritis	16.5	4.0
Membranous glomerulonephritis	13.0	4.6
Minimal change nephrotic syndrome	7.8	7.0
Focal proliferative/mesangiopathic glomerulonephritis	6.0	10.5
Diffuse proliferative glomerulonephritis	4.0	2.2
Chronic glomerulonephritis	4.0	7.0
Membranoproliferative glomerulonephritis	1.7	9.2
Glomerulosclerosis	13.0	10.5
Vasculitis	5.0	3.0
Amyloidosis	4.0	1.0
Wegener's granulomatosis	3.0	0.2
Systemic lupus erythematosus	1.7	13.8
Other systemic diseases	8.6	12.0
Miscellaneous	8.6	15.0

(From Moorthy AV, Zimmerman SW: Renal disease in the elderly: clinicopathologic analysis of renal disease in 115 elderly patients. Clin Nephrol 14:223, 1980.)

drome in the elderly is focal glomerulosclerosis (FGS). The histologic findings in FGS include focal segmental and global glomerulosclerosis affecting especially the juxtamedullary glomeruli. Immunofluorescence generally reveals granular deposits of IgM and C3 in the areas of segmental sclerosis. Although FGS usually occurs as a separate and distinct entity, it may also occur as the end result of various other glomerulopathies or systemic diseases, including diabetes and hypertension. Recently, the entity of physiologic hyperfiltration has been proposed to be the precursor of FGS in these disease entities.[17] In addition, FGS may also be associated with the increased age-related incidence of global sclerosis.[10]

Interestingly, the otherwise normal and healthy aged rat also has a histologic renal lesion very similar to that of human FGS with IgM and C3 deposition, which is accompanied by significant proteinuria.[77–79] In the rat, hemodynamic factors rather than immunologic factors seem to be responsible for this entity.[79] In humans, the age-related increase in the filtration fraction of the juxtamedullary glomeruli may also be responsible for the age-related development of glomerulosclerosis, but this remains to be established. Nevertheless, this is an important issue to consider in interpreting renal biopsies from elderly individuals. Clinically, FGS and the glomerulosclerosis associated with aging can usually be distinguished on the basis of the nonselective and significant proteinuria and hematuria that accompanies FGS.

Urinary Tract Infections

Urinary tract infections are an important problem in the elderly population. The reasons for the increased prevalence of urinary tract infections with advancing age are not known but may include changes in bladder function, pelvic musculature, prostate size, and impaired immune response, as well as concomitant illness. Although bacteriuria is found in less than 5 percent of middle-aged women and in less than 1 percent of middle-aged men, 20 percent of healthy men over the age of 65 have bacteriuria. The prevalence of bacteriuria in elderly men and women increases further to 25 percent of patients in extended care facilities, 30 percent in acute care hospitals, and over 35 percent in nursing facilities.[80] The increased prevalence of dementia and urinary and bowel incontinence further complicates the picture.

The elderly patients with bacteriuria may have a further significant decrease in creatinine clearance when compared with age-matched patients without bacteriuria.[81] The reason for the worsening of renal function is not clear but may indicate the presence of chronic pyelonephritis that eventually may be associated with focal segmental glomerulosclerosis. Bacteriuria may also be associated with a significant reduction in the survival rate of the elderly subjects, although a recent study did not find a difference in mortality between elderly male residents of a skilled nursing facility who were classified as nonbacteriuric, intermittently bacteriuric, or continuously bacteriuric during a 6-year follow-up.[81, 82] In the absence of renal disease, urinary tract abnormalities, and clinical evidence of sepsis, most agree that asymptomatic bacteriuria in the elderly should not be treated because the incidence of treatment failure and relapse is high.[83, 84] The efficacy of chronic suppressive therapy has not been determined, but one may anticipate problems with the emergence of highly resistant gram-negative infections, especially in the institutionalized and debilitated elderly patients.

SUMMARY

It is clear that aging is associated with significant changes in renal anatomy and function. The age-related decreases in renal blood flow, GFR, sodium conservation, maximal urinary concentration, maximal urinary dilution, and acidification are usually of no consequence to an otherwise healthy elderly individual. They have important implications for drug therapy and diagnostic tests, however, and during stress and disease, they may also predispose the elderly patients to life-threatening fluid and electrolyte disorders and acute renal failure. The medical student and house officer overseeing elderly patients should, therefore, recognize the presence and importance of the age-related alterations in renal function and take appropriate measures to maintain the fine balance that keeps the aging kidney functioning and surviving.

ACKNOWLEDGMENTS

The authors would like to thank Dr. Seymour Eisenberg for his critical comments and suggestions, Ms. Ginny Mitchell for expert secretarial assistance, and the Medical Media Department at the Dallas VAMC for the reproductions.

REFERENCES

1. Bichet DG, Schrier RW: Renal function and diseases in the aged. In Schrier RW, ed: Clinical Internal Medicine in the Aged. Philadelphia, WB Saunders Co, p 211, 1982.
2. Rowe JW: Aging and renal function. In Arieff AL, DeFronzo RA, eds: Fluid Electrolyte and Acid Base Disorders. New York, Churchill Livingstone, 1985, p 1231.
3. Brown WW, Davis BB, Spry LA, et al: Aging and the kidney. Arch Intern Med 146:1790, 1986.
4. Lindeman RD, Goldman R: Anatomic and physiologic age changes in the kidney. Exp Gerontol 21:379, 1986
5. Anderson S, Brenner BM: Effects of aging on the renal glomerulus. Am J Med 80:435, 1986
6. Meyer BR, Bellucci A: Renal function in the elderly. Cardiol Clin 4:227, 1986
7. Michelis MF, Davis BB, Preuss HG, eds: Geriatric Nephrology. (Monogr). New York, Field, Rich, and Associates, Inc, 1986.
8. Goldstein RS, Tarloff JB, Hook JB: Age-related nephropathy in laboratory rats. FASEB J 2:2241, 1988.
9. Levi M, Rowe JW: Aging and the kidney. In Schrier RW, Gottschalk CW, eds: Diseases of the Kidney. Boston, Little, Brown & Co, 1988, pp 2657–2679.
10. McLachlan MSF: The aging kidney. Lancet 2:143, 1978.
11. Ljungqvist A, Lagergren C: Normal intrarenal arterial pattern in adult and ageing human kidney. J Anat 96:285, 1962.
12. Takazakura E, Sawabu N, Handa A, et al: Intrarenal vascular changes with age and disease. Kidney Int 2:224, 1972.
13. Davies DF, Shock NW: Age changes in glomerular filtration rate, effective renal plasma flow, and tubular excretory capacity in adult males. J Clin Invest 29:496, 1950.
14. McDonald RK, Solomon DH, Shock NW: Aging as a factor in the renal hemodynamic changes induced by a standardized pyrogen. J Clin Invest 30:457, 1951.
15. Lee TD Jr, Lindeman RD, Yiengst MJ, et al: Influence of age on the cardiovascular and renal responses to tilting. J Appl Physiol 21:55, 1966.
16. Hollenberg NK, Adams DF, Solomon HS, et al: Senescence and the renal vasculature in normal man. Circ Res 34:309, 1974.
17. Brenner BM: Hemodynamically mediated glo-

merular injury and the progressive nature of renal disease. Kidney Int 23:647, 1983.

18. Lindeman RD, Lee TD Jr, Yiengst MJ, et al: Influence of age, renal disease, hypertension, diuretics, and calcium on the antidiuretic responses to suboptimal infusions of vasopressin. J Lab Clin Med 68:206, 1966.

19. Elema JD, Arends A: Focal and segmental glomerular hyalinosis and sclerosis in the rat. Lab Invest 33:554, 1975.

20. Tucker SM, Mason RL, Beauchene RE: Influence of diet and feed restriction on kidney function of aging male rats. J Gerontol 31:264, 1976.

21. Yu BPEJ, Masoro I, Murata HA, et al: Life span study of SPF Fischer 344 male rats fed ad libitum or restricted diets: longevity, growth, lean body mass and disease. J Gerontol 37:130, 1982.

22. Rowe JW, Andres R, Tobin JD, et al: The effect of age on creatinine clearance in men: a cross-sectional and longitudinal study. J Gerontol 31:155, 1976.

23. Luft FC, Fineberg NS, Miller JZ, et al: The effects of age, race, and heredity on glomerular filtration rate following volume expansion and contraction in normal man. Am J Med Sci 279:15, 1980.

24. Lindeman RD, Tobin J, Shock NW: Longitudinal studies on the rate of decline in renal function with age. J Am Geriatr Soc 33:278, 1985.

25. Levy SB, Talner LB, Coel MN: Renal vasculature in essential hypertension: racial differences. Ann Intern Med 88:12, 1978.

26. Cockcroft DW, Gault MH: Prediction of creatinine clearance from serum creatinine. Nephron 16:31, 1976.

27. Rowe JW, Andres R, Tobin JD, et al: Age-adjusted standard for creatinine clearance. Ann Intern Med 84:567, 1976.

28. Gral T, Young M: Measured versus estimated creatinine clearance in the elderly as an index of renal function. J Am Geriatr Soc 1:492, 1980.

29. Greenblatt DJ, Sellers EM, Shader RI: Drug disposition in old age. N Engl J Med 306:1081, 1982.

30. Epstein M: Effects of aging on the kidney. Fed Proc 38:168, 1979.

31. Macias Nunez JF, Garcia Iglesias A, Bonda Roman JL, et al: Renal handling of sodium in old people: a functional study. Age Ageing 7:178, 1978.

32. Tsunoda K, Abe K, Goto T, et al: Effect of age on the renin-angiotensin-aldosterone system in normal subjects: simultaneous measurement of active and inactive renin, renin substrate, and aldosterone in plasma. J Clin Endocrinol Metab 62:384, 1986.

33. Weidmann P, DeMytteraere-Burstein S, Maxwell MH, et al: Effect of aging on plasma renin and aldosterone in normal man. Kidney Int 8:325, 1975.

34. Weidmann P, deChatel R, Schiffmann A, et al: Interrelations between age and plasma renin, aldosterone and cortisol, urinary catecholamines, and the body sodium/volume, state in normal man. Klin Wochenschr 55:725, 1977.

35. Hegstad R, Brown RD, Jiang N-S, et al: Aging and aldosterone. Am J Med 74:442, 1983.

36. Macias Nunez JF, Garcia Igleias C, Tabernero Romo JM, et al: Renal management of sodium under indomethacin and aldosterone in the elderly. Age Ageing 9:165, 1980.

37. Anderson GH, Springer J, Randall P, et al: Effect of age on diagnostic usefulness of stimulated plasma renin activity and saralasin test in detection of renovascular hypertension. Lancet 2:821, 1980.

38. Lewis WH, Alving AS: Changes with age in the renal function in adult men. Am J Physiol 123:500, 1938.

39. Lindeman RD, Tobin J, Shock NW: Longitudinal studies on the rate of decline in renal function with age. J Am Geriatr Soc 33:278, 1985.

40. Lindeman RD, VanBuren HC, Maisz LG: Osmolar renal concentrating ability in healthy young men and hospitalized patients without renal disease. N Engl J Med 262:1306, 1960.

41. Dontas AS, Kasviki-Charvati P, Papanayiotou PC, et al: Bacteriuria and survival in old age. N Engl J Med 304:939, 1981.

42. Rowe JW, Shock NW, DeFronzo RA: The influence of age on the renal response to water deprivation in man. Nephron 17:270, 1976.

43. Miller JH, Shock NW: Age differences in the renal tubular response to antidiuretic hormone. J Gerrontol 8:446, 1953.

44. Helderman JH, Vestal RE, Rowe JW, et al: The response of arginine vasopressin to intravenous ethanol and hypertonic saline in man: the impact of aging. J Gerontol 33:39, 1978.

45. Rowe JW, Minzker KL, Sparrow D, et al: Age-related failure of volume-pressure-mediated vasopressin release. J Clin Endocrinol Metab 54:661, 1982.

46. Miller, PD, Krebs RA, Neal BJ, et al: Hypodipsia in geriatric patients. Am J Med 73:354, 1982.

47. Phillips PA, Phil D, Rolls BJ, et al: Reduced thirst after water deprivation in healthy elderly men. N Engl J Med 311:753, 1984.

48. Meier DE, Myers WM, Swenson R, et al: Indomethacin-associated hyperkalemia in the elderly. J Am Geriatr Soc 31:371, 1983.

49. Snyder NA, Feigal DW, Arieff AI: Hypernatremia in elderly patients. Ann Intern Med 107:309, 1987.

50. Beck LH, Lavizzo-Mowrey R: Geriatric hyponatremia. Ann Intern Med. 107:768, 1987.

51. Kleinfeld J, Casimir M, Borra S: Hyponatremia as observed in a chronic disease facility. J Am Geriatr Soc 27:156, 1979.

52. Sunderam SG, Mankikar GD: Hyponatremia in the elderly. Age Ageing 12:77, 1983.

53. Booker JA: Severe symptomatic hyponatremia in elderly outpatients: the role of thiazide therapy and stress. J Am Geriatr Soc 32:108, 1984.

54. Davis PJ, Davis FB: Water excretion in the elderly. Endocrinol Metab Clin North Am 16:867, 1987.

55. Adler S, Lindeman RD, Yiengst MJ, Beard E, et al: Effect of acute acid loading on urinary acid excretion by the aging human kidney. J Lab Clin Med 72:278, 1968.

56. Agarwal BN, Cabebe FG: Renal acidification in elderly subjects. Nephron 26:291, 1980.

57. Allen TH, Anderson EC, Langham WH: Total body potassium and gross body composition in relation to age. J Gerontol 15:348, 1960.

58. Sagild U: Total exchangeable potassium in normal subjects with special reference to changes with age. Scand J Clin Lab Invest 8:44, 1956.

59. Bengele HH, Mathias R, Perkins JH, et al: Impaired renal and extrarenal potassium adaptation in old rats. Kidney Int 23:684, 1983.

60. DeFronzo RA: Hyperkalemia and hyporeninemic hypoaldosteronism. Kidney Int 17:118, 1980.

61. Walmsley RN, White GH, Cain M, et al: Hyperkalemia in the elderly. Clin Chem 30:1409, 1984.

62. Mor R, Pitlik S, Rosenfeld JB: Indomethacin- and moduretic-induced hyperkalemia. Isr J Med Sci 19:535, 1983.

63. Meier DE, Myers WM, Swenson R, et al: Indomethacin-associated hyperkalemia in the elderly. J Am Geriatr Soc 31:371, 1983.

64. Kumar R, Hill CM, McGrown MG: Acute renal failure in the elderly. Lancet 1:90, 1973.

65. Moore RD, Smith CR, Lipsky JJ, et al: Risk factor for nephrotoxicity in patients treated with aminoglycosides. Ann Intern Med 100:352, 1984.

66. Byrd L, Sherman RL: Radiocontrast-induced acute renal failure: a clinical and pathophysiologic review. Medicine 58:270, 1979.

67. Rosenfeld JB, Shohat J, Grosskopf I, et al: Acute renal failure: a disease of the elderly? Adv Nephrol 6:159, 1987.

68. Lamy PP: Renal effects of nonsteroidal antiinflammatory drugs: heightened risk to the elderly? J Am Geriatr Soc 34:361, 1986.

69. Mukamel E, Nisenkorn I, Boner G: Occult progressive renal damage in the elderly male due to benign prostatic hypertrophy. J Am Geriatr Soc 27:403, 1979.

70. Oliveria DBG, Winerals CG: Acute renal failure in the elderly can have a good prognosis. Age Ageing 13:304, 1984.

71. Brynger H, Brunner FP, Chantler C, et al: Combined report on regular dialysis and transplantation in Europe X, 1979. In Robinson GHB, ed: Proc Eur Dialysis Transplant Assoc. London, Pitman Medical Press, p 88, 1980.

72. Smith MC, Ghose MK, Henry AR: The clinical spectrum of renal cholesterol embolization. Am J Med 71:174, 1981.

73. Montoliu J, Darnell A, Torras A, et al: Primary acute glomerular disorders in elderly. Arch Intern Med 140:755, 1980.

74. Potvliege PR, DeRoy G, Dupuis F: Necropsy study on glomerulonephritis in the elderly. J Clin Pathol 28:891, 1975.

75. Moorthy AV, Zimmerman SW: Renal disease in the elderly: clinicopathologic analysis of renal disease in 115 elderly patients. Clin Nephrol 14:223, 1980.

76. Fawcett IW, Hilton PJ, Jones NF, et al: Nephrotic syndrome in the elderly. Br Med J 2:387, 1971.

77. Bolton WK, Benton FR, Maclay JG, et al: Spontaneous glomerular sclerosis in aging Sprague-Dawley rats: Lesions associated with mesangial IgM deposits, I. Am J Pathol 85:227, 1976.

78. Couser WG, Stilmant MM: Mesangial lesions and focal glomerular sclerosis in the aging rat. Lab. Invest. 33:491, 1975.

79. Elema, JD, Arends A: Focal and segmental glomerular hyalinosis and sclerosis in the rat. Lab Invest 33:554, 1975.

80. Sherman FT, Tucci V, Libow LS: Nosocomial urinary tract infections in a skilled nursing facility. J Am Geriatr Soc 28:456, 1980.

81. Dontas AS, Marketos S, Papanyiouton P: Mechanisms of renal tubular defects in old age. Postgrad Med J 48:295, 1972.

82. Nicolle LE, Henderson E, Bjornson J, et al: The association of bacteriuria with resident characteristics and survival in elderly institutionalized men. Ann Intern Med 106:682, 1987.

83. Nicolle LE, Bjornson J, Hardin GKM, et al: Bacteriuria in elderly institutionalized men. N Engl J Med 311:753, 1984.

84. Boscia JA, Abrutyn E, Kaye D: Asymptomatic bacteriuria in elderly persons: Treat or do not treat? Ann Intern Med 106:764, 1987.

CARDIOVASCULAR AND PULMONARY PROBLEMS

CHAPTER 22

Syncope

Palmi V. Jonsson
Lewis A. Lipsitz

When on my sick-bed I languish,
Full of sorrow, full of anguish,
Fainting, gasping, trembling, crying,
Panting, groaning, speechless, dying, . . .
Methinks I hear some gentle spirit say,
Be not fearful, come away.
          THOMAS FLATMAN, *A Thought of Death*

Syncope is defined as transient loss of consciousness accompanied by loss of postural tone. Recovery is spontaneous, i.e., it does not require resuscitation. This common incident has multiple underlying causes and indicates increased risk of sudden death when the etiology is cardiac. Irrespective of etiology, syncope has potential adverse consequences, such as falls, fractures, subdural hematomas, and loss of independent function.

Seizures and hypoglycemia can present as syncope, although they are usually distinguishable on clinical grounds. Presyncope is the sensation of imminent loss of consciousness that usually precedes syncope.

EPIDEMIOLOGY

The information on incidence and prevalence of syncope is fragmentary. Studies of young people show a prevalence of syncope as high as 47 percent, which likely results from benign causes such as vasovagal reactions.[1] Data from the Framingham study show an increase in prevalence of syncope with age.[2] The proportion of different etiologies tends to change with age, and a greater fraction carries with it a risk of sudden death (Fig. 22–1). One percent of emergency ward evaluations and up to 3 percent of admissions to hospitals are attributed to syncope. Most of these hospital visits are by elderly patients. One nursing home study of very elderly patients revealed a 10-year prevalence of 23 percent and a 1-year incidence of 6 percent. The recurrence rate for syncope is about 30 percent.[3] Patients with cardiac causes of syncope are at the highest risk for death, with a 40 percent 2-year mor-

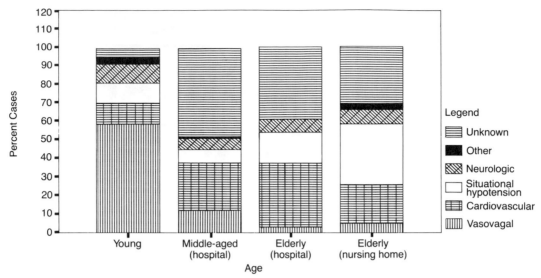

FIGURE 22–1. *Causes of Syncope According to Age (Adapted from Wayne HH: Syncope: physiological considerations and an analysis of the clinical characteristics in 510 patients. Am J Med 30:418, 1961; Kapoor WN, et al: A prospective evaluation and follow-up of patients with syncope. N Engl J Med 309:197, 1983; Kapoor WN, et al: Syncope in the Elderly. Am J Med 80:419, 1986; Lipsitz LA, et al: Syncope in an elderly, institutionalized population: prevalence, incidence, and associated risk. Q J Med 216:45, 1985.)*

tality. Patients with noncardiac causes of syncope have a 20 percent 2-year mortality, similar to that of syncope of unknown causes.[4, 5] Syncope is associated with a high mortality that most probably results from the underlying diseases rather than from an independent relationship between syncope and death. Recurrent syncope that is unexplained after thorough initial evaluation is not associated with excess mortality.[3, 6]

PATHOPHYSIOLOGY

Syncope results from inadequate energy delivery to the brain. The major energy substrates are oxygen and glucose. Significant hypoglycemia tends to result in coma rather than in syncope, and a prolonged cessation of oxygen delivery results in death. Thus, transient cerebral hypoxia from decreased cerebral blood flow is the final common pathway in most cases of syncope. Generalized hypoxemia and decreased oxygen-carrying capacity of the blood are risk factors for syncope, particularly in the elderly but are rarely the sole causes. Infrequently, focal stenosis of arteries supplying critical areas of the brain cause syncope.

Blood pressure is determined by the product of cardiac output and peripheral arterial resistance. A reduction in one variable without an increase in the other will lower blood pressure. Cardiac output may fall because of a reduction in stroke volume or because of extreme heart rates, either fast or slow. Reduced stroke volume may result from obstruction to flow within the heart or pulmonary vasculature, myocardial pump failure, or reduction in venous return. Venous return may decrease as a result of venous blood pooling or hypovolemia. Impaired arterial resistance can result from autonomic neural failure or medication effects. Triggered cardiovascular reflexes may cause syncope by decreasing vascular resistance and/or cardiac output.

Age-related and Disease-related Changes Predisposing to Syncope in the Elderly

One of the characteristics in the elderly that predisposes them to syncope is the presence of multiple clinical abnormalities.[7] Accumulation of age-related and disease-related conditions that threaten cerebral blood flow or reduce oxygen content in the blood may bring oxygen delivery close to the threshold needed to maintain consciousness. A situational stress that further reduces blood pressure, such as posture change or a Valsalva maneuver during defecation, may reduce cerebral oxygen delivery below the critical threshold and result in syncope. Several homeostatic mechanisms that normally preserve blood pressure and cerebral oxygen delivery during such stresses become impaired with age. These mechanisms include cerebral autoregulation, baroreflexes, and renal sodium conservation.

Cerebral blood flow declines with normal aging. In hypertension, which often accompanies advancing age, the threshold for cerebral autoregulation is shifted to higher levels of blood pressure, making the elderly patient with hypertension more vulnerable to cerebral ischemia from relatively small degrees of hypotension. Baroreflex sensitivity is also impaired with advanced age. This can be demonstrated by a blunted bradycardic response to hypertensive stimuli and diminished tachycardic response to blood pressure reduction. At the bedside, this is evident in the absent or modest cardioacceleration associated with posture change in the elderly patient.

With advancing age, the kidney's capacity to conserve salt also declines and predisposes the patient to hypovolemia. The older patient who stops eating or drinking because of an acute illness or who has limited access to food and fluids may continue to excrete some salt in the urine and therefore, may become dehydrated. This may be associated with age-related reductions in basal and stimulated renin secretion and reduction in plasma aldosterone concentration. Many elderly persons also have an impaired thirst response to hyperosmolality and thus may not consume enough fluids to prevent dehydration.

In addition to normal age-related physiologic changes, several diseases predispose to syncope. These include respiratory failure with hypoxemia, anemia, and gastrointestinal bleeding. Dyspnea may cause hyperventilation, which can reduce cerebral blood flow. Bleeding may simultaneously cause hypovolemia and reduce oxygen-carrying capacity of the blood. The elderly are particularly vulnerable to the hypotensive effects of a rapid heart rate. Because of progressive myocardial stiffness, impaired diastolic relaxation, and reduced early diastolic ventricular filling with advancing age, the aged heart becomes more dependent on atrial contraction to fill the ventricle and maintain cardiac output. A rapid heart rate further reduces the opportunity to adequately fill the ventricle with blood and therefore threatens cardiac output. During atrial fibrillation, the loss of atrial contraction further reduces cardiac output, independent of heart rate. This makes rapid atrial fibrillation particularly dangerous in the elderly patient.

ETIOLOGY

In Table 22–1 are shown the broad categories of conditions that can cause syncope, and Fig. 22–1 illustrates that the prevalence of different conditions causing syncope varies through the lifecycle. The relative frequency will also vary according to the patient's environment (e.g., community, emergency ward, hospital, nursing home).

Multiple studies have shown that 30 to 50 percent of syncopal episodes remain unexplained in spite of extensive evaluation.[8, 9] Of the diagnosable cases, 40 percent of nursing home patients to 60 percent of acute care hospital patients will have cardiac causes for syncope, depending on the setting.[3, 4] The most common cardiac causes are conduction disturbances, sinus node disease, tachyarrhythmias, and bradyarrhythmias. Small but significant numbers of people have aortic stenosis and myocardial infarction (MI). Carotid sinus syndrome is a treatable, but often overlooked, cause of syncope in 1 to 2 percent of patients.

Another 20 to 40 percent of cases are noncardiac in nature. One important condition leading to noncardiac syncope is orthostatic hypotension secondary to volume loss, use of medications, prolonged immobility, or autonomic insufficiency. In the elderly patient with impaired blood pressure homeostasis, syncope resulting from hypotension is also often provoked by other situational stresses such as eating, defecation, micturition, and cough.[3] Vasodepressor (or vasovagal) syncope secondary to pain or emotional stress is less common in the elderly than in the young.

TABLE 22–1. Causes of Syncope

Cardiac Disease (Decreased Cardiac Output)
Structural (Mechanical obstruction to flow)
Aortic stenosis
Mitral stenosis
Atrial myxoma
Cardiomyopathy
Pulmonary embolism
Myocardial
Acute myocardial infarction
Electrical
Tachyarrhythmias
Bradyarrhythmias (Conduction disturbance; Sinus node dysfunction)
Hypotension (Decreased volume or peripheral vascular resistance)
Orthostatic hypotension
Prolonged inactivity
Medications (vasodilator; antihypertensives; antidepressants; neuroleptics; diuretics)
Central nervous system disease (Shy-Drager syndrome; Parkinson's disease)
Peripheral autonomic neuropathies (Diabetes, Alcoholism, Amyloidosis)
Idiopathic
Postpranial Hypotension
Volume Depletion
Fluid or blood loss
Reflex (Decreased cardiac output or peripheral vascular resistance)
Vasovagal
Defecation
Micturition
Cough
Swallowing
Carotid Sinus Syndrome
Abnormal Blood Composition (Reduced energy substrates)
Hypoxemia
Hypoglycemia
Acute Anemia
Central Nervous System Disease
Seizures
Cerebrovascular Insufficiency

Occasionally, seizure disorders and strokes will masquerade as syncope. Although the literature suggests that 30 to 50 percent of cases remain unexplained after extensive evaluation, attention to situational causes in elderly patients is likely to leave the cause of fewer episodes unclear in that age group. A case in point is postprandial hypotension, which was only recently appreciated as an important cause of syncope.[10]

Syncope is also more likely to result from the coexistence of multiple pathologic abnormalities in the elderly that interact with one another to critically reduce cerebral blood flow to the threshold of cerebral ischemia.[7] Thus, the elderly patient with anemia, which results in a reduction in O_2 carrying capacity of the blood; chronic obstructive pulmonary disease (COPD), which causes a low PO_2; or cerebrovascular disease, which obstructs cerebral blood flow, has a significant compromise of oxygen delivery to the brain.

Any additional stress that reduces blood pressure or blood O_2 content such as posture change, a new drug, or the acute onset of pneumonia may produce global cerebral ischemia and result in syncope. For this reason, syncope may be the atypical manifestation of almost any disease process in the elderly patient.

EVALUATION

The history is the most important part of the evaluation and provides a diagnosis in up to 50 percent of cases where a cause is found. The physical examination gives a diagnosis in another 20 percent of cases.[11]

The history includes four key questions.[12] First, was there an obvious *precipitant?* Emotional stress, pain, cough, micturition, defecation, swallowing, effort (aortic stenosis), neck turning (carotid sinus syndrome), change in position, and recent meal or medication dose are all important clues. Second, were there any *associated symptoms*? Hunger, sweating, odd behavior, and slow onset and recovery may suggest hypoglycemia. Paresthesia may indicate hypocalcemia or hyperventilation. Flushing on recovery can reveal Stoke-Adams attack. Palpitations, dyspnea, or chest pain may disclose pulmonary embolism, angina pectoris, or MI. Dizziness may signify arrhythmia or hypotension. Focal neurologic symptoms suggest a neurologic disorder. Third, could *medications* have been responsible? Various antihypertensive and antianginal medications can cause hypotension. Digoxin can cause arrhythmias, and various antiarrhythmic medications can paradoxically cause arrhythmias. Fourth, *how long did the symptoms last?* If symptoms last for more than 15 minutes, one should consider transient ischemic attack, seizure, hypoglycemia, or hysteria.

Physical examination should focus on postural vital signs and cardiovascular and neurologic systems and on a search for trauma. Carotid sinus massage should be performed if it is not contraindicated by the presence of clinical or historic evidence of cerebrovascular disease or cardiac conduction abnormalities on the electrocardiogram (ECG). Blood pressure and heart rate are measured after at least a 5-minute rest in the supine position, then again after 1 minute and 3 minutes of standing. If the patient cannot stand, sitting will suffice but may lead to failure to diagnose orthostatic hypotension. A symptomatic fall in blood pressure focuses further evaluation on the causes for orthostatic hypotension. In the young patient, excessive acceleration of the pulse in response to posture change suggests that volume depletion, bleeding, or medications may be the cause of orthostatic hypotension; however, this finding is often absent in the elderly patient with baroreflex impairment. If pulse rate does not accelerate, autonomic dysfunction may also be the cause.

Careful evaluation of the carotid pulsations for their contour, amplitude and sound is important.[7] Although the carotid upstroke is characteristically delayed in aortic stenosis, a normal upstroke does not exclude the diagnosis of aortic stenosis in the elderly patient because of an age-related increase in vascular rigidity that increases the rate of rise of the carotid pulse. When aortic stenosis develops, the rate of the rise falls but the amplitude may feel normal for a younger patient. Also, a diminished carotid pulse or bruit may be suggestive of cerebrovascular disease, but its absence does not exclude a diagnosis of cerebral ischemia. Cardiopulmonary examination focuses on detection of obstructive cardiovascular disorders such as aortic stenosis, hypertrophic cardiomyopathy, and pulmonary embolism. Unfortunately, cardiac murmurs become exceedingly common with advanced age, and significant murmurs in the elderly may be atypical in character or location. Thus, associated clinical symptoms, such as congestive heart failure or angina pectoris, or signs, such as a diminished S2 or left ventricular hypertrophy, should heighten the suspicion of hemodynamically significant conditions and stimulate further studies such as a Doppler echo of the heart. Stools should be checked for blood, and a careful neurologic examination should include a search for focal deficits that may signify cerebral infarction, hemorrhage, or tumor.

Carotid sinus massage is an important test in the evaluation if cerebrovascular disease or cardiac conduction disturbances are not apparent. With the electrocardiogram operating and the head slightly extended and rotated to the opposite side, the carotid sinus is massaged for five seconds. The blood pressure is taken before and immediately after the procedure. Two to 3 minutes later, the procedure is repeated on the other side. Only symptomatic bradycardia or hypotension can be considered truly positive responses indicating carotid sinus hypersensitivity. However, there is general agreement that a systolic blood pressure decline of more than 50 mmHg (or an absolute value less than 90 mmHg) or a sinus pause of 3 seconds or longer is sufficient to produce syncope, particularly if the patient was in an upright position at the time of the syncopal event.

An ECG is indicated in all patients presenting with syncope, since it can provide diagnostic clues for MI, ischemia, or transient tachyarrhythmias or bradyarrhythmias. Multifocal and frequent atrial and ventricular ectopic beats are an indication for prolonged cardiac monitoring. In the electrocardiogram a short P wave to R wave interval on the surface EKG may indicate an accessory pathway. A Q wave to T wave interval prolongation on the surface EKG is associated with ventricular tachycardia and fibrillation. Sinoatrial pauses or inappropriate sinus bradycardia may indicate a sinus node disorder. The presence of atrioventricular conduction abnormalities or bundle branch block hints at transient heart block as the etiology of syncope.[7]

Because electrical cardiac disease is so common in elderly patients, continuous ECG monitoring is usually indicated— even without cues from the electrocardiogram—unless noncardiac causes are positively identified. Ambulatory cardiac monitoring is indicated in those syncope patients who are still suspected, after initial evaluation, in-hospital cardiac monitoring, or both, to have a symptomatic and safely treatable arrhythmia or conduction disturbance. Ambulatory monitoring should be performed while the patient is doing his usual daily activities to increase the diagnostic yield. When monitored for 24 to 48 hours, 10 to 40 percent of patients will have transient symptoms. Of these patients, an arrhythmic etiology can be confirmed or excluded in one half to three quarters.[13]

Laboratory tests are generally of low yield, but they are useful in the geriatric syncope patient without apparent etiology on history and physical examination because syncope may be the atypical presentation of several conditions evident only on laboratory testing. Cardiac enzymes should be obtained if there is any associated chest pain or ECG change, which raises the suspicion of MI. Evaluation of electrolytes, blood urea nitrogen (BUN) and serum creatinine is important both to determine volume status and to identify abnormalities that predispose to arrhythmias. Tests of arterial blood gases are indicated only if there are pulmonary symptoms. A hematocrit measurement is helpful to exclude anemia. Blood sugar should be measured in search of hypoglycemia and marked hyperglycemia, both of which may present as syncope in the elderly patient. Determining the drug levels of anticonvulsants, antiarrhythmics, digoxin, or broncodilators is useful to detect toxicity or undertreatment of a prior condition known to produce syncope.

The electroencephalogram (EEG) and a computed tomography (CT) scan of the head should be obtained only in the presence of focal neurologic abnormalities on physical examination or if signs and symptoms of seizures exist.[5] More invasive studies such as cerebral or coronary angiography are only indicated to confirm specific clinical diagnoses. Electrophysiologic studies of the heart are indicated in patients with cardiovascular disease and recurrent syncope in whom there is a high suspicion of sinus node dysfunction, conduction disturbance, or life-threatening arrhythmias. The benefits of any invasive procedure should be balanced against its risks and the potential adverse effects of therapy (including surgery and medications) before initiation in an elderly patient. The diagnostic approach to the elderly syncope patient is summarized in Figure 22–2.

THERAPEUTIC ISSUES

The purpose of treating an elderly patient with syncope is to prevent the morbidity and mortality associated with recurrent episodes. When the cause of a syncopal episode is readily apparent, specific therapy can be planned if potential morbidity of the treatment is less than that of recurrent syncope. Because therapeutic intervention may be toxic to elderly patients, it should be instituted with cautious attention to age-related and disease-related physiologic changes that may affect response to a treatment. No person should, however, be denied therapy on the basis of age alone.

When the cause of a syncopal episode is not clear, the therapy should be directed toward minimizing the risk of recurrence both by correcting age-related and disease-related impairments and by eliminating drugs that may incrementally contribute to a syncopal event.[7] For example, the risk of syncope in an older person may be substantially reduced by treating anemia with a blood transfusion, correcting hypoxemia with supplemental oxygen, improving cardiac ischemia with nitrates (observing for orthostatic hypotension), or preventing orthostatic hypotension with a high salt intake (observing for congestive heart failure), and support stockings.

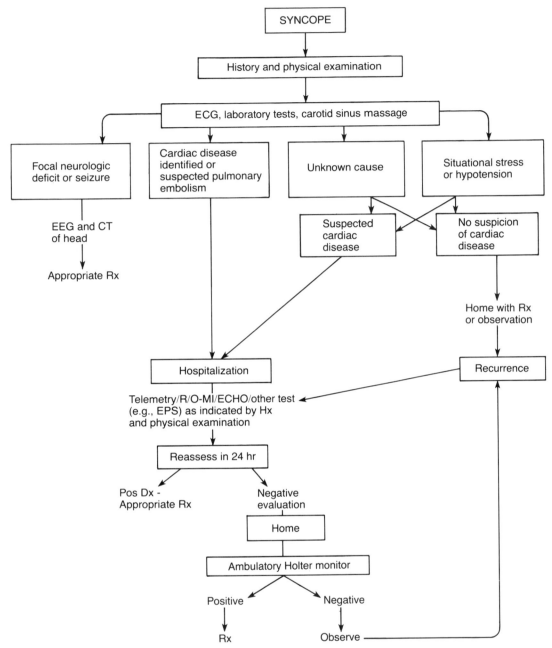

FIGURE 22–2. *Algorithm for the Diagnostic Evaluation of the Elderly Syncope Patient. EPS = electrophysiological stimulation; Rx = treatment; Dx = diagnosis; pos =positive; neg = negative.*

Before prescribing invasive therapy for a diagnosed condition, such as a pacemaker for symptomatic bradyarrhythmia or surgery for aortic stenosis, the safe, simple, common sense treatments should be implemented first. Such treatments include discontinuing potentially harmful drugs including digoxin, propranolol, and alpha methyldopa, which may predispose to carotid sinus hypersensitivity or sup-

press the sinus node; avoiding extreme neck rotation and tight collars when there is evidence of carotid sinus hypersensitivity; arising slowly from the supine position and dorsiflexing the feet a few minutes before standing in persons prone to postural hypotension; maintaining adequate intravascular volume through regular fluid intake in cognitively impaired or acutely ill patients; and urinating while sitting down in men with micturition syncope. Often a simple behavior change or drug elimination is the only therapy necessary to prevent recurrent syncopal episodes.

Antiarrhythmic medications should be prescribed for *symptomatic* rhythm disturbances only—and initially at one half of the usual dose—because of their prolonged half-life and the increased risk of toxicity in elderly patients.[7] Pacemakers are generally indicated for the amelioration of symptoms of bradyarrhythmias rather than for prolongation of life, except in patients with Stokes-Adams attacks, in whom they do improve longevity.[14] Indications for antiarrhythmic medications, pacemakers, and electrophysiologic studies are continually being reassessed, and the latest consensus should be sought and carefully considered prior to prescription in the elderly.

CONCLUSION

The presentation of syncope in the elderly patient is often different from that in the young because of important age and disease interactions. Usual age-related physiologic changes and multiple disease-related abnormalities predispose the geriatric patient to syncope. Thus, syncope may be the atypical manifestation of diseases or situational stresses not expected to produce it. Attention to situational stresses, such as posture change, food intake, or drug ingestion, is likely to increase the diagnostic yield and lead to simple therapy that can reduce the morbidity and potential mortality of recurrent episodes. Therapy should be directed toward minimizing the multiple risks for syncope, avoiding potentially toxic interventions, and treating specific *symptomatic* diseases, using underlying medical conditions, rather than age, as the criterion for invasive treatment.

ACKNOWLEDGMENTS

Supported by the Hebrew Rehabilitation Center for Aged, and by Grant #AG06443, and a NIA Teaching Nursing Home Award, AG04390, from the U.S. Public Health Service. Dr. Lipsitz was supported in part by a National Institute on Aging Academic Award, AG00213.

REFERENCES

1. Wayne HH: Syncope: physiological considerations and an analysis of the clinical characteristics in 510 patients. Am J Med 30:418, 1961.
2. Savage DD, Conwin L, McGee DL, et al: Epidemiologic features of isolated syncope: the Framingham Study. Stroke 16:626, 1985.
3. Lipsitz LA, Wei JY, Rowe JW: Syncope in an elderly, institutionalized population: prevalence, incidence, and associated risk. Q J Med 216:45, 1985.
4. Kapoor WN, Snustad D, Peterson J, et al: Syncope in the elderly. Am J Med 80:419, 1986.
5. Day SC, Look EF, Funkenstein H, et al: Evaluation and outcome of emergency room patients with transient loss of consciousness. Am J Med 73:15, 1982.
6. Kapoor WN, Peterson J, Wieand HS, et al: Diagnostic and prognostic implications of recurrences in patients with syncope. Am J Med 83:700, 1987.
7. Lipsitz LA: Syncope in the elderly. Am Intern Med 99:92, 1983.
8. Kapoor WN, Karpf M, Maher Y, et al: Syncope of unknown origin: the need for a more cost-effective approach to its diagnostic evaluation. JAMA 247:2687, 1982.
9. Silverstein MD, Singer DE, Mulley AG, et al: Patients with syncope admitted to medical intensive care units. JAMA 248:1185, 1982.
10. Lipsitz LA, Nyquist RP, Wei JY, et al: Postprandial reduction in blood pressure in the elderly. N Engl J Med 309:81, 1983.
11. Kudenchuk PJ, McAnulty JH: Syncope: evaluation and treatment. Mod Conc Cardiovasc Dis 54:25, 1985.
12. Ormerod AD: Syncope. Br Med J 288:1219, 1984.
13. Kapoor WN: Evaluation of syncope in the elderly. J Am Geriatr Soc 35:826, 1987.
14. Kunst M: Cardiac pacemakers. Med Clin North Am 57:1515.
15. Kapoor WN, Karpf M, Wieand S, et al: A prospective evaluation and follow-up of patients with syncope. N Engl J Med 309:197, 1983.

CHAPTER 23

Hypertension

Michael D. Cressman
Ray W. Gifford, Jr.

It gives me great pleasure to converse with the aged. They have been over the road that all of us must travel, and know where it is rough and difficult and where it is level and easy.

PLATO, *The Republic*

DEFINITIONS

Hypertension and *elderly* are generally defined numerically. Although these numerical definitions are not perfect and, indeed, are somewhat arbitrary, a discussion of hypertension in the elderly is difficult to present without these definitions. In this chapter, elderly refers to an individual who is at least 65 years old. The definitions of hypertension, summarized in the 1988 report of the Joint National Committee (JNC) on Detection, Evaluation, and Treatment of High Blood Pressure, are employed.[1] Individuals who have an average diastolic blood pressure (DBP) reading > 90 mmHg measured two or more times on each of three separate occasions have *diastolic hypertension*. Those with a systolic blood pressure (SBP) reading > 160 mmHg and a DBP < 90 mmHg have *isolated systolic hypertension* (ISH). Borderline ISH is present when the SBP is between 140 and 160 mmHg and the DBP is < 90 mmHg.

PREVALENCE

The prevalence of hypertension in the U.S. population has been estimated in individuals aged 6 through 74 years, using data from the second National Health and Nutrition Examination Survey (NHANES II) and other sources.[2] In NHANES II, three blood pressure measurements were obtained in a civilian noninstitutionalized population on a single occasion at 64 sample locations throughout the U.S. The average of these three measurements was used for analysis. Although the use of single occasion measurements probably overestimates the true incidence of hypertension, the NHANES II data clearly demonstrate that the incidence of hypertension in individuals aged 65 to 74 is very high (Table 23–1).[3] If a SBP > 140 mmHg and/or a DBP > 90 mmHg or reported use of antihypertensive medications is used to define hypertension, 76.1 percent of blacks and 63.1 percent of whites between the ages of 65 and 74 are hypertensive. The prevalence of diastolic hypertension is slightly higher in elderly women than in elderly men. These figures are similar to those obtained during screening for the Systolic Hypertension in the Elderly Program (SHEP), which is an ongoing treatment trial of elderly patients with ISH.[4] In this study, 68 percent of the individuals between 65 and 74 years old were hypertensive.

TABLE 23–1. Prevalence (%) of Diastolic Hypertension: 65- to 74-Year-Old Participants in NHANES II[3]

	BP > 160/ 95 (%)	BP > 140/ 90 (%)
Total (all races)	45.1	64.3
Total blacks	59.9	76.1
Total whites	43.7	63.1
Black women	72.8	82.9
Black men	42.9	67.1
White women	48.3	66.2
White men	37.5	59.2

Adapted from The Working Group on Hypertension in the Elderly: Statement on hypertension in the elderly. JAMA 256:70, 1986.

ments obtained from 20- to 24-year-old individuals.[18] The implication of these studies is that a rigid aorta would generate a higher SBP for a given stroke volume than a more elastic aorta.

Although the average SBP increases with age in most Western industrialized nations, the development of ISH is not a normal consequence of aging. Epidemiologic observations conducted in several nonindustrialized societies do not show an age-related rise in SBP.[19] Individuals in these societies tend to consume low-sodium, high-potassium, low-fat diets and remain lean and physically active throughout life.

Systolic hypertension resulting from rigidity of large arteries should be accompanied by a reduction in DBP (if total peripheral resistance remains normal). Even if this compensatory reduction in DBP occurs, cardiac work (CW) is increased because CW is a product of stroke volume (SV), heart rate (HR), and mean SBP (SBP), according the the formula:[20]

$$CW = SV \times HR \times SBP$$

For this reason, it is not surprising that certain complications of hypertension, such as congestive heart failure, are closely associated with elevation of SBP.

It should be pointed out that elderly individuals with diastolic hypertension often have a disproportionate elevation in SBP. As previously stated, 60- to 69-year-old participants in the HDFP had an average SBP that was 20 mmHg higher than that in 30- to 49-year-old participants, even though the DBP was virtually identical (101 mmHg) in both groups.[14] Koch-Weser defined disproportionate systolic hypertension as:[21]

$$SBP > (DBP - 15) \times 2$$

Diastolic Hypertension

Diastolic hypertension may be defined as primary (idiopathic, essential) or secondary to diseases such as renal artery disease, renal parenchymal disease, primary aldosteronism, Cushing's disease, and pheochromocytoma. Although detailed studies defining the prevalence of the secondary forms of hypertension in the elderly have not been performed, the vast majority of elderly patients with hypertension have primary hypertension. For this reason, a detailed laboratory investigation to identify secondary causes of hypertension in an older individual is usually not required. However, it should be recognized that the sudden onset of hypertension or the loss of control of previously controlled hypertension is an important clue to the presence of a secondary cause of hypertension. In this situation, atherosclerotic renal artery disease should be strongly considered. This is particularly true if the hypertension is severe or resistant to standard triple-drug therapy and the patient has evidence of generalized atherosclerosis on physical examination. Severe bilateral renal artery stenosis or severe stenosis in an artery to a solitary kidney should be considered in a patient who develops acute renal failure during treatment with an angiotensin converting enzyme (ACE) inhibitor.[22]

The neurohumoral and hemodynamic characteristics of diastolic hypertension are somewhat different between young and elderly patients. Elderly patients with hypertension, as a group, have lower cardiac output, higher peripheral vascular resistance, lower blood volume, lower plasma renin activity (PRA), and higher plasma catecholamine levels.[23] Messerli and coworkers reported that 60 percent of 30 elderly patients with hypertension had echocardiographic evidence of left ventricular hypertrophy (LVH); however, LVH was present in only 10 percent of the younger patients. The reduced cardiac output in elderly patients was caused by a reduction in both stroke volume and heart rate. Total peripheral vascular resistance was 40 percent higher in the older group, and total and central blood volume were lower in these patients.

Baroreceptor sensitivity is also decreased in the elderly.[24] Baroreceptor reflexes are primarily responsible for buffering excessive changes in blood pressure and are important in modulating the hemodynamic adjustments required to maintain blood pressure with changes in body position. When arising from a supine position, blood pressure in the upper thorax and head tends to fall. This results in reduced stimulation of high pressure carotid sinus and aortic baroreceptors. Reduced neural activity is sensed by the nucleus tractus solitarius and leads to stimulation of the vasoconstrictor center in the medulla and an inhibitory vagal response. Total peripheral resistance rises, and heart rate increases. Dysfunction in any portion of this reflex arc or an abnormality in the peripheral arterioles can lead to an excessive fall in SBP and DBP when the patient is upright. Orthostatic hypotension can produce unsteadiness, confusion, falls, or syncope in affected patients, particularly with use of certain antihypertensive drugs that interfere with these reflex responses. For this reason, peripherally acting sympatholytic agents such as guanethidine, guanadrel, prazosin, or terazosin should be used with great caution in the elderly. Overzealous diuretic treatment with its risk of volume depletion can also lead to orthostatic hypotension in these individuals.

In summary, elderly hypertensive patients have lower cardiac outputs and higher total peripheral vascular resistance levels than younger hypertensive patients. Blood volume and PRA levels also tend to be reduced in elderly compared with young hypertensive patients. Elderly hypertensive patients with reduced baroreceptor sensitivity are predisposed to orthostatic hypotension, which can be exacerbated when certain antihypertensive drugs are administered.

MANAGEMENT CONSIDERATIONS

Evaluation

The goals of the initial evaluation of any patient with hypertension are to confirm the presence of high blood pressure, assess the patient's overall health, evaluate the status of target organs, determine if other cardiovascular risk factors are present, and exclude secondary causes of high blood pressure.[1] Repeated blood pressure measurements are required to document the presence of sustained hypertension because blood pressure, particularly SBP, is often quite labile in elderly patients. In addition, concern has been raised about the accuracy of indirect blood pressure measurements in elderly patients with significant sclerosis of the brachial artery. Messerli and coworkers noted that

elderly patients with hypertension who were "Osler-positive" had indirect cuff blood pressure measurements that were 10 to 54 mmHg higher than direct intraarterial pressure measurements.[25]

A patient was classified as being Osler-positive if either the brachial artery or radial artery could definitely be palpated when occlusion of the artery was produced by increasing cuff pressure above SBP. Messerli found that 13 of 24 elderly hypertensive patients were Osler-positive. This spurious elevation in blood pressure, because of sclerosis of the large arteries, has been referred to as pseudohypertension. Other investigators have compared indirect measurements of blood pressure with direct arterial pressure measurements and found close correlations for SBP in patients up to 81 years of age.[26, 27] Irrespective of age, indirect blood pressure measurements overestimate DBP.

Nevertheless, one should consider pseudohypertension when (1) the blood pressure is elevated out of proportion to the degree of clinical evidence of target organ involvement, (2) blood pressure fails to respond to an appropriate antihypertensive regimen, and/or (3) symptoms suggestive of hypotension develop during drug treatment, despite persistence of measured blood pressure elevation.

Blood pressure should be measured at each visit while the patient is in the supine or sitting position and again while in the standing position because elderly individuals are more likely to have a significant orthostatic decrease in blood pressure and to develop symptoms of cerebral hypoperfusion that may include dizziness, unsteadiness, falls, and syncope. This is particularly important when pharmacologic therapy is administered.

The medical history and physical examination are used to detect associated conditions that frequently coexist with high blood pressure in the elderly. These conditions—and the medications used to treat them—may influence the choice of antihypertensive drugs. For example, agents with significant central nervous system (CNS) side effects (such as the beta-blockers or centrally acting sympatholytic agents) are best avoided in individuals with a history of depression or varying degrees of organic dementia. In addition, drugs such as the alpha$_1$ receptor-blockers (prazosin, terazosin) and the peripherally acting sympatholytic agents (guanethidine, guanadrel) should be avoided in individuals who have a history of stroke, significant extracranial or intracranial cerebrovascular disease, and significant orthostatic hypotension prior to initiation of drug therapy.

The status of the coronary circulation must be considered. Calcium channel-blockers and beta-blockers are particularly useful in the treatment of hypertensive patients with angina pectoris. However, beta-blockers and verapamil may further impair myocardial contractility in individuals with ischemic, idiopathic, or hypertensive cardiomyopathy. Beta adrenergic receptor-blockers should also be used with caution in patients with chronic obstructive pulmonary disease (COPD), particularly if a bronchospastic component is present. Renal blood flow and glomerular filtration rate (GFR) are often reduced in the elderly; for this reason, drugs with renal excretion should be used at a reduced dose. A large number of elderly hypertensive patients regularly use nonsteroidal anti-inflammatory drugs to treat various chronic arthropathies. These agents blunt the efficacy of most antihypertensive agents and may cause deterioration of renal function.

Treatment

NONPHARMACOLOGIC THERAPY

Although there are no long-term trials of nonpharmacologic therapy in the treatment of the elderly with high blood pressure, most physicians would agree that a 3- to 6-month trial of nondrug therapy is warranted in elderly individuals with mild diastolic hypertension or ISH. This is particularly true for ISH, since there is no evidence from treatment trials that drug therapy reduces cardiovascular mortality in this condition. Although there is a general impression that elderly individuals will not exercise, alter their diets, or attempt to reduce body weight, data from the Minnesota Heart Health Program suggest that a significant number of older individuals will make recommended lifestyle changes.[28]

Sodium intake can be very high in elderly patients, particularly in individuals who ingest large quantities of canned foods, processed meats, and snacks. Attempts to reduce sodium intake in these individuals are obviously desirable. Calcium intake is often inadequate in the elderly, and there has been increased enthusiasm for use of calcium supplements for the prevention of osteoporosis in postmenopausal women.[4] Some reports suggest that oral calcium supplementation has a beneficial blood pressure–lowering effect.[29] Finally, certain investigators advocate dietary supplementation of magnesium or potassium for the treatment of hypertension, and magnesium and potassium intake may be reduced in the elderly. However, one should recognize that the renal excretion of magnesium and potassium may be reduced in elderly patients with renal disease. Thus, this form of treatment is theoretically not without hazard. With these limitations and precautions in mind, a 3- to 6-month trial of nonpharmacologic therapy is reasonable in elderly hypertensive patients, except when moderate to severe diastolic hypertension or complications are present.

PHARMACOLOGIC THERAPY

DIURETICS. The JNC on Detection, Evaluation, and Treatment of High Blood Pressure report and the report of the Working Group on Hypertension in the Elderly recommended a diuretic as the first step in pharmacologic treatment for elderly patients with hypertension.[1, 3] Both of these reports suggested that small doses (e.g., 12.5 to 25 mg hydrochlorothiazide or equivalent) of diuretics should be prescribed initially. Diuretics were used in the elderly patients in the Australian Trial, the HDFP, and the European Working Party on High Blood Pressure in the Elderly Study.[16, 17, 30] As previously stated, chlorthalidone was given to elderly patients with ISH in the pilot phase of the SHEP trial.[4]

Hydrochlorothiazide was given in combination with triamterene in the European Working Party on High Blood Pressure in the Elderly Study.[17] This combination was quite effective in preventing diuretic-induced hypokalemia, but a slight increase in serum uric acid and creatinine and a reduction in glucose tolerance were observed in the diuretic-treated patients. Martin and coworkers reported that elderly patients receiving diuretics at the time of hospital admission had lower serum magnesium concentrations than elderly hospitalized patients who were not receiving diuretics.[31] Renal magnesium wasting was noted in hypomagnesemic subjects receiving either loop or thiazide-type diuretics. Wang and associates noted that hypomagnesemia was relatively common in hospitalized patients receiving diuretics and digitalis.[32] Because diuretics also cause hypokalemia, there is concern that the combination of hypokalemia and hypomagnesemia may increase the risk of digitalis-associated cardiac arrhythmias.

Despite these potential problems, diuretics are very useful agents because of their low cost, convenience, and proven efficacy. Patients with significant azotemia (serum creatinine above 2 to 3 mg/dl) may benefit from use of one of the newer thiazide-type diuretics such as indapamide or metolazone. Loop diuretics may be required in more severely azotemic individuals. These agents (furosemide, bumetanide, ethacrynic acid) generally require administration twice daily.

Some physicians routinely use a thiazide/potassium-sparing agent because of concern about the hypokalemic effect of the thiazides. There is, however, a risk of hyperkalemia, especially in elderly people receiving potassium-sparing diuretics such amiloride, spironolactone, or triamterene who also have renal insufficiency, diabetes mellitus, hyporeninemic hypoaldosteronism or are receiving a nonsteroidal anti-inflammatory agent, converting enzyme inhibitor, or potassium supplements. Because the risk of hyperkalemia is real and the thiazide/potassium-sparing agents do not always prevent hypokalemia, the serum potassium level must be monitored even if these agents are used. Our own preference is to reserve the use of thiazide/potassium-sparing drugs for those patients who develop diuretic-induced hypokalemia.

BETA-BLOCKERS. Beta-blockers are quite effective as single-agent therapy for hypertension in young individuals, but their efficacy seems to be reduced in the elderly. Buhler and colleagues noted an inverse relationship between age and the blood pressure–lowering response to beta-blocker monotherapy; an adequate response occurred in only 20 percent of patients aged 60 and older compared with a 75 percent response rate in individuals under 40 years of age.[33] The reduced antihypertensive response in the elderly may relate to the low renin status, reduced beta adrenergic receptor responsiveness, and/or the low cardiac output that has been described in these patients. However, there are elderly individuals who do respond to beta-blocker monotherapy, and these drugs are indicated in certain situations.

Beta-blockers are effective antianginal agents and have been shown to reduce the incidence of reinfarction and sudden death after an MI.[34, 35] Anderson and coworkers originally suggested that elderly patients did not benefit from postinfarction beta-blocker prophylaxis, based on the results of their relatively small study, using alprenolol.[36] Both the larger Norwegian trial (using timolol) and the Beta Blocker Heart Attack Trial (using propranolol) have shown a favorable response in older individuals.[34, 35] For this reason, it is rational to treat a hypertensive patient who has had an MI with a beta-blocker, since the protective effect of beta blockade seems to persist for several years after initiation of treatment.

It is important to recognize that absolute or relative contraindications to beta-blocker treatment, such as heart block greater than first degree, COPD, occlusive arterial disease, and diabetes mellitus, are more common in older than in younger individuals. Elderly individuals tend to have higher steady-state blood levels of beta-blockers than do younger patients treated with equivalent doses of these drugs because both hepatic and renal clearance of drugs are reduced in the elderly. In general, it is reasonable to initiate therapy with approximately one half the usual recommended dose of a given beta-blocker if one of these agents is used to treat hypertension in the elderly.

ALPHA$_1$ RECEPTOR-BLOCKERS. Prazosin and terazosin are post-synaptic alpha$_1$ receptor-blocking drugs that reduce blood pressure primarily by reducing peripheral vascular resistance. These agents also reduce preload as a result of their vasodilatory effects on the venous system. Although simultaneous reduction in preload and afterload is desirable in hypertensive patients with impaired myocardial pump function, there is a risk of developing orthostatic hypotension when these drugs are used to treat elderly patients with high blood pressure. For these reasons, they are not usually recommended as first line agents.

ALPHA/BETA-BLOCKER. Labetalol is a noncardioselective beta adrenergic receptor-blocker that also possesses prazosin-like alpha$_1$ receptor-blocking properties. The hemodynamic properties of labetalol in hypertensive patients differ somewhat from the profile of beta-blockers that lack alpha$_1$ receptor-blocking activity. Beta-blockers reduce blood pressure primarily by decreasing cardiac output. In contrast, labetalol's blood pressure–lowering effect is mainly caused by a reduction in peripheral vascular resistance. Cardiac output generally does not change. Since elderly hypertensive patients tend to have a low cardiac output and high peripheral vascular resistance, the hemodynamic profile of labetalol is theoretically desirable in the hypertensive elderly patient.[23] There is a limited body of information detailing the safety and efficacy of labetalol treatment in elderly hypertensives, but the drug appears to be effective and well tolerated.[37] It is prudent to initiate labetalol administration in low doses (100 mg once to twice daily) because of the risk of orthostatic hypotension, which is a theoretical problem with any drug that blocks alpha$_1$ receptors.

ANGIOTENSIN-CONVERTING ENZYME (ACE) INHIBITORS. Angiotensin-converting enzyme inhibitors (captopril, enalapril, lisinopril) have become popular antihypertensive agents in recent years. They reduce blood pressure by vasodilatation. Cardiac output may improve in patients with impaired myocardial pump function but does not change in individuals with normal cardiac output. The ACE inhibitors prevent the generation of the potent vasoconstrictor angiotensin II and also reduce angiotensin II–stimulated aldosterone secretion. The latter effect is responsible for the blunting of diuretic-induced hypokalemia, which has been observed when these agents are administered.[38] Diuretics also increase the antihypertensive efficacy of these drugs. Tuck and associates found that low-dose cap-

topril (25 mg twice daily) was effective as monotherapy in a group of elderly hypertensive patients.[39] Forette and colleagues were able to reduce blood pressure using enalapril to < 160/90 mmHg in 67 percent of elderly patients between 75 and 97 years of age after a period of 8 weeks.[40] Blood pressure fell to < 160/90 mmHg in 35 percent of patients receiving a placebo in this study.

There is evidence that the efficacy of the ACE inhibitors is reduced with age. Lijnen and colleagues found an inverse correlation between age and the reduction in SBP and DBP in hypertensive patients receiving captopril.[41] Similarly, Vidt noted that enalapril was more effective as monotherapy in patients under 55 years of age compared with older individuals.[42] Corea and coworkers compared the blood pressure–lowering effects of captopril (50 mg twice daily) to chlorthalidone (25 mg once daily) in 20 elderly patients.[43] The two regimens were equally effective in reducing blood pressure and were well tolerated. However, chlorthalidone caused a 0.5 meq/l decrease in serum potassium and a 5.5 mg/dl increase in fasting blood glucose. Captopril did not induce these biochemical changes.

The ACE inhibitors can cause acute renal failure in patients who have severe bilateral renal artery stenosis or severe stenosis in an artery to a solitary kidney.[22] This is of concern in elderly patients who have an increased incidence of atherosclerotic bilateral renal artery disease. The ACE inhibitors can also cause hypotension in individuals who are volume depleted, receiving diuretics, or have high plasma renin levels because of renovascular hypertension. Rash, nonproductive cough, and taste disturbance are probably the most frequent symptomatic side effects of captopril therapy. These agents are particularly useful in the treatment of hypertensive patients with chronic congestive heart failure, but treatment should be instituted cautiously in this setting. The cost of the ACE inhibitors may be prohibitive for many elderly patients who have limited incomes.

CALCIUM CHANNEL-BLOCKERS. There are three currently marketed calcium channel-blockers (diltiazem, nifedipine, nicardipine, and verapamil).[44] Nifedipine is the most potent vasodilating agent but may produce reflex tachycardia and profound blood pressure reduction after acute administration. Nifedipine does not produce any significant electrophysiologic effects on the heart and does not reduce cardiac output in vivo. In contrast, verapamil has potent suppressive effects on the cardiac conduction system and is quite useful in the management of supraventricular tachyarrhythmias.

Buhler and coworkers noted that verapamil was more effective in elderly than in younger hypertensive individuals.[33] Pool and associates reported the results of a multicenter trial using diltiazem.[45] Patients over age 60 had greater antihypertensive responses than did younger patients during the first 6 weeks of the trial, but by the end of 12 weeks, this age-related difference in efficacy was less apparent. It is of note, however, that enhanced efficacy of calcium channel-blockers in older individuals has not been confirmed in a number of other studies.[46, 47]

Verapamil and, possibly, diltiazem should be used with caution in patients receiving beta-blockers. Both classes of drugs reduce conduction through the atrioventricular node and reduce myocardial contractility. However, nifedipine has little electrophysiologic effects on the heart and does not usually produce a reduction in cardiac output. For these reasons, combination treatment with nifedipine and a beta-blocker seems reasonable.

Side effects of the various calcium channel-blocking drugs differ. Nifedipine and diltiazem can produce headache, palpitations, flushing, edema, and dizziness. Constipation is the most prominent side effect of verapamil. In addition, verapamil must be used with great caution in patients who have heart block greater than first degree. Calcium channel-blockers have been used in combination with a variety of other antihypertensive agents including diuretics, centrally acting sympatholytic agents, and ACE inhibitors.[48–50]

CENTRALLY ACTING SYMPATHOLYTIC AGENTS. Some centrally acting sympatholytic agents have been used to treat hypertension in elderly individuals for many years. These agents reduce blood pressure by stimulating alpha$_2$ receptors in the CNS. This results in a reduction of sympathetic outflow and a simultaneous reduction in plasma norepinephrine, blood pressure, and heart rate.

Messerli and associates reported that the hemodynamic response to monotherapy with methyldopa varied between young and elderly individuals.[51] In young patients, the antihypertensive response was due to a small simultaneous reduction in cardiac output and peripheral vascular resistance. In older individuals, the antihypertensive response was caused by a reduction in cardiac output. Peripheral resistance did not change significantly.

Fatigue, sedation, and dry mouth are the most frequent side effects associated with the centrally acting agents. These effects are particularly troublesome early in treatment but tend to diminish with time. The CNS side effects can be partially avoided by taking most of the total daily dose of these drugs an hour or two before bedtime. It is reasonable to initiate treatment with a single bedtime dose; if larger doses are required, we usually give approximately one third of the dose in the morning and two thirds of the dose before bedtime. It is prudent to avoid large doses of the centrally acting agents in the elderly. The reason for this is related to the possibility of a withdrawal rebound hypertension, which is characterized by a pheochromocytoma-like syndrome if the centrally acting agent (especially clonidine) is abruptly discontinued. This may occur in patients who forget to take their drugs or in those who cannot take medications because of an intercurrent illness.

Clonidine is available in a transdermal formulation that provides constant drug delivery over a period of approximately 7 days. This method of administration seems to reduce the incidence of side effects generally seen in patients receiving oral clonidine. However, skin rash can be a problem. The use of transdermal clonidine is theoretically attractive in individuals who have difficulty remembering to take medications daily.

CONCLUSIONS

The incidence of ISH or diastolic hypertension is very high in elderly individuals. Isolated systolic hypertension is associated with an increased risk of cardiovascular disease, but treatment trials demonstrating a reduction in cardiovascular mortality by treating ISH are currently not available.

In contrast, a number of trials have demonstrated that elderly patients with diastolic hypertension benefit from drug treatment and tolerate antihypertensive agents well.

The hemodynamic characteristics of essential hypertension differ between younger and older hypertensive patients, which may influence the response to drug treatment. The clinician must also consider the influence of medical conditions that coexist with hypertension in elderly patients and the large number of unrelated medications that elderly individuals often ingest.

Nonpharmacologic therapy, particularly weight reduction in obese patients and moderate sodium restriction, are useful starting points for treatment in elderly patients with ISH and mild diastolic hypertension. However, the patient must be followed closely to document the efficacy of these nonpharmacologic maneuvers. Low doses of thiazide-type diuretics (e.g., 12.5 to 25 mg hydrochlorothiazide or equivalent) are a logical first step of pharmacologic therapy in elderly patients with ISH or diastolic hypertension. These agents are inexpensive, convenient to administer, and well tolerated. It is prudent to monitor serum potassium levels after the maximum diuretic dose is reached, particularly in individuals with organic heart disease or in patients receiving digitalis preparations. Although beta-blockers tend to be less effective in older than in younger hypertensive patients, these agents may be useful in the treatment of individuals with coronary heart disease. This is particularly true in the first few years after an MI, provided that no contraindications to beta-blocker treatment exist.

Calcium channel-blockers are also effective antianginal agents and have become popular in the treatment of elderly individuals with high blood pressure. The ACE inhibitors can be used alone or in combination with diuretics, but acute renal failure can occur in patients with severe bilateral renal artery stenosis or severe stenosis of an artery to a solitary kidney. Centrally acting sympatholytic agents may also be useful but tend to produce sedation and dry mouth, particularly early in therapy. The alpha$_1$ receptor-blocking drugs and peripherally acting sympatholytic agents should be used with caution in elderly hypertensive patients because of the propensity to induce orthostatic hypotension.

It is prudent to initiate antihypertensive drugs at approximately one half of the usually recommended starting dose in older individuals. Increments in doses should be smaller than those in younger patients and should be made at longer intervals than usual. Blood pressure should be monitored in both the erect and sitting or supine postures. Evidence from treatment trials clearly demonstrates that elderly individuals with diastolic hypertension benefit from a carefully constructed and vigilantly monitored antihypertensive treatment regimen and tolerate these drugs well.[52]

REFERENCES

1. The 1984 Report of the Joint National Committee on Detection, Evaluation and Treatment of High Blood Pressure. Arch Intern Med 4:457, 1984.
2. Hypertension prevalence and the status of awareness treatment and control in the United States: final report of the subcommittee on Definition and Prevalence of the 1984 Joint National Committee. Hypertension 7:457, 1985.
3. The Working Group on Hypertension in the Elderly: Statement on hypertension in the elderly. JAMA 256:70, 1986.
4. Hulley SB, Furberg CD, Gurland B, et al: The systolic hypertension in the elderly program (SHEP): antihypertensive efficacy of chlorthalidone. Am J Cardiol 56:913, 1985.
5. Harlan W, Hull AL, Schmouder RL, et al: High blood pressure in older Americans: the first national health examination survey. Hypertension 6:802, 1984.
6. Garland C, Barrett-Connor E, Suarez L, et al: Isolated systolic hypertension and mortality after age 60 years: a prospective population-based study. Am J Epidemiol 118:365, 1983.
7. Kannel WB, Doyle JT, Ostfeld AM, et al: Optimal resources for primary prevention of atherosclerotic diseases: atherosclerosis study group. Circulation 70:153A, 1984.
8. Kannel WB, Gordon T, Schwartz MJ: Systolic versus diastolic blood pressure and risk of coronary heart disease. Am J Cardiol 27:335, 1971.
9. Kannel WB, Dawber TR, Sortie P, et al: Components of blood pressure and risk of atherothrombotic brain infarction: the Framingham study. Stroke 7:327, 1976.
10. Blood Pressure Study 1979. Chicago, Society of Actuaries and Association of Life Insurance Medical Directors of America, 1980.
11. Kannel WB: Implications of Framingham study data for treatment of hypertension: impact of other risk factors. In Laragh JH, Buhler FR, Seldin DW, eds: Frontiers in Hypertension Research. New York, Springer-Verlag, 1981, p 17.

12. Shekelle RB, Ostfeld AM, Klawans HL Jr: Hypertension and risk of stroke in an elderly population. Stroke 5:71, 1973.
13. Colandrea MA, Friedman GD, Nichaman MZ, et al: Systolic hypertension in the elderly: an epidemiologic assessment. Circulation 41:239, 1970.
14. Cressman MD, Gifford RW Jr: Clinicians' interpretation of the results and implications of the hypertension detection and follow-up program. Prog Cardiovasc Dis 29(3):89, 1986.
15. Hypertension, Detection and Follow-up Program Cooperative Group: Five-year findings of the hypertension, detection and follow-up program, II. Reduction in stroke incidence among persons with high blood pressure. J Am Med Assoc 247:633, 1982.
16. National Heart Foundation of Australia: Treatment of mild hypertension in the elderly: report by the management committee. Med J Aust 2:398, 1981.
17. Amery A, Birkenhäger W, Brixko P, et al: Mortality and morbidity results from the European working party on high blood pressure in the elderly trial. Lancet 1:1349, 1985.
18. Hallock P, Benson I: Studies on the elastic properties of human isolated aorta. J Clin Invest 16:595, 1937.
19. Page LB: Hypertension and atherosclerosis in primitive and acculturating societies. In Hypertension Update. Health Learning Systems, Inc, Bloomfield, NJ, 1980, p 1.
20. O'Malley K, O'Brien E: Management of hypertension in the elderly. N Engl J Med 302:1397, 1980.
21. Koch-Weser J: Management of hypertension in the elderly. N Engl J Med 302(25):1397, 1980.
22. Hricik DE, Browning PJ, Kopelman R, et al: Captropril-induced functional renal insufficiency in patients with bilateral renal artery stenoses or renal-artery stenosis in a solitary kidney. N Engl J Med 308:373, 1983.
23. Messerli FH, Sundgaard-Riise K, Ventura HO, et al: Essential hypertension in the elderly: haemodynamics, intravascular volume, plasma renin activity, and circulating catecholamine levels. Lancet 2:983, 1983.
24. Shimada K, Kitazumi T, Sadakane N, et al: Age-related changes of baroreflex function, plasma norepinephrine, and blood pressure. Hypertension 7:113, 1985.
25. Messerli FH, Ventura HO, Amadeo C: Osler's maneuver and pseudohypertension. N Engl J Med 312:1548, 1985.
26. O'Callaghan WG, Fitzgerald DJ, O'Malley K, et al: Accuracy of indirect blood pressure measurement in the elderly. Br Med J 286:1545, 1983.
27. Vardan S, Mookherjee S, Warner R, et al: Systolic hypertension. Direct and indirect BP measurements. Arch Intern Med 143:935, 1983.
28. Luepker RV, Jacobs DR, Gillum RF, et al: Population risk of cardiovascular disease: the Minnesota heart survey. J Chronic Dis 38:671, 1985.
29. Kaplan NM: Non-drug treatment of hypertension. Ann Intern Med 102(3):359, 1985.
30. Hypertension, Detection and Follow-Up Program Cooperative Group: Five-year findings of the hypertension, detection and follow-up program. II. Mortality by race, sex and age. J Am Med Assoc 242:2572, 1979.
31. Martin BJ, Milligan K: Diuretic-associated hypomagnesemia in the elderly. Arch Intern Med 147:1768, 1987.
32. Whang R, Oei TO, Watanabe A: Frequency of hypomagnesemia in hospitalized patients receiving digitalis. Arch Intern Med 145:655, 1985.
33. Buhler FR, Hulthen UL, Kiowski W, et al: β-blockers and calcium antagonists: cornerstones of antihypertensive therapy in the 1980s. Drugs 25(Suppl 2):50, 1983.
34. Beta-Blocker Heart Attack Trial Research Group: A randomized trial of propranolol in patients with acute myocardial infarction. I. Mortality results. JAMA 247:1707, 1982.
35. Norwegian Multicenter Study Group: Timolol-induced reduction in mortality and reinfarction in patients surviving acute myocardial infarction. N Engl J Med 304:801, 1981.
36. Anderson MP, Beschgaard P, Frederiksen J, et al: Effect of alprenolol on mortality among patients with definite or suspected acute myocardial infarction: preliminary results. Lancet 2:865, 1979.
37. Eisalo A, Virta P: Treatment of hypertension in the elderly with labetalol. Acta Med Scand (Suppl)665:129, 1984.
38. Weinberger MH: Influence of an angiotensin converting-enzyme inhibitor of diuretic-induced metabolic effects in hypertension. Hypertension 5(Suppl III):132, 1983.
39. Tuck ML, Katz LA, Kirkendall WM, et al: Low-dose captopril in mild to moderate geriatric hypertension. J Am Geriatr Soc 34:693, 1986.
40. Forette F, Handfield-Jones R, Henry-Amar M, et al: Traitement de l'hypertension arterielle du suject age par un inhibiteur de l'enzyme de conversion: enalapril. Presse Med 14:2237, 1985.
41. Lijnen P, Fagard R, Groeseneken D, et al: The hypertensive effect of captopril in hypertensive patients is age-related. Methods Find Exp Clin Pharmacol 5:655, 1983.
42. Vidt DG: A controlled multiclinic study to compare the antihypertensive effects of MK 421, hydrochlorothiazide, and MK 412 combined with hydrochlorothiazide in patients with mild to moderate essential hypertension. J Hypertens (Suppl 2):81, 1984.
43. Corea L, Bentivoglio M, Verdecchia P, et al: Converting enzyme inhibition vs diuretic therapy as first therapeutic approach to the elderly hypertensive patient. Curr Ther Res 36:347, 1984.
44. Spivak C, Ocken S, Frishman WH: Calcium antagonists: clinical use in the treatment of systemic hypertension. Drugs 25:154, 1983.
45. Poole PE, Seagren SC, Salel AF: Diltiazem as monotherapy for systemic hypertension: a multicenter, randomized, placebo-controlled trial. Am J Cardiol 57:212, 1986.
46. Hallin L, Andrén L, Hausson L: Controlled trial of nifedipine and bendroflumethiazide in hypertension. J Cardiovasc Pharmacol 5:1083, 1983.
47. Muiesan G, Agabiti-Rosei E, Castellano M, et al: Antihypertensive and humoral effects of verapamil and nifedipine in essential hypertension. J Cardiovasc Pharmacol 4(Suppl 3):325, 1982.
48. Aoki K, Kondo S, Mochizuki A, et al: Antihypertensive effect of cardiovascular Ca-antagonist in hypertensive patients in the absence and presence of beta-adrenergic blockade. Am Heart J 96:218, 1978.

49. Guazzi MD, Fiorentini C, Olivari MT, et al: Short- and long-term efficacy of a calcium antagonist agent (nifedipine) combined with methyldopa in treatment of severe hypertension. Circulation 61:913, 1980.

50. Guazzi MD, De Cesare N, Galli C, et al: Calcium channel blockade with nifedipine and angiotensin converting enzyme inhibition with captopril in the therapy of patients with severe primary hypertension. Circulation 70:279, 1984.

51. Messerli FH, Dreslinski GR, Husserl FE, et al: Antiadrenergic therapy: special aspects in hypertension in the elderly. Hypertension 3(Suppl II):226, 1981.

52. Curb JD, Borhani NO, Schnaper H, et al: Detection and treatment of hypertension in older individuals. Am J Epidemiol 121:371, 1985.

CHAPTER 24

Cardiac Arrhythmias

David E. Mann

The alarum watch, your pulse.
MATTHEW GREEN, *The Spleen*

Although there are no cardiac rhythm problems that occur exclusively in the elderly, the incidence of arrhythmias and conduction disturbances does increase with age. Arrhythmias occur frequently in the elderly not only because of a greater prevalence of heart disease in this population but also as a consequence of changes in the conduction system caused by the aging process itself. Loss of pacemaker cells in the sinus node and conduction fibers in the bundle branches occurs normally in the aging heart.[1] Sinus node dysfunction (the "sick sinus syndrome") and atrioventricular (AV) block, the most frequent causes of symptomatic bradycardia in the elderly, may both represent extreme forms of these "normal" processes. Amyloid deposition in the heart becomes increasingly common with age, appearing in 10 percent of patients over age 80 and in 50 percent of patients over age 90 in autopsy cases.[2]

Amyloid may be a frequent cause of cardiac conduction system disease in the elderly. Arrhythmias may also result from forms of heart disease that are also common in younger patients, such as coronary artery disease, valvular disease, hypertensive heart disease, and cardiomyopathy. In the case of elderly patients with chronic arrhythmias, the underlying pathophysiology is generally not reversible and has little relevance in managing the patient. The important issues in dealing with all patients with known or suspected arrhythmias are (1) establishing the nature of the rhythm problem, (2) determining whether the risk of allowing the problem to remain untreated outweighs the risk of treatment, and (3) if treatment is feasible, designing an appropriate treatment plan.

Arrhythmias may be symptomatic or asymptomatic. Symptoms may range from palpitations to syncope to sudden death. The mere presence of symptoms does not imply that treatment is necessary. The decision to treat should be based on whether the risk of treatment is justified by the severity of the symptoms. Ventricular ectopic beats causing only palpitations may be best treated with a dose of reassurance. On the other hand, syncope, which can result in broken bones in old people, will justifiably cause concern, and an arrhythmic cause should be treated.

It is important to demonstrate to the best of one's ability that a suspected arrhythmia actually caused the symptoms in question. In a patient being evaluated for syncope, an ambulatory electrocardiogram showing an asymptomatic episode of sinus bradycardia does not establish that a similar episode of bradycardia resulted in syncope, and such a finding does not justify implantation of a permanent pacemaker.

Treatment of asymptomatic arrhythmias in the elderly, as in all patients, is based on the assumption that such treatment will prevent serious symptoms or death in the future. In the elderly patient with asymptomatic arrhythmias, such an assumption may be difficult to support. As an example, no definite proof exists that treatment of asymptomatic ventricular ectopic beats with conventional antiarrhythmic drugs prevents sudden death. Given the high cost of antiarrhythmic drugs, the increased risk of toxicity and drug/drug interactions, and the intrinsic high mortality rate in the elderly, it is by no means a safe assumption that these drugs will eventually prove to be beneficial in the prevention of sudden death in this age group.[3] Nevertheless, they are widely prescribed for this indication, and recommendations for this usage can be found. If the benefit of therapy is unknown and there is a known risk of therapy, as is the case with antiarrhythmic drug treatment of ventricular ectopic beats, it is best that such therapy not be used, at least until further information to establish the risk benefit ratio is determined.

Many sophisticated devices and techniques have been developed for the detection and diagnosis of arrhythmias, including ambulatory electrocardiography (ECG), transtelephonic event recorders, esophageal electrodes, and, most definitive, electrophysiologic testing. Yet old people have more trouble filling out Holter monitor diaries and operating event records than do their younger counterparts.[4] They may not cooperate or be too frail for electrophysiologic testing. Aggressive new forms of arrhythmia treatment, including arrhythmia surgery, electrical ablation, and automatic implantable cardioverter defibrillator, also exist today. The problem for the physician is not whether a diagnosis can be made or a treatment found, but rather how far to go in pursuing the diagnosis and treatment of an individual elderly patient. Such a decision clearly depends on many factors unique to each patient. The guidelines for the diagnosis and treatment of arrhythmias given here should remain guidelines. How they apply to the individual patient is left to the discretion of the practicing physician.

SINUS NODE DYSFUNCTION

Sinus node dysfunction (sick sinus syndrome) can occur in all age groups, but it is most closely associated with old age. It is usually the result of degenerative disease of the sinus node. Normally, there is a loss of sinus node pacemaker cells with age, and the intrinsic sinus rate slows.[1] Asymptomatic sinus bradycardia is, thus, a common finding in the elderly and is usually of little hemodynamic consequence.[5] Electrophysiologically, abnormal sinus node function may result from either loss of automaticity, when the sinus node fails to depolarize at a proper rate (sinus arrest), or sino-atrial exit block, when impulses from the sinus node fail to conduct out of the node into the atrium. Clinically, the distinction is often impossible to make; the end result of both problems is sinus

pauses. Pauses over 3 seconds in duration often cause symptoms of dizziness or syncope. These pauses may occur spontaneously, or they may follow the abrupt termination of episodes of tachycardia, in particular atrial fibrillation or flutter. During the tachycardia, the sinus node is suppressed. When the tachycardia terminates, the sinus node must recover and begin firing again. When this recovery time is prolonged, symptomatic pauses may result. This clinical picture has been termed the "brady-tachy syndrome."[6]

In the electrophysiology laboratory, this syndrome can be mimicked by pacing the right atrium rapidly with a catheter. Upon cessation of pacing, the recovery time of the sinus node can be measured. An abnormal sinus node recovery time is fairly specific for sinus node dysfunction, but a normal sinus node recovery time does not exclude sinus node problems.[7, 8] Measurement of the sinus node recovery time is rarely necessary to establish the diagnosis of sinus node dysfunction. Ambulatory monitoring for 24 hours may detect abnormalities of sinus node function in patients with frequently occurring symptoms. Patient-activated event recorders that record an electrocardiogram for a brief period and then play the recording back over the telephone to a monitoring center can be useful to document the cause of infrequently occurring symptoms.

Sinus node dysfunction is frequently associated with other abnormalities of cardiac conduction.[9] Subsidiary cardiac pacemakers in the AV junction or ventricle may also be abnormal so that sinus pauses result in asystole. Atrial fibrillation may be present, sometimes with an abnormally slow ventricular response, implying associated abnormal AV node function. Asystole following cardioversion of tachyarrhythmias may be a manifestation of sinus node disease. Patients with known or suspected sinus node disease undergoing cardioversion should have a temporary pacemaker (either transvenous or transcutaneous) in position.[10] Hypersensitive carotid sinus syndrome, wherein episodes of syncope are precipitated by neck pressure, has been grouped with sick sinus syndrome. Syncope is caused by excessive vagal tone arising from carotid sinus pressure acting on a normal or abnormal sinus node. The diagnosis is suggested by a pause over 3 seconds following *gentle* carotid sinus massage. Vigorous massage should be avoided in the elderly, and the maneuver should not be performed if carotid artery disease is suspected.[11] Hypersensitive carotid sinus syndrome, as well as other hypervagatonic states, may cause vasodilation and sinus bradycardia; the resultant hypotension may not be fully reversed with permanent ventricular pacing. Dual chamber pacing may be of benefit in such patients.[12]

Sinus node dysfunction, although a cause of morbidity, is very infrequently a cause of mortality. In different studies of patients with sick sinus syndrome, the risk of death is variable; however, nearly all deaths have nonarrhythmic causes. Intervention with permanent pacemakers does not lower mortality; it does, however, ameliorate symptoms.[13–18] Because of this, permanent pacemakers are not recommended for asymptomatic patients with sinus node dysfunction. Their use should be reserved for patients in whom a definite connection between symptoms and sinus pauses can be established.

Drug-related sinus node dysfunction should be excluded before instituting pacemaker therapy. Many cardiac and noncardiac drugs can aggravate or precipitate sinus node dysfunction, including digoxin, beta-blockers, calcium channel-blockers, antihypertensive agents, and antiarrhythmic drugs. Sometimes, possible drug-related causes are subtle and are overlooked; for example, timolol (a beta-blocker) eye drops for glaucoma can be systemically absorbed and cause sinus node dysfunction. Situations in which continued drug therapy is mandatory may necessitate permanent pacing, although the sinus node dysfunction is drug-related. Such situations frequently occur in the brady-tachy syndrome, in which antiarrhythmic drugs used to treat the tachycardia also make the bradycardia worse.[6] Selection of an appropriate pacemaker for patients with symptomatic sinus node dysfunction is discussed subsequently.

ATRIOVENTRICULAR (AV) BLOCK

Atrioventricular block is another common cause of symptomatic bradycardia in the elderly. It is most frequently the result of degenerative fibrosis of the conduction system.[1] Whether this is diffuse throughout the bundle branches (Lengegre's disease) or involves only the proximal bundle branches (Lev's disease) is a pathologic distinction of little clinical importance.[19, 20] Other causes of AV block include coronary artery disease, cardiomyopathy, and calcification of the AV groove (mitral annular calcification).

First-degree AV block (PR interval > 0.2 sec) is a benign electrocardiographic finding and needs no intervention.[21] Bundle branch block, including bifascicular block (right bundle branch block and either left anterior or left posterior fascicular block or left bundle branch block), has a low risk of progressing to complete heart block—a risk of 1 to 2 percent per year, even in an elderly subset of patients.[22–24] Thus, permanent pacemakers are not indicated in asymptomatic patients with bifascicular block. In symptomatic patients with bundle branch block, further studies to establish a link between symptoms and intermittent heart block should be performed before considering permanent pacemaker implantation.

Patients with second-degree AV block associated with symptoms should receive pacemakers. Pacing in asymptomatic patients with second-degree AV block (i.e., intermittent blocked beats) is controversial. An attempt to localize the level of block in the conduction system should be made. Progressive prolongation of the PR interval prior to a blocked beat and shortening of the PR interval in the next conducted beat after the blocked beat is termed Mobitz I second-degree AV block (or Wenckebach block). It is usually associated with AV nodal block. A pattern of isolated nonconducted beats without changes in the PR interval before or after each blocked beat is termed Mobitz II second-degree AV block, and it is usually due to block distal to the AV node (that is, in the bundle of His or both bundle branches). Two to one, or higher, ratios of AV block may result from block in the AV node or distal to the AV node. Another clue to the anatomic site of block is the QRS pattern of the conducted beats; a narrow QRS implies that block is probably in the AV node, a wide QRS (bundle branch block) implies that block is distal to the AV node. The distinction between AV nodal and infranodal second-degree AV block may be important clinically because the latter site of block is associated with a high rate of progression to complete heart block and a poor prognosis.[25] Thus, pacing is usually not indicated in asymptomatic patients with second-degree AV block localized to the AV node, whereas pacing may be indicated in patients with infranodal second-degree AV block.[26] Occasionally, electrophysiologic testing, using a catheter to record a bundle of His electrogram, may be useful to establish unequivocally the site of block.

Complete, or third-degree, AV block may be caused by disease in the AV node, the bundle of His, or both bundle branches. Atrioventricular nodal block is usually associated with a narrow QRS complex escape rhythm, which arises in the AV junction (either distal AV node or proximal His bundle), and is often well tolerated. Infranodal complete AV block is associated with a slower and less reliable ventricular escape rhythm (with a wide QRS complex), which is frequently poorly tolerated. The survival in patients with complete heart block before the use of pacemakers was poor.[27, 28] Implantation of permanent pacemakers allows a survival rate comparable to the normal population and prevents recurrent syncope (e.g., Stokes-Adams attacks) and, in some cases, can improve congestive heart failure when it is caused by or exacerbated by bradycardia.[29] In the elderly, permanent pacemakers are indicated in nearly all patients who present with complete AV block, with or without symptoms.[26] Patients with the acute onset of third-degree AV block who are hemodynamically compromised need emergency temporary pacing. Atropine or isoproterenol can be administered until pacing can be instituted. In addition to the standard transvenous route for temporary pacing, transcutaneous pacing holds particular promise for the elderly because it can be instituted more quickly and is safer than transvenous pacing.[30]

SUPRAVENTRICULAR ARRHYTHMIAS

Premature atrial contractions are found in nearly all elderly subjects undergoing 24-hour Holter monitoring and are usually of no significance.[31, 32]

Atrial fibrillation and flutter are related arrhythmias, the incidence of which increases with age. Patients usually have underlying cardiovascular disease, commonly hypertension, valvular disease, or coronary artery disease.[33] These atrial arrhythmias may also be the presenting symptom of occult hyperthyroidism, which may be difficult to detect in the elderly.[34] Atrial fibrillation is associated with twice the mortality of age-matched controls and six times the risk of stroke.[33, 35] Patients with rheumatic mitral valve disease and atrial fibrillation are at the highest risk for stroke and usually should undergo oral anticoagulation therapy with warfarin (Coumadin). Patients with other forms of underlying heart disease and atrial fibrillation also have an increased risk of embolism, although it is lower than that in the rheumatic patient.[36]

The potential benefits of anticoagulation therapy must be weighed against the known risks in these patients. Patients without left atrial enlargement (assessed by echocardiography) or known heart disease have a low risk of embolization and do not require anticoagulation therapy. Patients who have already had an embolus have a 30 percent chance of recurrence and should undergo anticoagulation treatment. In patients with intermediate risk of emboli, the risk of anticoagulation agents (estimated to present a 0.2 to 2.5 percent chance of serious bleeding complications per year) must be considered. About 75 percent of systemic emboli are cerebral.[37] The risk of embolization in atrial flutter is unknown, but it is probably lower than the risk in atrial fibrillation.

The goal of treatment of atrial fibrillation may be the resumption and maintenance of sinus rhythm or, if that is not feasible, control of the ventricular rate. Conversion to sinus rhythm may be accomplished either with antiarrhythmic drugs or with electrical cardioversion. There is a 1 to 2 percent risk of embolization associated with both use of drugs and electrical cardioversion.[38, 39] Patients taking anticoagulants at the time of cardioversion have a lower risk of embolization.[39] Although no studies on the subject have been made, it is generally recommended that anticoagulation therapy be begun 1 to 2 weeks prior to cardioversion, presumably to allow loose clot to organize and become adherent to the atrial wall. Anticoagulation therapy should be continued for a few days following successful cardioversion, since there may be a delay before mechanical atrial systole is restored, accounting for emboli that are seen to occur a few days after cardioversion.

The decision to attempt cardioversion of atrial fibrillation is based on duration of fibrillation, left atrial size, presence of mitral valve disease, patient age, and results of previous attempts at cardioversion.[38] Generally, fibrillation lasting over 1 year, left atrial size over 4.5 cm (measured by echocardiogram), and mitral stenosis make maintenance of sinus rhythm for over 6 months unlikely.[40] Older patients generally have more atrial disease, and thus the chance of successfully maintaining sinus rhythm decreases with age. Cardioversion generally should not be repeated in an elderly patient in whom previous cardioversion did not result in sinus rhythm lasting for over 6 months. Clearly, more aggressive and repeated attempts may be made, despite these factors, in patients in whom the ventricular response is difficult to control with drugs or in those who have atrial fibrillation associated with congestive heart failure or recurrent emboli.

Electrical cardioversion should be performed electively with the patient under short-acting general anesthesia, with an anesthesiologist present. As noted in the foregoing discussion, a course of anticoagulation therapy of at least 1 week should precede cardioversion. If the patient is on digoxin, it should be withheld on the day that cardioversion is scheduled; electrical cardioversion should be delayed if there is any suspicion of digoxin toxicity or if digoxin blood levels are high. A minimum of 100 joules (J) should be delivered synchronously, and higher energy levels should then be tried if the first attempt fails. The immediate success rate of electrical cardioversion for atrial fibrillation is about 90 percent.[41] Pretreatment with quinidine or procainamide may increase the chance of successful conversion to and maintenance of sinus rhythm, as well as possibly converting the rhythm without the need for electricity. Occasionally, anterioposterior paddles may be useful in patients in whom the usual anterioapical paddle position is unsuccessful.

Chemical cardioversion can be achieved with various antiarrhythmic drugs, including quinidine, procainamide, disopyramide, flecainide, encainide, and amiodarone, although the last drug should be avoided because of high toxicity. In general, rate control should be attempted first with digoxin or other drugs to avoid acceleration of the ventricular response caused by the anticholinergic effects of some of these drugs, particularly quinidine. Digoxin alone may convert atrial fibrillation resulting from decompensated congestive heart failure, but it is ineffective in this role for other patients.[42] Chemical cardioversion should not be delivered any more cavalierly than electrical cardioversion because the incidence of systemic embolism is no different whichever method is used.[38]

To achieve rate control, AV node blocking drugs are used. These drugs include digoxin, verapamil, diltiazem, propranolol, and other beta-blockers. The goal of treatment should be to achieve a heart rate of less than 100 at rest and a heart rate with exercise that is commensurate with an expected exercise heart rate if the patient was in sinus rhythm.

Atrial flutter is nearly always associated with underlying heart disease. Generally, rate control is more difficult to achieve with atrial flutter than fibrillation. Patients usually present with 2:1 AV conduction, resulting in a ventricular rate of 150. In most cases, a form of cardioversion should be attempted. The aforementioned drugs for conversion of atrial fibrillation can be used for atrial flutter. Electrical cardioversion, with lower energy shocks than those used for atrial fibrillation, may be successful, with delivery starting at 25 J. If such low-energy shocks result in conversion to atrial fibrillation, a higher energy shock (100 J or more) should be tried immediately to achieve sinus rhythm. Atrial flutter can also be terminated using a pacing catheter in the right atrium, with pacing faster than the flutter rate (usually 300) thus interrupting the re-entry circuit.[43] With either atrial fibrillation or flutter, temporary atrial or ventricular pacing should be used prophylactically during electrical cardioversion to prevent sinus pauses following cardioversion, if there is any suspicion of sick sinus syndrome.

Paroxysmal supraventricular tachycardia (PSVT) occurs in all age groups, including the elderly. The major mechanisms of PSVT include re-entry within the AV node, re-entry involving the AV node and an accessory AV pathway capable only of retrograde (ventricle to atrium) conduction, and re-entry within the atrium.[44] The first two mechanisms require a one-to-one AV relationship; intra-atrial re-entry can continue despite AV block. Short runs of intra-atrial tachycardia appear frequently during Holter monitoring of elderly subjects and generally do not require treatment.[31] An episode of sustained PSVT should be treated first with vagal maneuvers (careful carotid sinus massage, the Valsalva maneuver, the diving reflex; that is, immersion of the face in cold water) and then with intravenous verapamil. Intravenous beta-blockers and digoxin also can be tried. Rarely, low-energy electrical cardioversion will be necessary if the tachycardia is poorly tolerated or resistant to medication.

It is important to differentiate PSVT with aberrant conduction (bundle branch block) from ventricular tachycardia (VT). The latter diagnosis is much more common in the elderly than in younger patients, and it is certainly a more serious diagnosis. Classification of tachycardia as PSVT versus VT, based on heart rate or whether or not the tachycardia is well tolerated is unreliable. AV dissociation, fusion beats, QRS interval greater than 0.14 sec, abnormal QRS axis, monophasic R wave in ECG lead V1, and a deep broad S in V6 are all characteristic of VT rather than of SVT.[45] Using IV verapamil as a diagnostic maneuver is dangerous because patients with VT may become hemodynamically unstable.[46, 47] Placing an esophageal electrode can help identify atrial activity and help make the diagnosis in difficult cases.[48] When in doubt, in the elderly patient, it is best to assume that a wide complex tachycardia is VT and to treat it accordingly.

Chronic treatment to suppress episodes of PSVT should be initiated in patients with frequently recurring, very symptomatic, or difficult to terminate episodes of PSVT. Drugs such as digoxin, verapamil, beta-blockers, quinidine, procainamide and others have been used successfully. Electrophysiologic testing to establish the mechanism of PSVT and to find a successful drug can be used in cases refractory to conservative treatment. Electrophysiologic testing is also mandatory if antitachycardia pacing is to be used. Antitachycardia pacemakers for PSVT can automatically recognize tachycardia when it occurs and pace the atrium in a preprogrammed fashion to interrupt the tachycardia. Such a pacemaker is a reasonable option even in an elderly patient, if he or she is refractory to or has side effects from antiarrhythmic drugs. Although rarely required, surgical or electrical ablation of an accessory pathway or even the AV node may be needed in certain patients with refractory supraventricular tachycardias.

The incidence of Wolff-Parkinson-White (WPW) syndrome decreases with age, probably because accessory AV pathways degenerate over time.[49] However, in a patient with WPW syndrome, the likelihood of atrial fibrillation increases with age. Rapid conduction down an accessory pathway during atrial fibrillation can cause sudden death in these patients. During atrial fibrillation in WPW, digoxin must be avoided because it is associated with an increased risk of degeneration of atrial fibrillation to ventricular fibrillation.[50] Selected patients with WPW and atrial fibrillation may need electrophysiologic testing and surgical ablation of the accessory pathway.[51]

VENTRICULAR ARRHYTHMIAS

The incidence of ventricular ectopic beats (VEB) increases with age.[31, 52] When they occur in patients with otherwise normal hearts, there is no prognostic significance.[53] Although VEB are associated with an increased risk of sudden death if underlying heart disease (particularly left ventricular dysfunction and congestive heart failure) is present, definitive studies showing that treatment of VEB is effective in preventing sudden death have not been performed.[54, 55] Antiarrhythmic drug therapy, however, is known to cause occasionally fatal exacerbations of arrhythmias.[56] There is also no evidence that treating patients with more complex ventricular ectopy (couplets or nonsustained runs of ventricular tachycardia) results in improved survival. Treatment of patients for up to 3 years following MI with beta-blocking drugs has been shown to modestly reduce the incidence of sudden death; however, it is not clear if the mechanism of this reduction relates to suppression of VEB or other actions of beta-blockers.[57, 58]

Sustained ventricular tachycardia and ventricular fibrillation are both emergency situations and causes of sudden cardiac death. Acutely, such arrhythmias require immediate treatment. If a patient presents in sustained ventricular tachycardia that is well tolerated hemodynamically, intravenous lidocaine or procainamide can be tried, followed by electrical cardioversion starting at 100 J if the arrhythmia persists. Hypotensive ventricular tachycardia or ventricular fibrillation require immediate electrical cardioversion or defibrillation with at least 200 J.

Chronic treatment of these arrhythmias (i.e., ventricular tachycardia and fibrillation) is difficult, but treatment is generally recommended because there is a high recurrence rate of about 30 percent per year.[59, 60] Patients with sustained ventricular tachycardia or ventricular fibrillation do not necessarily have frequent VEB on Holter monitoring, and even if they do, suppression of VEB with conventional antiarrhythmic drugs does not ensure a good outcome.[61] Electrophysiologic (EP) testing, using programmed electrical stimulation to artificially induce ventricular tachycardia or fibrillation, can be used in the majority of patients, and EP testing used serially to identify an antiarrhythmic drug effective in suppressing induction of VT is associated with improved survival.[62]

Patients in whom ventricular tachycardia cannot be induced in the EP lab to begin with or in whom ventricular tachycardia is refractory to conventional drugs can be treated with amiodarone. This is a potentially highly toxic drug with unusual pharmacokinetics that should be used only by experienced cardiologists.[63] A few patients are candidates for ventricular tachycardia ablation surgery, during which the focus of origin of the tachycardia is mapped out and excised.[64] Finally, the automatic implantable cardioverter defibrillator (AICD) holds promise for survivors of sudden death. This implantable device automatically senses ventricular tachycardia or ventricular fibrillation and then delivers an internal shock via electrodes attached to the heart. The AICD can be used with a low surgical mortality and the yearly survival rate of patients with this device is over 95 percent.[65] Problems with the AICD include large size, need for a thoracotomy to implant it, and short battery life. Future technologic advances, including subcutaneous electrodes that do not require a thoracotomy to implant, should expand the indications for this device.

PACEMAKER THERAPY

Over the years, pacemakers have become much more reliable and sophisticated. Routine features include the ability to program multiple functions, telemetry of pacer functions, small size, and long battery life. The transvenous route is preferred over the epicardial route because of its ease of insertion and low complication rate.

One decision the physician must make is whether to use a single- or dual-chamber device. Dual-chamber pacing provides atrioventricular (AV) synchrony and preserves the atrial kick that may account for up to 25 percent of the cardiac output at rest.[66, 67] Atrioventricular synchrony is less important in increasing cardiac output with exercise; increased cardiac output with exercise is achieved primarily by increased heart rate.[68, 69] Many patients requiring a pacemaker have sinus node dysfunction and, thus, cannot increase their atrial rate normally with exercise. Other patients have episodes of atrial fibrillation. These situations render dual-chamber pacemakers less useful. Dual-chamber pacemakers also have increased cost, increased complexity, increased failure rate, and decreased battery life.

Rate-responsive single-chamber pacemakers, which use other sensors than the atrial rate to determine the pacing rate, are important additions to the pacing armamentarium. Current devices can detect muscle movements and adjust the heart rate appropriately to the level of exercise.[70] The advantage over dual-chamber pacemakers is simplicity (i.e., only one chamber is paced) and slightly decreased cost. However, if a patient has a normal atrium and normal sinus node, a dual-chamber pacemaker will act as a fine rate-responsive pacemaker. Preservation of AV synchrony, even without a normal sinus node, should be considered in patients with stiff, noncompliant ventricles, such as those with aortic stenosis or hypertrophic cardiomyopathy. In such patients, cardiac output is more dependent on atrial contraction than it is in other patients. Rate-responsive and dual-chamber pacemakers have been shown to improve exercise tolerance both acutely and chronically in patients.[71-74] Such pacemakers should certainly be considered for patients with fixed heart rates, especially if congestive heart failure is present, and they should be considered particularly for active elderly patients. Single-chamber fixed rate ventricular pacing is appropriate in patients who are inactive or who have only intermittent bradycardia.

ANTIARRHYTHMIC DRUGS

Specific guidelines for antiarrhythmic drug use in the elderly have not been well documented. There is an increased incidence of adverse drug reactions, resulting both from altered metabolism with age and from increased use of polypharmacy, which lead to drug/drug interactions. Absorption, protein binding, volume of distribution, and hepatic and renal blood flow all change with age. Receptor changes may also alter the patient's sensitivity to drugs.[3] Some of the specific changes in individual drugs have been reviewed.[75]

It is not within the scope of this chapter to cover all the numerous antiarrhythmic drugs currently available. Because of the sometimes unpredictable metabolism of drugs in the elderly, it is best to follow serum drug levels to avoid both toxic and subtherapeutic responses. As emphasized above, the risk of toxicity is real with any of the antiarrhythmic drugs, especially in the elderly. Therefore, the prudent physician must expect a reasonable chance of benefit before using any of these drugs.

REFERENCES

1. Davies MJ: Pathology of the conduction system. In Caird FI, Dall JLC, Kennedy RD: Cardiology in Old Age. New York, Plenum Press, 1976, p 57.
2. Pomerance A: Senile cardiac amyloidosis. Br Heart J 27:711, 1965.
3. Goldberg PB, Roberts J: Pharmacologic basis for developing rational drug regimens for elderly patients. Med Clin North Am 67:315, 1983.
4. Dreifus LS: Clinical arrhythmias in the elderly: clinical aspects. Cardiol Clin 4:273, 1986.
5. Agruss NS, Rosin EY, Adolph RJ, et al: Significance of chronic sinus bradycardia in elderly people. Circulation 46:924, 1972.
6. Moss AJ, Davis RJ: Brady-tachy syndrome. Prog Cardiovasc Dis 16:439, 1974.
7. Mandel W, Hayakawa H, Danzig R, et al: Evaluation of sino-atrial node function in man by overdrive suppression. Circulation 44:59, 1971.
8. Gann D, Tolentino A, Samet P: Electrophysiologic evaluation of elderly patients with sinus bradycardia. Ann Intern Med 90:24, 1979.
9. Rosen KM, Loeb HS, Sinno MZ, et al: Cardiac conduction in patients with symptomatic sinus node disease. Circulation 43:836, 1971.
10. Ferrer MI: The sick sinus syndrome. Circulation 47:635, 1973.
11. Lesser LM, Wenger KM: Carotid sinus syncope. Heart Lung 5:453, 1976.
12. Morley CA, Perrins EJ, Grant P, et al: Carotid sinus syncope treated by pacing: analysis of persistent symptoms and role of atrioventricular sequential pacing. Br Heart J 47:411, 1982.
13. Fairfax AJ, Lambert CD, Leatham A: Systemic embolism in chronic sinoatrial disorder. N Engl J Med 295:190, 1976.
14. Wohl AJ, Blomqvist CG: Prognosis of patients permanently paced for sick sinus syndrome. Arch Intern Med 136:406, 1976.
15. Chokshi DS, Mascarenhas E, Samet P, et al: Treatment of sinoatrial rhythm disturbances with permanent cardiac pacing. Am J Cardiol 32:215, 1973.
16. Rubenstein JJ, Schulman CL, Yurchak PM, et al: Clinical spectrum of sick sinus syndrome. Circulation 46:5, 1972.
17. Krishnaswami V, Geraci AR: Permanent pacing in disorders of sinus node function. Am Heart J 89:579, 1975.
18. Gould L, Reddy CVR, Becker WH: The sick sinus syndrome: a study of 50 cases. J Electrocardiol 11:11, 1978.
19. Lenegre J: Etiology and pathology of bilateral bundle branch block in relation to complete heart block. Prog Cardiovasc Dis 6:409, 1964.
20. Lev M: The pathology of complete atrioventricular block. Prog Cardiovasc Dis 6:317, 1964.
21. Mymin D, Athenson FAL, Tate RB, et al: The natural history of primary first-degree atrioventricular block. N Engl J Med 315:1183, 1986.
22. McAnulty JH, Rahimtoola SH, Murphy E, et al: Natural history of "high-risk" bundle-branch block. N Engl J Med 307:137, 1982.
23. Dhingra RC, Wyndham C, Amat-y-Leon F, et al: Incidence and site of A-V block in patients with chronic bifascicular block. Circulation 59:238, 1979.
24. Dhingra RC, Wyndham C, Deedwania PC, et al: Effect of age on atrioventricular conduction in patients with chronic bifascicular block. Am J Cardiol 45:749, 1980.
25. Dreifus LS, Watanabe Y, Haiat R, et al: Atrioventricular block. Am J Cardiol 28:371, 1971.
26. Frye RL, Collins JJ, DeSanctis RW, et al: Guide-

lines for permanent pacemaker implantation. Circulation 70:331A, 1984.

27. Edhag O, Swahn A: Prognosis of patients with complete heart block or arrhythmic syncope who were not treated with artificial pacemakers. Acta Med Scand 200:457, 1976.

28. Rowe JC, White PD: Complete heart block: a follow-up study. Ann Intern Med 49:260, 1958.

29. Simon AB, Zloto AE: Atrioventricular block: natural history after permanent ventricular pacing. Am J Cardiol 41:500, 1978.

30. Zoll PM, Zoll RH, Falk RH, et al: External non-invasive temporary cardiac pacing: clinical trials. Circulation 71:937, 1985.

31. Fleg JL, Kennedy HL: Cardiac arrhythmias in a healthy elderly population: detection by 24-hour ambulatory electrocardiography. Chest 81:302, 1982.

32. Kantelip J-P, Sage E, Duchene-Marullaz P: Findings on ambulatory electrocardiographic monitoring in subjects older than 80 years. Am J Cardiol 57:398, 1986.

33. Kannel WB, Abbott RD, Savage DD, et al: Epidemiologic features of chronic atrial fibrillation. N Engl J Med 306:1018, 1982.

34. Forfar JC, Miller HC, Toft AD: Occult thyrotoxicosis: a correctable cause of "idiopathic" atrial fibrillation. Am J Cardiol 44:9, 1979.

35. Wolf PA, Dawber TR, Thomas HE, et al: Epidemiologic assessment of chronic atrial fibrillation and risk of stroke: the Framingham study. Neurology 28:973, 1978.

36. Hinton RC, Kistler P, Fallon JT, et al: Influence of etiology of atrial fibrillation on incidence of systemic embolism. Am J Cardiol 40:509, 1977.

37. Levine HJ: Which atrial fibrillation patients should be on chronic anticoagulation? Cardiovasc Med 6:483, 1981.

38. Goldman MJ: The management of chronic atrial fibrillation: indications for and method of conversion to sinus rhythm. Prog Cardiovasc Dis 2:465, 1960.

39. Bjerkelund CJ, Orning OM: The efficacy of anticoagulant therapy in preventing embolism related to D.C. electrical cardioversion of atrial fibrillation. Am J Cardiol 23:208, 1969.

40. Henry WL, Morganroth J, Pearlman AS, et al: Relation between echocardiographically determined left atrial size and atrial fibrillation. Circulation 53:273, 1976.

41. Morris JJ, Kong Y, North WC, et al: Experience with "cardioversion" of atrial fibrillation and flutter. Am J Cardiol 14:94, 1964.

42. Falk RH, Knowlton AA, Bernard SA, et al: Digoxin for converting recent-onset atrial fibrillation to sinus rhythm. Ann Intern Med 106:503, 1987.

43. Waldo AL, MacLean WAH, Karp RB, et al: Entrainment and interruption of atrial flutter with atrial pacing: studies in man following open heart surgery. Circulation 56:737, 1977.

44. Josephson ME, Kastor JA: Supraventricular tachycardia: mechanisms and management. Ann Intern Med 87:346, 1977.

45. Wellens HJJ, Bar FWHM, Lie KI: The value of the electrocardiogram in the differential diagnosis of a tachycardia with a widened QRS complex. Am J Med 64:27, 1976.

46. Buxton AE, Marchlinski FE, Doherty JU, et al: Hazards of intravenous verapamil for sustained ventricular tachycardia. Am J Cardiol 59:1107, 1987.

47. Stewart RB, Brady GH, Greene HL: Wide complex tachycardia: misdiagnosis and outcome after emergent therapy. Ann Intern Med 104:766, 1986.

48. Gallagher JJ, Smith WM, Kerr CR, et al: Esophageal pacing: a diagnostic and therapeutic tool. Circulation 65:336, 1982.

49. Wellens HJJ: The electrophysiologic properties of the accessory pathway in the Wolff-Parkinson-White syndrome. In Wellens HJJ, Lie KI, Janse MJ: The Conduction System of the Heart. Philadelphia, Lea & Febiger, 1976, p 567.

50. Klein G, Bashore TM, Sellers TD, et al: Ventricular fibrillation in the Wolff-Parkinson-White syndrome. N Engl J Med 301:1080, 1979.

51. Gallagher JJ, Pritchett ELC, Sealy WC, et al: The preexcitation syndromes. Prog Cardiovasc Dis 20:285, 1978.

52. Camm AJ, Evans KE, Ward DE, et al: The rhythm of the heart in active elderly subjects. Am Heart J 99:598, 1980.

53. Kennedy HL, Whitlock JA, Sprague MK, et al: Long-term follow-up of asymptomatic healthy subjects with frequent and complex ventricular ectopy. N Engl J Med 312:193, 1985.

54. Moss AJ, DeCamilla JJ, Davis HP, et al: Clinical significance of ventricular ectopic beats in the early post-hospital phase of myocardial infarction. Am J Cardiol 39:635, 1977.

55. Ruberman W, Weinblatt E, Goldberg JD, et al: Ventricular premature beats and mortality after myocardial infarction. N Engl J Med 297:750, 1977.

56. Velebit V, Podrid P, Lown B, et al: Aggravation and provocation of ventricular arrhythmias by antiarrhythmic drugs. Circulation 65:886, 1982.

57. Danforth J, Ports TA: Using beta blockers after MI in the elderly. Geriatrics 40(5):75, 1985.

58. Beta-blocker Heart Attack Study Group: A randomized trial of propranolol in patients with acute myocardial infarction. I. Mortality results. JAMA 247:1707, 1982.

59. Liberthson RR, Nagel EL, Hirschman JC, et al: Pre-hospital ventricular defibrillation: prognosis and follow-up course. N Engl J Med 291:317, 1974.

60. Schaffer WA, Cobb LA: Recurrent ventricular fibrillation and modes of death in survivors of out-of-hospital ventricular fibrillation. N Engl J Med 292:259, 1975.

61. Platia EV, Reid PR: Comparison of programmed electrical stimulation and ambulatory electrocardiographic (Holter) monitoring in the management of ventricular tachycardia and ventricular fibrillation. J Am Coll Cardiol 4:493, 1984.

62. Ruskin JN, DiMarco JP, Garan H: Out of hospital cardiac arrest: electrophysiologic observations and selections of long-term antiarrhythmic drug therapy. N Engl J Med 303:607, 1980.

63. Mason JW: Amiodarone. N Engl J Med 316:455, 1987.

64. Horowitz LN, Harken AH, Josephson ME, et al: Surgical treatment of ventricular arrhythmias in coronary artery disease. Ann Intern Med 95:88, 1981.

65. Echt DS, Winkle RA: Management of patients with the automatic implantable cardioverter/defibrillator. Clin Prog Electrophysiol Pacing 3:4, 1985.

66. Samet P, et al: Atrial contribution to cardiac output in complete heart block. Am J Cardiol 16:1, 1965.

67. Benchimol A: Significance of the contribution of atrial systole to cardiac function in man. Am J Cardiol 23:568, 1969.

68. Pehrsson SK: Influence of heart rate and AV synchronization on maximal work tolerance in patients treated with artificial pacemakers. Acta Med Scand 214:331, 1983.

69. Fananapazir L, Bennett DH, Monks P: Atrial synchronized ventricular pacing: contribution of the chronotropic response to improved exercise performance. PACE 6:601, 1983.

70. Benditt DG, Milstein S, Buetikofer J, et al: Sensor-triggered, rate-variable cardiac pacing. Ann Intern Med 107:714, 1987.

71. Kappenberger L, Gloor HO, Babotai I, et al: Hemodynamic effects of atrial synchronization in acute and long-term ventricular pacing. PACE 5:639, 1982.

72. Kruse I, Arnman K, Conradson T-B, et al: A comparison of the acute and long-term hemodynamic effects of ventricular inhibited pacing. Circulation 65:846, 1982.

73. Perrins EJ, Morley CA, Chan SL, et al: Randomised controlled trial of physiological and ventricular pacing. Br Heart J 50:112, 1983.

74. Kristensson B, et al: Physiological versus single-rate ventricular pacing: a double-blind cross-over study. PACE 8:73, 1985.

75. Marcus FI, Ruskin JN, Surawicz: Arrhythmias. J Am Coll Cardiol 10:66A, 1987.

CHAPTER 25

Coronary Artery Disease

Eugene E. Wolfel

A man is as old as his arteries.
Dr. Pierre J. G. Cabanis, *Epigram*

Cardiovascular disease is highly prevalent in the elderly population and is a cause of significant morbidity and mortality in this age group. Seventy-two percent of all cardiovascular deaths in the United States occur in patients over age 65, with 69 percent being related to complications from coronary artery disease. In fact, coronary artery disease is the most common cause of death in patients over 65 years of age. The prevalence of coronary artery disease has been estimated to be 50 to 60 percent in men at age 60. The impact of coronary artery disease in the elderly population is tremendous, and it definitely represents the most common cause of cardiac morbidity and mortality in this age group.

CORONARY ARTERY DISEASE

Epidemiology

Coronary atherosclerosis is an extremely common finding at autopsy in elderly patients. The incidence at autopsy has been reported to be 46 percent in the sixth decade and 84 percent in the ninth decade.[5] Autopsy material from routine cases in Olmstead County, Minnesota has shown that 60 percent of all patients over age 60 had at least one coronary artery with a 75 to 100 percent occlusion.[2] Pomerance has also shown that 48.5 percent of patients over age 75 with congestive heart failure had autopsy evidence of significant coronary artery disease.[6] In a study of routine autopsies in patients over 90 years of age, Waller and Roberts reported significant coronary artery disease in 39 of 40 patients.[7] The severity of coronary atherosclerosis did vary and was related to the serum cholesterol level in these patients.

These data suggested that coronary atherosclerosis may not be a necessary consequence of aging but may be related to coronary risk. In fact, other autopsy studies in the extreme elderly have shown only a one-third incidence of coronary artery disease. These high incidences of coronary artery disease at autopsy contrast sharply with the clinical incidence of disease in the elderly. At age 70, 15 percent of men and 9 percent of women have clinical evidence of coronary artery disease. At age 80, the incidence reaches 20 percent in both genders.[1] Results from the Framingham Study in patients age 65 to 74 also report a 20 percent incidence in men and a 15 percent incidence in women.[10] The prevalence of coronary artery disease is quite high in the elderly, with a 50 percent prevalence between 65–74 years of age and a 60 percent prevalence over 75 years of age.[4] Compared with a younger population, the prevalence and incidence of coronary artery disease in the elderly are similar for both men and women. The discrepancy between the autopsy and clinical evidence of coronary artery disease in the elderly suggests that the disease often goes undetected in this age group. The subtle presentation of coronary disease in the elderly, along with episodes of silent myocardial ischemia and infarction, contributes to the low rate of detection of coronary disease in this population.

Coronary Risk Factors

The decline in cardiovascular mortality in the last decade has been noted to a somewhat lesser extent in the elderly population. Although this decline may represent better medical care, reductions in coronary risk factors may also be involved. The Framingham study has shown that coronary risk profiles retain their predictive value for cardiovascular events in the elderly. Two percent of subsequent coronary artery disease cases were found in the lowest decile of risk factors, whereas 25 percent of coronary cases in men and 37 percent of cases in women were found in the highest risk decile.[9] An optimal risk group was defined as that with a systolic blood pressure of 105 mmHg, serum cholesterol of 185 mg/dl, no glucose intolerance, absence of cigarette smoking, and no electrocardiographic evidence of left ventricular hypertrophy. In this group, at age 70 only 10 percent of men and 9 percent of women developed clinical coronary artery disease. These results contrast to the high incidence of clinical disease in the poor-risk group, in which at age 70, 82 percent of men and 68 percent of women developed coronary artery disease. This poor-risk group was defined as having a systolic blood pressure of 195 mmHg, a serum cholesterol of 335 mg/dl, glucose intolerance, a history of current cigarette smoking, and electrocardiographic evidence of left ventricular hypertrophy.[10] The commonly recognized risk factors for coronary artery disease in the elderly are (1) elevated systolic blood pressure, (2) decreased high density lipoprotein (HDL), (3) elevated low density lipoprotein (LDL), (4) high LDL/HDL, (5) electrocardiographic left ventricular hypertrophy (LVH), and (6) diabetes mellitus, particularly in women.[9]

Although cigarette smoking has been shown to carry significant coronary risk in the elderly in one study, in general it has less predictive value than the other common risk factors.[3] As opposed to younger patients, serum cholesterol has minimal predictive value for coronary disease in the elderly. In contrast, high levels of LDL and low levels of HDL and their ratio retain significant predictive value for coronary risk in the elderly. Triglycerides are important only as they relate to the incidence of diabetes mellitus, especially in women. The effects of aging on serum lipids may explain the change in hierarchy of cardiovascular risk in the various lipid measurements.[11] Serum cholesterol does not rise after age 60 in men, although it

continues to rise until age 70 in women. At advanced age (i.e., age over 90) women have higher cholesterol values than men. LDL rises until age 60 and begins to decline by age 70. Again, women can have higher LDL values than men at advanced age. The protective effects of HDL do not appear to decline with age in men; however, HDL does decrease in elderly women, although their levels usually remain higher than those in men. Triglycerides also decline after age 50 in men but continue to increase in women, so that at age 70, women have higher levels than men. These lipid changes with aging in women may explain why the incidence and prevalence of coronary artery disease in elderly women is similar to men, unlike the situation at a younger age in which there is a striking preponderance in men. Systolic blood pressure elevation is a significant risk for cardiovascular disease and specifically coronary artery disease in the elderly. Clearly, levels greater than 180 mmHg are associated with a striking increase in coronary risk. Electrocardiographic LVH is associated with both systolic and diastolic hypertension in the elderly and constitutes evidence of end-organ damage.

Although these coronary risk factors have been well delineated, the role and safety of risk factor modification in the elderly is not well defined. Although systolic hypertension is strongly associated with both stroke and myocardial infarction (MI), there is minimal direct evidence that aggressive treatment will decrease the risk of MI and sudden death. Studies are currently being undertaken to test this hypothesis. At present, it seems reasonable to lower systolic blood pressure below 160 mmHg and diastolic blood pressure below 95 mmHg with pharmacologic agents, since the risks of therapy are relatively low. Clearly, diastolic hypertension needs to be controlled to levels below 95 mmHg.

The importance of decreasing coronary risk from lipid disorders is less clear. The Lipid Research Clinic study demonstrated that the lipid-lowering agent cholestyramine caused a 13 percent reduction in total cholesterol and a 25 percent reduction in LDL, which resulted in a decrease of 24 percent in cardiovascular mortality and a 19 percent decrease in nonfatal MI.[12] Subsequently, the Helsinki Heart Study also demonstrated that gemfibrozil, another lipid-lowering agent, caused an 8.5 percent reduction in cholesterol, an 8 percent reduction in LDL, and a 10 percent increase in HDL, which caused a 26 percent reduction in cardiovascular mortality and a 37 percent decrease in nonfatal MI.[8] Neither study demonstrated a decrease in total mortality, and neither study included elderly patients. It is not clear that results from these studies can be extrapolated to the elderly, particularly since some of the predictive value of lipid disorders changes with age. In addition, the side effects of cholestyramine and gemfibrozil may be more common in elderly patients. The value of the other lipid-lowering agents, such as lovastatin, nicotinic acid, and probucol, also has not been shown in elderly patients.

Because of these concerns, an attempt at dietary management and an increase in activity level seems to be a prudent and potentially productive initial approach. The diet should be low in saturated fat and cholesterol, should be rich in fiber, and contain a reasonable caloric intake. An increase in physical activity will help decrease body weight, which is closely related to other coronary risk factors in the elderly. Control of diabetes, especially in elderly women, may also modify coronary risk. The current approach to coronary risk factor modification in the elderly probably should be conservative, with an individualized approach. The potential psychologic and social impact of aggressive coronary risk-factor modification needs to be balanced against the potential improvement in longevity and the prevention of debilitating cardiovascular disorders in the elderly patient.

CHRONIC CORONARY ARTERY DISEASE

Angina is the most common presenting symptom of coronary artery disease in the elderly patient, occurring in 80 percent of this population. The history of classic exertional angina may be difficult to obtain. Many elderly patients have limited activity and do not develop symptoms until late in the course of their coronary artery disease, when rest angina or nocturnal angina become their first severe symptoms.

The description of chest pain may also be misleading because of the patient's inability to remember details of a recent painful episode or because of confusion with other medical disorders. Often, ischemic pain is thought to be a result of an arthritic problem in the shoulder or a gastrointestinal disorder such as peptic ulcer disease or esophagitis. The pattern of the chest pain syndrome and the factors precipitating its occurrence become the most important historic factors in determining whether ischemic pain is present. Dyspnea on exertion is a very common manifestation of coronary disease in the elderly. Aging causes an increase in stiffness of the left ventricle as well as an increase in end-diastolic volume with exercise.[24] These factors make the aged heart more susceptible to developing significant intraventricular pressure elevation produced by myocardial ischemia, thereby causing dyspnea with activity. Other symptoms that can be produced by myocardial ischemia in the elderly include episodes of weakness, unexplained diaphoresis, indigestion, and neck and shoulder pain.

Unstable angina, defined as rest angina, new onset angina, or rapidly progressive angina, occurs more frequently in the elderly. Data from patients in the registry of the Coronary Artery Surgery Study (CASS) indicated that 50 percent of all patients over age 65 with coronary artery disease had unstable angina compared with only 33 percent of patients under age 65. Coronary artery spasm may also contribute to anginal symptoms in the elderly. Vasomotor abnormalities in the coronary vascular bed could contribute to symptoms in elderly patients with known or suspected obstructive coronary disease who experience cold-induced angina, angina at rest, and angina occurring at a variable, unpredictable level of physical exertion. Finally, silent myocardial ischemia probably occurs in elderly patients, but its incidence as compared with younger patients is unknown. Patients with angina have been shown to have episodes of silent myocardial ischemia with activities of daily living.[19] Although elderly patients have been shown to have a higher incidence of silent MI, it remains to be proven that they have a high incidence of silent ischemia.[54]

Because the history of angina often can

be confusing in the elderly patient, other evidence is frequently necessary to confirm the diagnosis of coronary artery disease. Physical examination is usually not helpful because most elderly patients have fourth heart sounds resulting from altered ventricular compliance related to aging and a high prevalence of mitral murmurs caused by other cardiac disorders. The presence of carotid or peripheral vascular disease increases the likelihood of coronary disease but does not confirm the diagnosis. The resting electrocardiogram is usually abnormal in 50 percent of elderly patients, and by itself, it is not a specific indicator of coronary disease unless prior transmural MI is clearly demonstrated by the presence of Q waves. Echocardiography with Doppler ultrasonography can be useful to exclude noncoronary causes of cardiac chest pain, including valvular aortic stenosis, hypertrophic cardiomyopathy, pericardial disease, pulmonary hypertension, and mitral valve prolapse. The presence of regional left ventricular wall motion abnormalities is a good predictor of coronary artery disease, but it does not provide evidence as to the presence of ongoing myocardial ischemia. In order to determine if myocardial ischemia is present, some provocative method to stress the myocardium is usually necessary.

Diagnosis

Exercise testing has been the standard method employed in the diagnosis of coronary artery disease. Usually, a treadmill is used, with standard protocols modified for the decreased exercise capacity of most elderly patients.[32] Occasionally, bicycle exercise or arm ergometry is also used. The electrocardiogram (ECG) response to graded exercise has remained the most common variable analyzed for the presence of myocardial ischemia. The diagnostic accuracy of ST-segment depression during exercise as an indicator of myocardial ischemia depends on the sensitivity and specificity of the test, as well as on the prevalence of coronary artery disease in the population being studied.

According to Bayes' theorem, the pretest likelihood of disease is a strong determinant of whether an abnormal exercise ECG truly represents coronary artery disease. The higher prevalence of coronary disease in the elderly has a direct influence on the post-test likelihood of disease. Even elderly men 60 to 69 years of age with noncardiac pain still have a 28 percent pretest likelihood of disease compared with 14 percent in men aged 40 to 49 years (Table 25–1). The data are even more impressive in elderly women in whom a four- to six-fold greater likelihood of disease occurs with atypical symptoms, compared with younger women. The post-test likelihood of coronary disease in both men and women with 1.0 to 1.5 mm of ST-segment depression is clearly greater than in younger patients (see Table 25–1). Thus, in elderly patients, ST-segment analysis has the potential to be a more effective diagnostic tool than in younger patients, regardless of symptoms. In one study, the sensitivity of 1.0 mm of ST-segment depression in patients over age 65 was 63 percent, which was comparable to the 70 percent seen in younger patients.[31]

Difficulties arise with the specificity of abnormal ST-segment responses during exercise testing for coronary disease in the elderly. Often, the baseline ECG is abnormal, thereby greatly reducing the diagnostic accuracy of the test. Using ST-segment depression alone, Vasilomanolakis and colleagues found only a 29 percent specificity in patients over age 65 years due to the high incidence of an abnormal resting ECG.[31] The specificity of the test was greatly increased when other variables such as angina, R-wave amplitude, and Q-wave depth are included. Other standard exercise variables, including exercise duration, onset of signs or symptoms of ischemia, blood pressure responses, and heart rate responses, also provide diagnostic and prognostic information. Variables that indicate a poorer prognosis and a high likelihood of either significant left main coronary artery stenosis or severe three-vessel coronary disease include early onset of ST-segment depression, persistence of these changes beyond 7 minutes in the recovery period, a drop in systolic blood pressure > 10 mmHg during exercise, and widespread significant (≥ 2 mm) ST-segment depression. The presence of an abnormal exercise ECG response of ≥ 1 mm of ST-depression in elderly patients by itself also seems to be a predictor of subsequent cardiac mortality in this age group.[23]

TABLE 25–1. Effects of Age on the Diagnosis of Coronary Disease by Treadmill Testing

	Pretest Likelihood of Disease (%)					
	Nonanginal Pain		*Symptoms* *Atypical Pain*		*Classic Angina*	
Age	*Men*	*Women*	*Men*	*Women*	*Men*	*Women*
40–49 yrs	14	3	46	13	87	55
60–69 yrs	28	19	67	54	94	91
	Post-test Likelihood of Disease* (%)					
	Asymptomatic		*Nonanginal Pain*		*Atypical Angina*		*Typical Angina*	
	Men	*Women*	*Men*	*Women*	*Men*	*Women*	*Men*	*Women*
40–49 yrs	11	2	26	6	64	25	94	72
60–69 yrs	23	15	45	33	81	72	97	95

(Adapted from Diamond GA, Forrester JS: Analysis of probability as an aid in the clinical diagnosis of coronary artery disease. N Engl J Med 300:1350, 1979.)

*1.0 to 1.5 mm of ST-segment depression used as an indication of myocardial ischemia.

Because of the problems with sensitivity and specificity of routine exercise testing in the diagnosis of coronary disease, radionuclide methods have been used to improve the diagnostic accuracy of exercise testing. Thallium scintigraphy, using either qualitative or quantitative analyses, has increased the sensitivity of exercise testing from 58 percent (using ST-segment depression alone) to 83 to 92 percent. In addition, thallium scintigraphy has increased the specificity of the test from 82 to 90 percent.[14] There are no studies to determine whether this improvement in the diagnostic value of exercise testing with thallium also occurs in the elderly population. A recent study evaluating the role of thallium in exercise testing in 217 elderly patients found that abnormal myocardial perfusion in the setting of abnormal exercise responses influenced the decision to proceed with angiography.[20] Little diagnostic value was obtained from thallium if the routine exercise test was normal. It appears from this data that thallium scintigraphy can be a useful additional test in the diagnosis of coronary artery disease in the elderly if the patient has an abnormal resting ECG or equivocal ST-segment changes and chest pain or cannot complete the exercise protocol. Thallium scintigraphy has also be shown to increase the sensitivity and specificity of arm ergometry testing, which may be a useful approach in patients unable to perform leg exercise.[13]

The other radionuclide approach to improving the sensitivity and specificity of exercise testing for the diagnosis of coronary artery disease is the use of exercise radionuclide ventriculography. A failure to increase ejection fraction during exercise by ≥5 percent compared with the resting level and the development of regional wall motion abnormalities have been used as diagnostic criteria for the presence of myocardial ischemia during exercise. Using these criteria, the sensitivity and specificity of the exercise test in predicting coronary artery disease has been substantially improved.[14] Interpreting left ventricular events during exercise is more complex in the elderly patient because of the effects of aging itself on ventricular function. The expected increase in overall left ventricular ejection fraction to graded exercise is clearly reduced in older patients without cardiac disease.[29, 30] Because the global ventricular systolic responses to exercise can be influenced by a variety of factors in the elderly, the specificity of this response appears to be diminished, thereby limiting the usefulness of this test in the diagnosis of coronary artery disease.

The major limitations to exercise testing in the elderly relate to the inability of this group to perform adequate exercise. Often, these patients have significant musculoskeletal or respiratory symptoms that limit exercise performance. Many of these patients can attain only 85 percent of their age-predicted maximal heart rate, thereby decreasing the sensitivity of the exercise test. Thallium scintigraphy with intravenous dipyridamole may become a useful diagnostic study in these patients, thus avoiding the risks of coronary arteriography in patients who cannot perform an exercise study. Dipyridamole is a coronary vasodilator that promotes coronary vascular steal, thus producing a hypoperfused area of myocardium detectable by thallium scanning. Preliminary studies have shown that dipyridamole-thallium tests have a sensitivity of 90 percent and a specificity of 95 percent in younger patients with chronic coronary artery disease.[22] It has also been used in elderly patients to assess risk of perioperative MI and death in patients undergoing peripheral vascular surgery.[15] The safety and diagnostic value of this procedure has not been defined in elderly patients, but it has great potential as an important diagnostic tool. Because elderly patients are very sensitive to vasodilating drugs, the development of significant hypotension may limit the usefulness of dipyridamole as a diagnostic agent.

Twenty-four-hour ambulatory monitoring has also been used to diagnose silent myocardial ischemia in patients with coronary artery disease. Horizontal or downsloping ST-segment depression of ≥ 1 mm sustained for more than 60 seconds has been found to have a sensitivity of 55 percent and a specificity of 100 percent for myocardial ischemia and coronary artery disease.[18] The sensitivity of this test increases with longer periods of monitoring. The prevalence of an abnormal resting ECG in the elderly may limit the usefulness of asymptomatic ST-segment depression as an indicator of myocardial ischemia.

Coronary arteriography remains the definitive test for the diagnosis of coronary artery disease. Data from CASS indicates that elderly patients have a higher mortality and morbidity from this procedure.[38] The death rate was 1.9 per 1000 patients, with the incidence of nonfatal MI at 7.9 per 1000, vascular complications at 8.4 per 1000, embolic complications at 1.9 per 1000, neurologic complications (including stroke) at 3.7 per 1000, ventricular fibrillation at 4.2 per 1000, and an incidence of 23.8 per 1000 patients for one or more complications. Except for vascular complications, all of the other adverse effects of coronary arteriography were more frequent in elderly patients.

For these reasons, coronary arteriography should be reserved for elderly patients with more severe coronary artery disease, such as angina unresponsive to

medical therapy, severe unstable angina, myocardial ischemia presenting as pulmonary edema, and significant angina in the presence of left ventricular dysfunction, and for those patients with an exercise test suggesting a high-risk status. Because of the higher risks of coronary arteriography in the elderly patient, this test should not be routinely performed to exclude coronary artery disease in a stable patient with an atypical chest pain syndrome and a nondiagnostic noninvasive evaluation. In these patients, a therapeutic trial with sublingual nitroglycerin or empiric antianginal therapy may be warranted before exposing the patient to the increased risks of arteriography.

Treatment

All elderly patients with presumed or diagnosed coronary artery disease and chronic stable angina should be initially treated with medical therapy. Because of the increased morbidity and mortality of mechanical procedures in this age group, both coronary angioplasty and coronary bypass surgery should be reserved for patients with refractory symptoms or more severe disease. Anemia, hyperthyroidism, congestive heart failure, supraventricular and ventricular arrhythmia, and hypertension should be sought and treated, since they contribute to an increase in myocardial oxygen demand and may precipitate angina in an otherwise asymptomatic patient. In the patient with chronic stable angina, sublingual nitroglycerin remains the initial treatment. Elderly patients are particularly susceptible to the vasodilating effects of this drug, and they need to be carefully instructed in its proper use. For many patients with arthritis or poor vision, the sublingual spray will be easier to use than the standard sublingual tablets. If symptoms occur frequently, maintenance antianginal therapy is required. The currently available antianginal drugs and their mechanism of action and side effects are outlined in Tables 25–2 and 25–3.

In general, elderly patients should be treated with lower doses of all antianginal medications because of the higher incidence of side effects.[17] Nitrates remain the initial therapy for most patients with chronic stable angina, as well as those

TABLE 25–2. Medical Management of Angina in the Elderly—Mechanism of Action

Drug	Arterial Vasodilation	Venous Vasodilation	Coronary Vasodilation	Negative Inotropic	Negative Chronotropic	Negative Dromotropic
Nitrates, nitroglycerin	+	+ + +	+ +	0	− *	0
Beta-blockers	0	0	− †	+ +	+ + +	+ +
Calcium-blockers						
Nifedipine	+ + +	0	+ + +	+	− *	0
Verapamil	+	0	+ + +	+ +	+ +	+ +
Diltiazem	+ +	0	+ + +	+	+	+

Dromotropic properties refer to effects on left ventricular relaxation and filling.
*Both nitrates and nifedipine can increase heart rate by reflex sympathetic action.
†Beta blockade causes a reduction in coronary blood flow due to lower myocardial oxygen consumption and has been reported to cause coronary vasoconstriction in some patients.

patients with a component of vasospasm. Elderly patients are more sensitive to the vasodilating action of these drugs because of a decrease in plasma volume, a higher incidence of venous disease, a decreased sensitivity and responsiveness of the baroreceptor reflex, and a diminished cardiac response to catecholamine stimulation. Recent concerns about the development of pharmacologic tolerance to these drugs, especially the long-acting transdermal preparations, may limit the efficacy of these agents in patients with more severe symptoms. Elderly patients may also have more skin irritation from the preparation because of their transparent, fragile skin.

Beta-blockers continue to be the most effective therapy for exertional angina because of their effects on exercise heart rate, but the response to beta blockade is somewhat unpredictable. It can be more difficult to achieve effective beta-blocking effects, despite the higher blood levels of these drugs because of decreased metabolism. Elderly patients have a diminished chronotropic response to beta-adrenergic agonists, but the mechanism of attenuation of beta-blocking effects in some patients is unknown.[25] Hydrophilic beta-blockers (e.g., atenolol-nadolol) generally have fewer side effects than the lipophilic drugs, but their doses must be decreased in patients with a reduced creatinine clearance because they are excreted primarily by the kidney. Cardioselectivity is important in patients with diabetes and peripheral vascular disease. Interactions of beta-blockers with cimetidine and lidocaine necessitate a reduction in the dose or increasing the dosing interval of these drugs in the presence of beta-blockers. In general, the dose of beta-blocker should be titrated to produce a resting heart rate of between 50 and 60 beats per minute (bpm) and a peak exercise heart rate of less than 100 bpm.

Calcium blockers are becoming important agents in the therapy of both vasospastic and exertional angina. Although all three of the currently available drugs have vasodilating properties, they differ in their effects on cardiac conduction and ventricular function. Because of the higher prevalence of conduction defects and left ventricular dysfunction in the elderly, these patients are more susceptible to the side effects of calcium blockers. Initial doses of these drugs should be lower in elderly patients, with gradual titration to relief of symptoms or occurrence of side effects.

Combinations of antianginal drugs are

TABLE 25–3. Medical Management of Angina in the Elderly: Adverse Drug Effects

Drug	Adverse Effects
Nitrates, nitroglycerin	Orthostatic hypotension; headache; syncope; skin rash
Beta-blockers	Fatigue; depression; heart block; heart failure; symptomatic bradycardia; bronchospasm
Calcium-blockers	
Nifedipine	Orthostatic hypotension; flushing; edema; syncope
Verapamil	Constipation; heart block; heart failure; hypotension
Diltiazem	Heart block; edema; hypotension

reserved for patients with more severe symptoms. The risk of complications increases significantly in elderly patients on combination therapy; therefore, the initial dose of each drug should be low. The combination of verapamil and beta-blockers should be avoided because of a high incidence of either heart block or congestive heart failure. Diltiazem and beta-blockers need to be administered cautiously and at low doses because combined use increases the frequency of atrioventricular block. The combination of nitrates and nifedipine also should be used cautiously because the combined vasodilatory effects of these drugs may result in orthostatic hypotension or syncope. The role of antiplatelet agents in stable angina is unclear in elderly patients.

The treatment of unstable angina in elderly patients does not differ from that in younger patients. Initially, stabilization with intravenous nitroglycerin, beta-blockers, and calcium-blockers should be followed by a regimen of combined oral antianginal therapy. Aspirin has been shown in two studies to decrease the rate of infarction in patients with unstable angina and should be used early in the treatment course.[16, 26] In patients with refractory angina, intravenous heparin should be considered. The role of thrombolytic therapy in unstable angina remains unproven and represents a particularly hazardous form of therapy in elderly patients. Although intra-aortic balloon counterpulsation has been shown to be an effective form of therapy for refractory unstable angina in younger patients, this form of therapy should be used cautiously in elderly patients because of the higher morbidity from local vascular complications. Patients who have refractory symptoms will require coronary arteriography to assess their candidacy for coronary angioplasty or coronary bypass surgery. Fortunately, many patients are stabilized on medication. Results of two large randomized trials indicate that early coronary bypass surgery is not necessary in this group of patients because mortality and infarction rates are similar for both medical and surgical therapy.[27, 28]

Patients with three-vessel coronary artery disease and left ventricular dysfunction or those with refractory symptoms will benefit from early surgical intervention. The role of coronary angioplasty in elderly patients with unstable angina is unclear, but it may represent an alternative form of therapy at a lower risk than does coronary bypass surgery.

PERCUTANEOUS TRANSLUMINAL CORONARY ANGIOPLASTY IN THE ELDERLY

Elderly patients who present with severe unstable coronary artery disease or develop angina refractory to medical therapy become candidates for mechanical revascularization therapy. The risks of coronary bypass surgery are clearly higher in this patient population, with CASS registry data revealing a 4.6 percent mortality between 65 and 69 years of age and a 9.5 percent mortality in patients over age 75 years.[38] Percutaneous transluminal coronary angioplasty (PTCA) represents an alternative approach in these patients, with a reduced morbidity and mortality. Although the success rate of PTCA in elderly patients is less than that in younger patients, the results from several studies have been quite favorable. The initial concern about the inability to dilate the calcified, hardened atherosclerotic plaques in elderly patients has not been realized.

Data from the three published series involving PTCA in the elderly are presented in Table 25–4. The National Heart, Blood and Lung Institute (NHBLI) registry study represents an earlier multicenter experience with PTCA in the elderly.[34] The lower success rate may reflect the limitation of the catheter technology at that time. Subsequent technological developments, as well as better patient selection, are responsible for the higher success rates in more recent studies.[33, 35] Although the mortality and complication rates of PTCA in the elderly are higher than the rates in younger patients, the frequency of these adverse effects is lower than that in most series of coronary bypass surgery in the elderly. Of particular importance is the absence of significant neurologic complications with PTCA compared with coronary bypass surgery. The rates of restenosis are comparable to figures for PTCA in younger patients, and the continual

TABLE 25–4. Percutaneous Transluminal Coronary Angioplasty (PTCA) in the Elderly

	NHBLI (1984)	Taylor et al (1986)	Dorros et al (1986)
No. patients	370	35	109
Average age (yrs)	69	71	75.9
Success rate (%)	53	63	89
Emergency CABG (%)	2.8	8.6	0.9
Complications* (%)	19.5	NR†	15
Myocardial infarction (%)	5.6	0	2.8
Deaths (%)	2.2	2.9	1.8
Restenosis rate (%)	21.3	27	17
Improvement—1 yr (%)	74	86	92
Average hospital study (days)	4	3.4	3.4

(Adapted from Dorros G, Janke L, 1986; Mock MB, et al, 1984; Taylor GJ, et al, 1986.)
*Complications include arrhythmias, myocardial infarction, death, and emergency CABG.
†NR = not reported.

clinical improvement at 1 year after PTCA is striking. Although the effects of PTCA on morbidity and mortality of coronary artery disease have not been compared with either medical therapy or coronary bypass surgery in a comparable group of elderly patients, these initial, uncontrolled studies suggest that it represents an important form of therapy for more severe coronary artery disease in elderly patients.

CORONARY ARTERY BYPASS SURGERY IN THE ELDERLY

Early experience in the 1970s with coronary bypass surgery in the elderly indicated a surgical mortality between 3.7 and 19 percent. Because of these high surgical mortalities, surgery was performed mainly in elderly patients refractory to maximal medical therapy. With improvements in myocardial preservation techniques, the surgical mortality for coronary bypass surgery in elderly patients has dropped considerably. In carefully selected patient groups, mortalities of 1.6 to 3 percent have been reported in recent years.[40, 43] These lower surgical mortalities suggest that the role of coronary bypass surgery in the management of coronary artery disease in the elderly should be re-evaluated.

A more valid assessment of the risks of coronary bypass surgery in the elderly can be determined by reviewing the data from the CASS registry.[38] One thousand eighty-six patients over 65 years of age underwent coronary bypass surgery at various institutions. The overall perioperative mortality was 5.2 percent, compared with 1.9 percent in patients under age 65. The mortality rate increased with age, with a 4.6 percent mortality at ages 65 to 69 years, a 6.6 percent mortality at ages 70 to 74 years, and a 9.5 percent mortality in patients over age 75. Cardiogenic shock and refractory heart failure were the most frequent causes of death, and there were nine cerebrovascular accidents in the 1086 patients. Elderly patients also had longer hospital stays than did younger patients. The predictors of perioperative mortality in this elderly group were the presence of stenosis of 70 percent or greater of the left main coronary artery with a left dominant coronary circulation, a left ventricular end-diastolic pressure over 20 mmHg, a history of current cigarette use, presence of rales on lung examination, and one or more associated medical problems. There was a tendency for a slightly higher mortality in women (6.9 percent) compared with men (4.7 percent). When all 7658 patients who underwent coronary bypass surgery in the CASS registry were analyzed, age over 65 years became an independent predictor of mortality. The rank order of predictors for surgical mortality in the total population was (1) congestive heart failure score, (2) left main coronary stenosis with a left dominant circulation, (3) age over 65 years, (4) left ventricular wall motion score, (5) gender, and (6) a history of unstable angina. Thus, advanced age represented a significant risk for surgical mortality surpassed only by left ventricular dysfunction and left main coronary artery disease. Elderly patients with severe calcification of the ascending aorta also represent a high-risk group for neurologic complications and death and probably should not undergo coronary bypass surgery.[40]

With the higher risk of perioperative mortality in elderly patients, surgery is probably indicated less often for prolongation of survival alone than it is in younger patients. Clearly, patients who are refractory to medical therapy should be considered for surgery, especially if PTCA cannot be performed. Patients who present with acute pulmonary edema secondary to severe global ischemia and who have normal left ventricular function appear to benefit from coronary bypass surgery because they represent a high-risk group.[41]

Does coronary bypass surgery prolong life in elderly patients? The results of three randomized trials of coronary bypass surgery have shown that patients with three-vessel coronary disease and either severe symptoms, left ventricular dysfunction, or abnormal exercise performance have a lower mortality with surgical therapy.[36, 37, 42] None of these randomized studies included elderly patients; therefore, the data from these studies cannot be extrapolated to this patient population. An analysis of medical versus surgical therapy was performed in 1491 patients over age 65 in the CASS registry.[39] The overall 6-year survival rate was 79 percent in the surgically treated group, compared with 64 percent in the medically treated group. An analysis of survival in this study is shown in Table 25–5. Patients between the ages of 65 and 75 with two- or three-vessel disease, left ventricular dysfunction, and more severe symptoms had a lower mortality with surgical therapy. Surgery alone was found to be an independent predictor of survival. Patients with left main coronary disease and a left dominant coronary circulation were excluded from this analysis.

The results of this study must be interpreted with caution because the baseline characteristics of the two groups differed. The medically treated group included more women, more patients with other significant medical problems, and more left ventricular dysfunction, whereas the surgically treated group had more severe angina and more three-vessel disease. Despite these differences, the data does suggest that in higher-risk elderly patients, surgery may prolong life. Low-risk patients with stable angina and normal ventricular function did not benefit from surgical therapy, and these patients should be treated medically, unless they develop refractory angina.

ACUTE MYOCARDIAL INFARCTION IN THE ELDERLY

The mortality of acute MI in the elderly is substantially higher than in younger patients. The in-hospital mortality varies from 20 to 43 percent, and the 1-year mortality is 20 to 53 percent.[52, 55, 58] The high mortality in these patients is caused by the subtle early presentation of infarction, causing a delay in diagnosis and therapy as well as a high incidence of left ventricular dysfunction. Silent MI occurs in a significant number of elderly patients. Twenty-one percent of patients from a chronic care facility presenting with infarction had a silent MI.[45] The Framingham Study has also shown that 36 percent of men and 46 percent of women with a new MI on ECG had no symptoms, and a substantial number of these patients were over 65 years of age.[54]

The presenting symptoms of MI in the elderly can be quite atypical, especially in patients over age 80.[46] Although several studies have shown that chest pain is still a common presenting symptom, the incidence of this symptom is lower than in younger patients.[46, 52] Dyspnea is a very common early manifestation of MI in the elderly.[59] Other common presentations include mental confusion, syncope, neurologic disturbances, and gastrointestinal complaints. In contrast, diaphoresis is an uncommon manifestation of acute infarction in the elderly. In addition to an inexact history, other factors make the diagnosis of acute MI difficult in certain elderly patients. Many patients have conduction defects on the ECG that may mask the changes of acute transmural MI. The incidence of non–Q-wave MI appears to be higher in elderly patients, and the ECG changes may be subtle.[58, 61] Twenty percent of elderly patients with non–Q-wave

TABLE 25–5. Coronary Surgery in the Elderly—CASS Registry

	Medical Therapy	Surgical Therapy
Survival (%, 6 years)		
Overall	64	79*
65–69 yrs	67	81*
70–74 yrs	51	77*
> 75 yrs	56	75
One-vessel CAD	81	82
Two-vessel CAD	70	89*
Three-vessel CAD	47	75*
Normal LV function	83	87
Low-risk group	80	88
High-risk group	33	62*

(Adapted from Gersh BJ, Kronmal RA, Schaff HV, et al: Comparison of coronary artery bypass surgery and medical therapy in patients 65 years of age or older: a nonrandomized study from the Coronary Artery Surgery Study [CASS] registry. N Engl J Med 313:217, 1985.)

*Indicates significant difference at $p < 0.05$ level.

Low-risk group defined as mild angina, good left ventricular function, and no left main coronary disease. High-risk group defined as severe symptoms, usually unstable angina, left ventricular dysfunction, and severe three-vessel or left main coronary artery disease.

MI have "microinfarction."[51, 53] These patients have normal total creatine phosphokinase (CPK) levels, but elevated CK-MB fractions, and 20 percent of patients also developed a flip in the LDH_1/LDH_2, confirming that MI did occur. They usually have a clinical course consistent with MI and an increased in-hospital morbidity and mortality.

Elderly patients with MI have an increased incidence of pericarditis, supraventricular and ventricular arrhythmias, myocardial rupture, conduction disturbances, congestive heart failure, cardiogenic shock, cardiovascular accidents, pneumonia, phlebitis, and drug toxicity.[52, 55] The most common causes of death are severe congestive heart failure and shock, ventricular arrhythmias, sudden death, and myocardial rupture. The incidence of myocardial rupture in the elderly is much greater than that in younger patients, with a 28.6 percent incidence reported in one study.[55] Elderly women with hypertension who have a first MI appear to be at a particularly high risk for this complication. Univariate predictors of survival include age, prior infarction, diastolic hypertension, history of diabetes, history of congestive heart failure, presence of rales and a ventricular gallop, cardiomegaly on chest x-ray, Killip class (the presence and extent of rales on physical examination), and the use of diuretics or digoxin.[58] The only multivariate predictor

of survival is Killip class, indicating that left ventricular function is the most important predictor of survival after MI in the elderly.

Treatment

The therapy of acute MI in the elderly is similar to that in younger patients. Admission to the coronary care unit does seem to improve survival in most studies in this age group. Elderly patients have a lower incidence of ventricular fibrillation at the onset of their infarction, and because lidocaine toxicity is more common in the elderly, lidocaine prophylaxis is not indicated in the group. If lidocaine is required for ventricular arrhythmias, the loading dose should be 50 to 75 mg followed by an infusion at 25 µg/kg/min. Plasma levels should be used to monitor therapy. Because many elderly patients have abnormal gas exchange, oxygen therapy is extremely important to increase oxygen delivery. All elderly patients should receive low-dose subcutaneous heparin because of the high risk for venous thromboembolic disease in all patients at bed rest during MI. Full-dose anticoagulation therapy is often given to patients with anterior MI because of the high risk of mural thrombus and possible embolization. Because anticoagulation carries a substantial risk in this age group, all elderly patients should receive an echocardiogram within the first 48 hours of admission. If a pedunculated thrombus is seen, full-dose anticoagulation therapy is indicated (if there are no major contraindications). In patients of advanced age (over 80 years of age), the risks of this therapy probably outweigh the benefits.

The role of interventional therapy during the first few hours of MI has not been defined in the elderly. The GISSI study has shown a significant reduction in mortality with intravenous streptokinase during the first 3 hours of MI.[49] In patients over age 65 years, this benefit was not seen, and there was a higher incidence of bleeding complications. An analysis of intravenous streptokinase therapy in 24 elderly patients at Cedar Sinai Medical Center revealed an increased mortality in patients over age 75 years.[56] This increased mortality rate was directly related to a twofold increase in the incidence of major hemorrhagic complications, including an 8 percent incidence of intracranial hemorrhage. The risk was particularly high for women age 75 and older with a history of diabetes or hypertension. Only elderly men without diabetes or hypertension had a response comparable to that in younger patients. Tissue plasminogen activator (t-PA) has been shown to be a more effective thrombolytic agent, with the potential for less hemorrhagic complications. Its safety and efficacy in elderly patients are unknown. The role of acute PTCA in MI in the elderly is also unknown.

Since the 1-year mortality after MI in elderly patients is quite high, risk stratification should be performed, and these patients should be placed on therapy to decrease the likelihood of reinfarction and sudden death. Submaximal exercise testing should be performed in most patients prior to discharge. The presence of significant ST-segment depression, an abnormal blood pressure response, or development of angina are strong predictors of mortality, even in the elderly population.[60] Beta-blocker therapy has been shown in several large multicenter studies to decrease cardiac mortality after MI.[47, 57] In elderly patients, timolol has been shown to decrease mortality by 35.5 percent and reinfarction by 39.2 percent.[50] Several studies suggest that beta blockade may be especially protective in the elderly population. Patients with non–Q-wave infarction have been shown to have a higher early reinfarction rate, and diltiazem has been shown to reduce the risk of reinfarction at 2 weeks by 51 percent and the incidence of post-infarction angina by 49 percent.[48] A majority of patients in this study were over 60 years of age. Since non–Q-wave infarction seems to be more common in elderly patients, cautious use of diltiazem may play a major role in reducing future cardiac events. Antiplatelet therapy with aspirin also decreases the reinfarction rate in patients with non–Q-wave infarction.

The indications for PTCA and coronary bypass surgery after MI in elderly patients depend on the severity of symptoms, the degree of left ventricular dysfunction, and the severity of coronary disease. Surgery for acute mechanical complications of MI in the elderly has also been performed in selected patients with good results.[62]

Cardiac rehabilitation is an important aspect of post-MI therapy in elderly patients. The elderly are especially sensitive to the deconditioning effects of bedrest and require early mobilization to prevent a profound deterioration in functional capacity. The complications of orthostatic hypotension due to relative hypovolemia and thrombophlebitis due to circulatory stasis can thus be prevented. Elderly patients are able to increase their functional capacity with regular exercise by similar increments as do younger patients, although they start at a lower functional capacity.[44, 63] There is no increased risk of appropriately prescribed exercise in the elderly cardiac patient, and the attainment of a lower heart rate and blood pressure during submaximal exercise results in less myocardial oxygen demand during activities of daily living, thereby decreasing the likelihood of cardiac symptoms.

REFERENCES

GENERAL REVIEW AND EPIDEMIOLOGICAL STUDIES

1. Agner E: Epidemiology of coronary heart disease in the elderly patient. In Coodley EL, ed: Geriatric heart disease. Littleton, MA, PSG Publishing Co, 1985, p 114.
2. Elreback L, Lie JT: Combined high incidence of coronary artery disease at autopsy in Olmstead County, Minnesota, 1950–1979. Circulation 70:345, 1984.
3. Kennedy RD, Andrews GR, Caird FI: Ischemic

heart disease in the elderly. Br Heart J 39:1121, 1977.

4. Kennedy RD: Epidemiology of heart disease in old age. Israel J Med Sci 21:928, 1985.
5. Medalia LS, White PD: Disease of the aged: analysis of pathological observations in 1,251 autopsy protocols in old persons. JAMA 149:1433, 1952.
6. Pomerance A: Pathology of the heart with and without cardiac failure in the aged. Br Heart J 27:697, 1965.
7. Waller BF, Roberts WC: Cardiovascular disease in the very elderly: analysis of 40 necropsy patients aged 90 years or over. Am J Cardiol 51:403, 1983.

CORONARY RISK FACTORS IN THE ELDERLY

8. Frick MH, Elo O, Haapa K, et al: Helsinki Heart Study: primary-prevention trial with gemfibrozil in middle-aged men with dyslipidemia. N Engl J Med 317:1237, 1987.
9. Gordon T, Castelli WP, Hjortland MC, et al: Predicting coronary heart disease in middle-aged and older persons: the Framingham Study. JAMA 238:497, 1977.
10. Kannel WB, Gordon T: Evaluation of cardiovascular risk in the elderly: the Framingham Study. Bull NY Acad Med 45:573, 1978.
11. Kreisberg RA, Kasim S: Cholesterol metabolism and aging. Am J Med 82(Suppl 1B):54, 1987.
12. Lipid Research Clinics Program: The Lipid Research Clinics coronary primary prevention trial results. JAMA 241:351, 1984.

CHRONIC CORONARY ARTERY DISEASE—DIAGNOSIS AND MEDICAL THERAPY

13. Balady GD, Weiner DA, Rothendler JA, et al: Arm exercise-thallium imaging testing for the detection of coronary artery disease. J Am Coll Cardiol 9:84, 1984.
14. Beller G: Nuclear cardiology: current indications and clinical usefulness. In O'Rourke RA, ed: Current problems in cardiology 10(10), Chicago, Yearbook Medical Publishers, 1985, pp 1–76.
15. Boucher CA, Brester DC, Darling RC, et al: Determination of cardiac risk by dipyridamole-thallium imaging before peripheral vascular surgery. N Engl J Med 312:389, 1985.
16. Cairns JA, Gent M, Singer J, et al: Aspirin, sulfinpyrazone, or both in unstable angina: results of a Canadian multicenter trial. N Engl J Med 313:1369, 1985.
17. Covinsky JD: New therapeutic modalities for the treatment of elderly patients with ischemic heart disease. Am J Med 82(Suppl 1B):41, 1987.
18. Coy KM, Imperi GA, Lambert CR, et al: Silent myocardial ischemia during daily activities in asymptomatic men with positive exercise test response. Am J Cardiol 59:45, 1987.
19. Deanfield JE, Maseri A, Seluyn AP, et al: Myocardial ischemia during daily life in patients with stable angina: its relation to symptoms and heart rate changes. Lancet 2:753, 1983.
20. Detry JMR, Melin JA, Derwael-Barchy C, et al: Role of exercise testing and stress thallium scintigraphy in the management of old men with suspected or documented coronary artery disease. Eur Heart J 5(Suppl E):75, 1984.
21. Diamond GA, Forrester JS: Analysis of probability as an aid in the clinical diagnosis of coronary artery disease. N Engl J Med 300:1350, 1979.
22. Francisco DA, Collins SM, Go RT, et al: Tomographic thallium—201 myocardial perfusion scintigrams after maximal coronary artery vasodilation with intravenous dipyridamole: comparison of qualitative and quantitative approaches. Circulation 66:370, 1982.
23. Glover DR, Robinson CS, Murray RG: Diagnostic exercise testing in 104 patients over 65 years of age. Eur Heart J 5(Suppl E):59, 1984.
24. Lakatta EG, Mitchell JA, Pomerance A, et al: Human aging: changes in structure and function. In 18th Bethesda conference: cardiovascular disease in the elderly. J Am Coll Cardiol 10(Suppl A):42A, 1987.
25. Lakatta EG: Diminished beta-adrenergic modulation of cardiovascular function in advanced age. Cardiol Clin 4:185, 1986.
26. Lewis HD, Davis JW, Archibald DG, et al: Protective effects of aspirin against acute myocardial infarction and death in men with unstable angina: results of a Veterans' Administration cooperative study. N Engl J Med 309:396, 1983.
27. Luchi RJ, Scott SM, Deupree RH, et al: Comparison of medical and surgical treatment for unstable angina pectoris: results of a Veterans' Administration Cooperative Study. N Engl J Med 316:977, 1987.
28. National Cooperative Study Group: Unstable angina pectoris: National Cooperative Study Group to compare surgical and medical therapy. II. Am J Cardiol 42:839, 1978.
29. Port S, Cobb FR, Coleman RE, et al: Effect of age on the response of the left ventricular ejection fraction to exercise. N Engl J Med 303:1133, 1980.
30. Rodeheffer RJ, Gerstenblith G, Becker LG, et al: Exercise cardiac output is maintained with advancing age in healthy human subjects: cardiac dilatation and increased stroke volume compensate for a diminished heart rate. Circulation 69:203, 1984.
31. Vasilomanolakis E, Damian A, Mahan G, et al: Treadmill stress testing in geriatric patients. (Abstract) J Am Coll Cardiol 3(2):520, 1984.
32. Vasilomanolakis E: Geriatric cardiology: when exercise stress testing is justified. Geriatrics 40(12):47, 1985.

PERCUTANEOUS TRANSLUMINAL CORONARY ANGIOPLASTY IN THE ELDERLY

33. Dorros G, Janke L: Percutaneous transluminal coronary angioplasty in patients over the age of 70 years. Cathet Cardiovasc Diagn 12:223, 1986.
34. Mock MB, Holmes DR, Vliestra RE, et al: Percutaneous transluminal coronary angioplasty (PTCA) in the elderly patient: experience in the National Heart, Lung, and Blood Institute PTCA registry. Am J Cardiol 53:89C, 1984.
35. Taylor GJ, Rabinovich E, Mikell FL, et al: Percutaneous transluminal coronary angioplasty as palliation for patients considered poor surgical candidates. Am Heart J 111:840, 1986.

CORONARY ARTERY BYPASS SURGERY IN THE ELDERLY

36. CASS Principal Investigators: Coronary Artery Surgery Study (CASS): a randomized trial of coronary artery bypass surgery: survival data. Circulation 68:939, 1983.
37. European Coronary Surgery Study Group: Long-term results of prospective randomized study of coronary artery bypass surgery in stable angina pectoris. Lancet 2:1173, 1982.
38. Gersh BJ, Kronmal RA, Frye RL, et al: Coronary arteriography and coronary artery bypass surgery: morbidity and mortality in patients age 65 years or older: a report from the Coronary Artery Surgery Study. Circulation 67:483, 1983.
39. Gersh BJ, Kronmal RA, Schaff HV, et al: Comparison of coronary artery bypass surgery and medical therapy in patients 65 years of age or older: a nonrandomized study from the Coronary Artery Surgery Study (CASS) registry. N Engl J Med 313:217, 1985.
40. Knapp WS, Douglas JS Jr, Craver JM, et al: Efficacy of coronary artery bypass grafting in elderly patients with coronary artery disease. Am J Cardiol 47:923, 1981.
41. Kunis R, Greenberg H, Yeoh CB, et al: Coronary revascularization for recurrent pulmonary edema in elderly patients with ischemic heart disease and preserved ventricular function. N Engl J Med 313:1207, 1985.
42. Murphy ML, Hultgren HN, Detre K, et al: Treatment of chronic stable angina: a preliminary report of survival data of the randomized Veterans' Administration Cooperative Study. N Engl J Med 297:621, 1977.
43. Rahimtoola SH, Grunkemeier GL, Starr A: Ten-year survival after coronary artery bypass surgery for angina in patients aged 65 years and older. Circulation 74:509, 1986.

ACUTE MYOCARDIAL INFARCTION IN THE ELDERLY

44. Ades PA, Hanson JS, Gunther PG, et al: Exercise conditioning in the elderly coronary patient. J Am Geriatr Soc 35:121, 1987.
45. Aronow WS: Prevalence of presenting symptoms of recognized acute myocardial infarction and of unrecognized healed myocardial infarction in elderly patients. Am J Cardiol 60:1182, 1987.
46. Bayer AJ, Chadha JS, Farag RR, et al: Changing presentation of myocardial infarction with increasing age. J Am Geriatr Soc 34:263, 1986.
47. Beta-Blocker Heart Attack Trial Research Group: A randomized trial of propranolol in patients with acute myocardial infarction. JAMA 247:1707, 1982.
48. Gibson RS, Boden WE, Theroux P, et al: Diltiazem and reinfarction in patients with non–Q-wave myocardial infarction: results of a double-blind, randomized, multicenter trial. N Engl J Med 315:423, 1986.
49. GISSI Study Group: Effectiveness of intravenous thrombolytic treatment in acute myocardial infarction. Lancet 1:297, 1986.
50. Gundersen T, Abrahamsen AM, Kjekshus J, et al: Timolol-related reduction in mortality and reinfarction in patients ages 65–75 years surviving acute myocardial infarction. Circulation 66:1179, 1982.
51. Heller GV, Blaustein AS, Wei JY: Implications of increased myocardial isoenzyme level in the presence of normal serum creatine kinase activity. Am J Cardiol 51:24, 1983.
52. Hill RD, Glazer MD, Wenger NK: Myocardial infarction in the elderly. In Hurst JW, ed: Clinical Essays on the Heart, Vol 5. New York, McGraw-Hill Co, 1985, p 293.
53. Hong RA, Licht JD, Wei JY, et al: Elevated CK-MB with normal total creatine kinase in suspected myocardial infarction: associated clinical findings and early prognosis. Am Heart J 111:1041, 1986.
54. Kannel WB, Abbott RD: Incidence and prognosis of unrecognized myocardial infarction: an update on the Framingham Study. N Engl J Med 311:1144, 1984.
55. Latting CA, Silverman ME: Acute myocardial infarction in hospitalized patients over age 70. Am Heart J 100:311, 1980.
56. Lew AS, Hod H, Cercek B, et al: Mortality and morbidity rates of patients older and younger than 75 years with acute myocardial infarction treated with intravenous streptokinase. Am J Cardiol 59:1, 1987.
57. Norwegian Multicenter Study Group: Timolol-induced reduction in mortality and reinfarction in patients surviving acute myocardial infarction. N Engl J Med 304.801, 1981.
58. Olmsted WL, Groden DL, Silverman ME: Prognosis in survivors of acute myocardial infarction occurring at age 70 years or older. Am J Cardiol 60:971, 1987.
59. Pathy MS: Clinical presentation of myocardial infarction in the elderly. Br Heart J 29:190, 1967.
60. Pina IL, Smith EV, Castellanos A: Post-myocardial infarction exercise testing in elderly patients. Prac Cardiol 13(7):117, 1987.
61. Sugiuva M, Ohkawa S, Hiraoka K, et al: Clinicopathologic aspects of ischemic heart disease in the elderly. Japan Heart J 22:15, 1981.
62. Weintraub RM, Wei JY, Thurer RL: Surgical repair of remediable post infarction cardiogenic shock in the elderly: early and long-term results. J Am Geriatr Soc 34:389, 1986.
63. Williams MA, Maresh CM, Esterbrooks DJ: Early exercise training in patients older than age 65 years compared with that in younger patients after acute myocardial infarction or coronary bypass grafting. Am J Cardiol 55:263, 1985.

CHAPTER 26

Congestive Heart Failure

JoAnn Lindenfeld

Father Time is not always a hard parent, and, though he tarries for none of his children, often lays his hand lightly on those who have used him well.
                                    DICKENS, *Barnaby Rudge*

Congestive heart failure is an increasingly common cause of morbidity and mortality in the United States. It is a particular problem in the elderly, as 75 percent of all patients with congestive heart failure are over the age of 60.[1] The incidence of heart failure rises exponentially with age. New cases appear annually at the rate of 1.8 and 0.8 per 1000 in men and women, respectively, between the ages of 45 and 54, and the rate doubles with each succeeding decade.[2] Although the incidence of heart failure in the elderly primarily reflects the increasing incidence of underlying diseases such as coronary artery disease and hypertensive heart disease, the occurrence of heart failure carries a particularly bad prognosis whatever the underlying disease. The annual mortality for all patients with heart failure is 10 to 20 percent, and for those patients with symptoms of heart failure at rest (patients classified as New York Heart Association Class IV) the annual mortality is 50 percent.[3]

CARDIOVASCULAR CHANGES WITH AGING

Because a number of diseases increase in frequency with age, it has been very difficult to separate changes in the cardiovascular system that occur as a result of aging alone from those that result from underlying diseases. Disease processes may affect cardiovascular function by involving the heart directly or by affecting other organ systems, resulting in physical inactivity and cardiovascular deconditioning. Thus, although older studies reported a significant decline in cardiovascular function with age, more recent studies done carefully to exclude underlying diseases have reported little change caused solely by aging. Therefore, symptoms of congestive heart failure should not be attributed to age alone.

Age-related morphologic changes in the myocardium are few.[4] In general, experienced pathologists cannot discern age from microscopic examination of the myocardium. Macroscopic changes in the healthy elderly are nearly as subtle. Heart size is not changed with age alone, but there is a gradual, mild increase in left ventricular wall thickness, although it is not enough of a change to be classified as ventricular hypertrophy.[5] Systolic or contractile function does not appear to be significantly affected by aging. Mild changes in diastolic function do occur with a decrease in early diastolic filling, compensated for by an increase in late diastolic filling (the atrial portion of filling).[5, 6] These changes in diastolic filling have been postulated to result from diminished myocardial compliance, increased isovolumic relaxation time in the ventricle, and mild sclerosis of the mitral valve.

Age-related changes in the vascular bed are somewhat more prominent.[7] These changes appear first in the proximal aorta. There is gradual medial thickening, with fragmentation of elastic tissue and calcification of the media. The thickening of the media in the proximal aorta primarily results from the increased elastic lamina, whereas the media of the distal aorta enlarges because of smooth muscle proliferation. The changes in the wall of the aorta lead to progressive dilation and elongation. Elasticity is lost, and there is less contraction of the aorta during diastole. Thus, pulse pressure is increased, and the left ventricle faces an increased load with the larger volume of blood in the aorta in systole. This may explain the gradual thickening of the myocardial wall with age.

Resting heart rate does not change with age, but maximum heart rate declines by about one beat per year.[8] The maximum heart rate can be estimated by subtracting one's age from 220. Despite a diminished maximum heart rate, resting and exercise cardiac output do not decrease in healthy elderly subjects who have been carefully screened to exclude heart disease.[9] Increases in end-diastolic volume and stroke volume compensate for the decrease in heart rate. Earlier studies had shown a significant decrease in cardiac output with age caused by both the decreased maximum heart rate and a decline in stroke volume. However, in many of the elderly subjects in at least one of these studies, ejection fraction decreased below the resting value during exercise.[10] This was most likely a result of the presence of occult coronary disease, as shown by a more recent study in patients carefully screened for coronary disease with thallium exercise testing. In this study, ejection fraction actually increased with exercise, although the increase was not as great as that in younger subjects.[9] Despite the maintenance of cardiac output in the elderly, there is a fall in maximum exercise capacity as measured by maximum oxygen uptake (VO_{2max}) because of a decline in the arteriovenous oxygen difference ($A-VO_2$).

The elderly demonstrate alterations in functioning of the autonomic nervous system.[11] There is an attenuation of the baroreceptor reflex response with both hypotension and hypertension. In the normal individual, a fall in blood pressure is registered as a decrease in stretch of the baroreceptors in the carotid arteries. The response is a withdrawal of parasympathetic tone, with an increase in both heart rate and sympathetic activity. This causes an increase in heart rate and inotropic effect and vasoconstriction—all designed to maintain blood pressure and cerebral perfusion.[12] This system allows the normal person to stand up with only small increases in heart rate and little change in blood pressure.

In the elderly, the baroreceptor reflex is attenuated; thus, in some elderly patients, there may be a significant fall in blood pressure with standing. Despite this fall in blood pressure, heart rate does not increase as much as expected to compensate for the blood pressure decline. However, in the absence of other problems, many older people maintain a normal blood pressure with standing.[13] Baroreceptor attenuation is only manifest when there is an additional stress in the system such as volume depletion. The addition of even mild diuresis may result in significant orthostatic hypotension (Fig. 26–1).[13] The defect in baroreceptor function seems to be most closely related to the supine blood pressure; that is, the higher the supine blood pressure, the more significant the baroreceptor defect. This may be caused by the known baroreceptor dysfunction associated with atherosclerosis and hypertension.

In some elderly subjects, eating may result in orthostatic hypotension.[14] The exact cause of baroreceptor dysfunction in the elderly is not entirely clear and may be multifactorial, involving decreased vascular elasticity with decreased stretch of

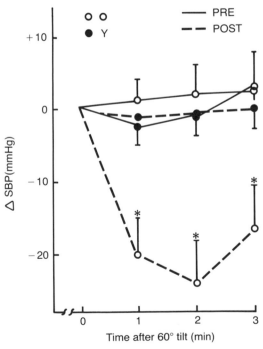

FIGURE 26–1. *Change in systolic blood pressure (SBP) during upright tilt (60°) in six young (Y) and six old (O) healthy adults before (PRE) and after (POST) modest diuresis. Asterisk indicates significant change from prediuresis values (P<0.02). (From Shannon RP, Wei JY, Rosa RM, et al: Hypertension 8:438, 1986; by permission.)*

the baroreceptors, altered parasympathetic activity, and decreased cardiovascular responsiveness to beta-adrenergic agonists.[11] The diminished responsiveness to beta-adrenergic agents has been demonstrated in the elderly in a number of situations and may be the reason for the smaller increase in ejection fraction with exercise in the healthy elderly subject than that in younger subjects.[9]

DEFINITION AND ETIOLOGY

Heart failure is not a disease itself, but a syndrome, or complex of signs and symptoms. It is most often defined as the inability (caused by a cardiac abnormality) to meet the oxygen demands of the body. Some patients, however, are primarily limited by symptoms resulting from pulmonary venous or systemic venous congestion. Thus, it is reasonable to expand the definition of heart failure to include patients who have symptoms of inadequate oxygen delivery, pulmonary or systemic venous congestion, or both. It is particularly important to realize that this complex of signs and symptoms recognized as heart failure may result from a number of diseases that affect the heart in different ways. Pressure or volume overload of the myocardium, loss of myocardium, diminished contractility of myocardium, or restricted filling of the myocardium may lead to heart failure individually or in combination.

In Table 26–1 are listed the most common causes of heart failure by disease

TABLE 26–1. Common Causes of Heart Failure in the Elderly

Ischemic heart disease

Hypertensive heart disease

Valvular heart disease
  Rheumatic
  Other
    Calcific degenerative aortic stenosis
    Calcification of the mitral annulus

Cardiomyopathy
  Idiopathic
  Hypertrophic
  Restrictive (amyloid)

Endocarditis
  Bacterial
  Nonbacterial

Cor pulmonale

process in the elderly. Hypertension and ischemic heart disease, alone or together, are found in about 90 percent of the elderly with heart failure.[1, 2, 15]

The prevalence of hypertension increases with age. The higher the systolic and diastolic pressures, the greater the cardiovascular morbidity and mortality, but in the elderly, elevated systolic pressure alone increases the risk of a major cardiovascular event. Hypertension is a risk factor for coronary artery disease, cerebral vascular event, renal failure, and peripheral vascular disease, as well as for heart failure. The development of left ventricular hypertrophy may lead to diastolic dysfunction and restricted filling of the ventricle.[16, 17] Eventually, the pressure overload on the myocardium may result in decreased contractility and systolic dysfunction.

The incidence of atherosclerotic coronary artery disease also increases in frequency with age. Coronary artery disease may lead to heart failure, with loss of myocardium following a myocardial infarction (MI). In addition, ischemia may result in diastolic dysfunction of the myocardium.

Rheumatic heart disease is still seen in elderly patients. Two other causes of valvular disease, however, are more specific to the elderly. Calcific degenerative aortic stenosis is seen with increased frequency as the population ages. Much less commonly, calcification of the mitral annulus may lead to significant mitral regurgitation.

Cardiomyopathies are generally divided into three types: congestive, hypertrophic, and restrictive.[18] Idiopathic cardiomyopathy seems to be less common in older patients than in younger patients, but it does occur.[18] Hypertrophic cardiomyopathy is not common in the elderly, but as with idiopathic cardiomyopathy, it cannot be excluded on this basis alone. Although infrequent, restrictive cardiomyopathy may be seen more in the elderly than in younger patients because of the increased incidence of amyloid heart disease. In pathologic studies, amyloid is seen frequently in the cardiovascular system of the elderly. However, it appears to be a cause of restrictive disease and heart failure only rarely. Amyloid may be seen in association with multiple myeloma.

In addition, there appear to be three distinct forms of senile amyloidosis with cardiovascular involvement.[19] *Senile atrial amyloidosis* involves only the atria with focal deposits of amyloid, whereas *aortic amyloid* involves only the aorta. The third form, *senile systemic amyloidosis*, involves the atria and ventricles as well as other organ systems, such as the lungs and liver. The specific diagnosis of senile systemic amyloidosis may be made with endomyocardial biopsy and immunohistochemistry.[20] Cor pulmonale is also seen in both elderly and the younger patients.

PATHOPHYSIOLOGY

An understanding of the patient with heart failure requires an understanding of the factors that determine cardiac performance, the compensatory mechanisms that occur when cardiac performance is inadequate, and the necessary balance between myocardial oxygen supply and demand.

Cardiac performance is determined by four major factors: preload, afterload, contractility, and heart rate.[21] As the resting length of myocardial fibers is increased, the force of contraction of these fibers increases. This is called the Frank-Starling effect. The length or stretch of the myocardial fibers is called the *preload*; that is, the load on the heart prior to contraction. It is not possible to measure the length of individual myocardial fibers in an intact patient; thus the intraventricular pressure at end-diastole (the end-diastolic pressure) is used as an estimate of the stretch or preload of the fibers. This is often graphically shown, using a left ventricular function curve in which a measure of the output of the heart is plotted against the end-diastolic pressure (Fig. 26–2A). The left ventricular end-diastolic pressure is frequently referred to as the left ventricular filling pressure. In clinical practice, the left ventricular filling pressure is often estimated by the pulmonary capillary wedge pressure, which is obtained using a Swan-Ganz catheter. As the left ventricular filling pressure increases, the cardiac output increases in both the normal and failing heart (see Fig. 26–2A). However, there is a point at which the left ventricular function curve reaches a plateau. At that point, an increase in preload or left ventricular filling pressure no longer results in an increase in cardiac output.

Afterload refers to the total load against which the heart must eject blood. The afterload is determined by a complex combination of factors, but it is best estimated by the myocardial wall stress, which is a function of the intraventricular pressure, and the ventricular radius divided by the ventricular wall thickness during contraction:

$$\text{wall stress} = P \times R/2h$$

where P is intraventricular pressure, R is the radius of the ventricle, and h is the thickness of the ventricular wall. Thus, wall stress or afterload increases as the intraventricular pressure increases or as the ventricular radius increases and decreases as the ventricular wall thickness increases. In actual practice, wall stress is difficult to measure, and systemic vascular resistance is used as an estimate of afterload in place of wall stress. As afterload or systemic vascular resistance increases, cardiac output decreases and vice versa (see Fig. 26–2B).

Contractility is the intrinsic force of contraction of the myocardial fibers. Myocardial contractility can be changed by many factors. For example, it can be increased by beta-adrenergic agonists, such as isoproterenol, or decreased by diseases that affect the myocardial fibers or by drugs with negative inotropic effects, such as verapamil. The effect of a primary change in contractility is shown in Figure 26–2C. Finally, if all other factors are held constant, cardiac output will increase as heart rate increases.

Typical ventricular function curves describing cardiac performance in a normal person and in patients with various degrees of heart failure are shown in Figure 26–3. (This figure is discussed further in the sections on symptoms and therapy.) It is important to note that in patients with heart failure, cardiac output is below normal at any given level of ventricular filling pressure; however, the determinants of cardiac performance still operate in the same general directions.

A fall in cardiac output initiates a number of compensatory mechanisms, both acute and chronic.[22, 23] There is increased activity of the sympathetic nervous system. This results in an increased *heart rate,*

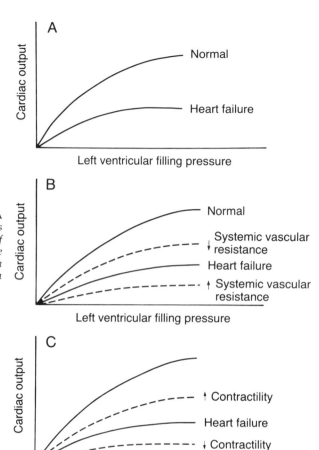

FIGURE 26–2. *Ventricular function curves. A shows a normal ventricular function curve and is described in the text. B demonstrates the effects of increased and decreased systemic vascular resistance on the ventricular function curve of a patient with heart failure. C shows the effects of changes in contractility.*

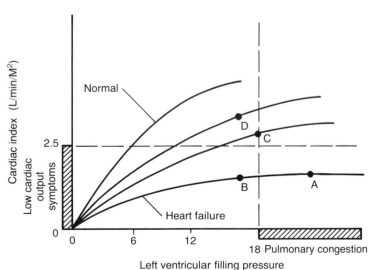

FIGURE 26–3. *Correlation of symptoms with hemodynamics and the effects of various therapeutic interventions in patients with heart failure as demonstrated by use of ventricular function curves. As cardiac index falls below 2.5 L/min/M² at rest, patients begin to note low output symptoms. Left ventricular filling pressures above 18 mm Hg are correlated with symptoms of pulmonary congestion. For description of points A-D see text. (From Miller RR: Ventricular afterload; reducing agents in congestive heart failure. In Mason DT, ed: Congestive Heart Failure. New York, Yorke Medical Books, 1976, p 358; by permission.)*

increased contractility of the myocardium, and increased vascular tone. The first two improve cardiac output, whereas increased vascular tone ensures that blood flow will be maintained to vital organs such as the brain. In general these compensatory events constitute a beneficial response, but increased heart rate and contractility can increase myocardial oxygen demand, whereas increased vascular resistance can increase afterload. Activity of the renin-angiotensin-aldosterone axis also increases in patients with heart failure, resulting in salt and water retention, as well as in vasoconstriction. With salt and water retention, preload is increased, thus increasing contractility of the heart. However, if preload increases too much, there may be pulmonary venous congestion resulting in dyspnea. Increases in other neurohumoral factors, such as vasopressin and atrial natriuretic peptide, may also be important in some patients.[24, 25] If the marked vasoconstriction that occurs in patients with heart failure can be decreased without causing a decrease in blood flow to vital organs, cardiac performance may improve. This is the basis for the use of vasodilators in heart failure.

When cardiac dysfunction and salt and water retention continue, ventricular dilatation may serve as an additional compensatory mechanism. As the ventricle dilates, the end-diastolic volume increases. This serves to maintain resting cardiac output, despite a decrease in ejection fraction. For example, the normal ventricle has an end-diastolic volume of 100 ml and an ejection fraction of 60 percent, thus the stroke volume is 60 ml. If the ventricle dilates to an end-diastolic volume of 200 ml and the ejection fraction is 30 percent, the stroke volume is still 60 ml.[26] However, just as with other compensatory mechanisms, ventricular dilatation may be detrimental. As the ventricular radius increases, so does ventricular wall stress. If the ventricle can hypertrophy, wall stress may return to normal, but some disease processes limit myocardial hypertrophy.

Finally, it is important to understand that there is a necessary balance between myocardial oxygen supply and demand. If demand increases without a concomitant increase in supply, myocardial function may worsen. Tachycardia, increased sympathetic activity, and ventricular dilatation all increase myocardial oxygen demands. Hypotension may limit myocardial oxygen supply. These factors assume particular importance in patients with coronary artery disease because myocardial oxygen supply is already limited by obstruction of the coronary arteries.

It is easy to see that compensatory mechanisms in heart failure may not always be beneficial. With a sudden fall in cardiac output, compensatory mechanisms may serve to maintain perfusion of vital organs, such as the heart and brain, while limiting flow to less vital organs. However, in the chronic situation, salt and water retention with pulmonary congestion and edema, vasoconstriction, and tachycardia all may impose an increased burden on the heart.

SIGNS AND SYMPTOMS

The symptoms of heart failure fall into three general categories—those of low output, those of pulmonary or systemic venous congestion, or both. Signs of low output occur when blood flow and thus oxygen delivery to various organs are limited. If blood flow to skeletal muscle is not increased with exercise, muscle fatigue results, and when blood flow to the brain is compromised, confusion and somnolence are seen. When ventricular end-diastolic pressure increases markedly, there is an increase in pulmonary venous pressures, causing pulmonary interstitial edema and dyspnea. Salt and water retention, combined with failure of the right ventricle and elevated systemic venous pressure, leads to peripheral edema and, if severe enough, to hepatic and splanchnic congestion. These symptoms can be better understood when superimposed on a ventricular function curve (see Fig. 26–3). Most patients with heart failure have symptoms of both low output and pulmonary congestion. However, patients may be more bothered by one set of symptoms than another, depending on the underlying disease, the duration of the disease, the compensatory mechanisms, the level of activity, and the treatment.

Early in heart failure, symptoms may occur only with significant exercise, but as heart failure progresses, symptoms may appear with mild exercise. Patients with severe heart failure may have symptoms at rest. This has led to a clinical classification of heart failure called the New York Heart Association Classification (Table 26–2).

A number of factors may obscure the symptoms of heart failure in the elderly. Older patients often have several diseases; thus, dyspnea may be caused by lung disease, and nocturia may result from benign prostatic hypertrophy. Limitations in physical activity because of arthritis or other problems may prevent exertional symptoms of heart failure. Elderly patients may have an altered respiratory drive and thus may not report dyspnea, but rather a chronic, nonproductive cough or other complaint. Finally, mental confusion is a common presenting sign of a variety of serious illnesses in the aged, and this may make it difficult to obtain an adequate history.[27]

The physical examination in heart failure is determined by the etiology and severity of the underlying disease as well as by compensatory mechanisms. The signs of heart failure are not particularly different between older and younger patients. There may be signs specific to the underlying disease, such as a murmur of mitral or aortic stenosis or the peripheral signs of endocarditis. A fourth heart sound is frequently heard in the elderly, reflecting the diminished compliance of the ventricle, but not necessarily indicating heart failure. A third heart sound is definitely abnormal in this age group and usually indicates heart failure. Rales and pleural effusion may be found. If there is right ventricular failure, gallop sounds may be heard over the right ventricle, usually along the left sternal border or in the subxiphoid area. These are usually accompanied by jugular venous distention. As heart failure progresses, various degrees of edema, ascites, and hepatomegally may occur. With severe heart failure, pulsus alternans or Cheyne-Stokes respiration may be observed.

DIAGNOSIS

The diagnosis of heart failure is usually made by the appropriate signs and symptoms. The electrocardiogram (ECG) is nonspecific, but it may give clues to the underlying diagnosis with Q waves or findings of left ventricular hypertrophy. The chest x-ray is often quite helpful by documenting pulmonary venous congestion and heart size. A number of other diagnostic tests can document underlying left ventricular dysfunction as well as provide clues to the specific disease process. Many of the patients who present with typical signs and symptoms of congestive heart failure have normal or near-normal left ventricular function.[28, 29] It is helpful to recognize these patients with diastolic dysfunction because therapy is often different than that in patients with systolic dysfunction. Radionuclide and echocardiographic-Doppler studies can differentiate systolic and diastolic dysfunction. These studies may also show specific localized ventricular wall motion abnormalities and ventricular aneurysms that suggest coronary artery disease. The echocardiographic-Doppler studies provide evidence for valve pathology, myocardial hypertrophy, and hypertrophic cardiomyopathy and, occasionally, may suggest amyloid

TABLE 26–2. New York Heart Association Functional Classification

Clinical Classification	Description of Symptoms
I	Patients with cardiac disease but without resulting limitations of physical activity. Ordinary physical activity does not cause undue fatigue, palpitation, dyspnea, or anginal pain.
II	Patients with cardiac disease resulting in slight limitation of physical activity. Patients are comfortable at rest. Ordinary physical activity results in fatigue, palpitation, dyspnea, or anginal pain.
III	Patients with cardiac disease resulting in marked limitation of physical activity. Patients are comfortable at rest. Less than ordinary physical activity causes fatigue, palpitation, dyspnea, or anginal pain.
IV	Patients with cardiac disease resulting in inability to carry on any physical activity without discomfort. Symptoms of cardiac insufficiency or of anginal syndrome may be present, even at rest. If any physical activity is undertaken, discomfort is increased.

infiltration.[30, 31] Exercise testing, with or without thallium-201, can document underlying coronary artery disease. In some patients, ambulatory ECG monitoring may give evidence of silent ischemia.[32] Cardiac catheterization will document coronary artery disease and restrictive or constrictive cardiac disease. Occasionally, myocardial biopsy is necessary to document infiltrative diseases of the myocardium.

MANAGEMENT

The approach to management of the patient with heart failure is outlined in Table 26–3. The first step is to diagnose the underlying disease; in some cases, surgical therapy can correct the underlying disease. Cardiac surgery, valvuloplasty, and coronary angioplasty are all feasible in many older patients. If surgical therapy is not appropriate, the next step is to correct any factors that may have precipitated the heart failure.[33] Potential precipitating factors for heart failure are listed in Table 26–4. Hypertension should be treated (see Chapter 23). Thyrotoxicosis may exacerbate heart failure and ischemia in the elderly, but the diagnosis may not be obvious because the usual associated noncardiovascular findings of thyrotoxicosis may not be evident in the elderly patient. Anemia may impose a volume burden on the heart while decreasing myocardial oxygen delivery. Endocarditis may be more subtle in the elderly than it is in the younger patient, and infections such as pneumonia or urinary tract infections may unmask moderate myocardial dysfunction by increasing myocardial oxygen demands. Arrhythmias, such as atrial fibrillation, should be controlled. As heart failure progresses, infections, arrhythmias, and pulmonary emboli all occur with increasing frequency.

TABLE 26–3. Management of the Patient with Heart Failure

Diagnose underlying disease
Correct precipitating factors
Reduced the workload on the heart
Restrict salt and water intake
Administer diuretics, vasodilators, digoxin
Intravenous dobutamine or amrinone or heart transplantation

TABLE 26–4. Precipitating Factors in Heart Failure

Increased sodium intake
Medication noncompliance
Medication interactions
Concurrent infections
Anemia
Thyroid disease

Increased cardiac workload
    Hypertension
    Increased physical activity
    Emotional stress

Hypoxia
Pulmonary embolism
Arrhythmias
Drug effects
Negative inotropic   Beta-adrenergic blockers; calcium channel blockers; disopyramide; flecainide; amiodarone; alcohol
Sodium retention   Steroids; estrogens; nonsteroidal, anti-inflammatory drugs
Myocardial damage   Anthracyclines

It is critical to ask patients to bring all their medications for inspection. Prescriptions may be confused or duplicated. In addition, there are a number of medications that may depress myocardial function or promote salt and water retention (see Table 26–4). Although it is well known that alcohol may cause a cardiomyopathy, it is less often appreciated that alcohol is a myocardial depressant and that moderate amounts may unmask latent myocardial dysfunction. Elderly patients often use a large number of medications, and interactions between these drugs may alter the pharmacokinetics and thus change the effects of a drug.

Once precipitating factors have been corrected, the next step is to decrease the workload of the heart. If the patient is obese, weight loss will be very helpful. Patients can be instructed to limit activity, but this can promote depression or feelings of isolation, particularly in the elderly. Instead, one or two rest periods each day may be helpful. If possible, emotional causes of stress should also be eliminated.

Therapy is next directed to correct salt and water retention. A careful dietary history may reveal excess sodium intake. Canned and packaged foods that are high in sodium are often a major part of the diet of the elderly. If the sodium content of the diet is high, it should be restricted to 4 grams per day (equivalent to no added salt); however, especially in the elderly, one must be careful that the diet does not become so unpalatable that nutrition is compromised. If sodium restriction is not adequate to relieve symptoms of heart failure, diuretics are extremely valuable.

There are four groups of diuretic drugs used in the treatment of heart failure (Table 26–5). A mild diuretic, such as a thiazide, is often used first. The thiazides cause less natriuresis, and thus less volume depletion, than the loop diuretics; however, they cause as much or more hypokalemia than the loop diuretics.[34] This may be a result of the longer duration of action of the thiazides. The natriuretic effect of thiazides decreases as glomerular filtration rate (GFR) falls below 50 ml/min, and they are ineffective below a GFR of 35 ml/min. It must be remembered that GFR often is decreased in the elderly without an increase in serum creatinine because of a loss of muscle mass.

If a thiazide is not potent enough, several loop diuretics are available. In general, the side effects of the loop diuretics are similar to those of the thiazides. Several factors make the elderly patient susceptible to diuretic-associated hypokalemia. Di-

etary sodium may be increased and dietary potassium decreased, and diuretic action may be prolonged by either diminished renal function or hepatic metabolism. Angiotensin-converting enzyme (ACE) inhibitors do decrease the incidence of hypokalemia in patients with heart failure. Changes in serum magnesium caused by diuretics generally follow changes in serum potassium. Diuretic-induced hyponatremia is also more common in the elderly population. Carbohydrate intolerance and hyperlipidemia are more problematic with thiazides than with the loop diuretics. Hyperuricemia is common with both groups but is rarely symptomatic. It is important to remember that the elderly patient is much more susceptible to orthostatic hypotension because of volume depletion caused by diuretics (see Fig. 26–1).

Part of the diuretic effect of loop agents is an increase in renal medullary blood flow, which is mediated by prostaglandins. Nonsteroidal anti-inflammatory drugs (NSAIDs) block prostaglandin synthesis and may significantly diminish the natriuretic effects of loop diuretics. In patients with very severe heart failure, NSAIDs may actually result in salt and water retention and azotemia.

Potassium-sparing diuretics are not generally used alone in patients with heart failure because they are not potent natriuretic agents. They are most often combined with the thiazides or loop diuretics

TABLE 26–5. Diuretics

Type	Maximum Filtered Na Excreted (%)	Duration of Action of Oral Drug (hr)	Hypokalemia (%)	Usual Dose (p.o.)
Thiazides				
Hydrochlorthiazide	5–8	6–12	5–30	25–100 mg/d
Chlorthiazide	5–8	6–12	5–30	500–1000 mg/d
Chlorthalidone	5–8	48–72	5–30	25–100 mg/d
Metolazone	5–8	12–24	20–30 or greater	5–10 mg/d
Loop				
Furosemide	20–25	4–6	5–15	20–1000 mg/d
Bumetanide	20–25	4–6	5–15	6–20 mg/d
Ethacrynic acid	20–25	6–8	5–15	50–150 mg/d
Potassium-Sparing				
Spironolactone	2–3	72–96	K-sparing	25–100 mg/d
Triamterene	2–3	7–9	K-sparing	100–300 mg/d
Amiloride	2–3	24	K-sparing	5–10 mg/d
Carbonic Anhydrase Inhibitors				
Acetazolamide	3–5	8–12	Unknown, but does occur	250–500 mg/d

(Modified from Puschett JB: Clinical pharmacologic implications in diuretic selection. Am J Cardiol 57:6A, 1986.)

to preserve potassium. They should be used carefully in the elderly, who are more susceptible to hyperkalemia and hypokalemia. If potassium-sparing diuretics are necessary, patients should be instructed to avoid potassium supplements and potassium-containing salt substitutes (which may have 50 to 60 meq of potassium per teaspoon). The combination of potassium-sparing diuretics and either ACE inhibitors or NSAIDs should be avoided because life-threatening hyperkalemia can result.

Acetazolamide is used primarily in patients with heart failure when a metabolic alkalosis complicates diuretic therapy, but significant salt and water retention persists. Often, only a few doses are necessary to restore acid-base balance.

The therapeutic benefit of diuretics in heart failure is a result of the decrease in salt and water retention, with a decrease in preload and symptoms of pulmonary and systemic venous congestion. This is demonstrated on a ventricular function curve as shown in Figure 26–3A and B. However, some data suggest that diuretics may actually lead to an improvement in left ventricular function by one of several mechanisms such as direct vasodilator action, improved oxygenation, decrease in vascular rigidity, and decrease in myocardial wall stress.

If moderate diuresis is not adequate, the next step is administration of either digitalis glycosides or vasodilators. The "right" choice is not automatic and depends on the underlying disease, the presence of atrial fibrillation, the patient's ability to take drugs frequently, the cost of the drugs, and the presence of associated diseases.

Digoxin has been used for years in the treatment of congestive heart failure. Its basic effect is to increase myocardial contractility, presumably through its effect on membrane $Na^+ - K^+$ ATPase.[35] Digoxin also slows conduction through the atrioventricular node; thus, digoxin is particularly useful in patients with atrial fibrillation and a rapid ventricular response. There is considerable controversy about the value of digoxin in patients with heart failure and normal sinus rhythm. If patients are chosen correctly (that is, if they have significant systolic dysfunction), they may experience a mild beneficial response.[36] However, patients with diastolic dysfunction or restricted filling are not likely to have a beneficial response.

Digoxin can be given once a day—a particular convenience in the older patients—but there are a number of factors that make digoxin more difficult to use in this age group. Lean body mass decreases with age, making the volume of distribution for digoxin lower. Renal function gradually declines with age, decreasing digoxin elimination. Thus, both the loading dose and maintenance dose of digoxin need to be decreased in the elderly. An average maintenance dose is 0.125 to 0.25 mg per day. Although some animal data suggest that the inotropic effect of digoxin may be reduced in the aged, it is not clear that this is true in humans. It does appear, however, that older patients are more susceptible to the toxic effects of digoxin. This is probably primarily caused by the decreased dosage requirements but may also be a result of the increased frequency of other factors that predispose to digoxin toxicity. An example is the larger number of drugs taken by older patients, thus increasing the possibility of drug interactions.

Factors that seem to predispose a patient to digoxin toxicity are listed in Table 26–6. Hypokalemia is a common problem in patients with heart failure because of diuretic use. If hypokalemia is present in a patient on digoxin, potassium replacement is mandatory. Diuretic-induced hypomagnesemia may also predispose to digoxin toxicity. Patients with chronic lung disease seem to have an increased incidence of digoxin toxicity, perhaps because of hypoxia or because drugs commonly used to treat this condition may sensitize the myocardium to the effects of digoxin. Patients with hypothyroidism are resistant to the

TABLE 26–6. Predisposing Factors for Digoxin Toxicity

Electrolyte abnormalities
Hypokalemia
Hypomagnesemia
Hyponatremia
Hyperkalemia
Renal failure
Pulmonary disease
Thyroid disease
Increasing age
Multiple drug therapy

effects of digoxin. Finally, patients with amyloid heart disease may be at particular risk for digoxin toxicity, possibly because digoxin binds to the amyloid fibrils.

Toxicity is most often manifested as an increase in arrhythmias. These may be of any variety, but they are often premature ventricular beats. Central nervous system symptoms such as confusion, hallucinations, or visual disturbances and gastrointestinal symptoms such as nausea or anorexia may suggest digoxin toxicity. If manifestations of digoxin toxicity are life-threatening, digoxin antibodies are a fast-acting and safe therapy.[35]

A number of drugs interact with digoxin to alter either the pharmacokinetics or the pharmacodynamics. In Table 26–7 are listed most of the drug interactions that affect the pharmacokinetic interactions of digoxin. All drugs that affect sinus node function or atrioventricular nodal function, alone or in combination with digoxin, may have greater than expected effects in the elderly.

In the last several years, there have been significant developments in the use of vasodilators for heart failure. These drugs have been shown to relieve symptoms, improve exercise capacity, and prolong

survival. Vasodilators can cause venous vasodilation, which increases venous capacitance and arteriolar vasodilation, which causes a decrease in systemic vascular resistance, or both. When vasodilators affect both the veins and arterioles, they are said to be mixed vasodilators. The effects of a vasodilator affecting primarily the venous system is shown in Figure 26–3, points A to B, and are similar to the effects of a diuretic. The average effect of a mixed vasodilator is represented in Figure 26–3, points A to D, and can be compared with the average effect of digoxin shown from points A to C.

Nitrates have effects on both the venous and arteriolar system but are predominantly venous vasodilators. Various forms of nitrates have been shown to be effective in reducing symptoms and prolonging exercise capacity in patients with heart failure. Recently nitrates, in combination with hydralazine, have been shown to improve mortality in patients with heart failure.[37] Almost any form of nitrate preparation may be used, but higher doses may be required in patients with heart failure than in patients with angina pectoris. Tolerance develops quickly to the hemodynamic effects of nitrates when transdermal patches

TABLE 26–7. Drug Interactions with Digoxin

Drug	Effect on Digoxin Pharmacokinetics	Change in Digoxin (%)	Suggested Remedy
Cholestyramine	Absorption	25	Give digoxin 8 hr before cholestyramine or use digoxin capsules
Kaolin pectate; Bran	Absorption	20	Separate by 2 hr
Antacids	Unknown	25	Separate by 2 hr
Neomycin; sulfasalazine; PAS	Unknown	18–22	Measure serum digoxin; increase digoxin dose if necessary
Erythromycin; tetracycline (10%)	Decreases intestinal metabolism	43–116	Measure serum digoxin; decrease dose; use digoxin capsules
Quinidine	Clearance—renal and nonrenal; volume of distribution and bioavailability	100	Decrease digoxin by 50%; measure serum digoxin at 1 week
Verapamil	Renal and nonrenal clearance	70–100	Same as for quinidine
Amiodarone	Renal and nonrenal clearance	70–100	Same as for quinidine
Diltiazem	Unknown renal clearance	0–22	None
Sprionolactone	Renal and nonrenal clearance	30	Measure serum digoxin
Triamterene	Nonrenal clearance	20	Measure serum digoxin

(Adapted from Marcus FI: Pharmacokinetic interactions between digoxin and other drugs. J Am Coll Cardiol 5:82A, 1985.)

are used, but tolerance also develops with other forms of nitroglycerin. Tolerance may be prevented by giving nitroglycerin at less frequent intervals. If patients have symptoms predominantly during one part of the day, nitrate therapy could be given for that time only. A drug-free interval of 8 to 12 hours seems to prevent the development of tolerance.

Hydralazine is a direct-acting vasodilator that has its effect on arterioles, thus decreasing vascular resistance. Hydralazine, when used alone, has not proven to be efficacious in the long-term management of patients with heart failure. When combined with nitrates, however, hydralazine does improve exercise capacity and survival. It is not clear whether hydralazine adds to the beneficial effects of nitrates. The effective dose of hydralazine varies widely among patients with heart failure, with effective doses of 25 to 300 mg four times a day. Side effects of hydralazine include hypotension, possible precipitation of ischemic events, and a lupus-like syndrome.

Prazosin, a peripheral alpha-1 adrenergic antagonist, has been widely used in the treatment of heart failure. A drawback is that tolerance appears to develop so commonly that long-term benefits in exercise capacity or mortality have not been clearly demonstrated.

Perhaps the most beneficial group of vasodilators in patients with heart failure is the ACE inhibitor. These drugs have shown consistent improvements in symptoms, exercise capacity, and mortality, with the fewest side effects.[37-39] A recent study with enalapril in patients with an average age of 70 years demonstrated their benefit even in older patients.[38] The most experience has been gained with captopril and enalapril. Captopril is not metabolized but is excreted by the kidneys. Its peak effect occurs in 1 to 2 hours, and its duration of action is 4 to 6 hours. The average dose in patients with heart failure is 25 to 50 mg three times a day. Enalapril requires hepatic conversion to enalaprilat, which is excreted by the kidneys. This prolongs its onset and duration of action. The average dose is 5 to 10 mg twice a day. Both drugs may require less frequent dosing and lower doses in elderly patients with abnormalities in hepatic and/or renal function. Angiotensin-converting enzyme in-

hibitors block the conversion of angiotensin I to angiotensin II, thus relieving vasoconstriction caused by angiotensin II. The decrease in angiotensin II decreases release of aldosterone, thus decreasing salt and water retention. As with most drugs used for the treatment of heart failure, the benefits of ACE inhibitors gradually increase over a period of weeks, and symptomatic improvement should not be expected immediately.

The major side effect of ACE inhibitors in heart failure is hypotension. The hypotension is often asymptomatic but can be a serious problem. Patients most likely to develop serious hypotension are those with the most severe heart failure, particularly those with hyponatremia. Hypotension can be minimized by avoiding volume depletion; thus, if possible, diuretics should be discontinued 24 hours before institution of ACE inhibitors. Other vasodilators should also be withheld while instituting an ACE inhibitor. Patients with severe heart failure should be started on a low dose of drug, either 6.25 mg of captopril or 2.5 mg of enalapril. Blood pressure should be monitored for 1 to 2 hours after the first dose of captopril and for 4 to 6 hours after the first dose of enalapril. Azotemia may also develop in 5 to 15 percent of patients, and renal function should be evaluated after therapy is instituted. Neutropenia and proteinuria are rarely problems in patients without collagen vascular diseases. Dysgeusia, cough, and skin rash are more common with captopril. Tolerance is not a significant problem with the ACE inhibitors.

Angiotensin-converting enzyme inhibitors improve hypokalemia in many patients with heart failure. Therefore, when an ACE inhibitor is instituted, potassium-sparing diuretics should be discontinued, and potassium supplements may need to be modified. NSAIDs may worsen hyperkalemia and azotemia.

Calcium blocking drugs all have vasodilator properties and have thus been tried in patients with heart failure. Verapamil has significant negative inotropic potential and should not be used in patients with severe systolic dysfunction. Nifedipine and diltiazem do not seem to be as beneficial as either ACE inhibitors or nitrates and hydralazine.

A number of experimental drugs with

inotropic and/or vasodilator effects are being evaluated in patients with heart failure. Amrinone is a phosphodiesterase inhibitor that has been approved for intravenous use in patients with heart failure. Its hemodynamic effects seem to be similar to those of dobutamine, but its onset and duration of action are significantly longer. Amrinone did not prove to be effective with long-term oral use. Many other oral phosphodiesterase inhibitors are being evaluated. Oral sympathomimetic drugs have not been proven beneficial in chronic long-term use, at least in part because of the tolerance that develops.

Levodopa (L-dopa) is converted to dopamine in the circulation, and one study has demonstrated both a short-term and a long-term benefit. However, the drug is difficult to use, has a high incidence of side effects, and may result in vasoconstriction in some patients. It should probably be used only in extreme circumstances in patients with heart failure. Other dopamine analogues are in various stages of testing.

When heart failure is refractory, several steps should be taken. There should be reconsideration of precipitating factors, including exacerbation of the underlying disease and drug interactions. Short-term dobutamine infusions may produce symptomatic improvement for several weeks. Heart transplantation has been expanded to include the elderly in some centers.

REFERENCES

1. Smith WM: Epidemiology of congestive heart failure. Am J Cardiol 55:3A, 1985.
2. McKee PA, Castelli WP, Mc Namara PM, et al: The natural history of congestive heart failure. N Engl J Med 285:1441, 1971.
3. Massie BM, Conway M: Survival of patients with congestive heart failure: past, present, and future prospects. Circulation (Suppl IV):11, 1987.
4. Pomerance A: Pathology of the myocardium and valves. In Caird FL, Dalle JLC, Kennedy RD, eds: Cardiology in Old Age. New York, Plenum Press, 1976, p 11.
5. Gerstenblith G, Frederiksen J, Yin FCP, et al: Echocardiographic assessment of a normal adult aging population. Circulation 56:273, 1977.
6. Miyatake K, Okamoto M, Kinoshira N, et al: Augmentation of atrial contribution to left ventricular inflow with aging assessed by intracardiac Doppler flowmetry. Am J Cardiol 53:586, 1984.
7. Yin FCP: The aging vasculature and its effects on the heart. In Weisfeldt ML, ed: The Aging Heart. New York, Raven Press, 1980, p 137.
8. Hossack KR, Bruce RA: maximal cardiac function in sedentary normal men and women: comparison of age-related changes. J Appl Physiol 53:799, 1982.
9. Rodeheffer RS, Gerstenblith G, Becker LC, et al: Exercise cardiac output is maintained with advancing age in healthy human subjects: cardiac dilation and increased stroke volume compensate for a diminished heart rate. Circulation 69:203, 1984.
10. Port S, Cobb FR, Coleman RE, et al: Effect of age on the response of the left ventricular ejection fraction to exercise. N Engl J Med 303:1133, 1980.
11. Lakatta EG: Age-related alterations in the cardiovascular response to adrenergic mediated stress. Fed Proc 39:3173, 1980.
12. Lindenfeld J: Syncope. In Horwitz LD, Groves BM: Signs and Symptoms in Cardiology. Philadelphia, JB Lippincott Co, 1985 p 51.
13. Shannon RP, Wei JY, Rosa RM, et al: The effect of age and sodium depletion on cardiovascular response to orthostasis. Hypertension 8:438, 1986.
14. Lipsitz LA, Nyquist RP, Wei JY, et al: Postprandial reduction in blood pressure in the elderly. N Engl J Med 309:81, 1983.
15. Pomerance A: Pathology of the heart with and without cardiac failure in the aged. Br Heart J 27:697, 1965.
16. Topol EJ, Traill TA, Fortuin NJ: Hypertensive hypertrophic cardiomyopathy of the elderly. N Engl J Med 312:277, 1985.
17. Massie BM: Myocardial hypertrophy and cardiac failure: a complex interrelationship. Am J Med 75:(3A)67, 1983.
18. Shah PM, Abelmann WH, Gersh BJ: Cardiomyopathies in the elderly. J Am Coll Cardiol 10:77A, 1987.
19. Cornwell GG III, Kyoe RA, Westermark P, et al: Frequency and distribution of senile cardiovascular amyloid: a clinicopathologic correlation. Am J Med 75:618, 1983.
20. Olson LJ, Gertz MA, Edwards WD, et al: Senile cardiac amyloidosis with myocardial dysfunction: diagnosis by endomyocardial biopsy and immunohistochemistry. N Engl J Med 317:738, 1987.
21. Braunwald E, Ross J, Sonnenblick E: Mechanisms of contraction in the normal and failing heart. Boston, Little, Brown & Co, 1976, pp 92–130.
22. Zelis R, Flaim SF: Alterations in vasomotor tone in congestive heart failure. Prog Cardiovasc Dis 24:437, 1982.
23. Francis GS, Goldsmith SR, Levine TB, et al: The neurohumoral axis in congestive heart failure. Ann Intern Med 101:370, 1984.
24. Szatalowicz VL, Arnold PE, Chaimovitz C, et al: Radioimmunoassay of plasma arginine vasopressin in hyponatremic patients with congestive heart failure. N Engl J Med 305:263, 1981.
25. Raine AEG, Erne P, Bürgisser E, et al: Atrial natriuretic peptide and atrial pressure in patients with congestive heart failure. N Engl J Med 315:533, 1986.
26. Lindenfeld J, Hammermeister K: Cardiovascular disease. In Schrier R, ed: Medicine: Diagnosis and Treatment. Boston, Little, Brown & Co, 1988, pp 55–56.
27. Howell TH: Causation of diagnostic errors in

octogenarians: a clinico-pathological study. J Am Gerintr Soc 14:41, 1966.

28. Soufer R, et al: Intact systolic function in clinical congestive heart failure. Am J Cardiol 55:1032, 1985.

29. Dougherty AH, Naccarelli GV, Gray EL, et al: Congestive heart failure with normal systolic function. Am J Cardiol 54:778, 1984.

30. Feigenbaum H: Echocardiography. Philadelphia, Lea and Febiger, 1986, pp 514–547.

31. Nishimura RA, Miller FA Jr, Callahan MJ, et al: Doppler echocardiography: theory, instrumentation, technique, and application. Mayo Clin Proc 60:321, 1985.

32. Cohn PF: Silent myocardial ischemia: dimensions of the problem in patients with and without angina. Am J Med 80:(Suppl 4C)3, 1986.

33. Sodeman WA, Burch GE: The precipitating causes of congestive heart failure. Am Heart J 15:22, 1938.

34. Flamenbaum W: Diuretic use in the elderly: po-

tential for diuretic-induced hypokalemia. Am J Cardiol 57:38A, 1986.

35. Smith TW: Digitalis glycosides. Orlando, Grune & Stratton, Inc, 1986, pp 5–27.

36. Arnold SB, Byrd RC, Meister W, et al: Long-term digitalis therapy improves left ventricular function in heart failure. N Engl J Med 303:1443, 1980.

37. Cohn JN, Archibald DG, Ziesche S, et al: Effect of vasodilator therapy on mortality in chronic congestive heart failure: results of a Veterans' Administration cooperative study. N Engl J Med 314:1547, 1986.

38. Captopril Multicentre Research Group: A placebo controlled trial of captopril in refractory heart failure. J Am Coll Cardiol 2:755, 1983.

39. Consensus Trial Study Group: Effects of enalapril on mortality in severe congestive heart failure: results of the Cooperative North Scandinavian Enalapril Survival Study (CONSENSUS). N Engl J Med 316:1429, 1987.

CHAPTER 27

Peripheral Vascular Disease

William R. Hiatt
Judith G. Regensteiner

AGE: its weakness and miseries
Old people have fewer diseases than the young, but
their diseases never leave them.
                    HIPPOCRATES, *Aphorisms*

Peripheral vascular disease (PVD) of the lower extremities is a manifestation of the atherosclerotic disease process. Associations with coronary and cerebral vascular diseases result in an increased mortality in these patients. Clinically, PVD is an important cause of disability in symptomatic patients. This disability may range from limited walking tolerance to limb loss. The loss of functional capacity that results from such disability can be highly detrimental to quality of life, since both leisure and work activities may be severely curtailed. Therefore, because of both the functional limitations that PVD can impose on a patient and the cardiovascular complications, this disease provides the physician with a unique set of patient management problems.

Although the symptom most often associated with PVD is intermittent claudication, more severe forms of the disease may present with other symptoms such as pain in the limb at rest, ischemic ulceration, and gangrene. Claudication, like angina, is an exercise-induced symptom of aching or cramping, but unlike angina, it presents in the calf, thigh, or buttock. With rest, the symptom is relieved within minutes, then is reproducibly brought on again by exercise. The severity of claudication and limitation of exercise performance is directly related to the decrease in leg blood flow caused by atherosclerotic occlusions.[1] With restoration of flow, claudication is relieved and exercise performance returns to normal.[2]

EPIDEMIOLOGY

As with all forms of atherosclerosis, the prevalence of PVD increases with age and is most common in individuals over the age of 55. The average annual incidence for intermittent claudication was 26 in 10,000 for men and 12 in 10,000 for women. This incidence was 25 percent of the rate for new coronary artery disease and therefore represents a substantial number of new cases each year.[3] In a population of retired individuals with an average age of 66, the prevalence of PVD determined by objective noninvasive tests is 12 percent, but increases to 20 percent for subjects over the age of 75.[4] In this same population, the average prevalence of claudication was 6 percent, indicating that many patients with atherosclerosis are asymptomatic or have atypical symptoms.[4, 5]

DIAGNOSIS

Most patients with PVD present to the physician with the symptom of intermittent claudication. Claudication defined by a standard series of questions, however, has a low sensitivity (albeit a high specificity) for PVD, with a positive predictive value of only 50 percent.[7] Pain in the extremities with exercise due to arthritis or musculoskeletal disorders is common in the elderly, and thus a patient with a symptom complex suggesting claudication may or may not have arterial occlusive disease.

On physical examination, the physician should listen for femoral bruits and palpate the femoral artery in the groin and the dorsalis pedis and posterior tibial pulses in the feet. Pulses should be graded as present or absent. Clinically, an absent posterior tibial pulse has the highest sensitivity for PVD, but the predictive value of this finding is similar to that of the symptom of claudication.[7] Other findings on examination such as hair loss, muscle atrophy, and thickened nails are not accurate in the diagnosis of PVD.

The noninvasive vascular laboratory diagnosis of PVD is highly accurate and generally obviates the need for angiography, except for patients who are candidates for surgery or angioplasty. These tests are based on the observation that a hemodynamically significant stenosis or arterial occlusion will result in a drop in pressure (and flow) across the lesion. Thus, in a normal supine individual, the pressure in the ankle should equal the pressure in the arm, whereas in a patient with PVD, the pressure in the ankle is reduced compared with that in the arm. Systolic pressures in the arm and ankle are determined by using a Doppler ultrasonic instrument. To normalize these pressures, a ratio is formed of the ankle to arm systolic pressure. Studies have shown that normal subjects have ratios greater than 0.95, and those with PVD have ratios below this value.[8] In patients with mild PVD, the ankle pressure may be normal at rest, but will become abnormal with walking exercise. Thus, exercise testing is often employed to enhance the sensitivity of the ankle/arm ratio in detecting PVD.[9, 10] These ratios have a sensitivity of 97 percent and a specificity of 96 to 100 percent for angiographically diagnosed PVD.[11] In addition, pressures taken in the thigh and calf can accurately localize the site of disease with nearly 100 percent accuracy.[12]

In summary, the symptom of intermittent claudication and the finding of a femoral bruit or an absent pedal pulse is not always associated with the presence of PVD. Patients with these signs or symptoms should have noninvasive studies performed to obtain both an objective diagnosis of PVD and an assessment of disease severity. The measurement of the ankle systolic pressure with Doppler ultrasonography can be performed by any physician in a clinic setting using inexpensive equipment.

The functional assessment of patients with PVD is based on several factors. Patients may describe the limits of their exertion by the number of blocks walked before claudication pain forces them to stop. This form of assessment has been found to be subjective and poorly reproducible such that treadmill testing is commonly employed for the functional assessment. In this setting, patients walk at a constant workload at a treadmill speed ranging from 1.5 to 3.0 mph and a grade of 10 to 12 percent. During the test, the time of pain onset and time of maximal claudication pain are recorded; thus, the results of an intervention can be judged by whether the patient can walk further without pain as a result of the treatment.[13–15] In our laboratory, we have modified these procedures so that the patient walks on a treadmill with a graded increase in workload until maximal claudication is achieved.[16] Further, in our studies, the measurement of oxygen consumption provides an objective marker of exercise performance. With this approach, objective, highly reproducible information on patient performance and functional status is obtained.

RISK FACTORS

The risk factors for atherosclerosis differ slightly for coronary, cerebral, and peripheral vascular disease. For PVD, the most important factors are diabetes and cigarette smoking, with hypertension and hyperlipidemia assuming roles of lesser importance than with coronary or cerebrovascular disease.

Diabetes

Diabetes is associated with a two-fold increased risk for coronary and cerebrovascular disease but with a four- to five-fold increased risk for PVD.[17] In the diabetic patient, the prevalence of PVD increases 7.5 percent with each decade of disease, and the risk is further magnified in the presence of hypertension, hyperlipidemia, or smoking.[18] Interestingly, the risk of PVD is not affected by the degree of blood sugar control.[19]

The diabetic patient with PVD often has a more distal distribution of atherosclerosis than the nondiabetic patient in that arterial occlusions are often seen in the popliteal and infrapopliteal arteries.[20] Because proximal and distal arterial occlusions are often coexistent, the diabetic patient may present with more severe arterial disease than the nondiabetic patient. There is, however, no evidence that the patient with diabetes has a unique microvascular lesion in the peripheral circulation.[20, 21] Diabetic patients are at an increased risk of developing foot ulcers, infection, and gangrene largely because of the combined insult of neuropathy and arterial occlusive disease.[21]

Cigarette Smoking

The second major risk factor for PVD is smoking. In some series, 60 to 90 percent of patients with severe PVD are smokers.[22, 23] The Framingham Study demonstrated that the risk for PVD is increased two-fold in patients who smoke two packs per day and three-fold in those who smoke more than two packs per day.[24] The rate of progression of arterial occlusions is greatly increased in smokers, whereas the prognosis improves for those who quit.[25]

Hyperlipidemia

A high low-density lipoprotein (LDL) cholesterol and a low high-density lipoprotein (HDL) cholesterol are the traditional lipid patterns associated with coronary artery disease. For PVD, an elevated triglyceride, rather than cholesterol, level is associated with angiographic disease severity.[26] Patients with PVD should have fasting plasma lipids assessed, with particular attention given to the triglyceride level. Further evidence to support this recommendation is the finding that regression of early femoral atherosclerosis is associated with the lowering of plasma triglycerides.[27] Therefore, elevated triglycerides have pathogenic significance for the development of PVD.

Hypertension

An elevated blood pressure is associated with the development of atherosclerosis, particularly in the coronary and cerebral circulation. In the patient with severe PVD, however, a high pressure may help to maintain perfusion across a stenosis. However, given the attendant risks of stroke or congestive heart failure in the hypertensive patient, every attempt must be made to lower the blood pressure, although this treatment may worsen claudication.

NATURAL HISTORY

Patients with PVD often have diffuse atherosclerosis and therefore are at a three- to five-fold increased risk of having concomitant coronary artery disease.[3] The 5-year survival rate in these patients is 74 percent, and the 10-year survival rate is 40 to 60 percent.[28, 29] The risk of a myocardial infarction or stroke is 20 percent at 5 years and 40 percent at 10 years, with the majority of deaths during this time resulting from cardiovascular disease. In a patient with PVD (determined by noninvasive studies), there is a four-fold increased risk of cardiovascular mortality.[30]

Despite the increase in mortality, patients with PVD follow a relatively stable clinical course in terms of their symptoms of claudication. In patients not treated with surgery, 80 percent remain stable, with less than 10 percent progressing to a mandated operation for ischemic pain at rest, ulceration, or gangrene when followed for a period of 5 to 8 years.[25, 31] The number of patients who require surgery for disabling claudication varies from study to study, but it is on average only 20 percent of all patients followed over time. The rate of clinical deterioration is higher in patients who are diabetic, older, have more severe disease, or who continue to smoke.[25]

MEDICAL THERAPY

Risk Factors

All patients with PVD need to be evaluated for the presence of cardiovascular risk factors. Risk factor modification may delay the progression of peripheral atherosclerosis and decrease the risk of coronary and cerebrovascular events.

The diabetic patient should strive for optimal glycemic control, particularly to prevent infection and the progression of distal neuropathy. Coexistent risk factors in the diabetic patient, such as hypertension and hyperlipidemia, may be more than additive for disease progression and must be treated aggressively. Cigarette smoking is highly associated with both the pathogenesis and disease progression of PVD. Although difficult, cessation of smoking is central to the management of these patients. Elevations of both cholesterol and triglycerides should be treated in patients with PVD, but particular attention should be given to elevated triglycerides. Modest to moderate elevations of triglycerides can be treated with a low-calorie diet and weight loss, although more severe elevations may require drug therapy. Finally, patients with hypertension should strive for normalization of the blood pressure, even if claudication is worsened by this therapy. The primary goal is to prevent stroke and congestive heart failure.

Drug Therapy

The pharmacologic treatment of PVD is limited. Vasodilators were once popular and included papaverine, niacin, and isoxsuprine as direct-acting agents and tolazoline, reserpine, and guanethidine as sympatholytic agents. However, these drugs were ineffective in relieving the symptoms of claudication or rest pain and did not result in an increased walking distance in controlled trials.[32] Although these drugs effectively dilate arterioles, they do not dilate large vessels occluded with atherosclerosis or the collaterals. Therefore, patients do not respond to these drugs because there is no increase in total blood flow to the extremity.

Aspirin is a drug commonly used to treat certain manifestations of coronary and cerebrovascular disease. In PVD, there is no role for aspirin, except in the postsurgical patient in whom some trials suggest that this drug may help maintain graft patency.[33] In this setting, aspirin is often combined with low-dose warfarin in patients at risk for graft occlusion.

A class of drugs that have been shown to be effective are those agents that alter blood hemorrheology. Historically, it has been shown that walking distance can be increased when patients with PVD undergo phlebotomy to a hematocrit of 35 percent with replacement of blood volume with saline.[34] Pentoxifylline is a drug that lowers blood fibrinogen, improves red cell deformability, and has antiplatelet effects. Although the mechanism of action is not well established, the drug may improve flow through alterations in viscosity. In a large multicenter trial, pentoxifylline produced a modest, but significant, improvement in walking performance compared with placebo.[13] This is the only drug approved for treatment of intermittent claudication and, as such, should be considered in the treatment of patients with moderate to severe PVD.

SURGICAL THERAPY

For patients with severe PVD who fail to improve with medical therapy, surgery should be considered. Several factors must be carefully evaluated in the potential PVD surgical candidate. The primary indication is the occurrence of manifestations of peripheral ischemia such as pain in the limb at rest, ulceration, or gangrene. Patients with severe ischemia may be at risk for tissue loss and, therefore, are operated on for limb salvage.

In the patient with intermittent claudication who does not have ischemic signs or symptoms, the indication for surgery would be to relieve disability. In this setting, disability would exist when claudication significantly impairs either work or leisure activities. Usually, the physician should first attempt medical therapy and exercise conditioning prior to surgical intervention.

Risk factors for surgery must be carefully assessed in the patient with PVD. Diabetes, hypertension, and chronic obstructive pulmonary disease are common coexisting conditions in these patients that increase the risks posed by surgery. In a series of 1000 patients studied with cardiac catheterization prior to vascular surgery, 32 percent had mild to moderate coronary artery disease, and 60 percent had severe coronary disease.[35] Although coronary artery disease is common, it may be asymptomatic in patients with PVD who are inactive as a result of claudication. Because of the high frequency with which perioperative complications occur in these patients, several clinical predictors of outcome have been evaluated. A prior history of myocardial infarction, congestive heart failure, abnormal electrocardiogram, poor functional class, and old age are all predictors of an increased risk of cardiovascular complications.[36, 37]

For the patient with proximal aortoiliac occlusive disease, surgical therapy is usually very successful. The operative mortality ranges from 2 to 4 percent, but it may be as high as 12 percent in patients over age 70.[38–40] The initial patency rates are 98 to 100 percent, and at 5 and 10 years, rates are 80 to 90 percent and 70 to 80 percent, respectively. If the patient has adequate distal runoff (i.e., the distal vessels are patent), generally this operation provides excellent relief of ischemic signs and symptoms, as well as of claudication.

Surgery for distal occlusive disease (femoropopliteal and infrapopliteal disease) is technically difficult and is performed on patients with greater disease severity than is the case for proximal disease. In general, these patients have surgery on a limb-salvage basis. The operative mortality is approximately 3 percent, but it is higher in diabetic patients.[40–42] Initial patency rates are 90 percent, which is less than rates for proximal disease surgery. When the operation is performed for claudication, patency rates are 74 percent at 5 years and 45 percent at 10 years.[38, 41] When performed for limb salvage, however, the 5-year patency rate is 46 percent, and the 10-year rate is 14 percent.[41] Diabetic patients with femoropopliteal disease have worse patency rates than patients without diabetes and generally are at a higher surgical risk.[42] Therefore, the decision to operate on a diabetic patient is often delayed.

There are several other types of operations available for patients with difficult anatomy for bypass or who are poor surgical risks. The extra-anatomic bypass is most often used in the patient with aortoiliac disease in whom abdominal surgery is contraindicated. For this indication and others, the axillary artery is grafted to the femoral artery via a long subcutaneous graft. Patency rates are less than rates associated with aortoiliac surgery. The in situ bypass is used to treat patients with severe ischemia of the lower extremity who have distal obstructions in the popliteal or infrapopliteal arteries. For this operation, the saphenous vein is used in situ by removing the valves prior to the bypass. The vein is then grafted from the common femoral to the posterior tibial, anterior tibial, or peroneal arteries. Patency rates are generally very acceptable for this operation.

ANGIOPLASTY

Percutaneous transluminal angioplasty is a less invasive procedure than surgical bypass and has become an accepted form of therapy. The indications for this procedure are similar to those for surgery and include patients with both claudication and ischemic signs and symptoms. Often, angioplasty is performed as the initial intervention, with surgery reserved for angioplasty failures and for patients with more extensive and severe disease.

The mortality from angioplasty is less than 0.5 percent. There are few complications, and hospital stay is less than that with surgery.[40, 43] However, initial and 5-year patency rates are lower than rates with surgery performed for a similar disease distribution.[40, 44–46] A number of patients require multiple dilations to maintain patency. The best results occur in patients who have short, proximal lesions.[45] Patients who do not respond well to angioplasty include the elderly, diabetic patients, and patients with distal, extensive disease.[46]

Angioplasty is less effective than surgery, but it is also less expensive and has fewer complications. On a cost-effective basis, angioplasty should be the initial intervention of choice, followed by surgery in the cases not appropriate for angioplasty and for angioplasty failures.[40]

This combined approach would minimize morbidity and mortality and produce acceptable patency rates.

EXERCISE REHABILITATION

Walking exercise has been recommended as a treatment modality for patients with PVD for the past century but has only been systematically used in the last two decades.[47] Numerous studies have now demonstrated the efficacy of exercise conditioning in increasing walking tolerance.[14, 48, 49]

Although all patients with PVD can potentially benefit from walking exercise, it is primarily indicated for those patients who are disabled by their claudication. Before enrolling a patient with PVD in an exercise program, a complete evaluation should be made of health status and fitness level. Generally, a screening history, physical examination, and resting lead-12 electrocardiogram should be performed to determine if there are medical conditions that contraindicate exercise. Patients with PVD should not participate in an exercise program if they have unstable angina, acute myocardial infarction, decompensated congestive heart failure, severe aortic stenosis, complex arrhythmias, pulmonary embolus, systemic infection, or any other severe disorder.

A supervised treadmill walking program has been found to be the most efficacious form of exercise conditioning for persons with peripheral vascular disease. To define the exercise prescription, a graded treadmill test to maximal claudication pain should be performed as previously described.[16] Maximal heart rate cannot be the basis for the prescription because claudication pain typically forces cessation of exercise before the maximum rate is reached.

The exercise intensity for optimal conditioning is based on the treadmill workload that brings on *moderate* claudication pain. In a supervised setting, the patient walks on a treadmill for a time sufficient to reach this pain intensity, rests until the pain subsides, then repeats the exercise at the same workload up to the same pain intensity. An exercise session should begin and end with 5 to 10 minutes of warm-up and cool-down time. During the session, patients should exercise on the treadmill repeatedly for 30 to 40 minutes. To provide maximum benefit, exercise should be carried out three to five times a week, with patients encouraged to take walks at home on days that they are not in the supervised exercise setting. Over a 3- to 6-month period, typically, a two- to six-fold improvement in walking distance is obtained.[14, 48, 49]

The mechanisms by which exercise conditioning benefits patients with PVD are not well established.[47] However, exercise may increase walking efficiency, pain tolerance, and oxygen delivery (blood flow). However, most evidence suggests that an improvement in muscle metabolism and oxygen extraction accounts for the improvements in exercise performance. In addition, exercise conditioning may improve the hemorrheologic properties of blood.[50]

An improvement in walking distance is seen in almost all patients with PVD after an exercise conditioning program.[49] As a result, these patients can carry out their daily activities with greater ease, which can mean the difference between a normal lifestyle and one that is severely limited. Walking therapy has therefore provided a successful nonsurgical intervention for patients with PVD.

In summary, patients diagnosed with PVD should initially have cardiovascular risk factors identified and treated. Pharmacologic therapy would consist primarily of using pentoxifylline in selected cases. In patients with severe PVD, angioplasty or surgery would be considered. Finally, all patients with disability from claudication should be evaluated for an exercise rehabilitation program.

REFERENCES

1. Sorlie D, Myhre K: Lower leg blood flow in intermittent claudication. Scan J Clin Lab Invest 38:171, 1978.
2. Pernow B, Saltin B, Wahren J, et al: Leg blood flow and muscle metabolism in occlusive arterial disease of the leg before and after reconstructive surgery. Clin Sci Mol Med 49:265, 1975.
3. Kannel WB, Skinner JJ, Schwartz MJ, et al: Intermittent claudication: incidence in the Framingham study. Circulation 41:875, 1970.
4. Criqui MH, Fronek A, Barrett-Connor E, et al: The prevalence of peripheral arterial disease in a defined population. Circulation 71:510, 1985.
5. Marinelli MR, Beach KW, Glass MJ, et al: Non-

invasive testing vs clinical evaluation of arterial disease: a prospective study. JAMA 241:2031, 1979.

6. Rose G, Blackburn H: Cardiovascular survey methods. WHO Monograph Series, No 56, 1968.

7. Criqui MH, Fronek A, Klauber MR, et al: The sensitivity, specificity and predictive value of traditional clinical evaluation of peripheral arterial disease: results from noninvasive testing in a defined population. Circulation 71:516, 1985.

8. Carter SA: Clinical measurement of systolic pressures in limbs with arterial occlusive disease. JAMA 207:1869, 1969.

9. Carter SA: Response of ankle systolic pressure to leg exercise in mild or questionable arterial disease. N Engl J Med 287:578, 1972.

10. Osmundson PJ, Chesebro JH, O'Fallon WM, et al: A prospective study of peripheral occlusive arterial disease in diabetes. II. Vascular laboratory assessment. Mayo Clin Proc 56:223, 1981.

11. Ouriel K, McDonnell AE, Metz CE, et al: A critical evaluation of stress testing in the diagnosis of peripheral vascular disease. Surgery 91:686, 1982.

12. Rutherford RB, Lowenstein DH, Klein MF: Combining segmental systolic pressures and plethysmography to diagnose arterial occlusive disease of the legs. Am J Surg 138:211, 1979.

13. Porter JM, Cutler BS, Lee BY, et al: Pentoxifylline efficacy in the treatment of intermittent claudication: multicenter controlled double-blind trial with objective assessment of chronic occlusive arterial disease patients. Am Heart J 104:66, 1982.

14. Larsen OA, Lassen NA: Effect of daily muscular exercise in patients with intermittent claudication. Lancet 2:1093, 1966.

15. Strandness DE: Functional results after revascularization of the profunda femoris artery. Am J Surg 119:240, 1970.

16. Hiatt WR, Nawaz D, Regensteiner JG, et al: The evaluation of exercise performance in patients with peripheral vascular disease. J Cardiopulmonary Rehabil 12:525, 1988.

17. Kannel WB, Skinner JJ, Schwartz MJ, et al: Intermittent claudication: incidence in the Framingham Study. Circulation 41:875, 1970.

18. Strandness DE, Beach KW: Vascular disease of the lower extremities. Mt Sinai J Med 49:241, 1982.

19. Beach KW, Strandness DE: Arteriosclerosis obliterans and associated risk factors in insulin-dependent and non–insulin-dependent diabetes. Diabetes 29:882, 1980.

20. Strandness DE, Priest RE, Gibbons GE: Combined clinical and pathologic study of diabetic and nondiabetic peripheral arterial disease. Diabetes 13:366, 1964.

21. LoGerfo FW, Coffman JD: Vascular and microvascular disease of the foot in diabetics: implications for foot care. N Engl J Med 311:1615, 1984.

22. Beach KW, Brunzell JD, Strandness DE: Prevalence of severe arteriosclerosis obliterans in patients with diabetes mellitus: relation to smoking and form of therapy. Arteriosclerosis 2:275, 1982.

23. Zimmerman BR, Palumbo PJ, O'Fallen WM, et al: A prospective study of peripheral arterial occlusive disease in diabetes. I. Clinical characteristics of the subjects. Mayo Clin Proc 56:217, 1981.

24. Kannel WB, Shurtleff D: The Framingham study: cigarettes and the development of intermittent claudication. Geriatrics 28:61, 1973.

25. Jonason T, Ringquist I: Changes in peripheral blood pressures after five years of follow-up in non-operated patients with intermittent claudication. Acta Med Scand 220:127, 1986.

26. Davignon J, Lussier-Cacan S, Ortin-George M, et al: Plasma lipids and lipoprotein patterns in angiographically graded atherosclerosis of the legs and in coronary heart disease. Can Med Assoc J 116:1245, 1977.

27. Blankenhorn DH, Brooks SH, Selzer RH, et al: The rate of atherosclerosis change during treatment of hyperlipoproteinemia. Circulation 57:355, 1978.

28. Boyd AM: The natural course of arteriosclerosis of the lower extremities. Angiology 11:10, 1960.

29. Lassila R, Lepantalo M, Lindfors O: Peripheral arterial disease—natural outcome. Acta Med Scand 220:295, 1986.

30. Criqui MH, Coughlin SS, Fronek A: Noninvasively diagnosed peripheral arterial disease as a predictor of mortality: results from a prospective study. Circulation 72:768, 1985.

31. Imparato AM, Kim GE, Davidson T, et al: Intermittent claudication: its natural course. Surgery 78:795, 1975.

32. Coffman JD: Vasodilators in peripheral vascular disease. N Engl J Med 300:713, 1979.

33. Clowes AW: The role of aspirin in enhancing arterial graft patency. J Vasc Surg 3:381, 1986.

34. Yates CJ, Andrews V, Berent A, et al: Increase in leg blood-flow by normovolaemic haemodilution in intermittent claudication. Lancet Jul 28; 2(8135):166–168, 1979.

35. Beven EG: Routine coronary angiography in patients undergoing surgery for abdominal aortic aneurysm and lower extremity occlusive disease. J Vasc Surg 3:682, 1986.

36. McPhail N, Menkis A, Shariatmadar A, et al: Statistical prediction of cardiac risk in patients who undergo vascular surgery. Can J Surg 28:404, 1985.

37. Cooperman M, Pflug B, Martin EW, et al: Cardiovascular risk factors in patients with peripheral vascular disease. Surgery 84:505, 1978.

38. Thompson JE, Garrett WV: Peripheral-arterial surgery. N Engl J Med 302:491, 1980.

39. Crawford ES, Bomberger RA, Glaeser DH, et al: Aortoiliac occlusive disease: factors influencing survival and function following reconstructive operation over a twenty-five-year period. Surgery 90:1055, 1981.

40. Doubilet P, Abrams HL: The cost of underutilization: percutaneous transluminal angioplasty for peripheral vascular disease. N Engl J Med 310:95, 1984.

41. DeWeese JA, Rob CG: Autogenous venous grafts ten years later. Surgery 82:775, 1977.

42. Reichle FA, Rankin KP, Tyson RR, et al: Long-term results of femoroinfrapopliteal bypass in diabetic patients with severe ischemia of the lower extremity. Am J Surg 137:653, 1979.

43. Health and Public Policy Committee, American College of Physicians: Percutaneous transluminal angioplasty. Ann Intern Med 99:864, 1983.

44. Spence RK, Freiman DB, Gatenby R, et al: Long-term results of transluminal angioplasty of the iliac and femoral arteries. Arch Surg 116:1377, 1981.

45. Collins RH, Voorhees AB, Reemtsma K, et al: Efficacy of percutaneous angioplasty in lower extremity arterial occlusive disease. J Cardiovasc Surg 25:390, 1984.
46. Rooke TW, Stanson AW, Johnson CM, et al: Percutaneous transluminal angioplasty in the lower extremities: a 5-year experience. Mayo Clin Proc 62:85, 1987.
47. Saltin B: Physical training in patients with intermittent claudication. In Cohen LS, et al: Physical Conditioning and Cardiovascular Rehabilitation. New York, John Wiley & Sons, 1981, p 181.
48. Ericsson MD, Haeger K, Lindell SE: Effect of physical training on intermittent claudication. Angiology 21:188, 1970.
49. Jonason T, Jonzon B, Ringqvist I, et al: Effect of physical training on different categories of patients with intermittent claudication. Acta Med Scand 206:253, 1979.
50. Ernst EE, Matrai A: Intermittent claudication, exercise, and blood rheology. Circulation 76:1110, 1987.

CHAPTER 28

Acute and Chronic Pulmonary Disease

Talmadge E. King, Jr.

*My diseases are an asthma and a dropsy, and what
is less curable, seventy-five.*
        SAMUEL JOHNSON, *Letter to W.G. Hamilton*

It is clear that lung function declines
with increasing age. This change occurs
so gradually that in the absence of disease,
breathing remains effortless. Throughout
life, however, the respiratory system is
continually exposed to factors such as pulmonary infection or environmental pollutants that may alter its function. Thus, in
the elderly, it is often a major challenge to
differentiate the "normal" decline in lung
function (i.e., the changes attributed to
the aging process itself) from the decline
that results from disease or the external
environment.

In general, there have been an inadequate number of longitudinal or cross-
sectional studies of large numbers of elderly persons, either normal or those
with specific pulmonary diseases. Consequently, a discussion of the acute and
chronic pulmonary diseases of the elderly
is based on an impression of the important
processes relative to the elderly rather
than to that determined by firm scientific
data. This chapter focuses on what is
known regarding the effect of aging on
the lung, those pulmonary diseases that
appear either more often in this age group
or represent particular diagnostic or management problems for the practicing physician, and finally on an often neglected
area—cardiopulmonary rehabilitation.

STRUCTURE AND FUNCTION OF THE RESPIRATORY TRACT

Morphologic Changes of Aging

Aging induces several changes in the
respiratory system that collectively result
in a decline in lung function (Table 28–1).
The anteroposterior diameter of the chest
increases, and skeletal deformities such as
kyphoscoliosis frequently develop with
age. Also, osteoporosis of the ribs and
vertebrae, calcification of the costal carti-
lages, decreased respiratory muscle
strength, progressive increase in chest
wall stiffness, and progressive enlargement of the respiratory bronchioles and
alveolar ducts, all contribute to the reduced pulmonary function that underlies
the increased susceptibility to cardiopulmonary diseases and diminishes the capacity for stress and exercise.[1, 2]

The chief physiologic manifestations of
aging on lung functions, however, are
related to the changes that occur in lung
and chest wall compliance. The chest wall
becomes stiffer with age, resulting in a
steady decline in chest wall compliance.
In addition, the muscles of respiration
(i.e., diaphragm, intercostal muscles, and
accessory respiratory muscles), like other
skeletal muscles, demonstrate a consistent
decline in strength and endurance with
age. This results in decreases in both maximal inspiratory and maximal expiratory
pressures when compared with a younger
age group.[2]

Conversely, as the chest wall stiffens
and the muscles that move it weaken, an
opposite and roughly equal process affects
the lung parenchyma and conducting airways. There is a progressive loss of lung
elastic recoil with age. The lung normally
is able to collapse when the chest wall is
opened (e.g., surgically or when a pneumothorax occurs) as a result of its elastic
recoil. This diminution in static elastic recoil with senescence results in an increased expansibility. In other words, the
compliance of the lung increases. (Compliance is defined as the change in volume

TABLE 28–1. Effects of Aging on the Respiratory System

Respiratory Abnormality	Physiologic Basis	Clinical Disorders
Decline in bellows function	Increased chest wall stiffness Loss of elastic recoil Decreased respiratory muscle strength Increased airway collapsibility	"Aging lung"
Abnormal gas exchange	Ventilation/perfusion mismatch Reduced diffusing capacity for carbon monoxide	Arterial hypoxemia
	Increased alveolar-arterial oxygen gradient	Decreased exercise tolerance
Abnormal breathing pattern	Diminished responsiveness to hypoxemia and hypercarbia	Cheyne-Stokes breathing
	Changing setpoint for ventilation caused by fluctuating level of wakefulness	Periodic breathing
Upper airway obstruction	Decreased airway muscle tone caused by loss of wakefulness stimulus, decreased metabolic respiratory drive	Snoring, sleep apnea, hypopnea, oxygen desaturation
Altered lung-host defense	Decreased ciliary action Impaired cough mechanisms Decreased IgA production Decreased phagocytic function of alveolar macrophages	Increased susceptibility to infection (pneumonia and chronic bronchitis)

per unit of change in pressure.) The decreased elastic recoil forces are believed to result from alterations in the connective tissue components of the lung. However, studies of age-related changes in collagen, elastin, and proteoglycans have yielded conflicting results.[1] There is no evidence that the surface-active lining material of terminal respiratory units, a second determinant of elastic recoil, is altered with aging. One could expect, however, that the loss of alveolar surface area accompanying aging would result in a reduction of the surface tension forces normally present and thereby result in some degree of loss of lung recoil. Consequently, the loss in elastic recoil of the lung, the stiffer chest wall, and the weaker respiratory muscles combine to make breathing more difficult for the elderly.

Changes in Dynamic Properties With Aging

Although the vital capacity (i.e., the amount of air that can be expelled from the lungs after a maximal inspiration) declines with age, the total lung capacity remains constant. The reason total lung capacity is not affected by aging is that although the elastic recoil of the lung decreases (i.e., the lung becomes more distensible), the concomitant reduced muscle strength and chest wall stiffness prohibit an increase in the maximum volume of the thorax. Therefore, the reduction in vital capacity results from an increase in the residual volume (i.e., the amount of air remaining in the lungs after a maximal expiration) (Fig. 28–1). This increase in residual volume (and functional residual capacity) results from the collapse of small airways that occurs at higher lung volumes as age increases. Residual volume increases nearly 50 percent between early adulthood and age 70.

In addition, standard spirometric measurements of lung function (i.e., forced expiratory volume in 1 sec, peak expiratory flow rate, maximal midexpiratory flow rate, and maximal expiratory flow volume) have been demonstrated to decline with age (Fig. 28–2). In fact, forced expiratory volume in 1 sec shows a steady decline of about 30 ml per year in healthy adult men. This results mainly from the diminished elastic recoil that occurs with aging (Fig. 28–3). However, other non–age-related factors that affect airway geometry and resistance also play a role in this decline with age.[3–6] In particular, cigarette smoking accelerates the age-related declines in flow rates.

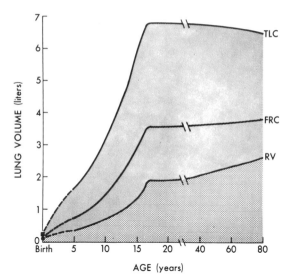

FIGURE 28–1. *Total lung capacity (TLC), functional residual capacity (FRC), and residual volume (RV) as a function of age from birth to 80 years for a male of "average" body build. (From Murray JF: The Normal Lung, Philadelphia, WB Saunders Co, 1976, p 312; by permission.)*

Alveolar Gas Exchange

The matching of ventilation and perfusion within the lung is critical for adequate gas exchange. Older persons have less uniform ventilation than young adults when breathing at moderate tidal volumes. With deep breathing, however, the elderly have the ability to improve the uniformity of ventilation, thereby eliminating the difference between the two groups. The nonuniformity of ventilation at low lung volumes is felt to result from closure of the small airways in the dependent portions of the lung during tidal

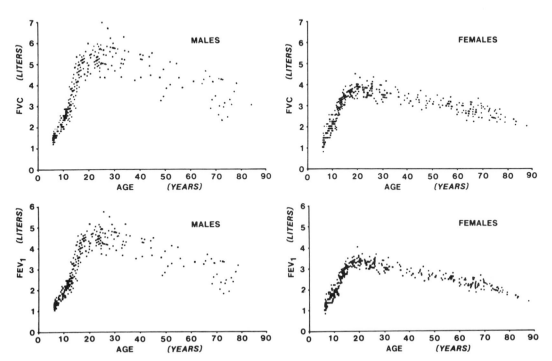

FIGURE 28–2. *Predicted values for forced vital capacity (FVC) and forced expiratory volume in 1 second (FEV$_1$) for males and females in the reference population (TOP = FVC; BOTTOM = FEV$_1$). (From Knudson RJ, Lebowitz MD, Holberg CJ, Burrows B, eds: Changes in the normal maximal expiratory flow-volume curve with growth and aging. Am Rev Respir Dis 127:725, 1983; by permission.)*

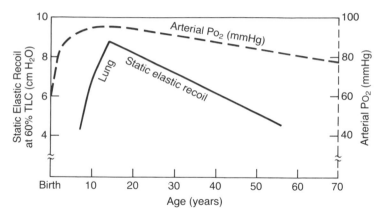

FIGURE 28–3. Static elastic recoil at 60 percent TLC (solid line) and arterial PO_2 as a function of age (broken line). Both increase from birth to maturity followed by a gradual decline with advancing age. These two variables are believed to be related through the effects of elastic recoil on airway caliber and therefore the uniformity of ventilation. (From Young RC Jr, Borden DL, Rachal RE, eds: Aging of the lung: pulmonary disease in the elderly. Age 10:138, 1987; by permission.)

breathing, which results in a ventilation and perfusion mismatch throughout the lung.

In addition to the changes in ventilation that occur with age, there are also changes in the pulmonary circulation. Although pulmonary capillary blood volume and total lung perfusion remain normal, there is a progressive decline in the alveolar capillary surface area, which can be measured by a parallel decline in the single breath-diffusing capacity for carbon monoxide (D_LCO). There is a progressive reduction in D_LCO ranging from 0.20 to 0.32 ml/min/mmHg per year of adulthood for men and 0.06 to 0.18 ml/min/mmHg per year for women.[7] This change does not appear to be of clinical importance in an otherwise healthy individual.

The arterial oxygen tension slowly declines with age, at the rate of approximately 4 mmHg per decade (see Fig. 28–3). This results predominantly from the imbalance in ventilation and perfusion caused by small airway closure in dependent lung zones that occurs during tidal breathing.[8] This imbalance is particularly marked in the recumbent position. In addition, cardiac output and mixed venous O_2 content also decline with aging, and therefore contribute to the fall in arterial PO_2 seen in the elderly. In contrast, arterial PCO_2 and pH do not change with age. The PCO_2 remains normal, despite an increase in the physiologic dead space, because minute ventilation increases with age.

Ventilatory Control

Normally, ventilation is regulated by a central controller in the brain that coordinates information fed to its various centers and modulates the activity of the respiratory muscles. There are two major sensors: the central chemoreceptors and the peripheral chemoreceptors. The central chemoreceptor is located in the medulla and has a slower response time than the peripheral chemoreceptor. This central receptor increases ventilation in response to acidosis, causing a lowering of arterial PCO_2. It is responsible for three fourths of the ventilatory response to CO_2. The peripheral chemoreceptors are located in the carotid bodies at the bifurcation of the common carotid arteries and in the aortic bodies above and below the aortic arch. The carotid body chemoreceptors are the most important in humans. The carotid body chemoreceptors respond to decreases in arterial PO_2 and pH by increasing alveolar ventilation. These receptors are solely responsible for the increase in ventilation that accompanies arterial hypoxemia.[9]

Although studies are limited, it appears that respiratory control becomes less precise with age.[1, 10] Elderly subjects have a blunted response to hypoxemia and hypercapnia when compared to young adults. The exact mechanism and the reason for these changes with aging are unknown. The CO_2 response appears to be predominantly centrally mediated.

Recently, considerable interest has been centered on sleep and the control of breathing. Numerous respiratory irregularities occur in adults during sleep, with apnea, hypopnea, and desaturation being common, and may occasionally be severe in the elderly.[11–13]

Lung Host-Defense

In addition to the respiratory activity identified above, the lung has important nonrespiratory functions, including purification of the inspired air and maintenance of an infection-free lung tissue.[14] No systematic evaluation of host defenses has been reported in elderly persons. It appears likely, however, that the nonspecific components of lung defenses have an age-related decline similar to that in other organ systems and their components.

Cell-mediated immunity and humoral antibody formation declines with age in some individuals; however, it has not been documented that this immune dysfunction is clearly involved in many disease processes in older adults. Autoantibody formation increases with age (i.e., antinuclear antibodies, antithyroglobulin antibodies, and rheumatoid factor). The importance of these types of changes remains to be clarified. In addition, several defense mechanisms are altered in the aged and are thought to be responsible for the increased susceptibility of the elderly to chronic bronchitis and pneumonia. These alterations include (a) impaired cough mechanism; (b) ineffective ciliary action so that inhaled particles are not cleared readily from the tracheobronchial tree; (c) decreased IgA (the secretory immunoglobulin of nasal and respiratory mucosal surfaces with neutralizing activity against viruses); and (d) defective alveolar macrophages, or phagocytic cells, that ingest foreign material that reach the alveolar space, especially in smokers.

RESPIRATORY DISEASES ASSOCIATED WITH AGING

Manifestations of Pulmonary Disease

Cough, often associated with sputum production, and shortness of breath (dyspnea) are the most common manifestations of respiratory disorders. Hemoptysis, chest pain, cyanosis, and an abnormal breathing pattern are less common manifestations of chest disorders.

COUGH

Cough plays a major role in host defense because of its ability to remove particles such as bacteria from the airways. In the elderly, the cough mechanism is frequently altered, in large part because of the age-related changes in lung mechanics (e.g., decreased elastic recoil) and the decreased respiratory muscle strength. Chronic cough with or without wheezing, should prompt careful attention to several important causes in the elderly. Chronic bronchitis, acute respiratory tract infection, asthma, and postnasal drip are the most common causes of chronic cough. In this age group, it is very important to exclude other causes such as gastroesophageal reflux or other mechanisms of aspiration, congestive heart failure, bronchogenic or metastatic carcinoma, interstitial lung disease, environmental irritant (e.g., tobacco smoke, noxious gases, dusts), foreign body in the airways, and pleural disease. Because cough is an important protective reflex, its suppression should only be attempted when the underlying cause has been addressed or when it is important to prevent other complications of cough, such as rib fracture, muscle strain, significant sleep deprivation, urinary incontinence, or hernias. Codeine (10 to 30 mg orally Q 4 to 6 hours, not to exceed 120 mg/day) is the most popular antitussive drug. In the elderly, cough suppression may result in the retention of respiratory secretions or lead to atelectasis, airway obstruction, or respiratory failure. Codeine may cause constipation, sedation, nausea, vomiting, dizziness, palpitation, pruritus, or agitation.[15]

DYSPNEA

Breathlessness, or dyspnea, is one of the most frequent complaints in the elderly patient and is commonly registered in patients with pulmonary, pleural, or cardiovascular processes. Unfortunately, dyspnea is a nonspecific sensation that may be extremely difficult for elderly patients to describe. Common expressions are an inability to get enough air, difficulty taking a deep breath or to breathe more rapidly, a smothering sensation, or a choking feeling. In a study of 70-year-old people, 45 percent of the study population had exertional dyspnea. Interestingly, of those who complained of exertional dyspnea, 64 percent of the men and 48 percent of the women suffered an identifiable illness of the cardiopulmonary system.[16] In the pulmonary diseases, dyspnea results from the increased work of breathing that commonly occurs in the aged lung and is worsened by the disease process itself.[17] Importantly, many elderly persons suffer significant breathlessness as a result of inactivity and thus deconditioning.

HEMOPTYSIS

The coughing up of blood, hemoptysis, varies from blood-tinged sputum to moderate or massive hemorrhage. It is sometimes difficult in the elderly to accurately determine where the blood being "coughed up" originates, such as from the nose or throat as a result of hematemesis (vomited blood) or from a portion of the bronchial tree. There are many causes of hemoptysis. Blood-streaked sputum is frequently seen in chronic bronchitis and upper respiratory infection and is an early finding in lung cancer. Massive hemoptysis (greater than 600 ml in 48 hours) most commonly occurs in lung cancer, pulmonary tuberculosis (both active and inactive), bronchiectasis, and lung abscess. A general rule is that the occurrence of hemoptysis before age 45 is most likely to result from mitral stenosis, tuberculosis, pneumonia, or bronchiectasis. After age 45, bronchogenic carcinoma, bronchitis, tuberculosis, and pulmonary embolus with infarction are more common causes of hemoptysis. Massive hemoptysis is a medical emergency that can result in hypotension, anemia, cardiovascular collapse, and asphyxiation. Supportive measures to maintain vital functions are important (e.g., volume replacement, oxygenation, and treatment with vasopressors). Control of the airway with endotracheal intubation should be carried out immediately, if required. The patient should be positioned with the bleeding side facing downward to prevent aspiration of blood into the contralateral lung. Localization of the bleeding site(s) by chest roentgenography and fiberoptic bronchoscopy is an absolute preoperative requisite, and prompt surgical resection is the treatment of choice. Contraindications to surgery include diffuse lung disease causing diffuse bleeding, coagulation abnormalities that may be associated with diffuse bleeding (e.g., anticoagulant therapy), inoperable lung cancer, and lung disease of such severity that the patient may not have adequate pulmonary reserve to survive resection of functioning lung tissue (i.e., a predicted $FEV_1 < 1.0$ liter after the procedure). In inoperable cases, bleeding can be controlled by tamponade of the bronchial segment with a Fogarty balloon catheter or by embolization of the arterial supply to the bleeding segment. The latter technique is usually unsuccessful because the systemic bronchial circulation is the source of the bleeding. Recent data suggest that embolization of both the bronchial and pulmonary vessels is effective in controlling bleeding in some patients.[18]

CHEST PAIN

Chest pain in the elderly patient is not always caused by myocardial ischemia. In fact, it may result from numerous causes and can present a difficult exercise in differential diagnosis.[19] Pleuritic pain caused by irritation of the parietal layer of the pleura complicates many pulmonary diseases. Pneumonia in a portion of the lung adjacent to the visceral pleural surface and pulmonary infarction are two important causes of pleurisy in the elderly. Rib fracture, costochondritis, pulmonary hypertension, post-herpetic neuralgia, and muscle pain (following severe coughing) are other causes of chest pain in the geriatric population.

BREATHING PATTERN

The presence of an abnormal breathing pattern can be an important clue to the presence of disease in any patient, especially in the elderly. Considerable attention has been focused recently on sleep and the control of breathing and is discussed later in this chapter.

Normal people at rest breathe eight to 16 times per minute, with a tidal volume of 400 to 800 ml. Several abnormal patterns of breathing have been characterized and may be helpful diagnostic clues.

1. Kussmaul's breathing, a form of hyperpnea characterized by a regular pattern, moderate rate, and large tidal volume, with little apparent effort, is suggestive of metabolic acidosis.

2. Obstructed breathing is seen in patients with chronic obstructive pulmonary disease (COPD) and is characterized by a

slow rate and increased tidal volume; often, wheezing is present.

3. Restricted breathing is characterized by small tidal volume and rapid rate and is seen in patients with restrictive lung diseases, especially the interstitial lung diseases.

4. Gasping respirations consist of irregular, quick inspirations associated with extension of the neck and followed by a long expiratory pause. It is characteristic of severe cerebral hypoxia and is a common pattern in patients with severe cardiac failure.

5. Cheyne-Stokes respiration (an extreme form of periodic breathing) describes a cyclic pattern of alternating apnea and hyperpnea. It is sometimes seen in healthy elderly persons but is generally found during sleep in patients with COPD, cardiac failure, or cerebrovascular insufficiency.

6. Hypoventilation is often difficult to identify and may be missed if not specifically sought, often with grave consequences for the elderly patient. It frequently results from severe obstructive lung disease, especially that associated with CO_2 narcosis, and from abnormalities in the control of breathing caused by cerebral vascular accidents, head trauma, oversedation, or narcotic administration.

Chronic Obstructive Pulmonary Disease (COPD)

Obstructive pulmonary diseases are characterized by alterations in ventilation that result from a limitation of expiratory flow. They are second only to heart disease as a cause of disability. Chronic obstructive pulmonary diseases include localized disease of the upper airway, bronchiolitis, cystic fibrosis, bronchiectasis, asthma, bronchitis, and emphysema. Of these, bronchitis and emphysema are primarily diseases of later life, with peak incidence in the sixth and seventh decades. Bronchiolitis is seldom recognized after age 4; cystic fibrosis usually results in death by the second or third decade; and bronchiectasis, although seen at any age, is primarily a disease of middle age.[20]

Despite this broad range of causes of airway obstruction, the term chronic obstructive pulmonary disease is most often applied to patients who have peripheral airway disease, emphysema, chronic bronchitis, or a mixture of the three, with or without airway hyper-reactivity.

EMPHYSEMA

The indiscriminate use of the term "emphysema" when referring to lower airway obstruction has resulted in considerable confusion about its exact definition. In addition, the separation of emphysema and bronchitis into two separate entities is occasionally misleading. The two diseases coexist frequently; consequently, it is often difficult to differentiate them clinically. Emphysema is defined as "a condition of the lung characterized by abnormal, permanent enlargement of airspaces distal to the terminal bronchiole, accompanied by the destruction of their walls, and without obvious fibrosis."[21] Destruction in emphysema is further defined as nonuniformity in the pattern of respiratory airspace enlargement so that the orderly appearance of the acinus (the respiratory airspaces arising from a single terminal bronchiole) and its components are disturbed and may be lost. Consequently, only a presumptive diagnosis of emphysema can be made in the living patient. Obstruction to airflow is frequently present to some degree in emphysema and predominantly results from a decrease in the elastic recoil of the lungs and collapsible airways. Three anatomic subtypes of emphysema are recognized, based on the portions of the acinus primarily involved.[22]

Panacinar emphysema is characterized by distention and destruction of all alveoli within the respiratory lobule. This type of emphysema has no definite regional preference, although the lower lobes may be more often affected. Interestingly, this form is associated with the primary emphysema seen in alpha-1-antiprotease deficiency (a familial disease with clinical manifestions occurring by age 40 in those who are homozygous for the Z gene).

Centriacinar emphysema is characterized by the destruction of the central part of the lobule; the proximal part of the acinus (respiratory bronchiole) is predominantly involved with the peripheral alveolar ducts and the alveoli are unaffected. There are two subdivisions of this form of lesion.

The first, known as centrilobular emphysema, is classically associated with cigarette smoking. Most of the lung changes in centrilobular emphysema occur in the apices of the upper lobe, but spread downward as the disease progresses. This type is rare before the age of 40 and occurs without clinical manifestations in about one fourth of people who die with no history of lung disease and a normal chest radiograph. In fact, one half of individuals over 70 years of age at autopsy have a mild form of centrilobular emphysema—the so-called aged lung—usually without disability. The second form is referred to as focal emphysema and occurs in individuals exposed to the inhalation of coal dust (i.e., coal pneumoconiosis) and other mineral dust. This lesion is relatively uniform in distribution in the lungs and is characterized by the dilation of respiratory bronchioles, with the intense accumulation of dust-laden macrophages in and around the respiratory bronchioles.

Distal acinar emphysema involves the distal part of the acinus, alveolar ducts and sacs, which abuts the pleura, vessel and airways, thus the emphysema is worse in these regions. Mild airflow obstruction, despite extensive bullous emphysema, and the spontaneous pneumothorax of young adults are the clinical associations of this form of emphysema.[21]

The pathogenesis of emphysema remains unknown. The protease-antiprotease imbalance concept remains the dominant hypothesis. Several recent reviews discuss these issues.[23-25]

DIAGNOSIS. It is unusual to find a patient with "pure" emphysema. Although emphysema alone can result in a crippling and fatal disease, when hypoxemia and cor pulmonale supervene, it is almost invariably associated with chronic bronchitis. The diagnosis of emphysema in life is made indirectly by the collective changes found in the clinical, radiologic, and functional status. The clinical manifestations are predominantly breathlessness, with or without cough, that progresses to severe disability as a result of unrelenting dyspnea. Early in the disease, the clinical examination may be of little value. As the severity increases, the physician is confronted by an anxious, thin, occasionally emaciated patient who demonstrates pursed-lip breathing with prominent use of accessory muscles of respiration because of his or her need to further inflate an already inflated chest. Breath sounds are markedly diminished, and the heart sounds are faint.

The chest radiograph is suggestive but not specific for the diagnosis of emphysema (Fig. 28–4). The presence of hyperinflation (low, flat diaphragm and large retrosternal air space); cardiovascular changes (a narrow vertical heart, prominent pulmonary trunk, and large hilar vessels with tapering peripheral vessels); and signs of local vessel loss (bullae that are demarcated by a thick, white line or with no definite margins [i.e., bullous area]) increases the diagnostic accuracy of the plain chest film. Few cases of mild emphysema can be recognized radiographically.[26] Computerized tomography (CT) is suggested as a useful radiographic technique for detecting the morphologic changes of emphysema in life.[27]

A combination of physiologic tests are necessary to indicate the presence of emphysema. In general, when a patient has airway obstruction, increased total lung capacity, diminished elastic recoil, increased static compliance, and a decreased carbon monoxide diffusing capacity, clinically significant emphysema is very likely to be present.[28]

CHRONIC BRONCHITIS

Chronic bronchitis is defined by the presence of a symptom: sputum production. It is characterized by cough, sputum production, airways obstruction, and chronic or recurrent bacterial infections. Simple chronic bronchitis is defined as mucus hypersecretion with resultant cough and expectoration on most days for at least 3 months of the year for 2 successive years when no other cause is present. Morphologic changes are primarily hypertrophy of mucous glands in the large bronchi and evidence of chronic inflammatory changes in the small airways. Although multiple factors have been implicated in the etiology of chronic bronchitis, the most common association is with cigarette smoking. Atmospheric pollution and occupational exposure have also been implicated.

CLINICAL PICTURE. A typical presentation of chronic bronchitis is that of a

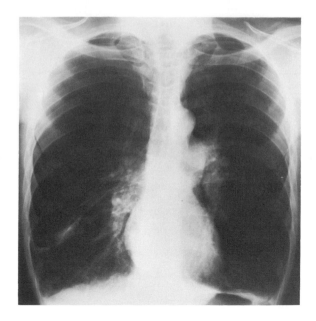

FIGURE 28–4. Pulmonary emphysema, PA view. Both lungs are hyperradiolucent and associated with a flat diaphragm and an enlarged pulmonary trunk and its right and left main branches. A large bulla is present in the right upper lobe.

middle-aged or elderly man who has had a history of a productive cough for several years. The patient invariably is or was a cigarette smoker for many years. He usually has had a decline in exercise tolerance because progressive dyspnea severely limits his exertional efforts. Several factors are responsible for the exercise limitation seen in these patients (Table 28–2). Frequently, episodes of acute purulent bronchitis supervene, and with time these episodes become more frequent.

The clinical examination usually reveals a stocky or overweight man with a dusky complexion. Cyanosis may or may not be apparent at this time, but invariably these patients become "blue and bloated." Chest examination reveals mild to moderate diminution of breath sounds, with scattered rales and rhonchi. Evidence of

right ventricular dysfunction with fluid retention i.e., jugular venous distention and pedal edema is usually present.

DIAGNOSIS. The chest radiograph demonstrates a normal position of the diaphragm and lung fields that are normal or have increased bronchovascular markings. Cardiac enlargement may be present (Fig. 28–5).

Physiologic studies generally reveal airway obstruction with normal lung volumes and elastic recoil. The diffusing capacity for carbon monoxide is not diminished as it is in emphysema. The arterial blood gases are frequently abnormal, revealing hypercapnia and hypoxemia. With prolonged hypoxemia, erythrocytosis may be present, with hematocrits as high as 70 percent.

TABLE 28–2. Factors Leading to Exercise Limitation in Patients with COPD*

Abnormal pulmonary mechanics

Impairment of pulmonary gas exchange

Abnormal perception of breathlessness and ventilatory control

Presence of impaired cardiac performance resulting from cor pulmonale or occult coronary artery disease

Poor nutritional status

Development of respiratory muscle fatigue

*(Adapted from Loke J, Mahler D, Man SFP, et al: Exercise impairment in chronic obstructive pulmonary disease. Clin Chest Med 5:121, 1984.)

Complications of COPD
(Table 28–3)

COR PULMONALE

Cor pulmonale is defined by the World Health Organization as "hypertrophy of the right ventricle from diseases affecting the function and/or structure of the lung, except when these pulmonary alterations are the result of diseases that primarily affect the left side of the heart, or of congenital heart disease."[29] The incidence of this form of heart disease is unknown. Although less than 50 percent of patients

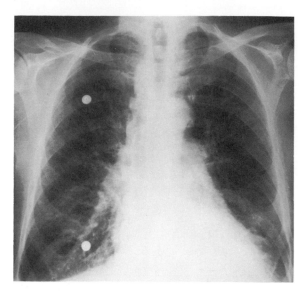

FIGURE 28–5. Chronic bronchitis, PA view. Increased vascular markings are prominent throughout the lung, and there is enlargement of the hilar pulmonary arteries. Left lower lobe pneumonia is also present.

with COPD manifest right ventricular hypertrophy at autopsy, chronic cor pulmonale most often results from COPD.[30] Elevation of the pulmonary artery pressure is the prerequisite for the development of cor pulmonale. The significance of pulmonary hypertension in COPD cannot be overstated because its occurrence is clearly an important determinant of the quantity and quality of life in these patients.[30] Patients with COPD frequently develop pulmonary arterial hypertension as a result of hypoxemia, hypercapneic acidosis, and an increased red cell mass (secondary polycythemia). Hypoxemia and acidosis induce pulmonary hypertension by the production of vasoconstriction. In addition, irreversible anatomic destruction or restriction of pulmonary vessels occurs in

TABLE 28–3. Complications of COPD

Chronic hypercarbia

Chronic cor pulmonale, peripheral edema

Supraventricular and ventricular arrhythmias

Secondary erythrocytosis

Sleep disorders and hypoxemia, neuropsychologic dysfunction

Pulmonary embolism

Spontaneous pneumothorax

Peptic ulcer disease

Acute respiratory failure

Side effects or adverse reaction to drug therapy

Malnutrition

patients with emphysema, thereby contributing to an increase in pulmonary vascular resistance. Polycythemia, usually seen in patients with hypoxemic bronchitis, increases pulmonary arteriole resistance as a result of increased blood viscosity. Also, the hypervolemia associated with polycythemia increases cardiac output, further complicating the pulmonary hypertension. Consequently, one or more of these factors set the stage for the development of cor pulmonale. Thus, long-standing, significant pulmonary hypertension produces right ventricular systolic and diastolic dysfunction by elevating afterload and reducing right ventricular myocardial oxygen supply relative to demand. This leads to subsequent dilation and hypertrophy and, finally, to cor pulmonale, with or without right ventricular failure.[31]

Generally, the presentation of cor pulmonale is dominated by the manifestations of the underlying lung disease. In the elderly, coexisting coronary artery disease makes the distinction between right and left ventricular dysfunction important, since therapeutic decisions depend on the accurate assessment of the relative role of each disease. In this regard, it is important to note that left ventricular dysfunction is rare in uncomplicated COPD.[32] Syncope and precordial pain are classic symptoms of pulmonary hypertension but are infrequent. Severe cyanosis, unexplained drowsiness, engorged neck veins, hepatomegaly, and fluid retention with dependent edema are often presenting findings. The presence of tachycardia, a right ventricular lift, a loud pulmonic component of the second heart sound, an atrial gallop, and a Graham Steell murmur (a soft, blowing, high-pitched diastolic murmur of pulmonic insufficiency) are extremely helpful in diagnosing pulmonary hypertension with cor pulmonale. The chest radiograph usually demonstrates enlargement of the central pulmonary arteries. Two chest radiographic measurements—the right descending pulmonary artery and left descending pulmonary artery diameters—are sensitive indices of pulmonary hypertension in COPD patients. A right descending pulmonary artery of greater than 16 mm is more specific and more accurate than an enlarged left descending pulmonary artery (greater than 18 mm). If both are enlarged, however, the combined sensitivity is 98 percent, and an accuracy of 90 percent for the presence of pulmonary artery hypertension is achieved.[33] Right ventricular hypertrophy (RVH) is difficult to diagnose on plain film of the chest. Also, the sensitivity and specificity of the electrocardiogram (ECG) in the diagnosis of RVH is low. Autopsy studies reveal that 25 to 40 percent of patients with COPD and RVH have no associated electrocardiographic changes at the time of death.[34] Nonetheless, it is extremely important that the presence or evolution of changes on the ECG consistent with right ventricular enlargement be identified because they signal the need for arterial blood gas analysis and the institution of supplemental oxygen therapy. The electrocardiographic findings of cor pulmonale may be present, including peaked P waves in leads II, III, and AVF, right axis deviation, RVH, and right bundle branch block. Continuous, long-term oxygen therapy helps ameliorate the effects of pulmonary hypertension and cor pulmonale in many patients with COPD and is discussed later in this chapter.[36]

ARRHYTHMIAS

Supraventricular and ventricular arrhythmias are common complications of COPD, particularly during the stage of cor pulmonale and acute respiratory failure.[37] Metabolic disturbances associated with respiratory failure are suspected as the cause of these arrhythmias. Consequently, arterial hypoxemia, hypercapnia, acidosis, and deficits in potassium, calcium, or magnesium must be treated aggressively. In addition, when these patients require mechanical ventilation, respiratory alkalosis secondary to overventilation occurs and may also trigger serious arrhythmias. Except in life-threatening situations, the use of antiarrhythmia drugs is appropriate only after all the possible causes of the arrhythmias have been corrected.

POLYCYTHEMIA

Secondary polycythemia, with hematocrits as high as 70 percent, occur because of the elevated renal erythropoietin that results from chronic hypoxemia. Polycythemia represents a mechanism that allows greater oxygen delivery to compensate for the chronically low arterial PO_2. The effectiveness of this response in COPD remains unclear. Supplemental oxygen to treat the hypoxemia present in these patients is the most important treatment modality. Occasionally, phlebotomy is indicated in patients who manifest congestive cor pulmonale with polycythemia.

SLEEP HYPOXEMIA

It has been estimated that over 80 percent of patients with COPD have serious nocturnal oxygen desaturation.[38] Many of these patients, however, do not have the classic features of sleep deprivation such as daytime hypersomnolence or right heart failure. Obesity and increasing age, especially in males and postmenopausal women, are strongly associated with episodes of nocturnal desaturation.[11, 39, 40] The causes of the hypoxemia noted during sleep are shown in Table 28–4.

The importance of identifying and managing the potentially severe nocturnal oxygen desaturation that occurs in patients with COPD cannot be overemphasized. Smolensky and coworkers reported several years ago that patients with chronic lung disease die more often in the middle of the night.[41] Furthermore, studies have demonstrated a relationship between nocturnal oxygen desaturation in the development of episodic pulmonary vasocon-

TABLE 28–4. Causes of Sleep Hypoxemia

Alveolar hypoventilation

Ventilation-perfusion mismatch

Prolonged central apneas

Upper airway obstructive apnea

Mucus hypersecretion and accumulation

Disordered breathing and altered controls of ventilation

Nocturnal bronchoconstriction

striction and pulmonary hypertension and have suggested this as a possible mechanism for the progression to cor pulmonale and the blue and bloated syndrome.[42, 43] Equally important has been the demonstration that severe nocturnal oxygen desaturation in patients with COPD correlates with cardiac arrhythmias and other electrocardiographic evidence of myocardial hypoxia.[44, 45] The clinical manifestations and management of disordered respiratory function during sleep are discussed later in this chapter.

PULMONARY EMBOLISM (PE)

Pulmonary embolism is a significant complication in COPD; a 20 to 60 percent incidence has been reported. Inactivity and right heart failure are felt to be the primary risk factors. Lippmann and Fein[46] and Fanta and colleagues[47] have suggested the following guidelines for the diagnosis of pulmonary embolism in patients with COPD (Fig. 28–6).

1. Clinical manifestations are generally not helpful. However, any patient who develops severe tachypnea (greater than 30 breaths per minute) and the clinical manifestations of cor pulmonale in the absence of infection or other cause and who is unresponsive to conventional bronchodilator therapy should be suspected of having PE. Typically, patients with COPD and cor pulmonale are not tachypneic to this degree because of their desire to minimize the work of breathing.

2. As a corollary, an increase in alveolar ventilation (decreased $PaCO_2$) in a previously hypercapneic patient is also suggestive of PE. Patients who develop cor pulmonale on the basis of COPD alone typically present with both hypoxemia and carbon dioxide retention (mean $PaCO_2$ of 53 mmHg). In patients with recurrent pul-

monary emboli as the cause of their cor pulmonale, the mean $PaCO_2$ was 32 mmHg.[46, 47]

3. Lung function tests in pulmonary emboli-induced cor pulmonale may not be impaired severely enough to explain the development of cor pulmonale in a COPD patient. It is uncommon for patients with a 1 second forced expiratory volume (FEV_1) greater than 1.5 l to develop cor pulmonale on the basis of COPD alone.

4. Radioisotopic studies are not useful in differentiating PE from worsening obstruction. Often, the patient cannot breath-hold long enough to perform an adequate ventilation scan. Because the emboli are frequently small, the resolution of the scan cannot adequately distinguish between the changes caused by COPD from those of emboli.

5. When possible, angiography should be undertaken to confirm the diagnosis of PE.

RESPIRATORY FAILURE

Respiratory failure is a common complication in patients with COPD. Often, respiratory failure occurs in combination with or as a result of many of the aforementioned problems. Acute respiratory failure is defined as arterial hypoxemia (PaO_2 less than 50 mmHg). The precipitating causes of respiratory failure in this setting include (a) respiratory infection; (b) CO_2 narcosis secondary to respiratory depression caused by the administration of oxygen; (c) oversedation (sedatives, narcotics, tranquilizers), which causes a reduction in the cortical "drive" to breathe and, consequently, depresses respiration; (d) left ventricular dysfunction, primary or secondary to silent myocardial infarction; (e) thoracic cage abnormalities (e.g., flail chest); (f) pneumothorax; and (g) PE.

ADULT RESPIRATORY DISTRESS SYNDROME

Finally, another cause of acute respiratory failure is the adult respiratory distress syndrome (ARDS). This is not considered a complication of COPD. In fact, the presence of any major chronic inflammatory or fibrotic pulmonary disease specifically excludes these patients from this disease category. However, ARDS is a

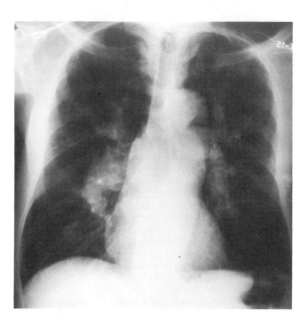

FIGURE 28–6. Recurrent pulmonary emboli in a patient with COPD; confirmed at autopsy. Note the markedly enlarged pulmonary arteries.

catastrophic event, especially in the elderly.[48, 49] It is characterized by severe dyspnea, refractory hypoxemia (arterial PO_2 of less than 150 mmHg on an FIO_2 of 100 percent) and diffuse bilateral pulmonary infiltrations, "stiff lung", right to left intrapulmonary shunting, usually normal or increased alveolar ventilation, increased physiologic dead space, and a pulmonary arterial wedge pressure of less than 10 mmHg. The mainstay of management is mechanical ventilation with positive end-expiratory pressure and close hemodynamic monitoring of cardiac output and fluid balance. Despite appropriate and aggressive treatment, the mortality rate is extremely high (average 65 percent) and can reach 90 to 100 percent in the presence of another organ failure.[49] This problem has been recently reviewed.[50–52]

A detailed discussion of the intensive care management of acute and chronic respiratory failure is beyond the scope of this chapter.[50, 53] Many of the basic principles of management are detailed below, and Table 28–5 outlines the many complications associated with respiratory failure and its management. It is important to understand that the aggressive management of respiratory failure in the elderly patient is justified. Although the long-term prognosis from COPD after respiratory failure is poor, the short-term prognosis in patients presenting with acute respiratory failure is better. In fact, a study of ventilatory management in the geriatric

population revealed a 51 percent recovery rate for patients over the age of 70.[50] Recent studies emphasize an improved survival rate.[54]

OTHER COMPLICATIONS

Spontaneous pneumothorax is a rare complication of COPD. However, it can have serious consequences when it occurs in the geriatric patient. Spontaneous pneumothorax, infection, and massive hemorrhage are important complications of bullous emphysema. Peptic ulcer disease occurs with greater frequency in patients with COPD (10 to 35 percent) than in the normal population (3 percent). Sexual dysfunction is relatively common in men with COPD and may be related to progression of the disease itself and not to associated illnesses (depression, cerebrovascular, cardiovascular, or peripheral vascular impairment) or to aging.[55]

Management of the Patient with COPD (Table 28–6)

Realistically, although we have divided this group of diseases into chronic bronchitis and emphysema, most patients with COPD have a combination of the two. In addition, many of these patients have wheezing (bronchospasm) as a prominent component and appear to be asthmatic.

Therapy of COPD is primarily directed

TABLE 28–5. Complications Associated with Acute Respiratory Failure and its Management*

Complications Associated with Intubation and Extubation
  Insertion trauma (laryngeal injury)
  Improper tube placement (esophagus or right mainstem)
  Cuff complications (tracheal stenosis, erosion or dilation, tracheoesophageal fistula,
    erosion of the innominate artery)
  Postextubation obstruction (supraglottic or subglottic edema)
  Gastric aspiration
  Airway obstruction (mucus, endotracheal tube)
  Endotracheal tube dislodgement (extubation)

Complications of Ventilatory and Monitoring Procedures
  Pulmonary barotrauma (pneumothorax, pneumomediastinum, subcutaneous
    emphysema)
  Acid-base disturbances (alkalosis)
  Cardiovascular problems
    Arrhythmias (multifocal atrial tachycardia)
    Hypotension and low cardiac output
  Machine failure (patient disconnected, alarm malfunction)
  Flow-directed, balloon-tip catheterization
    Pulmonary infarction
    Pulmonary hemorrhage
    Arrhythmias
  Deconditioning (respiratory muscle failure)

Metabolic Complications
  Syndrome of inappropriate antidiuretic hormone (SIADH)
  Electrolyte imbalances
    Hypokalemia and hypochloremia
    Severe hypophosphatemia and hypomagnesemia

Renal
  Fluid retention
  Renal failure

Gastrointestinal
  GI hemorrhage
  Ileus
  Gastric distention
  Pneumoperitoneum

Infection
  Sepsis
  Nosocomial pneumonia

Hematologic
  Anemia
  Thrombocytopenia
  Disseminated intravascular coagulation

Other Problems
  Pulmonary embolism
  Drug toxicity (theophylline, digitalis)
  Oxygen toxicity
  Malnutrition
  Psychiatric disturbances ("ICU psychosis," depression, agitation)

*(From King, TE Jr: Acute respiratory failure. Schrier, RW ed: Current Medical Therapy. New York, Raven Press, 1984, p 141; by permission.)

at controlling the symptoms and complications. Although both diseases can be treated with the same basic regimen, it is occasionally a grave error to oversimplify the management. In the author's practice, it is not uncommon for even the most precise and discriminating physician to lump these diseases and treat in a "cookbook" fashion. Consequently, patients with symptoms that are predominantly associated with emphysema, with no reversible bronchospasm, and with relative normoxia are overmedicated with bronchodilators, corticosteroids, and antibiotics. On the other hand, the true bronchitic patient with significant bronchospasm is undertreated and suffers needless morbidity. Therefore, every "chronic lunger" deserves a careful evaluation to determine, as specifically as possible, the predomi-

TABLE 28–6. Management of COPD

Strongly urge smoking cessation

Patient and family education

Reduce work of breathing caused by airway
 obstruction
  Relieve bronchospasm (aerosol or oral
   sympathomimetic bronchodilators, with or
   without corticosteroids)
  Reduce secretions (remove all possible irritants,
   control infection, initiate appropriate
   antimicrobial therapy, administer influenza
   vaccine annually, and pneumococcal vaccine
   once in a lifetime)

Chest physiotherapy
  Postural drainage and chest percussion
  Breathing retraining
  Exercise reconditioning

Low-flow oxygen therapy

---

nant pathologic process, and careful attention must be paid to those components of the disease that are potentially reversible. Comprehensive reviews of the management of COPD have been previously published.[51, 53] We will emphasize the key principles of treatment in the stable patient. When to hospitalize a patient with COPD is often a difficult decision. In Table 28–7 are provided some useful guidelines.

PATIENT EDUCATION

Patient education is unquestionably the most important aspect of a treatment program. Chronic obstructive pulmonary disease management requires patient and family cooperation and participation. The patient must be taught the basics of respiratory anatomy and physiology as well as how to deal with the psychologic stresses of a chronic illness. The most important lesson must be smoking cessation. A steady stream of evidence clearly implicates COPD as a specific complication of smoking. In a 20-year follow-up of British physicians, it was demonstrated that a 15-year abstinence from cigarette smoking resulted in a reduction of the risk of dying of COPD from 36 times that of nonsmokers to 8 times.[56] In addition, although low-tar, low-nicotine cigarettes may reduce the risk of lung cancer, there is no evidence that these cigarettes will reduce the incidence of COPD. The gestalt of most physicians is that once a patient presents with symptoms of COPD, it is too late to do any good. Recent data, however, suggest that this nihilistic attitude is not appropriate.[57] Normal persons lose 20 to 30 ml per year in their FEV_1. Patients susceptible to the effects of smoking have an annual FEV_1 decrement of 50 to 100 ml.[58–60] In addition, it has been demonstrated that the cessation of smoking results in a definite and rapid beneficial response, especially the reduction of cough and sputum production. Therefore, every patient, regardless of age, should be encouraged to stop smoking (Fig. 28–7).

BRONCHIAL HYGIENE

An attempt to maintain or improve airway clearance of bronchial secretions is important. Many patients with advanced

---

TABLE 28–7. Principal Indications for Hospitalization of the Patient with COPD*

Acute exacerbation of symptoms unresponsive to outpatient treatment (e.g., markedly increased dyspnea, cough, sputum production) especially in presence of marked fatigue or exhaustion†

Acute respiratory failure characterized by respiratory distress, hypercarbia, worsening hypoxemia, or impaired mental status

Acute cor pulmonale with dependent edema, further impairment of exercise capacity, and hypoxemia

Complications of COPD, such as acute bronchitis or pneumonia

Performance of invasive diagnostic procedures on the lung, such as bronchoscopy, transbronchial biopsy, or needle aspiration of nodules

Need for surgery or other procedures that require significant amounts of analgesics or anesthesia

Diseases that may not require hospitalization in themselves but that in the presence of severe COPD, represent a significant risk to the patient

*(Adapted from American Thoracic Society Statement. Standards for the diagnosis and care of patients with chronic obstructive pulmonary disease (COPD) and asthma. Am Rev Respir Dis 136:225, 1987.)

†When evaluating a patient during an acute exacerbation, it is important to get information from the family regarding the baseline level of function (mental and physical). Also, previous arterial blood gas measurements (especially baseline, asymptomatic values), pulmonary function tests, and response to treatment should be sought, since they can often guide current management.

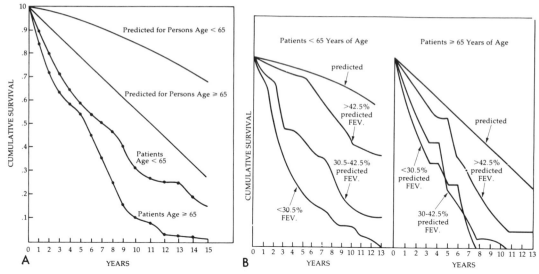

FIGURE 28–7. Cumulative survival of 200 patients with chronic bronchitis and emphysema. A, According to age; B, According to age and pulmonary function. (From Dodge R, Burrows B, eds: Chronic bronchitis and emphysema. In Fries JF, Ehrlich GE eds: Prognosis. Contemporary Outcomes of Disease. Bowie, Maryland, Charles Press Publishers, 1981, p 228.)

disease have considerable difficulty mobilizing airway secretion. Consequently, adequate hydration, humidification of inspired gases, a regular program of postural drainage, breathing exercises, and assisted cough are felt to be useful adjuncts.[22] Intermittent positive pressure ventilation (IPPB) has been demonstrated to have no benefit in hospitalized or ambulatory COPD patients and may be disadvantageous.[61] The use of so-called expectorants has never been proven effective.

THERAPEUTIC AGENTS

Bronchodilator drugs are the mainstay in the management of patients with reactive airway disease. Because most patients with COPD have some component of bronchospasm complicating their disease, all patients are given a defined trial of these agents. Appropriate subjective and objective evaluation of the results and side effects of bronchodilators is essential. The drugs should be withdrawn if some modification in dyspnea, bronchopulmonary secretions, or pulmonary function cannot be demonstrated.

The drugs most commonly employed are the methylxanthines and beta-adrenergic agonists. Theophylline, usually given orally as a sustained-release formulation, has not been clearly proven to be of value in patients with COPD.[22, 62] These drugs

are frequently used by clinicians because they produce bronchodilation, stimulate respiration, improve diaphragmatic function, and have cardiotonic and diuretic properties. Theophylline is the most commonly used methylxanthine. The use of theophylline preparations in the elderly is not without the potential for significant problems. A number of factors affect theophylline clearance including many drugs (e.g., cimetidine, erythromycin), environmental conditions (e.g., diet, illness), smoking, congestive heart failure, and liver disease. Some patients develop intolerance to theophylline regardless of the dose administered and often in the absence of a change in a previously acceptable dose. Toxicity to theophylline is usually manifested by restlessness, insomnia, tremor, nausea or vomiting, often at serum levels within the therapeutic range (i.e., 8 to 20 mcg/ml). Severe complications, such as cardiac arrhythmias and seizures, occur when the serum levels exceed 25 to 30 mcg/ml. Therapeutic drug monitoring is important in the elderly if dosage optimization is to be achieved.[63]

The sympathomimetics, especially those with a more selective beta$_2$-stimulating effect such as metaproterenol, albuterol, bitolterol, and terbutaline, are very effective drugs and are the keystone of therapy in patients with obstructive airway disease. These drugs are best given via metered-dose inhaler (MDI). Unfortunately, many elderly patients are unable to use the MDI optimally even after the repeated instructions that should be given to all patients using them. Worse still, many physicians and nurses do not take the time to properly instruct the patient or are not knowledgeable of the proper technique for using a nebulizer or MDI with or without a spacer. Elderly patients should be encouraged to use a large-volume reservoir to increase the amount of drug deposited in the lungs, while decreasing the amount of oropharyngeal deposition. This probably helps improve compliance by reducing the systemic side effects. Also, some patients require the use of a powered nebulizer unit for best results. Oral preparations are to be discouraged, if the aerosol preparation can be used effectively, because they require larger doses of the drug and cause more side effects.

The anticholinergics, such as atropine or ipratropium bromide, which block cholinergic stimulation and decrease intracellular cyclic GMP, have been improved such that the side effect of desiccation of secretions is less of a problem, and their use (usually in association with beta$_2$-adrenoceptor agonists) has increased in the management of chronic bronchitis associated with bronchospasm.[64]

Corticosteroid therapy has hitherto played a controversial role in the management of patients with chronic bronchitis and emphysema.[65] Despite this, it has long been recognized that a small proportion of patients with COPD have a considerable degree of reversible bronchospasm. Petty estimates that this type of patient represents approximately 10 percent of the total.[66] It has been noted that some patients given corticosteroids improve despite the inability to demonstrate reversible airway disease by pulmonary function tests. Several recent studies have demonstrated an objective response to corticosteroid therapy in COPD and acute respiratory insufficiency.[67–71] The following appear to be useful objective parameters of potential steroid responsiveness: (a) sputum and blood eosinophilia, with sputum eosinophilia being a better indicator of steroid responsiveness; (b) improvement in the FEV$_1$ of 30 percent or more over the baseline value in response to administration of beta-adrenergic agonists or an increase in

the FVC following a trial course of the drug; and (c) improvement in exercise tolerance, as well as general subjective improvement.

Current data do not support a role for inhaled corticosteroids.[72] It is extremely important that the physician (and patient) undertake a defined trial with objective measurements (i.e., vital capacity and FEV$_1$ measurements) before and after the institution of corticosteroids. The patient must have received optimal therapy (bronchodilator therapy, smoking cessation, physical rehabilitation, oxygen, and so forth) and demonstrate continued symptomatic and/or progressive disease before this corticosteroid trial is instituted. A reasonable regimen is 40 mg of prednisone or its equivalent once daily for 2 to 3 weeks. If improvement in flow rates or lung volumes is observed, the corticosteroid dose is tapered as rapidly as possible, while monitoring for any decline in lung function. The lowest effective daily dose or alternate-day therapy should be the goal. In acute exacerbations of COPD, the addition of intravenous corticosteroids (0.5 mg/kg every 6 hours for 72 hours) may be beneficial.[68] Because of the number and severity of side effects of corticosteroids, the therapy must be discontinued in the absence of objective improvement[73] (Table 28–8). Furthermore, many clinicians recognize that a small number of patients with COPD who are started on corticosteroids demonstrate little objective response yet are unable to have the drug discontinued. The mechanism of their subjective benefit is not clear.

Antibiotics are important agents in the treatment, as well as in the prophylaxis, of acute exacerbations of COPD.[74] Exacerbation of COPD is commonly characterized by increases in breathlessness and cough and sputum production with increased purulence in sputum. Respiratory infections are a primary cause of increased morbidity and mortality in patients with COPD. Most exacerbations appear to be initiated by viral infections (e.g., myxovirus, rhinovirus) or mycoplasma and then become secondarily infected by bacteria (most commonly *Hemophilus influenzae* or *Streptococcus pneumoniae*). Ampicillin, amoxicillin, tetracycline, erythromycin, and trimethoprim/sulfamethoxazole are the antibiotics currently prescribed. The

TABLE 28–8. Potential Complications of Corticosteroid Therapy in the Elderly*†

Short Term, High Dose (May be of Sudden Onset)

Mental and CNS disturbances including mood swings (euphoria to depression), jitteriness, severe psychosis (rare); pseudotumor cerebri (rare)

Sodium and fluid retention

Impaired glucose tolerance, hyperosmolar nonketotic coma (especially in presence of parenteral feedings)

Hypokalemic alkalosis, systemic arterial hypertension, glaucoma, pancreatitis, peptic ulceration and gastrointestinal hemorrhage, proximal myopathy (rare)

Long Term, Daily Steroids for Months or Years

Suppression of the hypothalamic-pituitary-adrenal axis, with adrenal insufficiency

Cushing's syndrome

Osteoporosis with vertebral compression and multiple bone fractures, aseptic necrosis of bone

Proximal myopathy

Increased susceptibility to opportunistic infections

Impaired wound healing, dermal atrophy

CNS manifestations—depression, lability of mood, anxiety, seizures

Posterior subcapsular cataract formation

---

*(Adapted from Chang SW, King TE: Corticosteroids. In Cherniack RM, ed: Drugs for the Respiratory System. Orlando, Grune & Stratton, Inc, 1986, p 112; by permission.)

†A number of these side effects are controversial and unproven.

TABLE 28–9. Criteria for the Institution of Home Oxygen Therapy

Severe and persistent hypoxemia (PaO_2 55 mmHg or less)*

Evidence of chronic hypoxemia (PaO_2 59 mmHg or less) associated with mental impairment, markedly deteriorating exercise capacity, pulmonary hypertension, cor pulmonale or right ventricular failure, polycythemia (hematocrit 55% or greater)

Sleep hypoxemia (PaO_2 55 mmHg or less), especially if associated with above complications†

Selected patients with hypoxemia during exercise (PaO_2 55 mmHg or less) and exercise intolerance (see text)

---

*In patient receiving optimal medical management, measured at least two times, 3 weeks apart.

†Following documented improvement during hospitalization

duration of treatment must be individualized, since recovery is usually prolonged. Most physicians treat patients with oral antibiotics for 7 to 14 days. Sputum cultures are not absolutely necessary for the institution of therapy in this setting because the so-called normal flora (i.e., normal oropharyngeal bacteria) are cultured, and there is little relationship between the organism identified and the response to antibiotics. Therefore, self-administration of antibiotics is desirable and safe in the properly instructed patient.

Oxygen therapy has an important role in the management of selective hypoxemic COPD patients (Table 28–9). There is no question of the usefulness of appropriate oxygen therapy in the management of acute respiratory failure. Its role in outpatient therapy has been recently clarified.[75–78] The details of oxygen therapy, as well as of other important management modalities, are discussed in the section on cardiopulmonary rehabilitation in this chapter.

Repeated phlebotomy for the management of secondary polycythemia is not frequently indicated. The appropriate management of the hypoxemia with oxygen will control the hematocrit below 55 percent.

Annual prophylaxis against influenza and a single-dose pneumococcal vaccine are recommended, especially in the elderly, with or without chronic lung disease. Amantadine hydrochloride is a tricyclic amine that inhibits an early state of replication of the influenza A virus. In the event of an epidemic, prophylaxis therapy should be seriously considered in elderly individuals who are unvaccinated, have serious coexisting medical illnesses, or are institutionalized. The recommended dosage is 100 mg twice daily and should be continued until the epidemic has passed or until 2 weeks after the patient has been vaccinated. In patients with suspected influenza, amantadine may reduce both the duration of the illness and the respiratory complications. In the elderly, the dose should be reduced to 100 mg daily after an initial loading dose of 200 mg because of the presence of renal insufficiency in this group. Furthermore, although side effects are not common (3 to 7 percent of treated individuals), they include confusion, disorientation, ataxia, tremors, and convulsions, especially in the elderly.

Bronchial Asthma

Asthma is a chronic disease characterized by episodic shortness of breath, usually accompanied by wheezing and cough, resulting from hyperirritable airways and reversible airflow obstruction. The airflow obstruction is caused by bronchial smooth muscle spasm, mucosal inflammation and edema, and mucus hypersecretion, with subsequent narrowing and plugging of the bronchial tree. Acute and chronic forms of asthma occur in the geriatric population. Elderly patients presenting for the first time with wheezing are uncommon and may present a diagnostic dilemma leading to delayed recognition and treatment.[79] In over 85 percent of asthmatic patients, the onset of illness occurs before age 40. Only 3 percent present after age 60, and less than 1 percent develop new onset asthma after the age of 70.[80] Many elderly patients with airway hyper-reactivity are labeled chronic bronchitics because of cough and sputum production without wheezing and may fail to receive appropriate therapy, especially treatment with corticosteroids. Most symptomatic asthmatic episodes are precipitated by nonallergenic stimuli such as viral respiratory infection, environmental irritants (e.g., sulfur dioxide), exercise, and cold air. In some patients, environmental allergens, emotional distress, and drugs such as aspirin will tend to precipitate symptoms. In elderly patients, the precipitating factor(s) may go undetected. Braman and Davis identified a group of elderly asthmatic patients in an outpatient clinic and demonstrated that approximately one half of the group had developed asthma after age 65.[81] The investigators noted that when asthma developed at an advanced age, it was often severe and required continuous bronchodilator therapy, including corticosteroids, to control the symptoms.

Finally, one is reminded that wheezing is not pathognomonic of asthma and that particularly in the elderly, it can result from congestive heart failure, pulmonary emboli, and recurrent aspiration. When wheezing is unilateral, a bronchial obstruction caused by bronchogenic carcinoma or foreign body aspiration, should be suspected. The widespread use of beta-blockers in the management of systemic arterial hypertension and glaucoma may result in reduced pulmonary function and bronchospasm in previously "normal" adults and in patients with asthma.[82, 83] Asthma management is similar to that of COPD, with bronchodilators and corticosteroids being the mainstay of treatment.

Sleep-Disordered Breathing in the Elderly

Recently, attention has been drawn to the fact that apnea (cessation of breathing for 10 seconds or longer), underventilation, and oxygen desaturation (a decrease of 4 percent or greater in the oxygen saturation as measured by ear oximetry) occur commonly during sleep and may be responsible for potentially serious psychologic and physiologic consequences, especially in the elderly. It is beyond the scope of this chapter to examine in detail sleep and breathing relationships; however, this topic has been extensively reviewed.[84–86]

Sleep is divided into two broad phases based primarily on the electroencephalographic (EEG) wave changes that occur. Body functions also change during these phases. Quiet or nonrapid eye movement (nonREM) sleep is characterized by EEG wave slowing, with increased wave amplitude. NonREM sleep (also called desynchronized or active sleep) is divided into four stages, representing progressively deeper stages of sleep. During stages 1 and 2 of nonREM sleep, the pattern is cyclical, with periods of Cheyne-Stokes breathing. As sleep becomes established, breathing stabilizes and is typically regular. In nonREM sleep, chemical control mechanisms determine ventilation. Periodic breathing during nonREM sleep increases with age. Active or rapid eye movement (REM) sleep is marked by EEG patterns of low-voltage, high-frequency waves indicative of intense cerebral activity. During REM sleep, heightened autonomic and metabolic activity occur, with increases in metabolic rate, body temperature, systolic blood pressure, and heart rate. Breathing becomes rapid and irregular, with associated periods of apnea as long as 15 to 20 seconds in normal adults. Similarly, airway smooth muscle tone also fluctuates during REM sleep. Intercostal muscle activity is decreased and results in a paradoxical movement of the rib cage and decreased functional residual capacity. Although these findings produce mild degrees of hypercapnia and hypoxemia, they are of little consequence in the healthy adult. In the presence of cardiac, neurologic, or pulmonary diseases, however, these episodes may be life-threatening. Many studies have now demonstrated that these presumably "normal" changes occur with greater frequency and severity in the elderly and in patients with COPD. The clinical significance of the oxygen desaturation is evident when one considers that nocturnal cardiac arrhythmias, pulmonary hypertension, and even sudden death are seen in these patients.

SLEEP-APNEA SYNDROME

Both sleep and respiration are disturbed during the sleep apnea syndromes. Patients with this syndrome exhibit a constellation of clinical signs and symptoms that resolve when the problem is appropriately treated (Table 28–10). Sleep apneas are classified depending on the presence or absence of respiratory efforts as central, obstructive, or mixed apneas (Fig. 28–8). In each instance, air flow at the nose and mouth are absent, indicating apnea. In central apnea, respiratory efforts are not detected. In upper airway obstructive apnea, respiratory efforts are present but are not accompanied by airflow at the mouth or nose. Mixed, or complex, apnea resembles central apnea early in the episode and obstructive apnea as the episode

TABLE 28–10. Sleep Apnea Syndrome— Signs and Symptoms

Nocturnal insomnia (restless sleep or violent body movements)

Daytime somnolence

Intellectual and personality changes (depression)

Sexual dysfunction

Morning headache and/or nausea

Hallucinations, automatic behavior

Dyspnea

Noisy snoring (obstructive apnea)

Obesity

Systemic hypertension

Pulmonary hypertension, cor pulmonale, heart failure

Polycythemia

Edema

Cardiac arrhythmias

Unexplained nocturnal death

progresses. All these situations result in alveolar hypoventilation, oxygen desaturation (decrease greater than 4 percent is considered abnormal), and sleep deprivation. Most often, obstructive or mixed apneas occur. Diagnosis of this syndrome frequently requires a searching inquiry when a patient presents with the symptoms and/or signs outlined in Table 28–10. Massively obese patients; those with COPD, stroke, and chronic heart disease; men; postmenopausal women; and patients with anatomic variations of the upper airway (e.g., hypognathia, nasal obstruction, and tongue or tonsillar enlargement) are predisposed to the sleep apnea syndrome.

The major pulmonary abnormalities occurring in this setting are (a) disordered breathing, with oxygen desaturation, especially during naps and prolonged nocturnal sleep, usually of short duration (i.e., less than 60 seconds); (b) ventilation-perfusion mismatching that occurs during REM sleep, producing periods of oxygen desaturation that last for longer periods (i.e., greater than 5 minutes); (c) pulmonary hypertension; (d) decreased mucociliary clearance and cough depression, which may be particularly important in patients with COPD who have excess airway secretions; (e) decreased intercostal muscle contraction with resultant paradoxical movement of the chest wall; and (f) bronchoconstriction.

OTHER SLEEP DISTURBANCES
(Table 28–11)

Before the clinician assumes that the aforementioned symptoms are related to sleep apnea syndromes, one must carefully rule out the "natural" changes in sleep pattern that occur with aging, especially the facts that apparently healthy older individuals may require a longer time to fall asleep, may awaken more often during the night, and need less sleep overall.[87–91] Furthermore, it is common that sleep disturbances occur in these patients as a result of concomitant illnesses such as depression, alcoholism, chronic use and dependence on sleeping pills, chronic pain syndrome, organic brain syndrome, and bereavement or situational insomnia. In the elderly, it is particularly difficult to distinguish between the normal variability

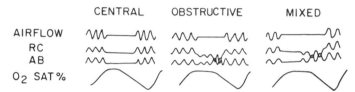

FIGURE 28–8. *Diagrammatic representation of the three patterns of apnea identified during sleep. In each, air flow at the nose and mouth is absent, indicating apnea. In central apneas, respiratory efforts, indicated in this instance by rib cage (RC) and abdominal (AB) displacement, are absent. During an obstructive apnea, efforts by the chest wall muscles are present throughout the entire episode of apnea. In mixed apneas, both central and obstructive patterns are present in the same apnea. Oxygen saturation ($O_2SAT\%$) will fall according to the general degree of oxygen saturation and the length of the apnea. (From Strohl KP, Cherniack NS, Gothe B, eds: Physiologic basis of therapy for sleep apnea. Am Rev Respir Dis 134:791, 1986; by permission.)*

of breathing during sleep and pathologic apnea.[91] Aged men, especially those who are overweight, are more prone to impaired respiration during sleep than are aged women.[40] The natural history and significance of the apneas found during sleep in the elderly is unclear.[40, 92]

Three additional points require emphasis. First, it is not always easy to predict the magnitude of the sleep disturbance on clinical grounds because the clinical findings, blood gas analysis, and pulmonary function tests during wakefulness may be misleading. The important features that should alert the physician to examine the patient for the possibility of sleep-related disturbances are (a) pulmonary hypertension or cardiac failure in excess of that expected from the awake pulmonary function tests and arterial blood gases, and (b) a poor response to the standard measures of treatment and rehabilitation in COPD. Secondly, the administration of nocturnal oxygen is a principal treatment modality for sleep hypoxemia. Recent data suggest, however, that there is a subgroup of patients with predominantly obstructive apneas for whom low-flow oxygen results in a prolongation of the apneic periods, with a dramatic rise in the $PaCO_2$ and resultant acidosis. Importantly, cardiac dysrhyth-

mias occurred more frequently in this setting.[93] How to determine which patients may suffer this deleterious effect of oxygen therapy from those who will not is unclear. Further, Martin and coworkers suggest that among this subset are patients who will benefit from oxygen therapy with a reduced total amount of apneic time and the number of cardiac arrhythmias.[94] Thirdly, not only does sleep aggravate gas exchange disturbances in patients with COPD, but COPD may aggravate sleep, such that these elderly patients develop changes in daytime behavior and performance, such as daytime somnolence, intellectual deterioration, impotence, depression, and essential hypertension.[95]

MANAGEMENT

Management of sleep apnea syndrome is important because many of the manifestations are reversible.[86] Obstructive sleep apnea requires measures that will maintain the patency of the upper airway during sleep. Weight reduction is the primary mode of therapy in morbidly obese patients. Agents that enhance ventilatory responsiveness, such as medroxyprogesterone acetate 20 mg three times a day or protriptyline 20 mg, p.o., at bedtime, have met with limited success in a few patients with obstructive sleep apnea. The application of continuous positive pressure (CPAP) by a face mask has been reported to be a useful method to keep the upper airway open. When life-threatening cardiorespiratory events occur during sleep, however, tracheostomy is required. Surgical correction (i.e., removal of tonsillar and adenoid tissue) may improve the syndrome.

In patients with central apneas, dia-

TABLE 28–11. Common Sleep-Related Complaints in the Elderly

Difficulty initiating and maintaining sleep

Frequent arousals

Abnormalities in time spent asleep and excessive time spent in bed

Restless legs and periodic movements in sleep

Frequent use of sedative-hypnotics, including alcohol

Night wandering, frequent micturition

phragmatic pacing via the phrenic nerve or a rocking bed may be helpful. The long-term efficacy of this approach remains to be fully evaluated. Patients with primary alveolar hypoventilation occasionally respond to medroxyprogesterone. The role of nocturnal oxygen therapy has been discussed above. Sedatives and alcohol should be avoided in these patients.

Interstitial Lung Diseases

The interstitial lung diseases are a heterogenous group of diseases that are progressive, generally fatal processes characterized by an interstitial and intra-alveolar inflammatory process, interstitial fibrosis, and revision of the distal lung architecture. Although these diseases are denoted as interstitial (i.e., involving that area bounded by the alveolar epithelial and endothelial basement membrane), it is important to realize that the entire lung parenchyma can be involved. This heterogenous group of disorders can be classified together because of common clinical, roentgenographic, physiologic, and pathologic features. Approximately two thirds of these diseases have no known cause and are, therefore, classified by their clinical and/or pathologic features[96] (Table 28–12). The most common causes of the interstitial lung diseases are those related to occupational and environmental exposures, especially to inorganic dust. Sarcoidosis is the most prevalent interstitial lung disease of unknown etiology, but it occurs uncommonly in the elderly. Idiopathic pulmonary fibrosis (IPF), with or without associated connective tissue disease, is also common, whereas most other conditions associated with interstitial lung disease are rare.

PATHOGENESIS

A common pathogenetic sequence underlies the majority of interstitial lung diseases regardless of etiology. The initial step appears to be injury to lung cells as a result of (a) direct toxicity to endothelial or epithelial cells from drugs or poisons; (b) generation of toxic oxygen radicals such as superoxide anion and hydrogen peroxide; (c) release of mediators and enzymes such as collagenase, elastase, beta

TABLE 28–12. Etiologic Classification of the Interstitial Lung Diseases

Category	Examples
Idiopathic	Idiopathic pulmonary fibrosis Synonyms: Hamman-Rich syndrome Cryptogenic fibrosing alveolitis Honeycomb lung Bronchiolitis obliterans, with or without organizing pneumonia
Connective tissue	Progressive systemic sclerosis Rheumatoid arthritis Polymyositis/dermatomyositis Systemic lupus erythematosus (SLE)
Occupational and environmental exposures	Inorganic dust diseases (silicosis, asbestosis, coal worker's dust) Hypersensitivity pneumonitis Farmer's lung Malt-working–induced
Drug-induced	Drug-induced SLE Immunosuppressive and cytotoxic agents (bleomycin, methotrexate, busulfan, BCNU, radiation therapy, gold salts) Antimicrobial agents (nitrofurantoin, sulfonamides, penicillin) Vasoactive and neuroactive agents (heroin, methadone, barbiturates)
Primary diseases	Sarcoidosis (third stage) Pulmonary histiocytosis X Lymphangitic carcinomatosis Vasculitides Chronic infection, especially tuberculosis Chronic pulmonary edema Chronic gastric aspiration Pulmonary amyloidosis

glucoronidase from inflammatory cells (macrophages and neutrophils); and (d) alterations in the immune system, with deposition of immune complexes in the lung (vasculitic syndromes, IPF, some connective tissue diseases, and histiocytosis-X). Following this injury to lung cells, several responses occur including (a) endothelial cell injury, resulting in the proliferation of neighboring cells; (b) damage on the alveolar surface, causing type II epithelial cells to proliferate; and (c) in both instances, influx of inflammatory and immune effector cells, resulting in alveolitis. The precise pathway leading from acute injury to fibrosis is not known. The major mechanism appears to be continued exposure to the inciting agent. In the presence of this chronic alveolitis, derangement in the interstitium occurs and eventually leads to loss of alveolar gas-exchanging units because of fibrosis and honeycombing.

CLINICAL PICTURE

The typical patient with interstitial lung disease is age 55 or older and presents with the insidious onset of breathlessness with exercise and nonproductive cough.[97] Other clinical manifestations are dependent on the underlying process and include constitutional symptoms such as fever, weight loss, fatigue, and myalgias and arthralgias. Physical examination commonly reveals bibasilar and end-inspiratory dry rales ("velcro" rales). Clubbing of the fingers is common in some patients (idiopathic pulmonary fibrosis) and rare in others (sarcoidosis). Signs of pulmonary hypertension and cor pulmonale are generally seen only in advanced disease.

DIAGNOSIS

An elevated erythrocyte sedimentation rate and hypergammaglobulinemia are commonly observed. Positive antinuclear antibodies, rheumatoid factors, and circulating immune complexes have been identified in many of these patients, even in the absence of a defined connective tissue disorder, which simply may be a reflection of the higher incidence of autoantibodies found in the elderly.[98, 99] The chest roentgenogram is useful in suggesting the presence, but not the stage, of interstitial lung disease and may be normal in as many as 10 percent of these patients. The most common radiographic abnormalities are a reticular or a reticulonodular pattern. A coarse reticular pattern or multiple cystic areas (honeycombing) is a late roentgenographic finding and portends a poor prognosis (Fig. 28–9). Radiographic evidence of pleural disease is uncommon in idiopathic pulmonary fibrosis, and its presence suggests a concomitant second process, e.g., a connective tissue disease, as the underlying cause of the interstitial lung disease.

Pulmonary function abnormalities are common. The classic findings are consistent with a restrictive impairment (i.e.,

vital capacity and total lung capacity are reduced), and unless there is a complicating airway disease such as bronchiolitis obliterans, endobronchial sarcoidosis, or COPD, flow rates are well maintained. Occasionally, patients with associated obstructive airway disease or diffuse cystic disease will have normal (sarcoidosis and rheumatoid disease) or increased (advanced histiocytosis X or lymphangioleiomyomatosis) total lung capacity. The diffusing capacity (corrected for alveolar volume and hemoglobin concentration) is reduced as a result of effacement of the alveolar capillary units and may precede or follow abnormalities in lung volumes. The resting arterial blood gas may be normal or reveal hypoxemia (secondary to a mismatching of ventilation to perfusion) and respiratory alkalosis. Commonly, blood gas abnormalities may only be elicited or accentuated by exercise. Despite the frequent presence of hypoxemia, erythrocytosis is uncommon. Serial lung function testing (especially exercise testing) is helpful in following the course and response to therapy.

The most important step in the evaluation of a patient with interstitial lung disease is a carefully taken clinical history. Particular emphasis should be placed on possible occupational and environmental exposures. A strict chronologic listing of the patient's employment, including specific duties and known exposures to organic and inorganic dusts, gases, and chemicals, is important. Review of the home environment, especially as it relates to pets, air conditioners, and so forth, is valuable.

Following the initial evaluation, the next most important issue is to confirm the diagnosis and determine the stage of disease so that decisions as to prognosis and therapy can be made. In many cases, open lung biopsy is required because a larger quantity of tissue, usually from two sites (i.e., an area of obvious abnormality and one that appears normal) is necessary to adequately define the process, especially in idiopathic pulmonary fibrosis. This approach decreases the sampling error that often occurs with transbronchial lung biopsy and allows the clinician to distinguish between active inflammation and end-stage fibrosis. It is often difficult to decide whether or not to obtain a tissue

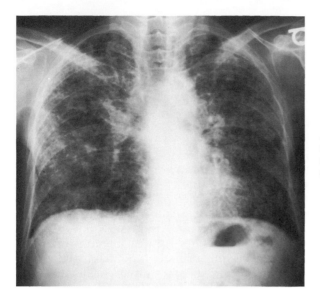

FIGURE 28–9. Idiopathic pulmonary fibrosis. Patient with longstanding disease with diffuse, coarse reticular infiltrates, roentgenographic honeycombing, and pulmonary hypertension.

diagnosis in elderly patients. Many clinicians opt for empiric treatment. Open lung biopsy is a low morbidity procedure in experienced hands, and therefore we recommend tissue diagnosis if there are no other contraindications to anesthesia or surgery and if treatment with corticosteroids or cytotoxic agents is contemplated. Fiberoptic bronchoscopy with transbronchial lung biopsy may be the initial procedure of choice in many cases, especially when sarcoidosis, lymphangitic carcinomatosis, eosinophilic pneumonia, Goodpasture's syndrome, or infection is suspected.

MANAGEMENT OF THE INTERSTITIAL LUNG DISEASES

Many of the interstitial lung diseases are not responsive to therapy, therefore, it is extremely important that all treatable possibilities be given careful consideration. Because therapy will not reverse fibrosis, the major goals are (1) early identification and aggressive treatment directed at suppressing the acute and chronic inflammatory process to prevent further lung damage; (2) permanent removal of the offending agent, when known; and (3) palliation of complications. Unfortunately, there are no accurate or specific methods available to stage the intensity of the alveolitis in a serial fashion. Open lung biopsy is both sensitive and specific for the evaluation of the alveolitis, but it is

generally only used once during the disease course. Symptoms, chest roentgenograms, pulmonary function tests, blood studies, gallium scanning, and bronchoalveolar lavage appear to reveal little information that is sensitive to or specific for the inflammatory process within the lung that actually define disease "activity" (especially in an individual patient). In general, the "responsive" patient will (1) report a decrease in symptoms; (2) demonstrate radiographic improvement; (3) demonstrate physiologic improvement such as increased total lung capacity (TLC) and diffusion (D_LCO) or have an improvement in the exercise-induced oxygen desaturation; or (4) show no further decline in lung function or other parameter of disease activity.

Corticosteroids remain the mainstay of therapy for suppression of the "alveolitis" present in these processes, but the success rate is low. In idiopathic pulmonary fibrosis, 40 to 50 percent of patients experience subjective improvement, but only 20 to 30 percent have objective improvement. Frequently, elderly patients with idiopathic pulmonary fibrosis are not treated because of both their poor underlying condition and the hazards of corticosteroid therapy. When treated, only 32 percent of those over age 65 are likely to obtain a satisfactory response, with improvement in breathlessness and chest x-ray. This is compared with 95 percent of those under age 45, 62 percent of those between ages

45 and 54, and 48 percent of those between ages 55 and 64.[100] High oral doses of prednisone (e.g., 80 to 100 mg per day for 6 to 12 weeks), followed by a slow tapering off of 5 to 10 mg every 2 to 3 weeks, is required to induce a response in most patients with idiopathic pulmonary fibrosis.

There is little evidence that corticosteroids influence the natural course of pulmonary manifestations in the connective tissue diseases, except in patients with polymyositis-dermatomyositis in whom approximately one half will have decreased dyspnea, clearing of the chest roentgenogram, and improved pulmonary function tests. In addition to the immediate removal from the etiologic agents in occupational and environmental processes, corticosteroid therapy is generally recommended for symptomatic patients with acute inorganic dust exposure, acute radiation pneumonitis, and drug-induced disease. In organic dust disease, corticosteroids (prednisone 60 to 80 mg per day in tapering doses administered over 6 to 12 weeks) are recommended for both the acute and chronic stages. Cyclophosphamide (1 to 2 mg/kg/day), with or without corticosteroids, results in dramatic improvement in the majority of patients with classic Wegener's granulomatosis. Cyclophosphamide, with or without prednisone, appears to lead to improvement in selected patients with idiopathic pulmonary fibrosis. Objective response to prednisone and cytotoxic drugs commonly takes 6 to 12 weeks to occur in most forms of interstitial lung disease. Consequently, a treatment trial should not be less than this time period, unless complications or side effects occur. Most patients have relapses so that life-long treatment is frequently required. If the patients demonstrate clinical and physiologic improvement and the medication is discontinued, careful monitoring on a 6- or 12-month basis is essential to identify relapses.

PROBLEMS IN MANAGEMENT

Significant side effects can result from corticosteroid therapy. These include increased appetite and weight gain; salt and water retention with exacerbation of cardiovascular disease, especially in elderly patients; hyperglycemia and/or overt dia-

betes mellitus; depression, hyperexcitability, or frank psychosis, especially in elderly women; osteoporosis and joint destruction; peptic ulcer disease; immunosuppression leading to opportunistic infections. Other side effects (e.g., hypokalemia, hypertension, renal lithiasis, poor healing, cataracts, ecchymosis, phlebitis, and hirsutism) may also occur.

On the other hand, steroid withdrawal may result in serious symptoms and morbidity such as fatigue, weakness, arthralgia, anorexia, nausea, desquamation of skin, orthostatic dizziness and hypotension, and fainting and hypoglycemia.

Cyclophosphamide's side effects include bone marrow suppression, which requires that therapy be aimed at inducing a modest leukopenia with a total white cell count greater than 3000/mm^3; hemorrhagic cystitis, which may be prevented with "forced" fluids and frequent bladder emptying; gastrointestinal symptoms such as anorexia, nausea, and/or vomiting; bone marrow suppression; azoospermia or amenorrhea; infection; development of hematologic malignancies; and interstitial lung disease itself. Therapy should be altered in the event of renal insufficiency. Consequently, if stabilization or clinical improvement cannot be documented, corticosteroid and/or cyclophosphamide therapy should be stopped, since significant adverse reactions can occur.

Severe hypoxemia (PaO$_2$ less than 55 torr) at rest and/or with exercise should be managed by supplemental oxygen. Patients with only exercise-induced hypoxemia should be given supplemental oxygen for use during exercise and possibly during sleep. Failure to do this often leads to progressive reduction in the patient's level of activity and hastens the onset of right heart failure. With the appearance of cor pulmonale, diuretic therapy and phlebotomy may occasionally be required. Pneumothorax, which is characteristic of eosinophilic granuloma of the lung, may also occur in other interstitial lung diseases. This may be extremely difficult to treat because the lung is stiff and difficult to re-expand. Prolonged chest tube drainage with high levels of negative pressure (20 to 40 mmHg) may be necessary. Acute pulmonary embolism is an occasional cause of clinical deterioration in this group of patients. Sudden worsening of dyspnea, with unexplained deterioration in arterial blood gases and without evidence of superimposed infection, should prompt the clinician to consider lung scan and/or pulmonary angiography. Malignancy (particularly adenocarcinoma) develops in idiopathic pulmonary fibrosis with increased frequency.[101]

Selected Interstitial Lung Diseases

COAL WORKER'S PNEUMOCONIOSIS

Of the occupational lung diseases, coal worker's pneumoconiosis, silicosis, and asbestosis are the most common inhalation exposures that result in predominantly fibrosis and restrictive lung disease. Coal worker's pneumoconiosis usually occurs in association with silicosis. Two forms of disease predominate, which are simple pneumoconiosis, represented by small opacities (less than 1 cm in diameter) predominantly in the upper lung zones and complicated pneumoconiosis or progressive massive fibrosis (opacity 1 cm or more in diameter). The prevalence rate among coal miners is approximately 10 percent, of which 0.4 percent develop progressive massive fibrosis. Pulmonary function abnormalities occur in simple coal worker's pneumoconiosis, usually in the presence of a history of cigarette smoking, regardless of the extent of radiographic involvement.

SILICOSIS

Silicosis is found in miners, sandblasters, glass manufacturers, quarry workers, stone dressers, foundry workers, and boiler scalers. Radiographically, silicosis appears as multinodular rounded densities predominantly in both upper lung zones. The radiographic changes almost always occur before the clinical and functional abnormalities. Progression from simple to progressive massive fibrosis occurs in a minority of patients. Patients with silicosis are highly susceptible to infection by *Mycobacterium tuberculosis* and other atypical mycobacteria. Furthermore, scleroderma and rheumatoid arthritis are unusually prevalent in silicotics.

ASBESTOSIS

Asbestos exposure is widespread because it is used extensively as an insulation material, a fire retardant, and a noise-reduction agent in many public facilities. Workers previously or currently employed in the shipyard, automotive, insulation, cement, textile, and asbestos mining industries are at greatest risk. There is a long latent period between exposure and the development of lung diseases, therefore, most of the cases occur in middle-aged or elderly persons. Smoking appears to facilitate the damaging effects of asbestos inhalation. Bilateral pleural thickening along the lower or midthoracic walls, calcified pleural plaques, and hazy infiltrates composed of irregular or linear small opacities, especially in the lower lung zones, are the most common roentgenographic changes. Asbestos is also carcinogenic. Pleural and peritoneal mesotheliomas and bronchogenic carcinoma are recognized complications of asbestos exposure.

HYPERSENSITIVITY PNEUMONITIS

The hypersensitivity pneumonitides are associated with repeated intense inhalation of finely dispersed organic dusts that produce diffuse patchy interstitial and/or alveolar infiltrates following the formation of antigen-antibody complexes (Arthus's reaction). Farmer's lung (exposure to moldy hay containing fungal spores) is the prototype, although air conditioner or humidifier lung disease (due to fungal overgrowth and aerosolization) and bird fancier's lung are more common in urban areas. The disease can present in two forms. The first is an acute reaction following heavy exposure characterized by the abrupt onset (4 to 6 hours later) of fever, chills, malaise, nausea, cough, chest tightness, and dyspnea without wheezing that subsides over hours or days. Diffuse, fine rales throughout the chest, mild hypoxemia, and a restrictive ventilatory defect accompanies these symptomatic episodes. A fleeting, micronodular, interstitial pattern in the lower and midlower zone may be identified on chest roentgenogram. Removal from exposure usually results in complete resolution. Pathologically, this stage is characterized by noncaseating interstitial granulomatous pneumonitis.

The second type is an insidious form that results if repeated acute episodes or continued low-level antigen exposure occurs. A patient with chronic hypersensitivity pneumonitis may not have any acute episodes. This form of disease is particularly difficult to diagnose and manage. It appears to occur more commonly in middle-aged and elderly individuals, especially among bird fanciers. Disabling and frequently irreversible respiratory findings such as pulmonary fibrosis are characteristic. Hypoxemia, decreased diffusing capacity, and pulmonary function studies consistent with a combined obstructive and restrictive defect are frequently present. The chest film shows progressive fibrotic changes with less nodular densities and loss of lung volume with shrinkage of the upper lobes. In addition to the granulomatous pneumonitis, biopsy specimens at this stage reveal bronchiolitis obliterans with distal destruction of alveoli (honeycombing) in association with densely fibrotic zones. The diagnosis of hypersensitivity pneumonitis is important because it is a reversible disease when diagnosed early. It often requires intensive detective work to uncover the source of the antigen. The serum can be tested against common antigens (the thermophilic actinomycetes, especially *Micropolyspora faeni* and *Thermoactinomyces vulgaris*), but the presence of precipitins does not make a definite diagnosis.

CONNECTIVE TISSUE DISEASES

The most common form of pulmonary involvement in the connective tissue diseases is a chronic interstitial pattern that is indistinguishable from idiopathic pulmonary fibrosis. Pleuropulmonary disease may be the initial manifestation in patients with previously undiagnosed connective tissue disease. Moreover, these findings may be a major cause of morbidity and mortality in these disorders. Rheumatoid arthritis is associated with (1) pleurisy, with or without effusion; (2) interstitial pneumonitis; (3) necrobiotic nodules (non-pneumoconiotic intrapulmonary rheumatoid nodules), with or without cavities; (4) Caplan's syndrome (rheumatoid pneumoconiosis); (5) pulmonary hypertension secondary to rheumatoid pulmonary vasculitis; (6) bronchiolitis obliterans; (7) upper airway obstruction due to arytenoid arthritis. Pulmonary lesions are commonly found in patients with progressive systemic sclerosis (scleroderma) and consist mainly of interstitial pneumonitis. Pulmonary function tests usually reveal a restrictive pattern, with reduced lung compliance and impaired diffusing capacity, often before any clinical or radiographic evidence of lung disease appears. Pulmonary vascular disease, alone or in association with pulmonary fibrosis, pleuritis, recurrent aspiration pneumonitis, and bronchiolar carcinoma, also occur. The interstitial lung disease and pulmonary hypertension associated with scleroderma are strikingly resistant to current modes of therapy.

The pleuropulmonary manifestations of systemic lupus erythematosus are (1) pleurisy, with or without effusion; (2) atelectasis; (3) interstitial pneumonitis (less than 5 percent of patients), which exists in two forms—acute interstitial pneumonitis (tachypnea, dyspnea, high fever, cyanosis, and pulmonary hemorrhage that can be fatal) and chronic interstitial pneumonia (dyspnea, nonproductive cough, pleuritic chest pain, hypocapnia, impaired diffusing capacity and a restrictive ventilatory defect); (4) uremic pulmonary edema; (5) diaphragmatic dysfunction, with loss of lung volume; and (6) infectious pneumonia. Predominance in females is striking. Sjögren's syndrome (keratoconjunctivitis sicca, xerostomia, and recurrent swelling of the parotid gland), polymyositis and dermatomyositis may be associated with chronic diffuse interstitial pneumonitis and fibrosis.

PULMONARY VASCULITIS

The pulmonary vasculitides are a heterogeneous group of disorders that have the common feature of necrotizing inflammation of blood vessels. The pathogenesis of pulmonary vasculitides is unknown. Most, if not all, are probably mediated by immune complex deposition in blood vessels, although cell-mediated immune processes may also be involved in some types. Wegener's granulomatosis most commonly occurs in the fifth decade of life and is characterized by the triad of (1) necrotizing granulomatous vasculitis of the upper respiratory tract (profuse rhinorrhea with sinus pain, epistaxis, and saddle nose deformity) and of the lower respiratory tract (cough, hemoptysis, and nodular, often cavitary, densities on chest roentgenogram); (2) disseminated vasculitis (leukocytoclastic vasculitis common); and (3) glomerulitis (azotemia, hypertension, and proteinuria). Lymphomatoid granulomatosis, a disease that occurs in men in the fifth to sixth decade of life, is clinically similar to Wegener's granulomatosis. They differ, however, in that (1) involved organs are infiltrated by a pleomorphic mass of invasive atypical lymphocytes and plasmacytoid cells, which is accompanied by a granulomatous reaction in an angiocentric and angiodestructive pattern; (2) septal and palatal perforations occur; (3) glomerulitis is rare; and (4) there is a tendency to progress to malignant lymphoma in untreated patients. The hypersensitivity vasculitides (Henoch-Schönlein purpura, cryoglobulinemia) are primarily systemic, with skin and visceral involvement. Although lung involvement is uncommon, it appears to occur more frequently in the elderly. Unlike the granulomatous vasculitides that involve the medium-sized vessels, these diseases primarily affect venules, arterioles, and capillaries.

DRUG-INDUCED LUNG DISEASE

The elderly take more drugs per capita than does the population as a whole, and the incidence of adverse drug reactions increases with age to the extent that patients in the eighth and ninth decades of life have three times the incidence of drug reactions than that observed in people under the age of 50. Chemotherapeutic agents are the most common culprits in drug-induced interstitial disorders. Unfortunately, the diagnosis is often missed or delayed because of the clinician's search for an opportunistic infection in these immunocompromised patients. Bleomycin, busulfan, chlorambucil, cylophosphamide, melphalan, and uracil mustard appear to cause fibrosis in a dose-dependent manner. The patient's age, number of cycles and cumulative dose, past history of lung disease, hematologic abnormalities, combination chemotherapy, and, most importantly, the concomitant use of radiation therapy or oxygen (FIO_2 greater than 40)

appear to exert synergistic or additive effects. Nitrofurantoin is the most common of the antibiotics to produce lung disease and may cause either an acute, spontaneously resolving pneumonitis associated with peripheral eosinophilia or a chronic interstitial pneumonitis that is pathologically indistinguishable from idiopathic pulmonary fibrosis.

IDIOPATHIC PULMONARY FIBROSIS

Idiopathic pulmonary fibrosis is a perplexing disease characterized by the insidious onset of dyspnea, clubbing, interstitial infiltrates on the chest x-ray, pulmonary function tests that reveal a restrictive impairment (decreased static lung volumes), impaired diffusing capacity for CO and arterial hypoxemia exaggerated or elicited by exercise. The mean survival is 4 to 6 years; however, the clinical course is quite variable. The pathogenesis of idiopathic pulmonary fibrosis is unknown, and open lung biopsy is required for the diagnosis and staging of this disease.

Pulmonary Embolism

Pulmonary embolism (PE) is responsible for approximately 140,000 deaths yearly, and about 600,000 patients suffer nonfatal PE each year in the U.S.[102] In 60 percent of these, the diagnosis of PE is not suspected.[103] Pulmonary embolism results from venous thrombi that become lodged in the pulmonary arterial circulation. The elderly patient is at significant risk for the development of venous thrombosis. They are more likely to be inactive, at bedrest, and have concurrent clinical phlebitis, congestive heart failure, venous insufficiency, or carcinoma. The older patient is also at greater risk in the postoperative state (especially following pelvic or hip surgery) because of prolonged immobilization. In addition, because of already compromised cardiac and pulmonary function, PE represents a dangerous and often fatal event for the older patient.[104] The diagnosis and management of venous thrombosis and PE has been recently reviewed.[105]

CLINICAL PICTURE

The clinical picture of PE is dictated by both the size and extent of the embolic episode and the pre-existing cardiopulmonary reserve. It is clear from autopsy studies that the majority of PE go unrecognized (Fig. 28–10). This may result from failure of the medical profession to suspect this diagnosis or from the relative absence of symptoms and signs. With massive PE, sudden syncope, chest pain, and acute dyspnea are common. Physical examination may reveal hypotension and signs of pulmonary hypertension such as increased pulmonic component of second heart sound, tricuspid insufficiency, and distended neck veins. With medium-sized PE, pleuritic chest pain, dyspnea, and hemoptyses are seen. Physical examination may be nonrevealing or demonstrate a pleural friction rub or findings of a pleural effusion. Mild temperature elevations may occur but not above 39°C.[106] In the hospitalized geriatric patient, symptoms and signs may be limited to tachypnea, tachycardia, and a changing mental status. Diffuse wheezing is heard in a small percentage of patients and may be associated with pulmonary edema.[107]

The third syndrome is insidious and is caused by recurrent episodes of small emboli that occlude the pulmonary arterial microvasculature, resulting in a picture of slowly progressive cor pulmonale. This syndrome is very difficult to differentiate from primary pulmonary hypertension, although the latter is more common in younger females with concomitant Raynaud's phenomenon and a familial predisposition.[108] In all patients with suspected PE, a search for deep venous thrombosis must be undertaken. More often than not, signs of deep venous thrombosis including edema, unilateral calf enlargement, tenderness, positive Homan's sign, and palpable cord are absent.

DIAGNOSIS

When PE is suspected, the diagnosis must be pursued in a logical sequence. Routine laboratory tests should be obtained to eliminate the many other possible diagnoses. Approximately 30 percent of patients with suspected PE on clinical grounds are actually proven positive. Whereas, 60 percent have an abnormal ventilation-perfusion scan, only around 50 percent of patients have documented PE (i.e., 50 percent false-positive).

Arterial blood gases usually reveal mild to moderate hypoxemia, a widened $P(A-a)O_2$ gradient, and hypocarbia. A normal arterial blood gas, however, does not exclude the diagnosis of PE. The ECG is usually normal, but an $S_1Q_3T_3$ pattern, evidence of right ventricular strain, right atrial abnormalities (P pulmonale), and supraventricular arrhythmias—particularly atrial fibrillation—may be present. However, tachycardia and nonspecific ST-T wave changes are most commonly present. The chest roentgenogram is usually normal or may have varying combinations of subtle or gross findings, including elevated hemidiaphragm, regional oligemia, pleural effusion, pleural-based infiltrate (Hampton's hump), subsegmental atelectasis, changes in the size of the pulmonary arteries, and right ventricular enlargement. Pneumothorax should be excluded. The next diagnostic test is usually a perfusion lung scan with at least four views. A normal perfusion scan excludes the diagnosis of PE. If a perfusion defect is present, a ventilation scan should be performed, with particular attention given to the views that clearly show the perfusion defects. Matched ventilation-perfusion defects are characteristic of parenchymal

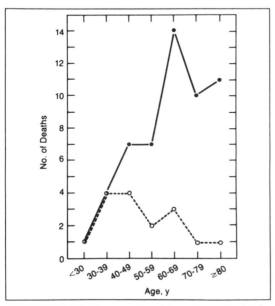

FIGURE 28–10. *Correct ante mortem diagnosis of pulmonary embolism versus patient age. Solid line indicates all patients; broken line indicates patients with correct ante mortem diagnosis. (From Gross JS, Neufeld RR, Libow LS, et al, eds: Autopsy study of the elderly institutionalized patient: review of 234 autopsies. Arch Intern Med 148:173, 1988; by permission.)*

diseases, whereas "mismatched" defects such as normal ventilation in zones of reduced perfusion are characteristic of vascular obstruction. Therefore, a high-probability scan (i.e., greater than 87 percent frequency of PE) is characterized by perfusion defects substantially larger than the radiographic abnormalities, one or more large segmental defects, or two or more moderate-size ventilation-perfusion mismatches, without a corresponding radiographic abnormality. The clinical relevance of matched and mismatched subsegmental defects and multiple small perfusion defects is unknown. Many of these patients are found to have PE as confirmed by angiography.

If a high index of suspicion remains in the presence of a low-probability or indeterminate ventilation-perfusion scan, lower extremity venography, pulmonary angiography, or both should be performed. Venography has fewer complications than does angiography, but 20 percent to 30 percent of patients with documented PE have negative venograms. If the venogram reveals proximal deep vein thrombosis (above the knee), full anticoagulation is recommended. The venogram may be negative because the source of the thrombosis may be from the deep pelvic veins, the renal veins, the right atrium, or the vena cava.

Pulmonary angiography is considered the "gold standard" of tests and should be performed whenever doubt exists as to the correct diagnosis or when major therapy is contemplated (e.g., thrombolytic therapy, inferior vena caval ligation, or embolectomy) (Fig. 28–11). Approximately 50 percent of patients suspected of having PE require angiogram, of which only one third are found to be positive. A normal angiogram excludes the diagnosis of PE. The combined morbidity and mortality from pulmonary angiography is 1 to 2 percent. The role of digital subtraction pulmonary angiography remains to be confirmed.

TREATMENT

Pulmonary embolism is a complication of venous thrombosis. Therefore, prevention is the key to successful management of PE. High-risk patients should be carefully monitored for the development of deep venous thrombosis. Useful techniques include fibrinogen leg scanning, impedance plethysmography, and contrast venography. Prophylactic therapy (e.g., low-dose heparin 5000 U, subcutaneous, every 12 hr) is effective in preventing venous thrombosis in selected high-risk patients. Treatment with aspirin and sulfinpyrazone appears to reduce the likelihood of deep venous thrombosis following hip replacement, especially among women. Early ambulation and elastic stockings are not protective in the prevention of deep venous thrombosis. Supportive care aimed at the treatment of hypoxemia (using oxygen therapy), hypotension, and reduced cardiac output is of first importance. Heparin is the drug of choice in the vast majority of patients with PE. It should be started as soon as the diagnosis is suspected on clinical grounds; it can be discontinued later if the workup is negative. It prevents further clot formation, but it cannot prevent detachment of pre-existing venous thrombi. The ideal heparin regimen for PE is unknown. A useful regimen is to begin anticoagulation with a large intravenous bolus (5000 to 20,000 U), followed by a continuous infusion of 1000 to 1500 U/hr, or enough to prolong the whole-blood clotting time or the activated partial thromboplastin time (PTT) 1½ to 2 times control.

Full-dose heparin is usually maintained for at least 7 to 10 days. Most patients are maintained on anticoagulation therapy for at least 3 months, unless persistent risk factors are present that would prolong the therapy. Warfarin (adequate to prolong the prothrombin time 1½ to 2 times the control value) or subcutaneous heparin (7500 U every 12 hr) are the two options for prolonged anticoagulation protection. Long-term heparin therapy represents a serious potential problem for the elderly.[109] Complications include bleeding in up to 8 percent of patients, reversible thrombocytopenia, hyperkalemia, osteoporosis, and interaction with other drugs.[110, 111]

In the presence of contraindications to anticoagulation, such as high risk of bleeding, recurrent emboli despite adequate anticoagulation, or severe embolization such that a recurrence may be fatal, *surgical interruption of the inferior vena cava is indicated.* This is accomplished by vena caval plication, clipping, ligation, or insertion of

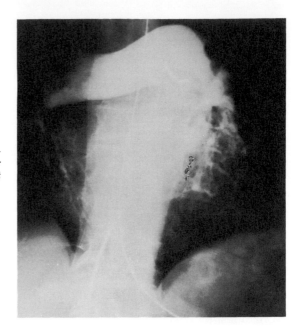

FIGURE 28–11. Pulmonary angiogram; massive pulmonary embolism. Note the filling defect in the left lower lobe artery and the abrupt cutoff of flow to the right upper and lower lung.

a Mobin-Uddin umbrella or Greenfield filter. Documentation of proximal deep venous thrombosis should be obtained before surgical interruption is performed.

Thrombolytic therapy warrants consideration in patients with massive pulmonary emboli (i.e., involvement of more than two lobar arteries), pulmonary emboli accompanied by shock, submassive pulmonary emboli superimposed on underlying cardiopulmonary dysfunction leading to physiologic decompensation, and iliofemoral thrombosis to prevent chronic postphlebitic problems. It does not replace the heparin therapy but is instituted for 24 to 48 hr before heparin to accelerate clot resolution. Absolute contraindications include active internal bleeding and cerebrovascular disease or a surgical procedure performed within the previous 2 months. Thrombolytic therapy is administered by giving a loading dose, followed by a constant infusion dose intravenously. Therapeutic monitoring is performed by measurement of the whole-blood euglobulin lysis time, the thrombin time, or the PTT 4 to 6 hr after institution of the thrombolytic agent to identify and confirm activation of the fibrinolytic system. Further laboratory monitoring is not required once systemic fibrinolysis has been established. The PTT should be measured before starting anticoagulation therapy. These thrombolytic agents are extremely expensive and have not been proven to have a positive impact on morbidity, mortality, or recurrence. Complications include bleeding (severe in 5 to 25 percent of patients), urticaria (approximately 5 to 15 percent), and low grade fever (approximately 25 percent).

Acute embolectomy is indicated in patients with angiographically proven massive embolism and persistent shock despite medical therapy. Selected patients with chronic pulmonary emboli may benefit from thromboendarterectomy.

In the presence of antithrombin III deficiency, heparin therapy is ineffective, and oral anticoagulation is required. Some experts feel that the antithrombin III levels should be determined as part of the initial evaluation of every patient in whom anticoagulation therapy is contemplated and should be followed in assessing the response to therapy. Patients with familial antithrombin III deficiency probably should be treated with anticoagulants for life.

Pulmonary Aspiration

Aspiration of foreign material into the airways represents a debilitating and life-threatening problem for the elderly patient. Conditions predisposing to aspiration in this age group include altered level of consciousness, diminished or absent gag and cough reflexes, anesthesia, endotracheal intubation, the use of nasogastric tubes, tracheotomy during resuscitative attempts, and alcoholism.[112] In a study of nursing home residents with the diagnosis of acute myocardial infarction (MI), autopsy revealed a 33 percent incidence of aspiration pneumonia.[113] In these subjects, the aspiration was considered to be the cause of death. In general, aspiration has a high mortality (40 to 60 percent), which correlates with the amount of material aspirated and to the age and underlying general condition of the patient.

TYPES OF ASPIRATION

ACID ASPIRATION (MENDELSON'S SYNDROME). The single most important factor in aspiration of gastric contents is the pH of the gastric juice. The pH of normal fasting gastric juice is between 1.5 and 2.4.[114] A pH below 2.5 appears to be critical in terms of resultant lung destruction.[115] The pathologic picture is one of ARDS. There are areas of hemorrhage and atelectasis and an outpouring of protein-rich fluid. This progresses to destruction of the alveolar spaces, which become filled with necrotic debris and inflammatory cells.[116] During the first 24 hours, the lung is sterile; however, if the patient survives several days, superinfection can occur.[117]

Clinically, there is marked respiratory distress characterized by tachypnea, wheezing, cyanosis, and change in mental status. Hypoxemia is severe and unresponsive to high oxygen concentrations, indicating a large right to left shunt. Arterial hypotension is seen in 25 percent of cases. The chest radiograph demonstrates diffuse alveolar infiltrates with a normal cardiac silhouette (Fig. 28–12). If aspiration of food particles accompanies the acid aspiration, bronchoscopy and removal are indicated, usually after endotracheal intubation. Corticosteroids and prophylactic administration of antibiotics are unproven modes of therapy and should not be begun empirically. Superimposed bacterial pneumonia in patients with acid aspiration, however, carries considerable morbidity and mortality, therefore, recurrence of fever, purulent sputum, leukocytosis, new or expanding pulmonary infiltrates, unexplained clinical deterioration, increasing hypoxemia, and pathogens in sputum should prompt appropriate antimicrobial

therapy. Positive-end expiratory pressure may be required to correct the hypoxemia. Because of the tremendous outpouring of plasma into the lung, hypovolemia will result, and careful attention must be given to fluid replacement. Because there may be pre-existing cardiac disease in the elderly, fluid replacement should be monitored with a Swan-Ganz catheter in place.

ASPIRATION OF SOLID PARTICLES. The clinical manifestations that follow aspiration of solid particles are determined by the size of the particles. Occlusion of the large upper airways may cause acute suffocation and be immediately relieved by the Heimlich maneuver (a quick upward thrust over the abdomen causing a sudden elevation of the diaphragm that forces air through the trachea). Smaller objects reach and occlude more peripheral airways, resulting in eventual atelectasis and bacterial superinfection with abscess formation. Unexplained atelectasis is a definite indication for bronchoscopy (Fig. 28–13). Failure to remove the obstructing object within 2 to 3 weeks may result in recurrent pneumonitis, bronchiectasis, lung abscesses, and/or empyema. Patients aspirate large volumes of inert fluids such as barium, saline, and nasogastric feeding solutions, causing transient, self-limited hypoxemia and simple mechanical obstruction. Immediate tracheal suctioning usually results in immediate resolution, and further therapy should be aimed at prevention.

CHRONIC ASPIRATION OF GASTRIC CONTENTS. This usually results from mechanical or neuromuscular problems. Disorders that interfere with the mechanical properties of swallowing include esophageal strictures, esophageal diverticula, hiatal hernias, nasogastric tubes, tracheostomy, and esophageal carcinoma. Neuromuscular problems include a myotonic esophagus and absent or poor gag reflex caused by a number of neurologic diseases. Continued aspiration often occurs at night, and the patient may report nocturnal dyspnea and wheezing. In most cases, the patient is seen for an infectious complication of chronic aspiration. They present with an infectious pneumonia, usually found in the dependent portions of the lung (i.e., the posterior segments of the upper lobes and the superior segments of the lower lobes). If the patient sleeps in

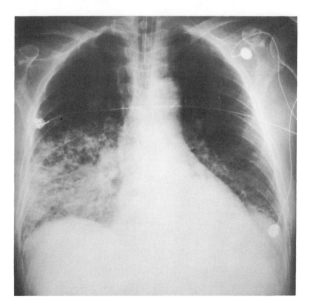

FIGURE 28–12. *Aspiration of gastric contents.*

the upright position, the basilar segments of the lower lobes are involved. The pneumonia may progress to lung abscess and empyema. Occasionally, recurrent and small aspirations, particularly with hiatal hernia, can result in lower zone pulmonary fibrosis without the history of recurrent pneumonia.[118] Treatment consists of careful attention to oral hygiene because mouth flora, including anaerobes, are most often responsible for the infectious complications, proper use of antibiotics, and correction of the anatomic problem, if possible.

MINERAL OIL ASPIRATION. Aspirations from the injudicious use of mineral oils may take several forms. There may be an acute pneumonitis with cough, sputum, and basilar infiltrates on chest radiographs (Fig. 28–14). Fat-filled macrophages are present in the sputum. These patients may also be relatively asymptomatic except for progressive dyspnea and may develop lower zone interstitial markings or pulmonary nodules that pathologically are lipoid granuloma. In either case, the history of the use of oily nose drops is obtained, and discontinuing this practice may result in marked improvement.[119]

Lung abscess frequently is one of the late complications of pulmonary aspiration. The presentation often is insidious,

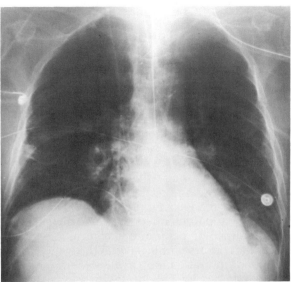

FIGURE 28–13. *Same patient as in Figure 28–12 after 24 hours. Partial atelectasis of the left lower lobe persists, although remarkable clearing of the infiltrate in the right lower lobe has occurred.*

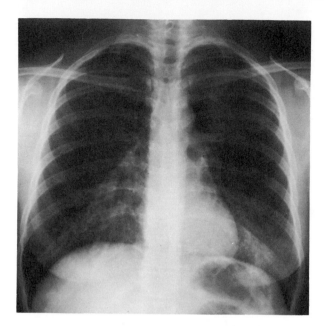

FIGURE 28–14. Mineral oil aspiration. Bilateral lower lobe infiltrates are present.

with weight loss, low-grade fever, and copious foul-smelling sputum production being the prominent findings. Diagnosis requires appropriate identification of the infecting agent through cultures taken of the material obtained from transtracheal aspiration, blood, pleural fluid, and occasionally transthoracic needle aspiration. Exclusion of other causes of cavitary lung disease such as tuberculosis, fungal infection, carcinoma, cavitary infarction (i.e., bland or septic embolism or vasculitis), infected cyst, or bullae must be determined. Fiberoptic bronchscopy should be used to exclude an obstructing endobronchial lesion (tumor or foreign body).

TREATMENT

Therapy demands drainage of the involved lung (postural drainage, steam inhalation, and, rarely, transthoracic needle aspiration or tube drainage) and antibiotic therapy. Penicillin is usually adequate. Patients with mild symptoms and no major medical problems can be given parenteral penicillin (procaine penicillin 600,000 U i.m., every 6 hr or aqueous penicillin G 5 to 20 million U/day, i.v., in divided doses) or oral penicillin (500 mg p.o., every 6 hr). Those given parenteral penicillin can be switched to oral penicillin if clinical improvement occurs within several days and continued on oral therapy until resolution of the cavity. In patients with severe

symptomatic disease, therapy with intravenous aqueous penicillin (2 million U, i.v., every 4 hr) may be required for 5 to 10 days. If empyema is present, chest tube drainage is required. Occasionally, thoracotomy with rib resection is necessary to drain loculated areas of pus. It should be noted that fever may persist for several days to 3 weeks despite adequate therapy, and it may take several more weeks for resolution of the cavity.

Carbon Monoxide Poisoning

Carbon monoxide is a colorless, odorless, highly toxic gas that binds avidly to hemoglobin (approximately 210 times greater than oxygen) so that oxygen transport in the body is markedly impaired and tissue hypoxia results. Acute exposure to high levels results in a well-documented clinical syndrome. On the other hand, the health effects of exposure to low levels is very controversial. One cannot help but wonder if the elderly are not predisposed to potential problems because exposure in the home is increasing as a result of efforts to make buildings air tight, the use of gas stoves for heating (a common practice among the urban poor in northern climates), and the use of kerosene and gas space heaters and wood stoves. Furthermore, the carbon monoxide levels may reach as much as twice the values identified in single-family residences. Although the health effects of low-level carbon monoxide exposure are controversial, it is nonetheless a syndrome that clinicians should recognize.[120] This is especially relevant when one considers that carbon monoxide poisoning is frequently misdiagnosed as food poisoning, psychiatric disorders, cerebrovascular disease, intoxication, and heart disease.

CLINICAL PICTURE

The manifestations are related primarily to the level of carboxyhemoglobin present. Associated disease, especially cardiac disease and other factors that influence oxygen demand and delivery, also determine the severity of the clinical findings. Diagnosis depends on measurement of the carboxyhemoglobin levels or oxygen content. Oxygen saturation should be measured directly and not calculated because the arterial PaO_2 usually is normal. At carboxyhemoglobin levels of 20 to 30 percent, headache, nausea, vomiting, weakness, dizziness, and diminished visual acuity are prominent symptoms. The finding of retinal hemorrhage on fundoscopic examination should alert the clinicians to possible carbon monoxide poisoning. At levels < 40 percent, there is little correlation between the symptoms and signs and the blood carboxyhemoglobin level. Characteristically, the manifestations are related to the brain, including coma, seizures, ataxia, and diffuse and fluctuating neurologic deficits, and to the cardiac system, such as syncope, ECG abnormalities, and myocardial ischemia/infarction. A level > 60 percent is associated with coma and death.

TREATMENT

The half-life of carboxyhemoglobin is 4 to 6 hr, but increased alveolar ventilation and high inspired oxygen concentrations will significantly alter the displacement of carbon monoxide. Therefore, the immediate institution of oxygen therapy (preferably 100 percent oxygen) is mandatory. This will improve tissue oxygen delivery and shorten the half-life of carboxyhemoglobin to 40 to 50 minutes. Intubation and mechanical ventilation may be required if the patient is hemodynamically unstable and/or hypoventilation is present. Hyperbaric oxygen will hasten the removal of carbon monoxide and is recommended in the treatment of life-threatening cerebral or coronary hypoxia. Appropriate steps should be taken to manage any factor that will reduce tissue oxygen delivery or increase tissue oxygen demand such as anemia, hypothermia, hypotension, fever, metabolic acidosis.

Bronchogenic Carcinoma

For the past century, the incidence of bronchogenic carcinoma has been steadily increasing. It is responsible for 100,000 deaths a year in the U.S. and represents the most common cause of cancer deaths for both men and women. The age-specific incidence of bronchogenic carcinoma increases dramatically with increasing age. Persons over age 65, when compared with those aged 45 to 64 years, have much higher incidence ratios (3.2 for men and 1.8 for women).[121] In fact, the group aged 65 and older constitutes roughly half of all lung cancer cases. Lung cancer is associated with a number of carcinogenic pollutants. Although cigarette smoke is by far the most important, others to keep in mind are asbestos, uranium, nickel, chlormethyl ether, and chromium. It appears that asbestos and uranium exposure act synergistically with cigarette smoke, thereby increasing the risk of developing bronchogenic carcinoma above that seen with cigarette smoking alone. In addition, scarring of the pulmonary parenchyma, secondary to diffuse insterstitial fibrosis, or localized scarring after tuberculosis predisposes to the development of a scar carcinoma.

CLINICAL PICTURE

There are five types of bronchogenic carcinoma. These include (1) epidermoid (squamous), (2) adenocarcinoma, (3) alveolar cell, (4) small cell (oat cell), and (5) large cell (undifferentiated). Most recent data suggest that adenocarcinoma and squamous carcinoma are the most common histologic types of lung cancer.[122] Clinically, the patient may be symptomatic or have an asymptomatic lesion discovered on a chest radiograph. In fact, recent data suggest that lung cancer is initially seen at a less advanced stage with increasing age.[122, 123] If the tumor is endobronchial in location, an irritative cough may be present. This is difficult to distinguish from a cough associated with chronic airway obstruction, which is also likely to be present in this patient. Streaky hemoptysis, a new onset of localized wheezing, worsening dyspnea, and chest pain are all symptoms of endobronchial disease. An endobronchial lesion may be heralded by an obstructive infectious pneumonia. If the chest wall is invaded, severe, deep bone pain may be present. Pleural invasion may be associated with pleuritic pain and progressive dyspnea as a pleural effusion develops. Mediastinal spread is indicated by hoarseness (recurrent laryngeal nerve paralysis), raised diaphragm on chest radiograph (phrenic nerve paralysis), difficulty in swallowing (esophageal obstruction), pericardial tamponade, and headache and facial swelling (superior vena cava obstruction).

Extrathoracic metastatic manifestations are commonly the first signs of bronchogenic carcinoma. This is particularly true of the small or oat cell variety. The most common sites of metastases are the CNS, bones, and liver. Symptoms may also be related to nonmetastatic extrathoracic manifestations, the paraneoplastic syndromes. The presence of a paraneoplastic syndrome indicates a poor prognosis. The endocrinopathies include inappropriate secretion of antidiuretic hormone (SIADH) seen with oat cell carcinoma, hypercalcemia secondary to parathyroid hormone-like material produced by squamous tumors, and adrenocorticotropic hormone (ACTH) production. Neuromuscular paraneoplastic syndromes include the Eaton-Lambert syndrome (reverse myasthenia gravis), peripheral neuropathy (sensory), and cerebellar degeneration. Patients with bronchogenic carcinoma may also present with dermatomyositis, pulmonary hypertrophic osteodystrophy (squamous cell), and acanthosis nigricans.

DIAGNOSIS

Chest radiography can be highly suggestive of the diagnosis of bronchogenic carcinoma. A hilar mass may be represented by unilateral hilar enlargement or increase in hilar density. This may be associated with a homogenous parenchymal infiltrate, which may represent either atelectasis or postobstructive pneumonia (Fig. 28–15). Mediastinal enlargement may be present (metastatic lymph nodes), and this may be associated with a paralyzed diaphragm (usually on the left) and an increase in size of the cardiac shadow, representing pericardial metastases with effusion. Lytic rib lesions, pleural effusions and masses, and diffuse lymphangitic carcinomatosis may also be seen (Fig. 28–16). A peripheral bronchogenic carcinoma may be associated with all of the above. If possible, it is important to obtain previous chest films to see if a "coin" lesion is new. Cavitation in a peripheral bronchogenic carcinoma is most often seen with squamous cell carcinoma (Fig. 28–17).

The staging of a potentially resectable bronchogenic carcinoma is still a matter of debate. To establish the diagnosis of central endobronchial lesions, sputum cytological examination is the initial step. If the cytology is positive for malignancy and the patient demonstrates no evidence of local spread to the mediastinum or chest wall or extrathoracic disease, fiberoptic bronchoscopy is then performed to determine the extent of the mucosal involvement. If cytology is negative, bronchoscopic examination is indicated, since this has been shown to be a well-tolerated, safe, and productive procedure, even in patients aged 70 and over.[124] Routine use of brain, bone, and liver-spleen scans has not been shown to be helpful unless there are symptoms or signs that may indicate metastatic spread to these organ systems.[125] Intrathoracic spread of bronchogenic carcinoma may be easily determined by chest radiography if mediastinal, bone, or pleural disease is present, and these would be definite contraindications to surgical intervention. Mediastinoscopy is indicated for all central (endobronchial) lesions. The use of mediastinoscopy for peripheral lesions is not as clear. In one study, nine of 46 patients with peripheral bronchogenic carcinoma had a positive mediastinal exploration. Seven of these, however, had positive chest radiographs for mediastinal enlargement. Compared with central carcinomas, 50 percent had negative chest radiographs and positive

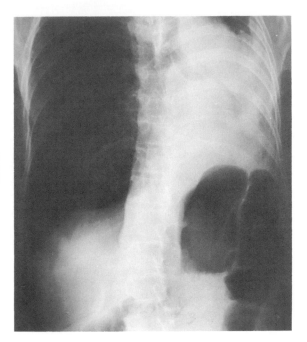

FIGURE 28–15. *Bronchogenic carcinoma. Atelectasis of the left lower lobe and lingual segment of the left upper lobe; an elevated diaphragm and left pleural effusion are present as a result of endobronchial disease.*

mediastinoscopy.[126] Gallium-67 scanning and CT of the chest have also been recommended to evaluate mediastinal spread.[127]

TREATMENT

Once all attempts are made to detect metastatic disease, the decision of whether surgery is indicated must be made. This is particularly important for patients 70 years and over because the overall operative mortality (10 to 14 percent) and morbidity

is increased.[128] Obviously, the mortality for pneumonectomy is greater than that for lobectomy or wedge resection. A diagnosis of oat cell carcinoma is a definite contraindication to surgery, and these patients should be treated with chemotherapy and, depending on the extent of the disease, such as CNS metastases, radiation therapy. The decision to operate on bronchogenic carcinoma in the elderly will depend upon the patient's underlying cardiovascular and pulmonary status. In the older patient, this is often a matter of clinical

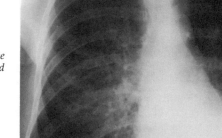

FIGURE 28–16. *Lymphangitic carcinomatosis. Note the left lower lobe mass with left pleural effusion and lymphangitic metastases to the right lung.*

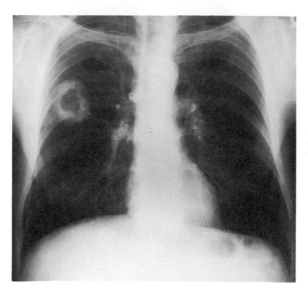

FIGURE 28–17. Squamous cell carcinoma of the lung with cavitation.

judgment. In the group aged 70 years and over, the major deterrent to resective pulmonary surgery is the presence of chronic airway obstruction. Severe physiologic disturbances, such as PO_2 less than 55 mmHg, PCO_2 greater than 40 mmHg, and FEV_1 less than 1.2 liters, are definite contraindications to resective surgery, and the patients are placed in another treatment protocol. There often is a group of elderly patients with whom the decision is not so clear, particularly those with small peripheral lesions and borderline physiologic status. In these patients with potentially curable lesions, much emphasis is placed on preoperative medical management, and a wedge resection should be considered. Recent evidence suggests that the results of wedge resection compares favorably with those of lobectomy, and the operative mortality and morbidity rates are less.[129]

Finally, it must be remembered that, despite the many therapeutic modalities available, the average survival of the majority of these patients is 6 to 8 months after diagnosis. Every effort should be made to provide comfort and support for the patient and his or her family. General supportive measures, such as correction of anemia, relief of pain, control of infection, and intensive psychosocial support, are important in these patients.

Tuberculosis

Although tuberculosis is no longer a major health hazard in industrialized countries, it still occurs and is a serious problem among the elderly[130] (Fig. 28–18). Because many geriatric patients have been exposed to tuberculosis infection (latent infection) as children, reactivation may occur during the adult years. It is estimated that in adults with negative chest films and positive tuberculin skin tests, the yearly infection rate will be 82 per 100,000 individuals.[131] Among the elderly confined to nursing homes, the rate for active tuberculosis can be extremely high. This rate is enhanced by alcoholism, malnutrition, diabetes, immunosuppressive drugs, neoplasia, and renal dialysis. These data indicate that tuberculosis will continue to be a major health hazard in the geriatric population, and thus it has been recommended that a high index of suspicion for the disease should be maintained, especially in elderly patients who present with multiple medical problems and nonspecific complaints.[132]

CLINICAL PICTURE

Tuberculosis is easily recognized in the patient who presents with fever, night sweats, weight loss, anorexia, and hemoptyses. Chest radiography will demonstrate upper zone infiltrates, with or without cavitation and a positive tuberculin skin test. Examination of the sputum will reveal acid-fast rods, making the diagnosis secure. Unfortunately, the typical clinical picture may not be seen in the elderly. In one study, of 31 geriatric patients who died of tuberculosis, a premortem diag-

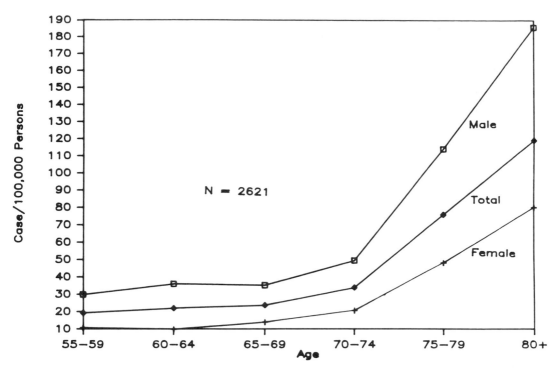

FIGURE 28–18. *Average age-specific tuberculosis case rates (cases/100,000 persons per year) in Arkansas from 1979 through 1985. A sharp increase is apparent at about age 70. (From Stead WW, To T, eds: The significance of the tuberculin skin test in elderly persons. Ann Intern Med 107:837, 1987; by permission.)*

nosis was made in only four.[133] Rather than demonstrating a well-defined clinical illness, the geriatric patient may show only weight loss and anorexia or fever of unknown origin as the major problem. Up to 20 percent of patients with active tuberculosis have a negative tuberculin reaction.[134] Instead of a typical chest radiograph demonstrating upper lobe infiltrative or cavitary disease, there may be single or multiple nodules (Fig. 28–19), pleural effusion, miliary spread (Fig. 28–20), or infiltrates in locations other than the upper lobes.[135] A virtually negative chest radiography may be present with active extrapulmonary sites. It becomes imperative, therefore, to consider the diagnosis of tuberculosis in all geriatric patients with a wide variety of symptoms in whom the diagnosis is not readily apparent.

DIAGNOSIS

All patients suspected of having tuberculosis should have an intradermal skin test with 5 U of purified protein derivative (PPD). A positive test (10 mm or more of induration) indicates prior infection, but,

as noted in the foregoing discussion, a negative test does not exclude the diagnosis.[136] A patient with a negative reaction may undergo a repeat test after 1 week. A positive test at this time indicates a previously diminished skin hypersensitivity that has been activated by further exposure to tuberculous protein.[137] Importantly, it has been shown that in the elderly, the first significant reaction may not be elicited until the third test with the same dose of antigen. Sputum, preferably an early morning specimen, is collected for 3 consecutive days. Induced sputums by the inhaled aerosol technique may be used for patients who are unable to voluntarily produce sputum. If these methods are ineffective, gastric aspiration or bronchoscopic specimens for culture may be obtained. If the patient has sterile pyuria, hematuria, and/or proteinuria, the morning urine specimen should be cultured for tuberculosis. An intravenous pyelogram may further define the extent of renal tuberculosis. If the chest radiograph is not helpful, extrapulmonary tuberculosis should be considered. A miliary pattern may not be apparent on the chest radiograph until the disease is far advanced.

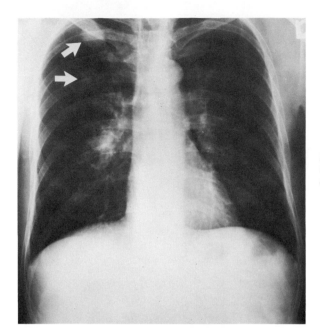

FIGURE 28–19. *Pulmonary tuberculosis. Multiple nodules are present in the right upper lung zone, and a single nodule is superimposed on the right hilum.*

Other sites that may be sampled, depending on symptoms, clinical findings, and laboratory results, include the bone marrow, spine (cold abscess), joints, meninges, liver, pericardium, and peritoneum.

TREATMENT

Modern chemotherapy is highly effective in the treatment of tuberculosis. The major challenge in the elderly is to select a therapeutic regimen that produces minimal adverse reactions, is easily administered, and is acceptable to the patient.[138]

Once active tuberculosis is diagnosed, therapy should be instituted in the hospital, and after 2 to 4 weeks, the patients are considered noninfectious and may be discharged. All positive cultures should be speciated to rule out atypical mycobacterial infections, and drug sensitivity studies should be performed because of the increased incidence of isoniazid (INH) resistant strains. This is especially true in both noncompliant patients and those who have received prior therapy.

The three first-line drugs for treatment of tuberculosis in the elderly are isoniazid,

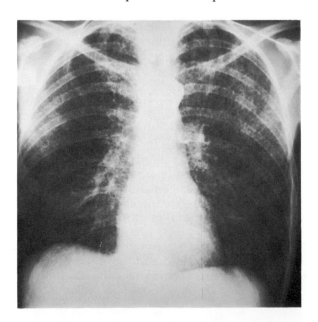

FIGURE 28–20. *Widespread miliary nodulation throughout both lungs.*

rifampin, and ethambutol. Isoniazid-induced hepatitis is a real problem in the elderly, particularly in those with active liver disease or impaired liver function. Because rifampin, in combination with isoniazid, increases the risk of further liver damage, streptomycin may be substituted for a total of 3 months. Streptomycin, however, should be avoided, if possible, because of its ototoxicity. This is particularly true in patients with impaired renal function. In low doses (15 mg/kg), the ocular complications of ethambutol are minimal (impairment of color vision and visual acuity). However, when ethambutol is used with isoniazid in a two-drug regimen, the recommended dosage is 25 mg/kg. At this dose, visual problems may occur, and the patient should receive monthly eye testing. For the usual patient, it is recommended to employ rifampin, isoniazid, and ethambutol for 3 months, and then to discontinue rifampin and continue with isoniazid and ethambutol for an additional year. Short-course chemotherapy with isoniazid and rifampin is currently recommended for pulmonary tuberculosis presumed to be due to fully susceptible organisms. The usual regimen is daily for 9 months or daily for 1 month, followed by an altered dose of the drug twice weekly for another 8 months.[139] If one is dealing with resistant organisms, second-line drugs can be instituted only after consultation with an expert in this area. Corticosteroids may occasionally be indicated in tuberculosis of the CNS, in tuberculous pericarditis, and in tuberculous peritonitis.[140, 141] Corticosteroids are thought to be effective in reducing fibrous adhesions.

Isoniazid prophylaxis for 1 year is recommended for those high-risk patients who have a positive skin test (induration of at least 12 mm) without culture evidence of active disease.[142] High-risk patients include those with recent conversion to skin test positivity and those with chronic debilitating disorders, such as chronic renal failure, chronic airway obstruction, gastric resection, diabetes, silicosis, and alcoholism. Recent experience indicates that preventive treatment in elderly persons is effective in reducing the incidence of tuberculosis and that the incidence of toxicity from isoniazid is small.[143]

Pneumonia

Lower respiratory tract infections are a major cause of morbidity among the elderly. In 1977, pneumonia (primarily bacterial) and influenza were the fourth leading causes of death in persons over age 65. This is presumably due to deterioration of the body's immunologic defenses and the presence of other chronic diseases, which further impair immunity and allow for colonization of the respiratory tract.[144] Hospitalized geriatric patients are at further risk, since the use of respiratory therapy equipment, immunosuppressive drugs, and broad-spectrum antibiotics allows the entrance and proliferation of potential pathogens into the respiratory tract.

CLINICAL PICTURE

The presentation of pneumonia in the elderly patient may differ markedly from that seen in younger age groups. High spiking fevers, productive cough, and an elevated white cell count may not be seen. Instead, altered mental status, tachypnea, and evidence of dehydration may dominate the clinical picture. Although an alteration in mental status may be the result of hypoxia, septicemia, or volume depletion, meningitis must be excluded. Approximately 20 percent of elderly patients with community-acquired pneumonia may be afebrile on admission.[145] The typical chest physical findings may not be heard because of an increase in the anterioposterior (AP) diameter. The characteristic radiographic appearance of lobar or segmental consolidation may be distorted by underlying emphysema, producing a pattern of incomplete consolidation (Swiss-cheese pattern) (Fig. 28–21). This may be confused with tuberculosis or abscess formation.

ETIOLOGY

When considering the etiology of pneumonia in the elderly, it becomes important to determine whether the disease was acquired in the community or in an institution such as the nursing home or hospital. *Streptococcus pneumoniae* and *Hemophilus influenzae* are the most frequent causes of community-acquired pneumonia, followed by *Legionella pneumophila* and enteric

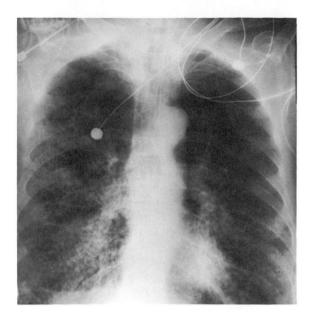

FIGURE 28–21. AP view; acute pneumonia superimposed on emphysema, incomplete consolidation.

gram-negative bacteria. Hospitalized and institutionalized persons are most commonly infected with *Klebsiella pneumoniae* and other enteric gram-negative bacilli, and *Legionella pneumophila* and *Streptococcus pneumoniae* are also etiologic agents in this setting.[146]

DIAGNOSIS AND TREATMENT

All attempts should be made to acquire sputum for Gram stain and culture. If the patient is obtunded and unable to voluntarily expectorate, catheter suction and suction traps should be utilized. Transtracheal puncture and aspiration should be considered for those patients in whom all other methods have been unsuccessful. Blood cultures should be obtained in all patients with pneumonia. Careful attention must be paid to gas exchange because many of these patients will have underlying cardiopulmonary disease and the insult of a superimposed pneumonia will cause respiratory failure. The choice of antibiotic will depend on the Gram stain results and may be modified after culture results are available.

VACCINATION

It is clear that vaccination against the influenza virus protects the high-risk elderly patient from influenza and its complicating pneumonia. The problem lies in the ability of the influenza A virus to antigenically shift about every 10 years. These shifts are often accompanied by a pandemic in a nonimmune population. The chronically debilitated elderly subject bears the brunt of this pandemic. Vaccines recommended for the particular year should be administered yearly to this high-risk population.[146] Amantadine hydrochloride, an antiviral compound for the prevention of illness and treatment of symptoms of respiratory tract infections from influenza A viral strains, is a recommended (but not proven) treatment in older persons.

Pneumococcal pneumonia is still a major cause of death in the elderly population in spite of effective antibiotic treatment. A vaccine prepared from purified capsular polysaccharide material from 23 types of pneumococci theoretically should be protective against 85 percent of the bacteremic pneumococcal pneumonias. After a single intramuscular dose, the resultant antibody responses are adequate enough to be 70 percent effective in those over 55 years of age. Unfortunately, this is not true for those patients who are already immunosuppressed. Unlike influenza vaccine, pneumococcal vaccine is given once in a lifetime. Mass immunization is not necessary because pneumococcal pneumonia does not occur as pandemics. Therefore, it is recommended for asplenic patients, patients with altered immunologic responses, individuals over age 65, and those with diabetes mellitus, chronic cardiorespiratory disease, or cirrhosis.[148]

CARDIOPULMONARY REHABILITATION

As noted, the capacity to perform physical tasks declines with age. Further, the geriatric patient with chronic pulmonary disease is particularly likely to experience these effects of aging on cardiorespiratory performance during exercise. Thus, it is not surprising that the most common and distressing symptoms in such patients is dyspnea, especially with exertion and fatigue. Consequently, a comprehensive care program is required to allow elderly patients to lead as complete a life as possible despite their disease.

A recent American Thoracic Society (ATS) statement reported that the objectives of pulmonary rehabilitation were to control and alleviate symptoms and pathophysiologic complications and to achieve optimal ability to carry out activities of daily living.[22] The physician plays a central role in recognizing the need for and establishing the type of rehabilitation program required by the patient. Thus, it is extremely important that the physician not only prescribe the medications that may control and alleviate the patient's symptoms, but he or she should pay particular attention to the physical and psychosocial factors that, when corrected or improved, will allow the elderly patient to re-establish an independent existence. The type of rehabilitation program must be individualized to each patient, but in general, the key elements include those outlined below. Pulmonary rehabilitation is most beneficial for patients with COPD; however, certain aspects of this program are appropriate for the majority of patients with any pulmonary disorder.

Education

Ongoing education of both the patient and family is one of the keys to successful management. It is important that the cognitive ability of each patient be assessed and the program of education tailored to maximize understanding and allow for any difficulties the patient and spouse may have with memory, eyesight, or hearing.

Psychosocial Support

Psychosocial support is required in many patients with COPD and is an essential component of any rehabilitation program.[22, 149] Fear, anxiety, depression, and problems with cognitive, perceptual, and motor activity are common manifestations of chronic pulmonary diseases, especially COPD. Therefore, psychosocial intervention provides the patient with improved acceptance of the physiologic limitations, optimizes strength, and clarifies reasonable goals and priorities. Thus, effective psychosocial approaches provide the patient with a sense of control and mastery of his or her disease and enhances the quality of life.[22] Many options are available for psychosocial intervention, including education, counseling, individualized psychotherapy, group sessions, vocational counseling, and psychiatric consultation. Antidepressant medication should be utilized when indicated.

Nutritional Support

Nutritional support is important because poor nutrition is a major problem in the elderly and in COPD patients, especially those patients with severe emphysema in whom approximately 30 percent will have significant protein-calorie malnutrition.[150] At present, the precise factors responsible for the malnutrition have not been identified, but elevated resting energy requirements appear to play a key role. It is apparent that insufficient protein/calorie intake may be responsible for the loss of weight and muscle mass (including that of the diaphragm and respiratory muscles) seen in patients with advanced COPD. The methods of nutritional assessment and management of malnutrition in COPD patients have been recently reviewed.[151, 152] The proper methods of nutritional assessment in the clinical setting and recommendations for nutritional support are described in Chapter 36.

Chest Physiotherapy

Chest physical therapy is frequently recommended for a patient with a variety of pulmonary problems. This encompasses the use of postural drainage, chest percussion and vibration administered by hand or mechanical percussion, and cough and deep breathing.[22] It appears to benefit those COPD patients who have excessive secretions (30 ml/day or greater) that are difficult to expectorate. Despite its widespread use at home and in most hospitals in the U.S., there is little objective evidence of its efficacy in other situations. Use of chest physiotherapy has not been shown to be effective in exacerbations of chronic bronchitis or in patients with pneumonia without large volumes of sputum or with status asthmaticus.[21, 153–155]

Results are optimized by giving bronchodilator therapy before chest physiotherapy. Complications are uncommon, but they include worsening hypoxemia (caused by positioning with the abnormal lung dependent) and bronchospasm. Even in those few situations in which chest physiotherapy is likely to be of benefit, it is difficult to establish in the home setting because it requires the patient and family members to undergo a complete educational program on the technique and goals. Trained respiratory care personnel, nurses, or physical therapists provide this instruction, and usually it requires several sessions and often home visit evaluations to ensure proper understanding and technique.

Oxygen Therapy

Frequently, the institution of oxygen therapy is viewed as the "final insult" in an otherwise proud and independent life. The physician should be compassionate, and it should be suggested at a time when the pros and cons of its use can be fully discussed. It is important that the physician, patient, and family members understand the role of oxygen therapy in the management of hypoxemic COPD patients. Long-term home oxygen use has been shown to improve exercise tolerance, alleviate pulmonary hypertension, reduce the red cell mass, promote general well-being so that some patients return to work, markedly improve neuropsychiatric function, and reduce the number of hospitalizations.[77]

Continuous oxygen therapy (at least 18 hrs/day) is more efficacious than nocturnal therapy, especially in those patients with severely altered pulmonary and cerebral function. Oxygen therapy is expensive, and in the elderly in whom limitations of financial and social resources are commonplace, its use should be guided by careful monitoring and objective assessment. This is important because it has been demonstrated that as many as 50 percent of the patients meeting the criteria for the initiation of oxygen therapy (such as those with hypoxemia, with PaO_2 of less than 55 mmHg) will have improvement in their hypoxemia following therapy directed at secretions, bronchospasm, and infection so that oxygen therapy is no longer necessary.[78]

SELECTION CRITERIA FOR PRESCRIBING HOME OXYGEN

Oxygen therapy should be instituted only after the patient has undergone at least a 3- to 4-week stabilization period during which aggressive management is employed to improve the hypoxemia (e.g., secretion control, relief of bronchospasm, and control of infection). Room air arterial blood gases should be obtained on at least two separate occasions and reveal a PO_2 of 55 mmHg or less or be consistently between 56 and 59 mmHg in the presence of evidence of an adverse response to hypoxemia such as cor pulmonale, impaired mental function, or erythrocytosis greater than 55 percent. A minority of patients with COPD and interstitial lung diseases will have only sleep hypoxemia (saturation less than 85 percent). The COPD patients are usually obese or have CO_2 retention, unexplained erythrocytosis, or, rarely, cor pulmonale. Therefore, measurement of PaO_2 during sleep or continuous monitoring of oxygen saturation is required to identify nocturnal hypoxemia. Oxygen therapy that is adequate to produce a minimum nocturnal oxygen saturation of approximately 90 percent is a reasonable therapeutic goal.[22] Patients with obstructive sleep apnea require additional treatment aimed at relieving the nocturnal upper airway obstruction (discussed below). Other patients may have only significant exercise-induced hypoxemia. Thus, a treadmill or bicycle exercise study or similar stress testing (walking in hall or up stairs), using oximetry to measure oxygen saturation, will identify patients with this problem. If it is demonstrated that exercise is limited by exercise-induced hypoxemia, or if cardiac arrhythmias occur only during ambulation, prescribing oxygen with exercise appears warranted. It has not been clearly documented that the use of supplemental oxygen in this setting has long-term benefit. In the elderly, deciding to use oxygen for exercise-induced hypoxemia can be difficult because many of these patients spend very little time exercising. Thus, it is difficult to believe that exercise-induced hypoxemia plays a prominent role in survival or function at rest. Nonetheless, in selected patients, the institution of oxygen therapy in this setting can result in a remarkable increase in the level of activity and sense of well-being, especially if this therapy is combined with defined exercise reconditioning programs, breathing retraining, instructions in work simplification, the use of energy conservation devices, and adequate nutrition.

METHODS OF OXYGEN DELIVERY AND TYPES OF OXYGEN SYSTEMS

Nasal prongs are by far the most practical way to deliver home oxygen to patients. Recently, oxygen-conserving devices that supply oxygen only during inspiration have been developed.[156] Also, a method of delivery of oxygen directly to the sublaryngeal trachea via a chronic transtracheal cannula has been developed.[157] These systems require further study before they can be comfortably recommended for general use.

Compressed gas in cylinders or tanks has been the usual source of oxygen. It has several advantages including widespread availability and cost-efficiency, especially during intermittent use, and storage ability for long periods without loss of oxygen, which can decrease the frequency of oxygen deliveries. The disadvantages are that (1) it is usually quite heavy and cannot be easily transported or moved; (2) it requires a pressure regulator; (3) its high pressure presents a rare, but potential,

explosive hazard; and (4) it holds a limited supply of oxygen. This system is most convenient for patients who are essentially housebound. Small tanks on small carts are available for those who have limited ambulatory ability.

Liquid oxygen systems permit the easy administration of oxygen during exercise and outside of the home. Because of its portability, it comes closest to enabling the patient to be on oxygen 24 hours a day. The reservoirs are more attractive than the cylinders. Its disadvantages are that (1) it is the most expensive of the systems available; (2) the oxygen is lost by venting when not used continuously; and (3) it requires frequent refilling. Nevertheless, it is preferred for patients who require the greatest range away from their stationary oxygen source. This system allows one to work several hours each day away from the home.

Oxygen concentrators are stationary machines that concentrate oxygen by using a molecular sieve to impede nitrogen and create 90 to 100 percent oxygen from room air. The advantages of this system are that (1) it provides a constant, inexhaustible home oxygen supply; (2) it is more attractive equipment than the others; and (3) it is very economical for long-term therapy. The disadvantages are that (1) it requires electrical power and thus will increase the monthly electrical bills; (2) it is somewhat noisy; (3) it requires periodic maintenance and back-up cylinder system in the event of a power failure or for travel.

Because ambulation is deemed extremely important in patients requiring oxygen therapy, the liquid system is preferred from an overall therapeutic point of view. The cost of oxygen, however, is expensive and varies between $250 and $500 per month, depending on location and the amount of oxygen used. The liquid system is the most expensive form of oxygen.

The oxygen prescription must provide the following documentation: (a) evidence that alternative therapies have been employed in an attempt to correct the hypoxemia (e.g., bronchodilators, corticosteroids, antimicrobials, physical therapy); (b) diagnosis (e.g., emphysema, chronic bronchitis, cor pulmonale, COPD, cystic fibrosis, interstitial lung disease, or bronchiectasis) for which home oxygen is appropriate therapy; (c) definite oxygen flow rate (usually 1 to 2 l/min via nasal cannula) and daily duration (usually continuously, 24 hours a day). Occasionally, documentation that hypoxemia drastically limits exercise or is accompanied by excessive tachycardia or cardiac arrhythmias or documentation of nocturnal hypoxemia must be provided; and (d) laboratory evidence of hypoxemia (PaO_2 less than 55 mmHg or oximetry oxygen saturation less than 85 percent) while stable and breathing room air. Renewal of the oxygen prescription often requires documentation of the clinical benefit by an increase in exercise performance and performance of other activities of daily living.

COMPLICATIONS OF OXYGEN THERAPY

There are few complications of low-flow oxygen therapy. On the other hand, the fear of significantly increasing hypercapnia and acidemia by oxygen administration in the acutely ill patient with COPD is well founded, but it need not be crippling. Modest increases in $PaCO_2$ can be considered an expected adaptive response and is usually well tolerated. There are no good criteria that allows one to predict which patients will develop a rising $PaCO_2$ with oxygen therapy. The chance of a patient requiring intubation and mechanical ventilation is markedly reduced by avoiding uncontrolled or injudicious use of oxygen, avoiding sedatives or other medication that may lead to respiratory or cough suppression, and monitoring the effect of oxygen therapy on $PaCO_2$ by measuring arterial blood gases. It must be remembered that severe hypoxemia causes death, whereas the disturbances associated with severe CO_2 retention are not usually lethal. Therefore, in an acutely ill and severely hypoxemic COPD patient, once oxygen is started, never discontinue its administration, even in the event of hypercapnia (i.e., add mechanical ventilation, but do not discontinue oxygen). The lower the dose of oxygen (less than 40 percent O_2), the lower the risk of CO_2 retention. The use of humidified gas will prevent drying of secretions and nasal irritation.

Physical Reconditioning

Most elderly people avoid regular exercise, and subsequently they become deconditioned, which contributes to the exertional breathlessness and easy fatigue they experience. Age is not a deterrent to physical conditioning. Therefore, physical training should be encouraged. Before an elderly patient with COPD or other chronic pulmonary disease is enrolled in a physical reconditioning program, optimal medical management of the disease should be achieved. Motivation is the key factor in the selection of patients for this program. Several lines of reasoning can be used to help motivate the elderly to exercise, including (a) quality of life issues such as the feeling of well-being, improvement in functional capacity, and performance of activities of daily living; (b) weight control, reduction of blood pressure, and probably reduced risk of coronary artery disease; and (c) reduction in medical care costs, chiefly due to savings as a result of a decreased number of hospitalizations.[149, 158] Selection of patients for pulmonary reconditioning requires screening, which should include spirometry, studies of arterial blood gases at rest and during exercise (exercise oximetry may be used to determine the presence of exercise arterial desaturation), and cardiac stress testing.

Although difficult to assess, it is generally felt that physical conditioning, inspiratory muscle training, breathing retraining, and energy conservation techniques are important modalities in the improvement of exercise performance that increases the dyspnea-limited level of activity or decreases the degree of dyspnea associated with the same level of activity.[22]

Exercise reconditioning and inspiratory muscle training to improve performance and reduce the dyspnea experienced by patients with COPD have been shown to be beneficial in this setting. The accepted benefits of exercise reconditioning include (a) increased endurance and exercise tolerance; (b) increased maximal oxygen consumption (generally small); and (c) increased skill in performance of a task, with decreased ventilation, oxygen consumption, and heart rate.[22] The type of exercise (stair climbing, walking, treadmill walking, or stationary bicycling) appear unimportant and is best determined by the individual patient's physical ability, preference, and economic resources. Even arm and leg exercises in a chair or wheelchair are useful in more impaired patients. The minimal duration and frequency required to improve performance appears to be 20 to 30 minutes, three to five times per week. Unfortunately, the beneficial effects of exercise conditioning last only as long as the patient continues the exercise program. Isocapneic hyperventilation (the patient ventilates maximally while CO_2 is added to the breathing circuit to maintain a normal PCO_2 tension) and inspiratory resistance training (added resistance applied during inspiration for 15 minutes twice daily to train the inspiratory muscles) are the currently available methods for ventilatory muscle training. The efficacy of this therapy is unknown, but it appears to offer promise for selected patients, especially those elderly patients who are unable to perform walking or bicycling exercise because of hip or knee problems that limit mobility.

Energy conservation is the planning and pacing of activities to improve performance. Therefore, instruction in work simplification and the use of energy conservation devices allow more independence and greater participation in activities of daily living.

Breathing retraining consists of teaching patients to utilize pursed-lip breathing, expiratory abdominal augmentation, synchronization of movement of abdomen and thorax, and relaxation techniques for the accessory respiratory muscles. This appears to allow patients to increase tidal volume, decrease respiratory rate, and lower functional residual capacity, thereby regaining control of symptoms. It also seems to permit patients to overcome attacks of hyperventilation precipitated by fear and anxiety and to speed recovery from dyspnea induced by mild exercise.

SUMMARY

The aging lung is structurally and functionally different from the younger lung; however, the clinical significance of the age-related changes in the lung is minor in an otherwise healthy older person. When lung disease supervenes, however, it may result in numerous problems, and in many instances, pulmonary diseases, especially respiratory failure and pneumonia, are terminal events. Nonetheless, the elderly patient with pulmonary disease can often lead a productive life if managed appropriately.

Patients require that the physician, nurse, and other allied health care professionals work collaboratively to develop a management plan that not only maximizes longevity but the quality of life. Through a comprehensive rehabilitation approach that is individualized to each patient, careful attention can be directed to the medical, physiologic, nutritional, and psychologic problems that these patients face. The goal should be to provide a treatment program that allows these patients to remain in their own environment and to be with their family and friends.

REFERENCES

1. Krumpe PE, Knudson RJ, Parson G, et al: The aging respiratory system. Clin Geriatr Med 1:143, 1985.
2. Mahler DA, Rosiello RA, Loke J: The aging lung. Clin Geriatr Med 2:215, 1986.
3. Knudson RJ, Clark DF, Kennedy TC, et al: Effect of aging alone on mechanical properties of the normal adult human lung. J Appl Physiol 43:1054, 1977.
4. Jones RL, Overton TR, Hammerlindl DM, Sproule BJ. Effects of age on residual volume. J Appl Physiol 44:195, 1978.
5. Knudson RJ, Lebowitz MD, Holberg CL, et al: Changes in the normal maximal expiratory flow-volume curve growth and aging. Am Rev Respir Dis 127:725, 1983.
6. Fowler RW, Pluck RA, Hetzel MR: Maximal expiratory flow-volume curves in Londoners aged 65 and over. Thorax 42:173, 1987.
7. Muiesan G, Sorbini CA, Grassi V: Respiratory function in the aged. Bull Physiopathol Respir 7:973, 1971.
8. Holland J, Milic-Emili J, Macklem PT, et al: Regional distribution of pulmonary ventilation and perfusion in elderly subjects. J Clin Invest 47:81, 1968.
9. Berger AJ, Mitchell RA, Severinghaus JW: Regulation of respiration. N Engl J Med 297:92, 1977.
10. Kronenberg RS, Drage CW: Attenuation of the ventilatory and heart rate responses to hypoxia and hypercapnia with aging in normal men. J Clin Invest 52:1818, 1973.
11. Block AJ, Boysen PG, Wynne JW, et al: Sleep apnea, hypopnea, and oxygen desaturation in normal subjects: a strong male predominance. N Engl J Med 300:513, 1979.
12. Naifeh KH, Severinghaus JW, Kamiya J: Effect of aging on sleep-related changes in respiration variables. Sleep 10:160, 1987.

13. Smith PL, Bleecker ER: Ventilatory control during sleep in the elderly. Geriatr Clin North Am 2:227, 1986.

14. Reynolds HY: Lung host defenses: a status report. Chest 75:239, 1979.

15. Cott GC: Drug Therapy in the Management of Cough. In Cherniack RM, ed: Drugs for the Respiratory System. New York, Grune & Stratton, Inc, 1986, p 165.

16. Landahl S, Steen B, Svanborg A: Dyspnea in 70-year-old people. Acta Med Scand 107:225, 1980.

17. Howell JBL, Campbell EJM: Breathlessness in pulmonary disease. Scand J Respir Dis 48:321, 1967.

18. Muthuswamy PP, Akbik F, Franklin C, et al: Management of major or massive hemoptysis in active pulmonary tuberculosis by bronchial arterial embolization. Chest 92:77, 1987.

19. Harris R: Evaluation of chest pain in the old age patient. Int Med 10:65, 1980.

20. Hogg JC, Williams J, Richardson JB, et al: Age as a factor in the distribution of lower-airway conductance and in the pathologic anatomy of obstructive lung disease. N Engl J Med 282:1283, 1970.

21. National Heart, Lung and Blood Institute, Division of Lung Diseases Workshop Report: The definition of emphysema. Am Rev Respir Dis 132:182, 1985.

22. American Thoracic Society Statement: Standards for the diagnosis and care of patients with chronic obstructive pulmonary disease (COPD) and asthma. Am Rev Respir Dis 136:225, 1987.

23. Hoidal JR, Niewoehner DE: Pathogenesis of emphysema. Chest 83:679, 1983.

24. Janoff A: Elastases and emphysema: current assessment of the protease-antiprotease hypotheses. Am Rev Respir Dis 132:417, 1985.

25. Flenley DC, Downing I, Greening AP: The pathogenesis of emphysema. Bull Eur Physiopathol Respir 22:245s, 1986.

26. Thurlbeck WM, Simon G: Radiographic appearance of the chest in emphysema. Am J Roentgenol 130:429, 1978.

27. Hruban RH, Meziane MA, Zerhouni EA, et al: High resolution computed tomography of inflations-fixed lungs: pathologic-radiologic correlation of centrilobular emphysema. Am Rev Respir Dis 136:935, 1987.

28. Petty TL, Silvers GW, Stanford RE: Mild emphysema is associated with reduced elastic recoil and increased lung size but not with airflow limitation. Am Rev Respir Dis 136:867, 1987.

29. Chronic cor pulmonale: report of an expert committee. Circulation, 27:594–615, 1963.

30. Stevens PM, Terplan M, Knowles J: Prognosis of cor pulmonale. N Engl J Med 269:1289, 1963.

31. Morrison DA: Pulmonary hypertension in chronic obstructive pulmonary disease: the right ventricular hypothesis. Chest 92:387, 1987.

32. Kachel RG: Left ventricular function in chronic obstructive pulmonary disease. Chest 73:286, 1978.

33. Matthay RA, Schwarz MI, Ellis JH Jr, et al: Pulmonary artery hypertension in chronic obstructive pulmonary disease: determination by chest radiography. Invest Radiol 16:95, 1981.

34. Nicholas WJ, Liebson PR: ECG changes in

COPD: what do they mean? Part 1, 2. J Respir Dis 8:13; 103, 1987.

35. Timms RM, Khaja FV, Williams GW, et al: Hemodynamic response to oxygen therapy in chronic obstructive pulmonary disease. Ann Intern Med 102:29, 1985.

36. Morrison DA, Henry R, Goldman S: Preliminary study of the effects of low flow oxygen on oxygen delivery and right ventricular dysfunction in chronic lung disease. Am Rev Respir Dis 133:390, 1986.

37. Hudson LD, Kurt TL, Petty TL, et al: Arrhythmias associated with acute respiratory failure in patients with chronic airway obstruction. Chest 63:661, 1973.

38. Wynne JW, Block AJ, Hunt LA, et al: Disordered breathing and oxygen desaturation during sleep in patients with chronic obstructive pulmonary disease (COPD). Am J Med 66:573, 1979.

39. Block AJ, Wynne JW, Boysen PG: Sleep-disordered breathing and nocturnal oxygen desaturation in postmenopausal women. Am J Med 69:75, 1980.

40. Bliwise DL, Feldman DE, Bliwise NG, et al: Risk factors for sleep disordered breathing in heterogeneous geriatric population. J Am Geriatr Soc 35:132, 1987.

41. Smolensky M, Halbert F, Sargent F II: Chronobiology of the life sequence. In Itah S, Ogata K, Yoshimura H, eds: Advances in Climatic Physiology. New York, Springer-Verlag, 1972, p 281.

42. Boysen PG, Block AJ, Wynne JW, et al: Nocturnal pulmonary hypertension in patients with chronic obstructive pulmonary disease. Chest 76:536, 1979.

43. Block AJ, Boysen PG, Wynne JW: The origins of cor pulmonale: a hypothesis. Chest 75:109, 1979.

44. Tirlapur VG, Mir MA: Nocturnal hypoxemia and associated electrocardiographic changes in patients with chronic obstructive airways disease. N Engl J Med 306:125, 1982.

45. Flick MR, Block AJ: Nocturnal vs diurnal cardiac arrhythmias in patients with chronic obstructive pulmonary disease. Chest 75:8, 1979.

46. Lippman M, Fein A: Pulmonary embolism in the patient with chronic obstructive pulmonary disease: a diagnostic dilemma. Chest 79:39, 1981.

47. Fanta CH, Wright TC, McFadden ER Jr: Differentiation of recurrent pulmonary emboli from chronic obstructive lung disease as a cause of cor pulmonale. Chest 79:92, 1981.

48. Fowler AA, Hamman RF, Zerbe GO, et al: Adult respiratory distress syndrome: prognosis after onset. Am Rev Respir Dis 132:472, 1985.

49. Bell RC, Coalson JJ, Smith JD, et al: Multiple organ system failure and infection in adult respiratory distress syndrome. Ann Intern Med 99:293, 1983.

50. King TE Jr: Acute respiratory failure. In Schrier RW, ed: Current Medical Therapy. 2nd ed. New York, Raven Press, 1989, pp 140–177.

51. Bone RC, ed: Symposium on respiratory failure. Med Clin North Am 67:549, 1983.

52. Hudson LD, guest ed: Adult respiratory distress syndrome. Semin Respir Med 2:99, 1981.

53. Chin R, Pesce R: Practical aspects in management of respiratory failure in chronic obstructive pulmonary disease. Crit Care Q 6:1, 1983.

54. Pierson DJ, Neff TA, Petty TL: Ventilatory management of the elderly. Geriatrics 28:86, 1973.
55. Fletcher EC, Martin RJ: Sexual dysfunction and erectile impotence in chronic obstructive pulmonary disease. Chest 81:413, 1982.
56. Doll R, Peto R: Mortality in relation to smoking: 20 years' observation on male British doctors. Br Med J 2:1525, 1976.
57. Postma DS, Burema J, Gimeno F, et al: Prognosis of severe chronic obstructive pulmonary disease. Am Rev Respir Dis 119:357, 1979.
58. Kanner RE, Renzetti AD Jr, Klauber MR, et al: Variables associated with changes in spirometry in patients with obstructive lung disease. Am J Med 67:44, 1979.
59. Bosse R, Sparrow D, Rose CL, et al: Longitudinal effect of age and smoking cessation on pulmonary function. Am Rev Respir Dis 123:378, 1981.
60. Clement J, Van de Woestrijne KP: Rapidly decreasing forced expiratory volume in one second or vital capacity and development of chronic airflow obstruction. Am Rev Respir Dis 125:553, 1982.
61. Intermittent Positive Pressure Breathing Trial Group: Intermittent positive pressure breathing therapy of chronic obstructive pulmonary disease: a clinical trial. Ann Intern Med 99:612, 1983.
62. Rice KL, Leatherman JW, Duane PG, et al: Aminophylline for acute exacerbations of chronic obstructive pulmonary disease: a controlled trial. Ann Intern Med 107:305, 1987.
63. Staib AH, Bodem G, Weisbach D: Theophylline pharmacokinetics in the aged: results of a dose finding study in 12 geriatric patients. Methods Find Exp Clin Pharmacol 9:199, 1987.
64. Mann JS, George CF: Anticholinergic drugs in the treatment of airways disease. Br J Dis Chest 79:209, 1985.
65. Sahn SA: Corticosteroids in chronic bronchitis and pulmonary emphysema. Chest 73:389, 1978.
66. Petty TL: Chronic bronchitis versus asthma - or what's in a name? (Editorial) J Allergy Clin Immunol 62:323, 1978.
67. Shim C, Storer DE, Williams MH Jr: Response to corticosteroids in chronic bronchitis. J Allergy Clin Immunol 62:363, 1978.
68. Albert RK, Martin TR, Lewis SW: Controlled clinical trial of methylprednisolone in patients with chronic bronchitis and acute respiratory insufficiency. Ann Intern Med 92:753, 1980.
69. Mandella LA, Manfreda J, Warren CPW, et al: Steroid response in stable chronic obstructive pulmonary disease. Ann Intern Med 96:17, 1982.
70. Blair GP, Light RW: Treatment of chronic obstructive pulmonary disease with corticosteroids. Chest 86:524, 1984.
71. Sahn SA: Corticosteroid therapy in chronic obstructive pulmonary disease. Prac Cardiol 11(No. 8):150, 1985.
72. Shim CS, Williams MH Jr: Aerosol beclomethasone in patients with steroid-responsive chronic obstructive pulmonary disease. Am J Med 78:655, 1985.
73. Chang S-W, King TE: Corticosteroids. In Cherniack RM, ed: Drugs for the Respiratory System. Orlando, Grune & Stratton, Inc, 1986, p 77.
74. Anthonisen NR, Manfreda J, Warren CPW, et al: Antibiotic therapy in exacerbations of chronic obstructive pulmonary disease. Ann Intern Med 106:196, 1987.
75. Nocturnal Oxygen Therapy Trial Group: Continuous or nocturnal oxygen therapy in hypoxemic chronic obstructive lung disease: a clinical trial. Ann Intern Med 93:391, 1980.
76. Medical Research Council Working Party: Long-term domiciliary oxygen therapy in chronic hypoxic cor pulmonale complicating chronic bronchitis and emphysema. Lancet 1:681, 1981.
77. Petty TL, Neff TA, Creagl CE, et al: Outpatient oxygen therapy in chronic obstructive pulmonary disease: a review of 13 years' experience and an evaluation of modes of therapy. Arch Intern Med 139:28, 1979.
78. Timms RM, Kaule PA, Anthonisen NR, et al: Selection of patients with COPD for long-term oxygen therapy. JAMA 245:2514, 1981.
79. Banerjee DE, Lee GS, Malik SK, et al: Underdiagnosis of asthma in the elderly. Br J Dis Chest 81:23, 1987.
80. Derrick EH: The significance of the age on onset of asthma. Med J Aust 1:1317, 1971.
81. Braman SS, Davis SM: Wheezing in the elderly: asthma and other causes. Geriatr Clin North Am 2:269, 1986.
82. Dunn TL, Gerber MJ, Shen AS, et al: The effect of topical ophthalmic instillation of timolol and betaxolol on lung function in asthmatic subjects. Am Rev Respir Dis 133:264, 1986.
83. Fraley DS, Bruns FJ, Segel DP, et al: Propranolol-related bronchospasm in patients without history of asthma. South Med J 73:238, 1980.
84. Cherniack NS: Respiratory dysrhythmias during sleep. N Engl J Med 305:325, 1981.
85. Edelman NH, Santiago TV, eds: Breathing Disorders of Sleep. New York, Churchill Livingstone, 1986.
86. Strohl KP, Cherniack NS, Gothe B: Physiologic basis of therapy for sleep apnea. Am Rev Respir Dis 134:791, 1986.
87. Reynolds CF III, Coble PA, Black RS, et al: Sleep disturbances in a series of elderly patients: polysomnographic findings. J Am Geriatr Soc 28:164, 1980.
88. Carskadon MA, Dement WC: Respiration during sleep in the aged human. J Gerontol 36:420, 1981.
89. Bixler EO, Kales A, Cadieux RJ, et al: Sleep apneic activity in older healthy subjects. J Appl Physiol 58:1597, 1985.
90. Naifeh KH, Severinghaus JW, Kamiya J: Effect of aging on sleep-related changes in respiratory variables. Sleep 10:160, 1987.
91. Knight H, Millman RP, Bur RC, et al: Clinical significance of sleep apnea in the elderly. Am Rev Respir Dis 136:845, 1987.
92. Bliwise DL, Pursley AM, Bliwise NG, et al: Impaired respiration in sleep is associated with mortality in an ambulatory, non-institutionalized aged sample. Sleep Res 15:104, 1986.
93. Guilleminault C, Cummiskey J, Molta J: Chronic obstructive airflow disease and sleep studies. Am Rev Respir Dis 122:397, 1980.
94. Martin RJ, Sander MH, Gray BA, et al: Acute and long-term ventilatory effects of oxygen administration in adult sleep apnea syndrome. Am Rev Respir Dis 125:175, 1982.

95. Phillipson EA: State of the art—control of breathing during sleep. Am Rev Resp Dis 118:909, 1978.

96. Schwarz MI, King TE Jr: Interstitial Lung Disease, Toronto, BC Decker, 1988.

97. Turner-Warwick M, Burrows B, Johnson A: Cryptogenic fibrosing alveolitis: clinical features and their influence on survival. Thorax 35:171, 1980.

98. Dreisin RB, Schwarz MI, Theofilopulos AN, et al: Circulating immune complexes in idiopathic interstitial pneumonias. N Engl J Med 298:353, 1978.

99. Quaranta JF, Cassuto JJP, Giacobi R, et al: Rheumatoid factor in the elderly. New Method Pathol Biol 26:656, 1980.

100. Turner-Warwick M, Burrows B, Johnson A: Cryptogenic fibrosing alveolitis: response to corticosteroid treatment and its effect on survival. Thorax 35:593, 1980.

101. Turner-Warwick M, Lebowitz M, Burrows B, et al: Cryptogenic fibrosing alveolitis and lung cancer. Thorax 35:496, 1980.

102. Dalen JE, Alpert JS: Natural history of pulmonary emboli. Prog Cardiovasc Dis 17:259, 1975.

103. Wilson JE: Pulmonary embolism diagnosis and treatment. Clin Notes Respir Dis 19:13, 1986.

104. Gross JS, Neufeld RR, Libow LS, et al: Autopsy study of the elderly institutionalized patient: review of 234 autopsies. Arch Intern Med 148:173, 1988.

105. Hirsh J, ed: Venous Thrombosis and Pulmonary Embolism: Diagnostic Methods. Edinburgh, Churchill Livingstone, 1987.

106. Murry HW, Ellis GC, Blumenthal DS, et al: Fever and thromboembolism. Am J Med 67:232, 1979.

107. Meth RF, Tashkin DP, Hansen KS, et al: Pulmonary edema and wheezing after pulmonary embolism. Am Rev Respir Dis 111:693, 1975.

108. Melmin RL, Braunwald E: Familial pulmonary hypertension. N Engl J Med 169:770, 1963.

109. Vieweg WUR, Piscatelli RL, Houser JJ, et al: Complications of intravenous administration of heparin in elderly women. JAMA 213:1303, 1970.

110. Bell WR, Rayall RM: Heparin associated thrombocytopenia: a comparison of three heparin preparations. N Engl J Med 303:902, 1980.

111. Glazier RL, Crowell EB: Randomized prospective trial of continuous vs intermittent heparin therapy. JAMA 236:1365, 1976.

112. Zavala DC: The treat of aspiration pneumonia in the aged. Geriatrics 32:46, 1977.

113. Rossman I, Rodstein M, Bornstein A: Undiagnosed disease in the aging population. Arch Intern Med 133:366, 1974.

114. Cameron JL, Mitchell WH, Zuidema GD: Aspiration pneumonia. Arch Surg 106:49, 1973.

115. Ribano CA, Grace WJ: Pulmonary aspiration. Am J Med 50:510, 1971.

116. Cameron JL, Anderson RP, Zuidema GD: Aspiration pneumonia: a clinical and experimental review. J Surg Res 7:44, 1967.

117. Spencer H: Pathology of the Lung. New York, Pergamon Press, 1962, p 122.

118. Mays EE, Dubois JJ, Hamilton GB: Pulmonary fibrosis associated with tracheobronchial aspiration. Chest 69:512, 1976.

119. Weill H, Ferrams VJ, Gay RM, et al: Early lipoid pneumonia; roentgenologic, anatomic, and physiologic features. Am J Med 36:370, 1964.

120. Samet JM, Marbury MC, Spengler JD: Health effects and sources of indoor air pollution. Part 1. Am Rev Respir Dis 136:1486, 1987.

121. Levin DL, et al: Cancer Rates and Risks, 2nd ed. US Dept HEW, PHS Publication No 75–691, Washington, DC, US GPO, 1974, p 3.

122. O'Rourke MA, Feussner JR, Feigl P, et al: Age trends of lung cancer stage at diagnosis: implications for lung cancer screening in the elderly. JAMA 258:921, 1987.

123. DeMaria LC Jr, Cohen MJ: Characteristics of lung cancer in elderly patients. J Gerontol 42:540, 1987.

124. Macfarlane JT, Storr A, Wart MJ, et al: Safety, usefulness and acceptability of fiberoptic bronchoscopy in the elderly. Age Ageing 10:127, 1981.

125. Hooper RG, Beechler CR, Johnson MC: Radioisotope scanning in the initial staging of bronchogenic carcinoma. Am Rev Respir Dis 118:279, 1987.

126. Whitcomb ME, Barham E, Goldman AL, et al: Indications for a mediastinoscopy in bronchogenic carcinoma. Am Rev Respir Dis 113:189, 1976.

127. DeMeester TR, Golomb HM, Kirchner P, et al: The role of gallium 67 scanning in the clinical staging and preoperative evaluation of patients with carcinoma of the lung. Ann Thorac Surg 28:451, 1979.

128. Kirsh MM, Rotman H, Bove E, et al: Major pulmonary resection for bronchogenic carcinoma in the elderly. Ann Thorac Surg 22:369, 1976.

129. Hoffman T, Ransdell HT: Comparison of lobectomy and wedge resection for carcinoma of the lung. J Cardiovasc Thorac Surg 79:211, 1980.

130. Stead WW, Lofgren JP: Does the risk of tuberculosis increase in old age? J Infect Dis 147:951, 1983.

131. 1975 Tuberculosis Statistics: No (CDC) 77–8249. Washington, DC, US Dept HEW, 1976, p 2.

132. Alvarez S, Shell C, Berk SL: Pulmonary tuberculosis in elderly men. Am J Med 82:602, 1987.

133. Fullerton JM, Dyer L: Unsuspected tuberculosis in the aged. Tubercle 46:193, 1965.

134. Holden M, Dubin MR, Diamond PH: Frequency of negative intermediate strength tuberculin sensitivity in patients with active tuberculosis. N Engl J Med 285:1506, 1971.

135. Chang S-C, Lee P-Y, Perng R-P: Lower lung field tuberculosis. Chest 91:320, 1987.

136. Rooney JJ, Crocco JA, Dramer S, et al: Further observations on tuberculin reactions in active tuberculosis. Am J Med 60:517, 1976.

137. Thompson NJ, Glassroth JL, Snider DE Jr, et al: The booster phenomenon in serial tuberculin testing. Am Rev Respir Dis 119:587, 1979.

138. Iseman MD: Tuberculosis in the elderly: treating the "white plague." Geriatrics 35:90, 1980.

139. Stratton MA, Reed MT: Short-course drug therapy for tuberculosis. Clin Pharm 5:977, 1986.

140. O'Toole RD, Thornton GF, Mukherjee MK, et al: Dexamethasone in tuberculous meningitis. Ann Intern Med 70:39, 1969.

141. Kopanoff DE, Kilburn JO, Glassroth JL, et al: A continuing survey of tuberculous primary drug

resistance in the United States: March 1975 to November 1977. Am Rev Respir Dis 118:835, 1978.

142. Stead WW, To T: The significance of the tuberculin skin test in elderly persons. Ann Intern Med 107:837, 1987.

143. Stead WW, To T, Harrison RW, et al: Benefit-risk considerations in preventive treatment for tuberculosis in elderly persons. Ann Intern Med 107:843, 1987.

144. Johanson WG, Pierce AK, Stanford JP: Changing pharyngeal bacterial flora of hospitalized patients: emergency of gram-negative bacilli. N Engl J Med 281:1137, 1969.

145. Gleckman RA, Bergman MM: Bacterial pneumonia: specific diagnosis and treatment of the elderly. Geriatrics 42:29, 1987.

146. Niederman MS, Fein AM: Pneumonia in the elderly. Geriatr Clin North Am 2:241, 1986.

147. Barker WH, Mullooly JP: Influenza vaccination of elderly patients. JAMA 244:2547, 1980.

148. Health and Public Policy Committee, American College of Physicians: Pneumococcal vaccine. Ann Intern Med 104:118, 1986.

149. Paine R, Mabe BJ: Pulmonary rehabilitation for the elderly. Clin Geriatr Med 2:313, 1986.

150. Hunter AM, Carey MA, Larsh HW: The nutritional status of patients with chronic obstructive pulmonary disease. Am Rev Respir Dis 124:376, 1981.

151. Wilson DO, Rogers RM, Hoffman RM: Nutrition and chronic lung disease. Am Rev Respir Dis 134:347, 1986.

152. NIH Workshop Summary: Nutrition and the respiratory system: chronic obstructive pulmonary disease (COPD). Am Rev Respir Dis 134:347, 1986.

153. Kirilloff LH, Owens GR, Rogers RM, et al: Does chest physical therapy work? Chest 88:436, 1985.

154. Mohsenifar Z, Rosenberg N, Goldberg HS, et al: Mechanical vibration and conventional chest physiotherapy in outpatients with stable chronic obstructive lung disease. Chest 87:483, 1985.

155. Graham WGB, Bradley DA: Efficacy of chest physiotherapy and intermittent positive-pressure breathing in the resolution of pneumonia. N Engl J Med 299:624, 1978.

156. Tiep BL, Lewis MI: Oxygen conservation and oxygen-conserving devices in chronic lung disease: a review. Chest 92:263, 1987.

157. Christopher KL, Spofford BT, Petrun MD, et al: A program for transtracheal oxygen delivery: assessment of safety and efficacy. Ann Intern Med 107:802, 1987.

158. Mahler DA, Cunningham LN, Curfman GD: Aging and exercise performance. Clin Geriatr Med 2:433, 1986.

MUSCULOSKELETAL DISEASES

CHAPTER 29

Osteoporosis and Other Metabolic Bone Diseases

Paul D. Miller

It is the soundness of the bones that ultimates itself in the peach-bloom complexion.
EMERSON, *Conduct of Life: Beauty*

INTRODUCTION AND THE "NEW" DEFINITION OF OSTEOPOROSIS

Osteoporosis, the most prevalent metabolic bone disease in the geriatric population, now requires our renewed attention and redefinition. This is because of the increased ability to diagnose osteoporosis at an earlier stage before fractures occur; the ability to initiate effective, preventive medication programs to maintain bone mass; and the current capabilities to increase bone mass in patients who have had fractures so that, hopefully, future fractures do not occur.

Previously, the medical community's attitude about osteoporosis had been one of frustration and hopelessness. Consequently, the problem had been ignored. This lack of interest on the part of the medical community about osteoporosis had been, and continues to be, interpreted by the public as meaning that osteoporosis is a normal, inevitable process of aging.

Elderly women, therefore, expect to lose height and to develop stooped posture with age.

The burden is on the newer generation of physicians to remove these attitudes. The expectations of the public need to be changed as well so that osteoporosis is detected before fractures occur. Hence, it is critical that physician and public awareness be directed to the fact that finally something can be done about osteoporosis and to the redefinition of the term "osteoporosis" in its entirety.

Osteoporosis has been defined as a loss of bone calcium of a sufficient magnitude to result in nontraumatic fractures of bone. Consequently, the disease process had to be far advanced before osteoporosis was recognized as being clinically present. It is vital to the issue of prevention of osteoporosis that we completely redefine this condition so that we can consider osteoporosis *before* fractures occur.

In this regard, many analogies can be made between the processes of osteoporosis and hypertension. Both are silent diseases which, if left unrecognized and untreated, the end result is the clinical manifestation of the final stage of that disease process. In the case of hypertension, the end result is the cerebrovascular accident (CVA), myocardial infarction (MI), or renal failure. In the case of osteoporosis, the end result is the fracture of a bone. Both disease processes are quite prevalent, and both disease processes can be detected in early stages. Hence, we need to redefine osteoporosis as a silent disease process of bone calcium loss of sufficient magnitude to render a patient *susceptible* to nontraumatic fractures of bone.

Bone calcium loss is a universal aging process that occurs in both males and females. Therefore, bone calcium loss could be viewed as a "normal" consequence of aging. However, the process results in fractures in nearly 50 percent of white and Oriental women over the age of 50.[1] Therefore, we should not accept a substantial reduction in bone mass as being normal any longer.

EPIDEMIOLOGY OF OSTEOPOROSIS

Osteoporotic fractures currently affect 24 million Americans in the U.S.[1] This figure represents the disease process in its final stages, in which fractures have already occurred. Because the vast majority of elderly white and Oriental female Americans have significant osteopenia and yet have not sustained fractures, we can justifiably state that osteoporosis may be present in nearly every elderly citizen in the U.S. In this regard, it may be the most prevalent geriatric disease.

Although not all Americans with significant osteopenia will develop fractures, a significant number will, and this results currently in 1.3 million new fractures annually. We have no method of predicting with certainty which individuals with significant osteopenia will ultimately develop fractures. Statistical relationships can be made from cross-sectional and, more recently, from longitudinal studies between bone mass (particularly of the axial skeleton) and the likelihood of a vertebral compression fracture;[2–4] and although a relationship exists between the bone mass of the hip and hip fractures,[5–7] in any individual patient who has significant osteopenia, certainty with regard to future fractures cannot be predicted. The fact that one

cannot predict, on an individual basis, which patients with asymptomatic high blood pressure will develop a high blood pressure–related complication does not negate the importance of the link between high blood pressure and cardiovascular disease. Similarly, the fact that not all patients with significant osteopenia will develop a fracture does not negate the importance of the relationship between osteopenia and fractures. Nontraumatic fractures do not develop without substantial osteopenia, and the cumulative risk of an age-related fracture is substantial.[4, 8]

It has been estimated that up to 33 percent of women and more than 17 percent of men could experience a hip fracture by the age of 90 years.[8] When average life expectancy is considered, the lifetime risk of a hip fracture is about 15 percent in women. This is a very high figure when considering the growing proportion of our elderly population.

Currently, 250,000 new hip fracture cases occur annually in the U.S. This figure is expected to double by the year 2000 because our population is getting older. Hence, the prevalence of osteoporosis-related fractures is increasing, in part, because of the growing size of the aging population. Currently, 11 percent of the population in the U.S. is 65 years of age or over, and this is expected to increase to 22 percent by the year 2000. The 1-year mortality related to hip fractures is nearly 20 percent, and nearly one half of the survivors end up in permanent nursing homes and institutionalized care facilities. Hence, the magnitude of the hip fracture problem is very great.

Although the fracture of the distal forearm, the proximal humerus, or the vertebral body is ordinarily not fatal, we should not minimize the importance of these fractures on morbidity, quality of life, and subsequent cost to society. An estimated one third of women over age 65 in Rochester, Minnesota, have had one or more vertebral compression fractures.[8] The National Institutes of Health Consensus Conference on Osteoporosis reported that as many as 50 percent of women in the U.S. over age 65 have had at least one nontraumatic vertebral compression fracture.[1]

The vertebral compression fracture problem has been minimized by many individuals in the medical community because it is a less dramatic consequence of osteoporosis than the hip fracture. For patients, however, vertebral compression fractures are quite important. Many are painful. A negative impact of vertebral compression fractures is the subsequent loss of height with compromised pulmonary function. Equally important are patients' concerns that their clothes do not fit correctly and that their abdomens protrude, causing social embarrassment. Self-esteem and body image deteriorate so that relationships with spouses become negatively affected.[9]

For the clinician responsible for managing patients with vertebral compression fractures, these are very important problems that frequently occur at an earlier age than problems associated with hip fractures. Vertebral compression fractures can be quite progressive and silent, as well.

The total economic consequence of these various fractures is very large. It is estimated that the cost of acute and long-term care for patients with fractures of the proximal femur alone now exceeds 10 billion dollars annually in the U.S., and although exact figures for the cost of fractures at other bone sites have not yet been determined in detail, in the aggregate, it is estimated to cost more than 18 billion dollars annually.[1, 8] Because the incidence of fractures as the result of osteoporosis is increasing from an age-related aspect, these costs are expected to increase as well.

An additional issue that needs to be addressed regarding osteoporosis epidemiology is that the prevalence of osteoporosis may also be increasing in the U.S. as a result of factors unrelated to age.

It seems that the attainment of a normal peak bone mass at the age 25 or 30 years is highly dependent on the dietary calcium intake during our building-block years of bone development (between the ages of 12 and 25 years); and on the degree of physical activity during bone growth.[10]

Recently, the U.S. Public Health Service estimated that more than 80 percent of the adolescent population currently do not consume nearly half of the recommended dietary allowance (RDA) for calcium, which is 1200 mg/day for this age group, and less than 74 percent can pass standard physical fitness tests.[11, 12]

There is concern that if peak bone mass is not attained in the current generation, the ultimate prevalence of osteoporosis will increase, caused by these factors not associated with age. Because we all begin to lose bone mass between the ages of 25 and 30 years, we are less likely to develop significant osteopenia and subsequent fractures if we begin with a higher peak bone mass than if we begin with a lower peak bone mass. Therefore, attention needs to be given to the physical activity and the nutritional requirements of the adolescent population.

Once peak bone mass is achieved, bone mass loss begins. The rate, initially, is the same in men and women (approximately 0.5 percent per year) and begins in the premenopausal years, in the axial skeleton, or areas with greater predominance of trabecular bone. Cortical bone mass is normally well maintained until the time of menopause.[5, 13–15]

At the time of menopause, trabecular bone loss accelerates so that it increases in women to rates of 2 to 3 percent per year.[14, 16] In the center of the axial skeleton, this rate may increase to as high as 6 to 8 percent per year for the first 5 to 10 years after the menopause.[17, 18] In addition, cortical bone mass begins to decline at menopause. For the first decade after menopause there is, consequently, a rapid slope of trabecular bone mass loss and the initiation of cortical bone mass loss. After approximately a decade of this estrogen-dependent bone mass loss, the rates at both skeletal sites begin to become less pronounced again so that by the age of 65 or 70 years, the rate of loss of bone mass in women is again approximately the same as in men, as it was in the premenopausal years. Hence, in the latter years of life, this age-dependent bone mass loss recurs. The cumulative effect, in women at least, is a 20 to 30 percent reduction in total skeletal mass over a period of approximately 20 years.[17]

Although there is a predictable decline in bone mass, not all elderly women or men will have osteopenia to levels that render them susceptible to fractures. There are differences in the degree of osteopenia. There is a large overlap for the population so that certain individuals will have a relatively well-preserved bone mass and will be much less susceptible to fractures. Thus, there may be value in the determination of the level of osteopenia, even in the elderly population, because decreased skeletal mass is the most important factor leading to fractures of bones resulting from osteoporosis.[18-22] Other factors that are related to fractures, such as the presence of osteomalacia, the propensity to fall, and altered bone quality, also are important considerations to the risk of sustaining fractures. It is felt that patients with osteoporotic fractures have, on the average, bone mass values below values in age-matched controls determined by various techniques, even though overlap exists between those who have sustained fractures and those who have not.[17] Hence, for the axial skeleton, a statistical "fracture threshold" exists for critical levels of bone mineral density that predict vertebral compression fractures.[2, 18, 20] Additionally, dual photon absorptiometry (DPA) and computerized axial tomography (QCT) measurements of bone mass have shown statistical relationships between increasingly low values of bone mineral density and increasing numbers of vertebral compression fractures.[23]

It has been argued by some that the similarities in bone mineral densities of the hip of those who have sustained hip fractures and those who have not make DPA of little value in predicting risk of hip fracture.[24] On the other hand, equally plausible arguments have been made justifying why this discrimination is important.[6, 7, 25] Evidence exists that assessing cortical bone mass may allow better discrimination between patients who are likely to fracture hips and those who are not.[17, 26, 27] The integrity and strength of the hip may depend more on the cortical bone mass than on its trabecular bone. Qualitative defects in bone, in addition to the quantitative reductions in bone mass, are also important in fracture susceptibility.[17, 22, 27] These latter qualitative factors have not been as well defined, so current focus has been on bone mass measurements in the management of osteoporotic fracture risk.

During the aging process, certain individuals will reach bone mineral densities of the spine or hip that are significantly lower than others of comparable age. It is not entirely understood why this occurs. In part, it is a result of the peak bone mass achieved and the subsequent rates of decline. Furthermore, although for the population at whole, there is a predictable rate of trabecular and cortical bone mass loss, a certain number of premenopausal females will be "rapid bone losers." This rapid bone loss may be related to lifestyle or to mechanical, nutritional, and genetic factors.[17] Hence, clinical assessment of bone mass allows an exact objective measurement of a patient's level of bone calcium content. Subsequent compliance with a preventive medication program or an active treatment program will be enhanced by obtaining this objective value of bone mass. Patients are often not convinced that they have a significant medical problem unless they are shown that a problem really exists. Therefore, clinicians can make a strong argument for the responsible detection of osteopenia by the newer, highly sensitive radiologic techniques.

DETECTION OF OSTEOPOROSIS

In any silent disease process, detection at a late stage is not difficult. With osteoporosis, detection before fractures occur would be very important.

Previously, physicians had to rely on plain x-rays in order to detect significant osteopenia. To detect significant osteopenia by plain lateral thoracic spine roentgenogram, an approximately 50 percent reduction in bone mass must have occurred before a very subjective conclusion with regard to osteopenia can be made.[28, 29] However, more precise and sensitive radiologic tests have been developed to help detect osteopenia at an earlier stage.

The very first noninvasive radiologic test developed was the single photon densitometer, which measures bone mass at the wrist using an ^{125}I radioisotope source. This technique will detect osteopenia, if it is present, by as low as 2 to 3 percent. The single photon densitometer represented the first major breakthrough in early detection.[28, 29]

The precision and reproducibility of the single photon absorptiometry (SPA) is also about 2 to 3 percent; thus its ability to detect changes in bone mass over time when following the patient longitudinally is also quite good. The major drawback of the SPA is that the wrist is predominantly cortical bone, which is, as previously discussed, ordinarily well-preserved in earlier stages of osteoporosis until the time of the menopause. Thus, as a method for detecting early trabecular bone osteopenia, it is less specific.

On the other hand, in the elderly population with concomitant cortical bone osteopenia, the SPA may be of value, although most clinical authorities in osteoporosis would advocate the simultaneous use of a measurement of trabecular bone as well in these situations. This is because trabecular bone has a higher metabolic turnover rate than solid, cortical bone and should, in most situations, reflect changes with preventive medication programs or active treatment programs more rapidly than cortical bone. This is not to negate the importance of measuring cortical bone mass or of monitoring bone mass at several sites in patients with either active disease or who are under therapy. Additionally, there are clinical circumstances in which cortical bone may be affected more rapidly and more significantly than trabecular bone. In such disease processes, the use of SPA to measure cortical bone may be quite important.[32] These circumstances include disease processes such as primary hyperparathyroidism, renal metabolic bone disease, certain pediatric metabolic bone diseases, and, potentially, the response to estrogen replacement therapy.[29]

Recently, SPA has been used for the early detection of trabecular bone osteopenia at the ultradistal site of the radius, which has more trabecular bone, and at the os calcis, which is also predominantly made of trabecular bone.[21, 31] However, the precision of the SPA declines at the ultradistal radius. The os calcis, which is subject to mechanical stresses, may respond differently over time from those sites that are encountered at the spine and the hip.

Three methods currently exist for measuring the trabecular bone mass of the axial skeleton where osteopenia can be detected at its earliest stages. These are DPA, QCT, and, most recently, dual-energy x-ray (DPX), or QDR.[28–30, 33] These methods are capable of measuring the bone mass of the spine, as well as of the hip, and were developed because of their ability to examine trabecular bone sites.

Because osteopenia begins first in the axial skeleton, these methods are currently the preferred and recommended techniques for the earliest detection of osteopenia. In addition, measurement of trabecular bone by DPA, QCT, or DPX/QDR should be the method utilized in most clinical settings when following a patient longitudinally.

DPA and QCT have equal degrees of sensitivity in the detection of osteopenia.[28, 29] The advantages of the DPA over the QCT are its precision and reproducibility. With good quality control, the precision and accuracy of the DPA is approximately 3 to 5 percent. In comparison, the precision and reproducibility of single-energy QCT may be as high as 10 to 15 percent.[28, 29] Hence, smaller changes over time can be better realized by use of DPA.

The disadvantages of DPA as compared with QCT are that DPA measures the entire vertebral body, including the pedicles and the spinous processes, which are often affected by calcification and osteophyte formation. These clinical circumstances, which occur quite frequently in the elderly population, will falsely elevate the readings of DPA. Since QCT technique measures the center of the vertebral body itself, it is not affected by osteophyte formation or calcification of the aorta.

The newest technique, DPX/QDR, uses x-rays rather than radioisotopes, and appears to be more precise than either DPA or QCT and because of greater resolution is not nearly as influenced by osteophyte formation or aortic calcification.[33] The DPX method may ultimately replace both of the previously used methods of measuring trabecular bone.

A basic question about bone mass measurements is: If axial osteopenia is detected and there has been no vertebral compression fracture, what does a single low bone mass measurement mean? This measurement could indicate one of several things, including (1) normal peak bone mass never may have been achieved, and a declining bone mass may not be occurring; (2) a normal bone mass was obtained, and rapid bone mass loss is taking place; or (3) a relatively normal bone mass was attained, was rapidly lost to a certain current level, and is now on a second slope of slow bone mass loss.

The distinctions between these various

possibilities can only be made by making longitudinal measurements over time. This is an important issue in the care of the patient with osteopenia. Thus, it is important to advise the patient that annual measurements should be made, using the same technique, in order to define the significance of a single low bone mass measurement in an individual without fracture. Additionally, unless an individual has a very low bone mass, it is inappropriate to cause excessive concern and alarm so that the patient alters his or her lifestyle when it is equally possible that this low bone mass may have been present for a number of years. Appropriate clinical evaluation to assess the mechanisms of the osteopenia are justified, and appropriate prevention medicine programs are certainly indicated; however, exaggerated conclusions should be avoided.

Another important issue concerning a patient with significant osteopenia is whether or not a wedging of the vertebral body has occurred. From a very practical, clinical point of view, assessment of potential vertebral compression can be performed by taking annual measurements of height of all patients in the office setting using a standard and reproducible method. This should be as routine as taking an annual body weight measurement. When this is done on a regular basis, one is often surprised at how frequently patients remark that they are actually taller than the physician has measured. If such a discrepancy is discovered, a lateral thoracic and lumbar spine x-ray is appropriate to determine whether or not there have been any vertebral compression wedging or deformities. If none are seen, the height loss, if real, could represent intervertebral disk disease. Alternatively, if vertebral compression fractures or wedging are observed, the significance of osteopenia increases. In a patient who has significant osteopenia of the axial skeleton without any loss of height, it is unlikely that significant wedging of vertebra has occurred.

Significant wedging of the vertebrae has generally required a reduction in the anterior height of the vertebrae of more than 20 percent as compared with the posterior height.[34] This should be measured very precisely, and, in patients on therapy, it should be followed on an annual basis to correlate any changes in bone mineral den-sity by the aforementioned radiologic techniques that measure the progression or nonprogression of compression fractures. Thus, the most important aspect of the preventive or treatment programs in osteoporosis is the prevention of fractures.

Finally, the development of new, noninvasive radiologic equipment for the detection of osteopenia has had its mixed blessings. As with all new medical technology, debate exists concerning the appropriate use of this equipment.[35–38] Extreme positions need to be avoided. The new radiologic techniques are developed for use in clinical medicine and should be employed in a very responsible way in the evaluation of patients with suspected osteopenia. Measurements should be carefully taken with full attention to quality control and in situations in which responsible, total clinical assessment of the patient can be performed with ongoing monitoring. Additionally, the indiscriminate mass screening of all perimenopausal women is not justified and would be irresponsible.

The following guidelines established by the Scientific Advisory Board of the National Osteoporosis Foundation indicate in which cases bone mass measurements should be performed.[29, 39]

1. In postmenopausal women in deciding whether or not to initiate estrogen replacement.

2. In objectively quantifying osteopenia in patients suspected on plain x-rays of having osteopenia.

3. In monitoring bone loss in patients with asymptomatic primary hyperparathyroidism and in deciding upon surgery.

4. In patients on chronic glucocorticoid therapy to monitor the efficacy of treatment.

5. In individuals who are on active treatment programs designed to pharmacologically increase bone mass.

It is important to be aware of risk factors for osteoporosis (Table 29–1), but the use of risk factors alone to predict osteoporosis will miss approximately 50 percent of the osteoporotic population.

Prevention requires detection, and efficacy of prevention requires measuring any change in bone mass. Thus the efficacy of pharmacologic therapy to increase bone mass requires longitudinal bone mass measurements to monitor such efficacy.

**TABLE 29–1. Major Risk Factors for
Primary Osteoporosis**

Age (advanced)

Sex (female)

Race (white and Asian)

Habitus (petite or thin)

Menopause (premature, surgically induced)

Family history (positive)

Lifestyle

  Cigarette smoking

  Alcohol abuse

  Limited physical exercise

  Inadequate calcium intake

The aforementioned radiologic tests can provide such valuable data.

Biochemical methods of determining significant osteopenia and the rapid bone loser are being examined as well in current research settings, but they are too new to be advocated at the current time.[40, 41]

Once significant osteopenia is detected, each patient needs to have a consideration of a differential diagnosis.

DIFFERENTIAL DIAGNOSIS OF OSTEOPENIA

A patient with osteopenia does not necessarily have osteoporosis. Although osteoporosis will be the cause of the osteopenia in the majority of cases, consideration as to whether a patient may also have concomitant osteomalacia is important. The exact prevalence of osteomalacia in subjects that have what appears to be otherwise pure osteoporosis is unknown.

There is evidence that in individuals who have femoral neck fractures, the incidence of osteomalacia may not be small.[42–44] Additionally, the data suggest that the prevalence of occult osteomalacia may also be present in a substantial number of individuals who have axial osteopenia with vertebral compression fractures.[45]

Osteomalacia may accompany osteoporosis and may be expected to be seen more often in the geriatric population than in the younger population because of the higher prevalence of nutritional vitamin D deficiency in the elderly.[46–49] In addition, intestinal diseases, including intestinal lac-

tase deficiency with concomitant malabsorption of calcium, or avoidance of dairy products, which provide the major source for vitamin D, is more prevalent in the elderly. The seemingly high prevalence of asymptomatic celiac disease in this population also leads to a greater chance for osteomalacia to be present.[50] It is quite important, therefore, to consider osteomalacia as a possibility in each and every osteopenic individual.

A number of historic and biochemical abnormalities should be considered when evaluating an individual with osteopenia, which, if present, increases the likelihood that osteomalacia may be present (Tables 29–2 and 29–3).

Some of the important biochemical tests that should be performed in addition to the serum calcium and phosphorus concentrations are the alkaline phosphatase and the 25 hydroxy vitamin D levels. The serum calcium and phosphorus concentrations and the serum 25 hydroxy vitamin D levels are normal in patients with osteoporosis. If these are low in any situation, the index of suspicion for osteomalacia has to be quite high. The alkaline phosphatase is normal in patients with osteoporosis, unless they have sustained a recent frac-

TABLE 29–2. Etiologies of Osteomalacia

Vitamin D Abnormalities

  Deficiency

    Nutritional

    Malabsorption or hemigastrectomy

    Hepatic disease

    Phenobarbital or Dilantin usage

    Decreased 1,25 vitamin D_3 production

  Resistance

    Normal or elevated 1,25 vitamin D_3 levels

    Chronic renal failure

Calcium Deficiency

Phosphorus Deficiency

Chronic Metabolic Acidosis

Drug-induced (aluminum, fluoride, lithium, diphosphonates)

Hyperalimentation

Tumor-associated Osteomalacia

Primary Hyperparathyroidism (postparathyroidectomy)

Beta-thalassemia

Postparathyroidectomy

TABLE 29–3. Clinical Setting to Increase Index of Suspicion that Osteomalacia is Present

Hypocalcemia and/or hypophosphatemia

Low serum calcium-phosphorus product (< 25 mg/dl)

Renal disease or renal tubular acidosis

Malabsorption states

Hemigastrectomy patients

Chronic Dilantin or phenobarbital use

Chronic antacid use

Osteopenia plus proximal muscle weakness

Osteopenia and/or bone pain with a sustained elevation of the bone alkaline phosphatase

Constant bone pain, particularly at rest

ture. The alkaline phosphatase increases in the plasma during the repair phase of a bone fracture and then returns to normal. This usually takes place over a period of 6 to 8 weeks. Therefore, if an elevated alkaline phosphatase level is sustained for more than several months and no interval fractures have occurred, the index of suspicion for osteomalacia must be increased.

The only reliable way to confirm a diagnosis of osteomalacia is by performing a very careful and precise quantitative histomorphologic evaluation of bone taken through an appropriate, nondecalcified bone biopsy technique.[51] Strict criteria for the diagnosis of histologic osteomalacia need to be maintained to totally distinguish osteomalacia from certain subhistologic varieties of osteoporosis.[52] Additionally, it is quite important that prior to a bone biopsy, double tetracycline labeling be done so that the proper quantitative hallmarks distinguishing osteomalacia from osteoporosis can be assessed.[51–53]

The hallmarks of osteomalacia include an accumulation of osteoid, accompanied by a decrease in the rate of bone mineralization.[51] The importance of precisely defining osteomalacia lies in the fact that if osteomalacia is diagnosed, an etiology for this distinct metabolic bone disease should be sought.

If it is determined that osteoporosis exists, the patient should have a differential diagnosis completed so that secondary causes of osteoporosis are not overlooked. Elderly patients will have the most common forms of osteoporosis, which are postmenopausal osteoporosis (type I os-

teoporosis) and/or age-related bone mass loss (type II osteoporosis).[54] The inclusive list for the differential considerations of the etiologies of osteoporosis are also shown in Table 29–4.

There are several causes for osteopenia in which, for the geriatric population, the index of suspicion has to be quite high. These include primary hyperparathyroidism, multiple myeloma, hyperthyroidism and/or the effects of thyroid hormone replacement in an otherwise euthyroid individual. Primary hyperparathyroidism is a very prevalent disease, particularly in the postmenopausal population.[55, 56] Whether this is a result of an actual increase in the prevalence of the disorder in this group or a result of the enhanced biologic expression of parathyroid hormone (PTH) in the estrogen-deficient state is unknown. Nevertheless, the prevalence of primary hyperparathyroidism is seen in the same group of individuals who also have the highest prevalence of both postmenopausal and age-related osteoporosis, namely, the elderly, postmenopausal woman.

Additionally, because PTH may have its most pronounced effect on cortical bone sites rather than on trabecular bone sites and the integrity of the hip may depend more on its cortical bone structure than on its trabecular bone structure, primary hyperparathyroidism is an important disease for which a high index of suspicion is maintained. This is true even if the patient is normocalcemic in the initial assessment. The routine measurement of PTH is, however, not appropriate for all postmenopausal or elderly subjects with osteoporosis without some other biochemical marker suggesting hyperparathyroidism, such as an elevated chloride/phosphate ratio or hypophosphatemia. However, if additional data do suggest that hyperparathyroidism may be present, PTH measurement becomes appropriate. The PTH level is often normal in cases of mild hypercalcemic-hyperparathyroidism. In these situations, bone histology may provide valuable information to help confirm the diagnosis.[57, 58]

Additionally, although a diagnosis of normocalcemic or intermittently mild hypercalcemic primary hyperparathyroidism is made in this group of patients, not all patients could or should have a parathy-

TABLE 29–4. Differential Considerations of the Etiologies of Osteoporosis

Primary Osteoporosis
      Juvenile
      Idiopathic (premenopausal women;
          middle-aged and young men)
      Involutional osteoporosis
Secondary Osteoporosis (partial list)

Endocrine Diseases	*Bone Marrow Disorders*
Hypogonadism including athletic amenorrhea	Multiple myeloma and related diseases
Ovarian agenesis	Systemic mastocytosis
Hyperadrenocorticism	Disseminated carcinoma
Hyperthyroidism	
Hyperparathyroidism	*Connective Tissue Diseases*
Diabetes mellitus	Osteogenesis imperfecta
Acromegaly	Homocystinuria
	Ehlers-Danlos syndrome
	Marfan's syndrome
Gastrointestinal Diseases	
Subtotal gastrectomy	*Miscellaneous Causes*
Malabsorption syndromes	Immobilization
Chronic obstructive jaundice	Chronic obstructive pulmonary disease (COPD)
Primary biliary cirrhosis	Chronic alcoholism
Severe malnutrition	Chronic heparin administration
Anorexia nervosa	Rheumatoid arthritis
Alactasia	

roidectomy.[59, 60] If surgery is not performed on such individuals with suspected primary hyperparathyroidism, there are potential alternative medical therapies for this condition.[61–64] Estrogen replacement and phosphorus are potentially useful in this regard. It is also important to follow longitudinally both cortical bone sites and trabecular bone sites by bone mass measurement techniques in individuals who undergo nonsurgical therapy.[65–67]

There is a higher prevalence of multiple myeloma in the elderly than in the younger population, and the disorder can present with diffuse osteopenia, with or without fractures. In the geriatric population, certainly a sedimentation rate and a serum protein electrophoresis are justified in the medical assessment of the osteopenic patient.

It is well known that hyperthyroidism will lead to accelerated bone mass loss. It has also been suggested recently that thyroid hormone replacement in the otherwise euthyroid individual may have a negative effect on bone metabolism as well.[68, 69] Patients undergoing thyroid hormone replacement therapy who otherwise appear clinically and biochemically euthyroid should undergo a measurement of bone mass.

If it is concluded that the secondary causes of osteoporosis are not present in the osteopenic patient, one can attend to the maintenance of bone mass in the aforementioned common forms of osteoporosis (i.e., postmenopausal and age-related bone mass loss).

PREVENTION OF OSTEOPENIA AND MAINTENANCE OF BONE MASS

The presence of osteopenia when no fracture has been sustained necessitates maintenance and preservation of the bone mass at that level. In most instances, particularly in the elderly population who have what appears to be truly age-related bone mass loss, the rate of change in bone mass over time will be quite slow. Even if the individual is a "rapid bone loser," the rate of bone loss over a period of 12 months, as assessed by two bone mass measurement determinations, will not likely be dramatic.

Maintenance of bone mass at any given level depends on education of the patient and compliance with a preventive program that includes (1) adequate exercise; (2) adequate calcium intake; (3) adequate vitamin D intake; and (4) in the appropriate situation, estrogen replacement therapy.

Exercise delays bone loss in the axial

skeleton and may increase bone mass, even in situations of age-related bone mass loss.[70, 72] The effects of exercise on bone turnover are complex and poorly understood, but we do know that immobilization of an otherwise healthy individual at bedrest will result in excessive bone resorption, hypercalciuria, and bone mass loss. Weightlessness in space also leads to accelerated bone mass loss. It is also known that bone loss caused by immobilization and weightlessness in space are completely reversible if weight-bearing exercise in an environment with gravity is initiated soon after the deficit occurs. Additionally, it is known that in normal, menstruating women, those who exercise in moderation have a bone mass that is higher than that of their nonexercising, eumenorrheic, age-matched counterparts.[73] Likewise, the bone mass in the wrist of the dominant arm is higher than that in the wrist of the nondominant arm. Hence, one of the simplest ways to try to alter bone metabolism is to encourage patients to walk at least 1½ miles 3 times a week. We know that immobilization is detrimental, and there may be a very positive effect from walking and other forms of impact-loading on the skeleton.

Additionally, studies suggest that a positive relationship exists between activity and hip bone density and that the relative risk for hip fracture is lowest among elderly patients who have the highest degree of physical activity.[74, 75]

It is vital, particularly for the geriatric population, that the prevention of falls is addressed.[76, 77] If we encourage increased mobility, attention to the risks of falls must be given as well. Individuals may be able to do more to prevent hip fractures by minor details such as tacking down and securing loose or unstable furniture in the home and using canes or walkers properly. If needed at all, physicians must administer the lowest doses of CNS sedative medications that may alter alertness and cause falls.[78]

Calcium is important not only to achieve a normal peak bone mass, but also to maintain a positive calcium balance and, potentially, to prevent the progression of osteopenia at certain skeletal sites.

The RDA of calcium for the adult, non-osteopenic population in the U.S. is currently 800 mg of elemental calcium per day.[1, 12] The NIH Consensus Conference recommended that postmenopausal patients or osteopenic patients of any age consume 1500 mg of elemental calcium per day.[1] It is known that estrogen-deficient individuals require 2000 mg of elemental calcium per day in order to maintain positive calcium balance.

Estrogen loss (type I osteoporosis) results in a deterioration of calcium balance caused, in part, by a decreased calcium absorption efficiency from the diet and from a decreased renal conservation of calcium. In the early postmenopausal years, as a result of increased bone resorption, PTH levels fall and thus so does the synthesis of 1,25 dihydroxy vitamin D. Hence, renal tubular resorption of calcium declines, as does the gastrointestinal absorption of calcium. In patients over the age of 65, there seems to be a further impairment of calcium absorption, again, particularly at lower dietary calcium intakes, so that the adaptation to increase the fractional absorption of calcium becomes lost with aging.[17, 79–81] In this situation of type II osteoporosis (age-related bone mass loss), PTH levels are elevated as a group, theoretically because of a larger deficit in gastrointestinal calcium absorption. Plasma 1,25 dihydroxy vitamin D levels are also decreased and calcium absorption efficiency declines. It is quite important, therefore, that patients with established osteopenia have higher intakes of elemental calcium per day, i.e., the 1500 mg of elemental calcium per day recommendation.

In fact, the average adult in the U.S. consumes only approximately 500 mg of elemental calcium a day, as shown by the Hanes I Survey.[12] This is probably even lower in the geriatric population because of their higher incidence of intolerance to milk products. Consequently, calcium supplements should be prescribed to make up the deficit between what is naturally being consumed and what is required. For the elderly population, the form of calcium supplement is important to consider. Calcium carbonate, the most prevalent and least expensive form of calcium that can be obtained has potential problems with bioavailability, particularly in the achlorhydric subject.[82, 83] Patients with achlorhydria may not absorb calcium carbonate adequately, although they do so if the supplement is taken with a meal. Patients who have achlorhydria, a problem of increasing importance in the geriatric population, or those individuals who may or may not have achlorhydria but cannot take calcium carbonates with a meal should be advised to utilize calcium citrate, which is well-absorbed independent of meal consumption.[83, 84]

Although it is felt that calcium supplementation alone will not prevent estrogen-dependent bone mass loss, particularly from trabecular bone sites, there does seem to be some degree of a positive effect of adequate calcium supplementation on total body calcium and cortical bone sites.[85–87] The effect is not as pronounced as the combination of calcium and estrogen replacement therapy; however, there is a beneficial effect. There is also reason to suspect that the integrity of the skeleton would be more severely compromised in those individuals who do not consume any calcium whatsoever.[12, 17] Intrapopulation studies have shown a relationship between calcium intake and fracture susceptibility.[88] It is likely that without even the recommended dietary calcium replacement, bone mass loss would be even more accelerated.

Attention to vitamin D is equally important. The current recommended dietary allowance for vitamin D is 400 IU per day. Most American adults do not consume this. The only natural source for vitamin D is through sunlight activation of the skin stores of vitamin D precursors and in fortified dairy products. Many individuals do get the RDA for vitamin D supplied in the usual over-the-counter multivitamin, most of which have at least 400 IU of vitamin D per tablet. However, for the geriatric population, milk consumption is often low or nonexistent, exposure to sunlight is often very limited, and basic nutritional status is often marginal. In those patients who reside in institutionalized care centers or who live alone and are more reclusive, there is a substantial prevalence of nutritional vitamin D deficiency.[46–49] Consequently, it has been determined that low plasma levels of 25 hydroxyvitamin D, the best indicator of the nutritional intake and absorption status of vitamin D in human beings, is often low in the elderly American population. Vitamin D supplementation of up to 800 to 1000 IU per day in order to ensure normal 25 hydroxyvitamin D levels are recommended for the geriatric population.

There are other nutritional factors that are important in the maintenance of normal bone mass. Excess dietary protein can lead to a negative calcium balance and increase urinary calcium excretion.[17] Additionally, high caffeine intake, chronic cigarette smoking, and chronic excessive alcohol consumption predispose to bone loss.[17, 89] Consequently, patients need to be instructed to modify these important health matters to try to maintain bone mass.

Estrogen replacement therapy in adequate doses, if started soon enough after menopause, can prevent postmenopausal bone mass loss.[90]

Exactly how estrogens inhibit bone resorption is unknown. Certainly, there is evidence that the initiation of estrogen replacement therapy within the first 5 to 10 postmenopause years will halt the bone mass loss that is linked to the estrogen-dependent component of this process. Additionally, retrospective studies suggest that estrogen replacement therapy decreases fracture rates.[90, 91]

Nevertheless, despite the apparent beneficial effects of estrogen replacement therapy on osteoporosis prevention and on decreasing cardiovascular mortality, it is not currently recommended that all individuals be placed on estrogen replacement therapy, even if it can be started at the most critical time (i.e., within the first 5 years of menopause). This is because estrogens do increase the chance of endometrial cancer, although this increased risk can be eliminated by the addition of progesterones.[17] The addition of progesterones, however, increases the incidence of abnormal vaginal bleeding and also obliterates, at least in most of the recommended doses (e.g., 10 mg of Provera), the favorable increase in high-density lipoprotein (HDL) that is created by the addition of estrogen replacement therapy. Preliminary evidence exists that low-dose continual Provera at 2.5 mg a day (administered on a daily basis along with .625 mg of conjugated estrogen) may be equally protective against endometrial cancer without inducing a menstrual cycle or negatively affecting HDL.[92]

Nevertheless, to protect against the risk

of endometrial cancer, the patient on estrogen replacement therapy should be advised to either cycle estrogen with adequate progesterone or, if on unopposed estrogen, to have an annual endometrial biopsy to monitor against any abnormal endometrial hyperplasia.

The current recommended dose of estrogen to prevent bone mass loss is 0.625 mg of conjugated estrogen taken from day 1 through day 25 of each month.[17, 93] Adequate data regarding any potential equal beneficial effects of parenteral or vaginal estrogens are unavailable. Because there have been no adequately confirmed studies showing the effect of estrogen receptors on bone and on the mechanism of how estrogens inhibit bone resorption, efficacy of these other preparations need to be demonstrated.

A woman with osteopenia at the time of menopause may become more convinced of the need for estrogen replacement therapy, if there is any reluctance to initiate such therapy. The physician has a stronger base for justifying the initiation of such replacement therapy in such a patient as compared with a woman who enters menopause with a perfectly normal bone mass. In those individuals who are either started on replacement therapy or who elect not to start estrogen replacement therapy, measurements of bone mass every year or two for a minimum of three measurements should be done to assess changes in reduced bone mass. It is anticipated that a certain percentage of women may not respond to adequate doses with good compliance to estrogen replacement therapy. This is probably a very small group of patients, but there are still objective methods of monitoring the efficacy of such a program once it is initiated.

It is unknown how long a patient should be maintained on estrogen therapy. It is known that if it is continued for up to 3 years, withdrawal of estrogen results in the same slope of declining bone mass that is seen immediately following menopause.[94] It is recommended that estrogen replacement therapy be maintained for a minimum of 10 years.[90] If it is decided to terminate estrogen at that time, annual bone mass measurements can be used to objectively decide whether or not estrogen therapy needs to be reinitiated.

The issue of the initiation of estrogen therapy in the elderly postmenopausal woman (i.e., over age 65) who has never received estrogen or who has been off estrogen for years is unresolved with little data to support or refute the efficacy. Recent data does suggest that even in the geriatric patient, including the elderly individual who has never received estrogen, the initiation of estrogen therapy may be of benefit at cortical bone mass sites.[95] In this regard, for the geriatric patient who potentially has a number of very active years to live, estrogen therapy may be a stronger consideration than for the biologically older patient with a very limited future. Whether to initiate estrogen in the elderly patient thus becomes an individualized decision to be made by the physician and patient at the appropriate time.

TREATMENT OF OSTEOPOROSIS

For individuals who have had reduction in bone mass of sufficient magnitude to result in bone fractures, it would be ideal to try to pharmacologically increase their bone mass to levels that either reduce or eliminate the risk of future fractures.

One of the difficulties with the pharmacologic manipulation of bone cells is the inherent coupling that occurs between cells that are responsible for bone resorption (osteoclasts) and the cells that are responsible for increasing bone formation (osteoblasts).[96]

Bone remodeling is a continuous process that is believed to be initiated by a number of local and systemic hormonal factors. Whereas mechanical loading or unloading alter bone metabolism through local mechanisms, the most important systemic initiator of bone remodeling is PTH.

By indirectly initiating osteoclastic activity, PTH starts the remodeling process through the formation of resorptive cavities at the bone surface. With the initiation of osteoclastic activity, the osteoclast simultaneously sends biochemical signals to the osteoblasts, which will induce osteoblastic activity.[96–98] With the initiation of bone remodeling and the resorption of bone, resorptive cavities are created by osteoclastic mediated bone resorption. After the osteoclast has created resorption cavities, the osteoblasts will then stimulate bone formation with a layer of nonmineralized bone (osteoid) that is then mineralized with calcium and phosphorus crystallization.

All along a bone surface there are bone remodeling units. At one site along the surface, certain areas are undergoing active resorption, other areas are undergoing active formation, and still other areas are quiescent. The exact reason for this nonsynchronization of packets of bone units is unknown, but within any given unit, this intimate relationship between osteoblasts and osteoclasts exists.[99]

Conceptually, one of the difficulties in the pharmacologic manipulation of bone cells is that whatever is done to increase osteoblastic activity may, in the long run, result in an equivalent increase in osteoclastic activity and thus result in no net change in bone mass. Similarly, if there is a pharmacologic inhibition of osteoclastic activity, one would expect an equivalent inhibition of osteoblastic activity as well. Hence, the uncoupling of this process to produce an increase in bone formation in place of bone resorption is what is attempted to effect a net increase in bone mass.

This pharmacologic manipulation to increase bone mass is being tried with a number of medications. The only compound that currently has Food and Drug Administration approval for the treatment of established postmenopausal osteoporosis is salmon calcitonin.[100-102] There are a few rigorous studies on the effect of salmon calcitonin in postmenopausal osteoporosis, but no fracture data has yet been published. It does appear that patients with high bone remodeling, as determined by biochemical markers of bone turnover, respond the best to calcitonin administration.[102]

In those patients who have already experienced established fractures, calcitonin administered on an every other day basis at 50 to 100 MRC units subcutaneously can be considered a pharmacologic method to potentially increase bone mass.

There is a belief that calcitonin also possesses an analgesic action in patients with painful fractures. However, this potential benefit has not been vigorously studied in controlled trials.

The side effects of calcitonin are that a significant number of patients develop nausea, and the medication is expensive. Additionally, it currently has to be administered in parenteral form. Other routes of administration of this compound are currently under investigation.

A number of investigators have demonstrated the ability of sodium fluoride to stimulate osteoblastic formation and increase bone mass.[103-107] At doses of 40 to 80 mg/day of sodium fluoride, bone mass of the axial skeleton increases within 12 months in those individuals who respond to fluoride. This response rate seems to occur in approximately 50 percent of individuals undergoing therapy and may be predicted by histologic changes in the bone osteoid.[108] Recent data also suggest that in responders this bone mass increase is sustained and is accompanied by a decrease in vertebral fracture rates.[106, 107]

The rather high incidence of gastrointestinal and rheumatologic side effects with fluoride use often precludes continued use.[109] Furthermore, there is concern that the histologic changes of osteomalacia may be seen in a substantial number of patients on long-term fluoride.[110] The clinical significance of this histologic alteration in bone mineralization is unknown, but it can be blunted to some degree by the concomitant administration of adequate doses of vitamin D and calcium. However, since there may be an increased incidence of hip fractures in patients on fluoride, this potential change in bone histology and, therefore, bone quality is a reason for concern.[108, 109]

Anabolic steroids inhibit bone resorption and may have some effect on increasing bone formation.[111-113] However, longitudinal studies showing major increases in bone mass or decreases in fracture rates have not been reported. Its side effects, such as potentially atherogenic changes in plasma lipoproteins, may ultimately limit the usefulness of anabolic steroids.

Because of the knowledge that stimulation or inhibition of one bone cell line is followed by an equivalent stimulation or inhibition of the opposite bone cell line, conceptually, it has been felt that the best way to effect a net increase in bone mass is to try to uncouple this normal process. Also, attempts to synchronize the normally unsynchronized individual bone remodeling units are considered. Consequently, the concept of ADFR therapy for the treatment of osteoporosis was created and hinges on the simultaneous activation and, hence, synchronization of bone remodeling at many sites by one pharmacologic agent (A), followed by depression of bone resorption (D), allowing bone formation to continue for a prolonged period of time (F), uncoupled with bone resorption that has been depressed pharmacologically by an agent that has a long-term effect on the osteoclasts. This cycle is then repeated periodically and sequentially approximately every 3 months (R), based on the hypothetical turnaround time of the remodeling cycle in any given bone remodeling unit.[114]

The sequential therapeutic regimen of ADFR is begun by initiating osteoclastic mediated bone resorption. This has been done with exogenous 1-34 amino acid PTH or indirectly with the administration of oral phosphate.[97, 115, 116] Phosphorus administration, by lowering the serum ionized calcium, stimulates endogenous PTH secretion, which then initiates the remodeling cycle. After the activation of osteoclasts to send their chemical messengers to the osteoblasts, osteoclastic bone resorption is depressed either with the use of etidronate disodium or with calcitonin. The etidronate disodium or calcitonin prevents the resorption phase from being completed and, because the signal for bone formation has already been sent to the osteoblasts, the osteoblasts can now continue to increase bone formation uncoupled with continual bone resorption.

Data are very encouraging that there can be a very rapid increase in bone mass in a substantial number of patients with this form of therapy.[117, 118] An alternative form of cyclical therapy with the diphosphonates without utilizing an activator of bone remodeling has also been shown to increase bone mass.[119, 120] Furthermore, continuous administration of diphosphonate has been shown also to augment bone mass.[121]

The means of actively treating osteoporosis in those patients who have had reductions in bone mass to levels that have already resulted in fractures may therefore be imminent. Additionally, these responses seem to be quite rapid, which is important because the osteopenic process in most circumstances has taken years to develop, and in the elderly population, we have only a few years to re-establish bone mass. The rapid increase in bone mass over a short period of time is what is being sought and appears to be realizable in preliminary studies. We certainly need to be able to offer hope to those individuals who have already had a substantial number of vertebral compression fractures, have a dowager's hump, or have had a hip fracture. In the appropriate and responsible clinical setting, these pharmacologic modalities to attempt to increase net bone mass and decrease future fractures can be employed.

It is important to emphasize that *prevention* of the decline in bone mass, in the long run, will be much more cost-effective and medically important than trying to reverse an already established process. In this regard, the keys to prevention are through efforts to increase public and physician awareness that osteopenia is no longer an acceptable process of aging, to increase the awareness of the techniques available to detect early osteopenia before fractures occur, and to educate with regard to the very important preventive methods that are available to halt the decline in bone mass.

If all of these issues are attended to and if the equally important issues of attaining normal peak bone masses through appropriate exercise and nutrition during the adolescent years of bone development are addressed as well, we have the ability to actually eliminate a very prevalent and costly disease process. Finally, for those with established fractures, we stand at the threshold of being able to pharmacologically increase bone mass so that these individuals can, hopefully, achieve good, strong bone and eliminate risk of future fractures.

REFERENCES

1. Consensus Conference: Osteoporosis. JAMA 252:799, 1984.
2. Riggs BL, Wahner HW, Dunn WL, et al: Differential changes in bone mineral density of the appendicular and axial skeleton with aging; relationship to spinal osteoporosis. J Clin Invest 67:328, 1981.
3. Ross PD, Wasnich RD, Vogel JM: Detection of prefracture spinal osteoporosis using bone mineral absorptiometry. J Bone Min Res 3:1, 1988.
4. Hui SL, Stemenda CS, Johnston CC Jr: Age and

bone mass as predictors of fracture in a prospective study. J Clin Invest 81:1804–1809, 1988.

5. Riggs BL, Wahner HW, Seeman E, et al: Changes in bone mineral density of the proximal femur and spine with aging: differences between the postmenopausal and senile osteoporosis syndromes. J Clin Invest 70:716, 1982.

6. Mazess RB, Barden H, Ettinger M, et al: Bone density of the radius, spine and proximal femur in osteoporosis. J Bone Min Res 3:13, 1988.

7. Melton LJ III, Wahner HW, Richelson LS, et al: Osteoporosis and the risk of hip fracture. Am J Epidemiol 124:254, 1986.

8. Melton LJ III, Riggs BL: Epidemiology of age-related factors. In Avioli LV, ed: The Osteoporotic Syndrome. Orlando, Grune & Stratton, Inc, 1987, p 1.

9. Swogger G Jr: The Emotional Effects of the Osteoporotic Syndrome. In Avioli LV, ed: The Osteoporotic Syndrome. Orlando, Grune & Stratton, Inc, 1987, p 143.

10. Kanders B, Dempster DW, Lindsay R: Interaction of calcium nutrition and physical activity on bone mass in young women. J Bone Min Res 3:145, 1988.

11. FDA-NIH Combined Special Topic Conference on Osteoporosis. October 1987.

12. Avioli LV: The Calcium Controversy and the Recommended Dietary Allowance. In Avioli LV, ed: The Osteoporotic Syndrome. Orlando, Grune & Stratton, Inc, 1987, p 57.

13. Riggs BL, Melton LJ III: Involutional osteoporosis. N Engl J Med 314:1676, 1986.

14. Riggs BL, Wahner HW, Melton LJ III, et al: Rates of bone loss in the appendicular and axial skeletons of women: evidence of substantial vertebral bone loss before menopause. J Clin Invest 77:1487, 1986.

15. Buchanan JR, Myers C, Lloyd T, et al: Early vertebral trabecular bone loss in normal premenopausal women. J Bone Min Res 3:583, 1988.

16. Nilass L, Borg J, Gotfredsen A, et al: Comparison of single- and dual-photon absorptiometry in postmenopausal bone mineral loss. J Nucl Med 26:1257, 1985.

17. Heaney RP: Prevention of Osteoporotic Fracture in Women. In Avioli LV, ed: The Osteoporotic Syndrome. Orlando, Grune & Stratton, Inc, 1987, p 67.

18. Genant HK, Ettinger B, Cann CE, et al: Osteoporosis: assessment by quantitative computed tomography. Orthop Clin North Am 16:557, 1985.

19. Smith DM, Khairi MRA, Johnston CC: The loss of bone mineral with aging and its relationship to risk of fracture. J Clin Invest 56:311, 1975.

20. Wahner HW, Dunn WL, Riggs BL: Noninvasive bone mineral measurements. Semin Nuc Med XIII:282, 1983.

21. Wasnich RD, Ross PD, Heilbrun LK, et al: Prediction of postmenopausal fracture risk with use of bone mineral measurements. Am J Obstet Gynecol 153:745, 1985.

22. Ott SM, Kilcoyne RF, Chesnut CH: Ability of four different techniques of measuring bone mass to diagnose vertebral fractures in postmenopausal women. J Bone and Min Res 2:201, 1987.

23. Reinbold WD, Genant HK, Reiser UJ, et al: Bone mineral content in early-postmenopausal and postmenopausal osteoporotic women: comparison of measurement methods. Radiology 160:469, 1986.

24. Cummings SR: Are patients with hip fractures more osteoporotic? Am J Med 78:487, 1985.

25. Mazess RB: Are patients with hip fractures more osteoporotic? Am J Med 78:A35, 1985.

26. Bohr H, Schaadt O: Bone mineral content of femoral bone and the lumbar spine measured in women with fracture of the femoral neck by dual photon absorptiometry. Clin Orthop 179:240, 1983.

27. Heaney RP: Osteoporotic fracture space: a hypothesis. Bone Min 6:1, 1989.

28. Kimmel PL: Radiologic methods to evaluate bone mineral content. Ann Intern Med 100:908, 1984.

29. Chestnut CH III: Noninvasive methods of measuring bone mass. In Avioli LV, ed: The Osteoporotic Syndrome. Orlando, Grune & Stratton, 1987, p 31.

30. Cummings SR: Bone mineral densitometry. Ann Intern Med 107:932, 1987.

31. Wahner HW, Eastell R, Riggs BL: Bone mineral density of the radius: where do we stand? J Nucl Med 26:1339, 1985.

32. Riis BJ, Christiansen C: Measurement of spinal or peripheral bone mass to estimate early postmenopausal bone loss? Clin Sci 84:646, 1988.

33. Mazess RB, Collick B, Trempe J, et al: Performance evaluation of a dual x-ray bone densitometer. Calcif Tissue Int 44:228, 1989.

34. Hedlund LR, Gallagher JC: Vertebral morphometry in diagnosis of spinal fractures. Bone Min 5:59, 1988.

35. Cummings SR, Black D: Should perimenopausal women be screened for osteoporosis? Ann Intern Med 104:817, 1986.

36. Ott S: Should women get screening bone mass measurements? Ann Intern Med 104:874, 1986.

37. Hall FM, Davis MA, Baran DT: Bone mineral screening for osteoporosis. N Engl J Med 316:212, 1987.

38. Davis MR: Screening for postmenopausal osteoporosis. Am J Obstet Gynecol 156:1, 1987.

39. Peck WA: Physician's Resource Manual on Osteoporosis. Washington, DC, National Osteoporosis Foundation, 1987, p 14.

40. Christiansen C, Riis BJ, Rodbro P: Prediction of rapid bone loss in postmenopausal women. Lancet 1:1105, 1987.

41. Podenphant J, Johansen JS, Thomsen K, et al: Bone turnover in spinal osteoporosis. J Bone Min Res 2:497, 1987.

42. Chalmers J, Conacher WD, Gardner DL, et al: Osteomalacia: a common disease in elderly women. J Bone Joint Surg 49B:403, 1967.

43. Jenkins DHR, Roberts JG, Webster D, et al: Osteomalacia in elderly patients with fracture of the femoral neck. J Bone Joint Surg 55B:575, 1973.

44. Aaron JE, Gallagher JC, Anderson J, et al: Frequency of osteomalacia and osteoporosis in fractures of the proximal femur. Lancet 1:229, 1974.

45. Miller PD, Huffer W, McIntyre D, et al: Axial osteopenia: the necessity of bone histology in distinguishing between osteoporosis and osteomalacia. First International Symposium on Osteoporosis. Copenhagen, October 1984.

46. Parfitt AM, Gallagher JC, Heaney RP, et al: Vitamin D and bone health in the elderly. Am J Clin Nutr 36:1014, 1982.
47. McKenna MJ, Freaney R, Meade A, et al: Prevention of hypovitaminosis D in the elderly. Calcif Tissue Int 37:112, 1985.
48. Clemens TL, Zhou XY, Myles M, et al: Serum vitamin D_2 and vitamin D_3 metabolite concentrations absorption of vitamin D_2 in elderly subjects. J Clin Endocrinol Metab 63:656, 1986.
49. Holick MF: Vitamin D requirements for the elderly. Clin Nutr 5:121, 1986.
50. Miller PD: Osteomalacia due to asymptomatic celiac disease presenting as axial osteoporosis. J Bone Min Res 1988 (article submitted).
51. Teitelbaum SL: Osteoporosis and the Bone Biopsy. In Avioli LV, ed: The Osteoporotic Syndrome. Orlando, Grune & Stratton, Inc, 1987, p 45.
52. Whyte P, Bergfeld MA, Murphy WA, et al: Postmenopausal osteoporosis: a heterogeneous disorder as assessed by histomorphometric analysis of iliac crest bone from untreated patients. Am J Med 72:193, 1982.
53. Frost HM: Tetracycline-based histological analysis of bone remodeling. Calc Tissue Res 3:211, 1969.
54. Riggs BL, Melton J III: Evidence for two distinct syndromes of involutional osteoporosis. Am J Med 75:899, 1983.
55. Mundy GR, Cove DH, Fisken R: Primary hyperparathyroidism: changes in the pattern of clinical presentation. Lancet 8182:1317, 1980.
56. Heath H III, Hodgson SF, Kennedy MA: Primary hyperparathyroidism. N Engl J Med 302:189, 1980.
57. Lufkin EG, Kao PC, Heath H III: Parathyroid hormone radioimmunoassays in the differential diagnosis of hypercalcemia due to primary hyperparathyroidism or malignancy. Ann Intern Med 106:559, 1987.
58. Miller PD: The value of bone histomorphometry in the diagnosis of the osteopenic primary hyperparathyroid patient. Arch Intern Med 1988 (article submitted).
59. Scholz DA, Purnell DC: Asymptomatic primary hyperparathyroidism: 10-year prospective study. Mayo Clin Proc 56:473, 1981.
60. Coe FL, Favus MJ: Does mild, asymptomatic hyperparathyroidism require surgery? N Engl J Med 302:224, 1980.
61. Editorial: Medical management of primary hyperparathyroidism. Lancet 1:727, 1984.
62. Marcus R, Madvig P, Crim M, et al: Conjugated estrogens in the treatment of postmenopausal women with hyperparathyroidism. Ann Intern Med 100:633, 1984.
63. Selby PL, Peacock M: Ethinyl estradiol and norethindrone in the treatment of primary hyperparathyroidism in postmenopausal women. N Engl J Med 314:1481, 1986.
64. Coe FL, Favus MJ, Parks JH: Is estrogen preferable to surgery for postmenopausal women with primary hyperparathyroidism? N Engl J Med 314:1508, 1986.
65. Leppla DC, Snyder W, Pak WYC: Sequential changes in bone density before and after parathyroidectomy in primary hyperparathyroidism. Invest Radiol 17:604, 1982.
66. Martin P, Bergmann P, Gillet C, et al: Partially reversible osteopenia after surgery for primary hyperparathyroidism. Arch Intern Med 146:689, 1986.
67. Kochersberger G, Buckley NJ, Leight GS, et al: What is the clinical significance of bone loss in primary hyperparathyroidism? Arch Intern Med 147:1951, 1987.
68. Coindre JM, David JP, Riviere L, et al: Bone loss in hypothyroidism with hormone replacement. Arch Intern Med 146:48, 1986.
69. Ross DS, Neer RM, Ridgway EC, et al: Subclinical hyperthyroidism and reduced bone density as a possible result of prolonged suppression of the pituitary-thyroid axis with L-thyroxine. Am J Med 82:1167, 1987.
70. Aloia JF, Cohn SH, Ostuni JA, et al: Prevention of involutional bone loss by exercise. Ann Intern Med 89:356, 1978.
71. Krolner B, Toft B, Pors Nielsen S, et al: Physical exercise as prophylaxis against involutional vertebral bone loss: a controlled trial. Clin Sci 64:541, 1983.
72. Dalsky GP, Stokek S, Ehsan AA, et al: Weight-bearing exercise training and lumbar bone mineral content in postmenopausal women. Ann Intern Med 108:824, 1988.
73. Heath H III: Athletic women, amenorrhea, and skeletal integrity. Ann Intern Med 102:258, 1985.
74. Pocock NA, Eisman JA, Yeates MG, et al: Physical fitness is a major determinant of femoral neck and lumbar spine bone mineral density. J Clin Invest 78:618, 1986.
75. Kreiger N, Kelsey JL, Holford TR, et al: An epidemiologic study of hip fracture in postmenopausal women. Am J Epidemiol 116:141, 1982.
76. Peck WA: Falls and hip fracture in the elderly. Hosp Pract 72A-72L, 1986.
77. Tinetti ME, Spechley R: Current concepts. Geriatrics: prevention of falls among the elderly. N Engl J Med 320:1055, 1989.
78. Ray WA, Griffin MR, Schaffner W, et al: Psychotropic drug use and the risk of hip fracture. N Engl J Med 316:363, 1987.
79. Heaney RP: Calcium intake requirement and bone mass in the elderly. J Lab Clin Med 100:309, 1982.
80. Bullamore JR, Wilkinson R, Gallagher JC, et al: Effect of age on calcium absorption. Lancet 2:535, 1970.
81. Gallagher JC, Riggs BL, Eisman J, et al: Intestinal calcium absorption and serum vitamin D metabolites in normal subjects and osteoporotic patients: effect of age and dietary calcium. J Clin Invest 64:729, 1979.
82. Heaney RP, Recker RR: Estimation of true calcium absorption. Ann Intern Med 130:516, 1985.
83. Recker RR: Calcium absorption and achlorhydria. N Engl J Med 313:70, 1985.
84. Harvey JA, Zobitz MM, Pak CYC: Dose dependency of calcium absorption—a comparison of calcium carbonate and calcium citrate. J Bone Min Res 3:253, 1988.
85. Christiansen LN, Rodbro P: Calcium supplementation and postmenopausal bone loss. Br Med J 289:1103, 1984.
86. Ettinger B, Genant HK, Cann CE: Postmenopausal bone loss is prevented by treatment with low-dosage estrogen with calcium. Ann Intern Med 106:40, 1987.

87. Riis B, Thomsen K, Christiansen C: Does calcium supplementation prevent postmenopausal bone loss? A double-blind, controlled study. N Engl J Med 316:173, 1987.

88. Matkovic V, Kostial K, Simonovic L, et al: Bone status and fracture rates in two regions of Yugoslavia. Am J Clin Nutr 32:549, 1979.

89. Bikle DD, Genant HK, Cann C, et al: Bone disease in alcohol abuse. Ann Intern Med 130:42, 1985.

90. Lindsay R: Estrogens in Prevention and Treatment of Osteoporosis. In Avioli LV, ed: The Osteoporotic Syndrome. Orlando, Grune & Stratton, Inc, 1987, p 91.

91. Ettinger B, Genant HK, Cann CE: Long-term estrogen replacement therapy prevents bone loss and fractures. Ann Intern Med 102:319, 1985.

92. Weinstein L: Efficacy of a continuous estrogen-progestin regimen in the menopausal patient. Obstet Gynecol 69:929, 1987.

93. Lindsay R, Hart DM, Clark DM: The minimum effective dose of estrogen for prevention of postmenopausal bone loss. Obstet Gynecol 63:759, 1984.

94. Christiansen C, Christiansen MS, Transbol IB: Bone mass in post-menopausal women after withdrawal of estrogen/gestagen replacement therapy. Lancet 1:459, 1981.

95. Quigley MET, Martin PL, Burnier AM, et al: Estrogen therapy arrests bone loss in elderly women. Am J Obstet Gynecol 156:1516, 1987.

96. Raisz LG, Kream BE: Regulation of bone formation. N Engl J Med 3309:29; 83, 1983.

97. Slovik DM, Neer RM, Potts JT Jr.: Short-term effects of synthetic human parathyroid hormone-(1-34) administration on bone mineral metabolism in osteoporotic patients. J Clin Invest 68:1261, 1981.

98. Dewhirst FE, Ago JM, Peros WJ, et al: Synergism between parathyroid hormone and interleukin 1 in stimulating bone resorption in organ culture. J Bone Min Res 2:127, 1987.

99. Frost HM: The origin and nature of transients in human bone remodeling dynamics. In Frame B, Parfitt AM, Duncan H, eds: Clinical Aspects of Metabolic Bone Disease. Amsterdam, Excerpta Medica, 1973, p 124.

100. Gennari C, Avioli LV: Calcitonin therapy in osteoporosis. In Avioli LV, ed: The Osteoporotic Syndrome. Orlando, Grune & Stratton, Inc, 1987, p 121.

101. Fatourechi V, Heath H III: Salmon calcitonin in the treatment of postmenopausal osteoporosis. Ann Intern Med 107:923, 1987.

102. Civitelli R, Gonnel S, Zacche F, et al: Bone turnover in postmeopausal osteoporosis: effect of calcitonin treatment. J Clin Invest 82:1268, 1988.

103. Riggs BL, Seeman E, Hodgson SF, et al: Effect of the fluoride/calcium regimen on vertebral fracture occurrence in postmenopausal osteoporosis. N Engl J Med 306:446, 1982.

104. Dambacher MA, Ittner J, Ruegsegger P: Long-term fluoride therapy of postmenopausal osteoporosis. Bone 7:199, 1986.

105. Bikle DD: Fluoride treatment of osteoporosis: a new look at an old drug. Ann Intern Med 98:1013, 1983.

106. Mamelle N, Dusan R, Martin JL, et al: Risk-benefit ratio of sodium fluoride treatment in primary vertebral osteoporosis. Lancet 1:361, 1988.

107. Pak CYC, Khashayar S, Zerwekit JE, et al: Safe and effective treatment of osteoporosis with intermittent slow release of sodium fluoride: augmentation of vertebral bone mass and inhibition of fractures. J Clin Endocrinol Metab 68:150, 1989.

108. Budden FH, Bayley TA, Harrison JE, et al: The effect of fluoride on bone histology in postmenopausal osteoporosis depends on adequate fluoride absorption and retention. J Bone Min Res 3:127, 1988.

109. O'Duffy JD, Wahner HW, O'Fallon WM, et al: Mechanism of acute lower extremity pain syndrome in fluoride-treated osteoporotic patients. Am J Med 80:561, 1986.

110. Lane JM, Healey JH, Schwartz E, et al: Treatment of osteoporosis with sodium fluoride and calcium: effects on vertebral fracture incidence and bone histomorphometry. Orthop Clin North Am 15:729, 1984.

111. Chesnut CH, Ivey JL, Gruber E, et al: Sanozolol in postmenopausal osteoporosis: therapeutic efficacy and possible mechanism of action. Metabolism 32:571, 1983.

112. Need AG, Morris HA, Hartley TF, et al: Effects of nandrolone decanoate on forearm mineral density and calcium metabolism in osteoporotic postmenopausal women. Calcif Tissue Int 41:7, 1987.

113. Johansen JS, Hassagen C, Podenphant J, et al: Treatment of postmenopausal osteoporosis: is the anabolic steroid nandrolone a candidate? Bone Min 6:77, 1989.

114. Frost HM: Treatment of osteoporosis by manipulation of coherent bone cell populations. Clin Orthop 143:227, 1979.

115. Slovik DM, Rosenthal DI, Doppelt SH, et al: Restoration of spinal bone in osteoporotic men by treatment with human parathyroid hormone (134) and 1,25-dihydroxyvitamin D. J Bone Min Res 1:377, 1986.

116. Silverborg SJ, Shane E, Delacruz L, et al: Abnormalities in parathyroid hormone secretion and 1,25-dihydroxyvitamin D_3 formation in women with osteoporosis. N Engl J Med 320:277, 1989.

117. Hodsman AB: Effects of cyclical therapy for osteoporosis using an oral regimen of inorganic phosphate and sodium etidronate: a clinical and bone histomorphometric study. Bone Min 5:201, 1989.

118. Miller PD, Neil BJ, McIntyre D, et al: Effect of cyclical coherence therapy (ADFR) on axial bone mass in post menopausal osteoporosis. In Christiansen C, Johansen JS, Riiss BJ, eds: Osteoporosis. Norhaven A-S, Viborg, Denmark, 1987, p 884.

119. Genant HG, Harris ST, Steiger P, et al: Effect of cyclical therapy (ADFR) on post menopausal osteoporosis. In Christiansen C, Johansen JS, Riiss BJ, eds: Osteoporosis. Norhaven A-S, Viborg, Denmark, 1987, p 1177.

120. Storm T, Thamsborg G, Sorensen OH, et al: Pulse dose therapy of osteoporosis utilizing cyclical etidronate. In Christiansen C, Johansen JS, Riiss BJ, eds: Osteoporosis. Norhaven A-S, Viborg, Denmark, 1987, p 1172.

121. Valkema R, Vismans FJ, Papapoulos SE, et al: Maintained improvement in calcium balance and bone mineral content in patients with osteoporosis treated with the bophosphonate APD. Bone Min 5:183, 1989.

CHAPTER 30

Foot Disorders

Stephen F. Albert
Gerit D. Mulder

Make your feet your friend.
J.M. BARRIE, Sentimental Tommy

In the past, medical attention was focused on acute, life-threatening diseases, the conquering of which extended man's lifespan. Chronic diseases then assumed greater importance, sometimes proving to be more difficult to manage and quite frequently affecting the quality of life. Chronic diseases affecting the feet can cause significant morbidity and, particularly in the elderly, can lead to loss of mobility and independence and a decline in physical and mental well-being. The foot in general has received less medical attention than other parts of the human anatomy, possibly because disorders of the foot are seldom the cause of mortality. The awareness of the importance of specialized foot care grew in concert with quality-of-life issues. Unfortunately, the importance of foot care is still not fully appreciated by many who care for the elderly. Williamson found that 35 percent of the elderly population living at home had significant foot disability that was unrecognized by their primary physician. Surprisingly, even when diagnosed, some patients failed to receive appropriate treatment.[1] This iceberg phenomenon perfectly describes the reality that for every known sufferer of foot problems, there exist many more unknown sufferers (Fig. 30–1). The failure to receive appropriate treatment may be more of a problem in Europe than in the U.S. because there is no comparable practitioner to the podiatrist, a medical/surgical specialist of the foot.

PATIENT DEMOGRAPHICS

In the U.S., individuals requiring foot care services clearly fit into distinct categories by age and gender. A Johns Hopkins research team, using both 1980 census data and information from the National Medical Care Utilization and Expenditure Survey, found that 70 percent of podiatric physician visits were made by females. The data on age revealed that 38 percent of the patients were over 65 years of age, with an additional 37 percent between ages 45 and 65.[2]

FREQUENCY AND TYPES OF FOOT CONDITIONS

A 1979 study conducted through the Veterans' Administration podiatric service, surveyed 5510 patient visits in an attempt to determine the types of conditions commonly encountered in V.A. foot clinics and the frequency of occurrence.[3] This survey continues to be one of the largest focused studies on foot pathology. Although it did not target specifically a geriatric population, the average age was 56.5 years; its results still bear relevance (Fig. 30–2).

CAREGIVERS OF FOOT CARE SERVICES—PODIATRISTS AND ORTHOPEDISTS

Who are the caregivers of foot care services in the U.S. and what strengths and weaknesses does each group possess? The majority of foot care services—approximately 65 percent—are provided by podiatrists. Podiatrists attend 4 years of professional school after completing prerequisite studies at the collegiate level and taking the Medical College Admission Test. Many, but not all, obtain additional

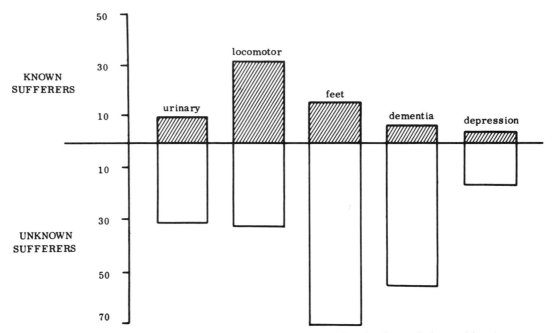

FIGURE 30–1. *Unknown disabilities in older persons. Where most of the iceberg is submerged, the practitioner's awareness of the disability is low.*

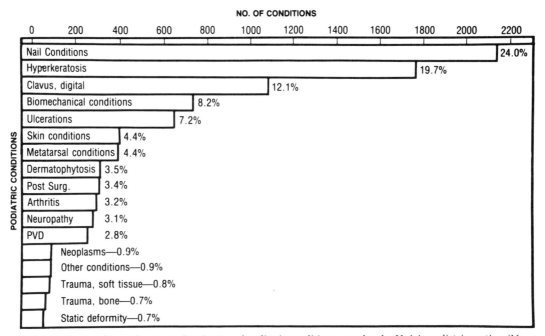

FIGURE 30–2. *Number and percent distribution of podiatric conditions seen by the V.A.'s podiatric section (No. = 8,927).*

postgraduate training in residency programs or fellowships. Podiatrists obtain a Doctorate of Podiatric Medicine degree and are licensed to independently diagnose and treat conditions of the foot. Podiatrists may hold hospital medical staff appointments, perform surgical procedures, and write prescriptions for the treatment of patients under their care. Podiatric medicine is the only health care profession that focuses exclusively on the foot. Podiatrists excel in treating bunion, hammertoe, corn/callus, nail disorders, and symptoms attributable to biomechanical dysfunction.[4]

Orthopedic surgeons specialize in disorders of the bones and joints throughout the human body. Having earned an M.D. degree and served a residency, orthopedists tend to focus on the larger bones and joints. When they do provide foot care, it seems to be in relation to trauma, particularly fractures and sprains, amputations, and congenital deformities.

OBSTACLES TO PROPER DIAGNOSIS AND TREATMENT

Obstacles to proper foot care for the elderly occur both inside and outside of this population group. Internal obstacles include the patient's own attitudes and assumptions regarding painful feet, available care and its cost. External obstacles include the attitudes and assumptions of the primary care practitioner, uncertainty by referring physicians as to who will best provide foot care, availability of specialists—both geographically and within a particular hospital or managed care delivery system—and the third-party (private insurance, Medicare, Medicaid and so forth) system.

One of the problems associated with providing foot care services is that many elderly persons accept foot pain as a normal consequence of aging and therefore fail to seek treatment. Some patients may have been disappointed with their initial physician's interest and approach to their problem and may feel that their foot problem is too trivial for the doctor or that nothing further can be done. Many frustrated patients, concerned over the cost of medical care, attempt to self treat, pur-

chasing the most expensive "special" shoes, over-the-counter remedies, or mail order "arch supports" and become fairly successful in wasting time, money, and delaying proper diagnosis and treatment.

And what about the providers that may present obstacles? Primary care physicians in general do not consistently inquire about foot problems and may never examine their patients' feet. Some podiatrists are all too quick to prescribe surgery as a quick, convenient way to solve a foot problem instead of exhausting conservative treatment options first. Some orthopedists are not interested in treating the foot, particularly the types of foot problems that geriatric patients experience, yet some do not want podiatrists to treat foot problems. Additionally, physicians in general are programmed to welcome patients that clearly fit into diagnostic patterns that they were trained to recognize and consciously or subconsciously communicate to patients where their medical interests lie. This interest rarely includes the foot.

Finally, the changes in the U.S. medical delivery system is impacting to a greater extent those services deemed elective and not life-threatening. Foot care services are being increasingly scrutinized and altered by policy more to the dictates of the financial bottom line rather than to meeting the health care needs of the elderly. Second opinion programs, preauthorization for procedures and hospitalization, and rigid rules requiring outpatient or office procedures all promise to cut health care expenditures but can place a disproportionate burden on the elderly.

COMMON FOOT DIAGNOSIS

Grouped by organ system, the following diagnostic possibilities for feet may prove beneficial for primary care physicians (Table 30–1).

Systemic Diseases Manifesting in the Foot

Three systemic diseases contribute to significant foot disability: diabetes mellitus, rheumatoid arthritis, and gout.

**TABLE 30–1. Common Foot Diagnoses
by Organ System**

Dermatologic
Xerotic (dry) skin with associated diffuse
  hyperkeratosis and fissures
Tinea pedis and/or tinea ungium
Nail hypertrophy, atrophy or incurvation, plantar
  fat pad atrophy and/or displacement
Hard/soft corns, intractable plantar keratomas,
  calluses, and other pedal hyperkeratoses
Plantar warts, psoriasis, dermal ulceration, and
  neoplastic diseases (i.e., Kaposi's sarcoma,
  squamous cell carcinoma, malignant melanoma)
Vascular
Arteriosclerosis obliterans
Microembolization (also called blue/purple toe
  syndrome)
Distal tibial vascular insufficiency and
  microangiopathy, especially in diabetics
Venous stasis/ulceration
Phlebitis/postphlebitic syndrome
Raynaud's disease/phenomenon; frostbite/frostnip
  vascular sequella
Neurologic
Physiologic, sensory, motor, and autonomic
  peripheral polyneuropathy as well as specific
  peripheral neuropathies (i.e., diabetic, alcoholic,
  nutritional, entrapment, ischemic, etc.)
Tarsal tunnel syndrome
Morton's neuroma
Distal symptoms of intervertebral disc protrusions
  and sciatica
Foot dysfunction secondary to gait abnormalities of
  extrapyramidal disease
Parkinson's disease, multiple sclerosis, and atrophic
  or spastic conditions of the lower extremities
Musculoskeletal
Subungual exostoses
Hammertoe
Mallet toe
Overlapping/varus rotated digits
Hallux rigidus or other pedal degenerative joint
  disease
Hallux valgus/bunion deformity
Tailor's bunion or bunionette
Dorsal metatarsal cuneiform exostoses
Heel spur/plantar fasciitis syndrome
Haglund's deformity
Foot biomechanical dysfunction secondary to varus
  or valgus positions of the forefoot or rearfoot
Pes planus or pes cavus
Ankle equinus
Proximal bone deformity
Joint dysfunction
Muscle dysfunction or limb length inequality

DIABETES MELLITUS

Approximately 20 percent of all hospital admissions by diabetic patients are primarily for foot problems, and between 50 and 70 percent of all nontraumatic amputations are performed on diabetic patients.[5] Vascular and immune system compromise, along with peripheral neuropathy, renders the foot of the diabetic patient prone to painless ulceration and infection. Therefore, lesser insults can result in major infections. Poorly fitting shoes, thermal injury, trauma, ingrowing toenails, pressure points, particularly those with hyperkeratosis or vesicle/bulla formation, all can be hazardous to the diabetic patient. Sometimes, early lesions are not detected, and the patient is unaware of a problem, because of neuropathy or retinopathy, until ulceration or infection has advanced. Additionally, some patients develop diabetic osteoarthropathy, commonly referred to as a Charcot joint, with ultimate destruction of the bone and joint architecture of the foot.

RHEUMATOID ARTHRITIS

Rheumatoid arthritis may manifest in the foot, leading to hallux valgus/bunion formation, hammertoes with fibular digital deviation, displacement of the plantar fat pad, and plantar prominence of often deformed metatarsal heads. In 1975 the Annals of Rheumatic Disease reported that 30 percent of the patients surveyed with rheumatoid arthritis had significant disease in their feet. Corns, calluses, and intractable plantar keratoses occur commonly, and shoe fitting becomes difficult because of the skeletal deformity that occurs primarily at the metatarsophalangeal joints. Pressure points can ulcerate, but more commonly they create foot pain with resultant immobility. If infections do develop, management may be hampered by the many immunosuppressant agents now used to treat rheumatoid arthritis.

GOUT

Gout may manifest in the foot acutely or as a chronic arthritis. The acute process results from intra-articular deposition of monosodium urate crystals during an episode of serum hyperuricemia. The symptoms include a sudden onset of severe pain, erythema, and edema at the first metatarsophalangeal joint at the base of the great toe. Even light touch provokes a painful response, and patients are frequently unable to tolerate bedsheets over the affected site. In the elderly, however, such a striking presentation may be lessened.

The chronic form of gout results in tophaceous deposits and gouty arthritis, characterized by subchondral joint erosions on plain radiographs. Symptoms may be chronic or subacute, articular or nonarticular, and with or without associated deformity. Gouty arthritis affecting the feet must be differentiated from rheumatoid arthritis and osteoarthritis.

SHOES AND THEIR ROLE IN FOOT PATHOLOGY

The adage, "They neither cause nor cure," applied to footgear is still, for the most part, true. There are obvious exceptions: shoe contact dermatitis, manufacturing defects, worn shoes, or improper size. However, for most conditions, the shoe serves as an aggravating factor for a deformity that has already developed. Helfand, during a 5-year longitudinal study of an elderly population, found that the patients' footgear was satisfactory over 93 percent of the time.[6]

In the elderly, two shoe-related problems are of importance. First, many elderly ignore the importance of having their foot measured for proper sizing. They assume that their foot size does not change, and they will ask the salesperson for a particular size and width that they have always worn. Too often, this results in a tight shoe that may go unrecognized, because of a physiologic decrease in sensory perception that occurs in the extremities with advancing age. The second shoe-related problem occurs with patients having diabetes mellitus and its associated peripheral polyneuropathy. The purchase of new shoes should be accompanied by a period of heightened observation so as to identify and correct any pressure points that may lead to blister formation, secondary infection, and ulceration. This precaution is particularly important if digital and metatarsal deformities are present.

THE SYSTEMATIC EXAMINATION OF THE FOOT (FOUR-PART EXAMINATION)

A consistent approach to examination of the foot ensures completeness and avoids missing subtle clues that may well lead to diagnosis. One method this author advocates is the four-part examination. This consists of a nonweight-bearing evaluation (with and without dependency), stance procedure, examination during gait, and inspection of footgear.

During the nonweight-bearing portion, attention should be given to the skin, the peripheral vessels and nerves, and the bones, joints, and muscles of the lower extremity. Seeking subtle clues would lead the examiner to assess the skin (particularly of the sole and toe webs), the peripheral vascular status (particularly the presence or absence of pedal pulses), the plantar pallor and temperature gradient from leg to foot, the peripheral nerve status (especially loss of or diminished sensation and/or motor function), and the musculoskeletal findings of diminished, painful, or altered joint range of motion. With dependency of the foot, evaluation of color return and venous filling and the presence of dependent rubor can be determined. A stance examination reveals what happens to the foot when loaded with body weight. It is crucial to determine if there is a collapse or elevation of the arch. A gait evaluation reveals dysfunction in locomotion and is vital in determining the need for functional orthoses, neurologic consultation, or further studies. Inspection of footgear should not be neglected. Shoes and their wear patterns can be revealing and may aid diagnosis.

ANCILLARY STUDIES

Certain ancillary studies are used to aid diagnosis of foot disorders, the most common being radiographs. Because the foot is a weight-bearing structure, standing radiographs provide a look at the osseous structures in a functional position and should often be performed unless contraindicated. Use of the clinical laboratory for urine, blood chemistry, hematologic, microbiological, and serologic examinations can aid in diagnosis of diabetes mellitus, rheumatoid arthritis, gout, and infectious, inflammatory, and other disorders to determine appropriate therapy and measure the effects of therapy. Noninvasive vascular studies play a very important role in assessing possible vascular insufficiency, healing potential, and amputation levels. Radioisotope scans (Gallium 67 Citrate, Technetium^{99m}, and Indium^{111}) assist in localizing and determining the magnitude of infectious processes, stress fractures, and changes in bone physiology. Nerve conduction studies and electromyograms (EMGs) assist in diagnosis of peripheral nerve and muscle pathology. Electrodynograms and pedobarographs provide information about the foot as it functions, discerning normal from abnormal pressure areas.

Magnetic resonance imaging and computerized axial tomography can also be helpful in diagnosing disease and injury of the foot.

SPECIFIC FOOT DISORDERS PREVALENT IN THE ELDERLY AND THEIR MANAGEMENT

Nail Disorders

Onychomycosis, onychauxis, onychogryphosis, and onychocryptosis are among the more common nail disorders seen in the elderly. Onychomycosis, or tinea ungium, is a superficial fungal infection of the nail. It commonly presents as a very thickened, brittle, and yellowish nail, with or without accompanying tinea pedis, or athlete's foot. The presence of onychomycosis can be determined by microscopic evidence of fungal parts on a KOH slide preparation of subungual nail scrapings or by a positive culture. Although topical antifungal agents are available, their effectiveness in onychomycosis has proven disappointing. Griseofulvin, an oral antifungal, can be effective, although commonly quoted cure rates of 16.7 to 41 percent[7, 8] should give those contemplating its use in the elderly reason to pause, particularly in light of its cost, duration of therapy, side effects, potential drug interactions, and recurrence rates after cessation of treatment. Clinical management, therefore, differs little from management of onychauxis, or hypertrophic nail plate, and onychogryphosis, or horny, thickened, deformed nails. Management focuses primarily on reduction of the thickened nail plate mechanically, chemically (with 40 percent urea paste), or nail

eradication. Onychocryptosis, or ingrown nail, most frequently involves either side of the great toenails and occasionally presents acutely as a result of a localized bacterial abcess secondary to nail penetration of the adjacent soft tissue. If causative factors such as tight shoes and improper cutting can be identified and remedied, the need for corrective nail surgery may be avoided. However, should the problem persist, the corrective chemomatricetomy nail procedures commonly used are relatively pain-free and effective with minimal morbidity. Contrary to past treatments, in which the whole nail was eradicated, current treatments have emphasized correcting only what is necessary to relieve symptoms and remove recurring deformity. The once popular orthopedic procedure of partial digital amputation, also called a terminal Syme procedure, is rarely, if ever, indicated for nail pathology.

Hyperkeratotic Foot Lesions

Hyperkeratotic lesions collectively accounted for 33 percent of all podiatric conditions seen in the Veterans' Administration study (see Fig. 30–2). These lesions can be divided into two groups: those seen on the digits and those located on the sole of the foot.

Hyperkeratotic lesions found on the digits are commonly referred to as clavi or corns and can be further subdivided into heloma dura, or hard corns, and heloma molle, or soft corns. Heloma dura characteristically occur on the dorsal, dorsolateral, or distal tips of digits and clinically exhibit as hard, oval, or circular cornified skin lesions, whereas heloma molle are found interdigitally, exhibiting a soft, macerated, whitish lesion of the skin that occasionally ulcerates.

Hyperkeratotic lesions found submetatarsally may appear as a discrete, centrally nucleated, cornified skin lesion, always located under a submetatarsal head called an intractable plantar keratoma, or as a diffuse cornified skin lesion on the sole, which may or may not be directly located under a submetatarsal head, called a shearing callus or tyloma.

The aforementioned hyperkeratotic lesions result from concentrated pressures and friction, which evoke a protective response by the skin. Treatment of clavi begins with evaluation of extrinsic factors—primarily of footgear—followed by an investigation of likely intrinsic factors, such as a change in or malposition of phalangeal bones. Historically, surgeons amputated digits because of painful clavi. Such radical procedures are rarely, if ever, necessary. Many senior citizens can live quite comfortably with periodic podiatric paring of the hyperkeratosis, supplemented with soft pads or custom fabricated orthodigital devices and extra depth shoes. In those patients in whom paring is necessary every two months or more, shoe fitting becomes problematic. If fixed digital deformities such as hammertoes, clawtoes, or mallet toes are present, and pain and dermal ulceration occur repeatedly, surgical correction may be indicated. Traditional procedures of digital interphalangeal arthrodesis and arthroplasty are now being supplemented with interphalangeal joint prostheses that aid in stability and alignment, allow more normal function, and provide an enhanced cosmetic result.

Treatment of shearing callus and intractable plantar keratoma is complicated by the need to differentiate the lesions from plantar warts. Plantar warts are virally induced skin lesions, which, when examined closely, have a cauliflower appearance that disrupts normal skin lines. They tend to bleed easily when pared. Paring of shearing callus and intractable plantar keratoma, when done professionally, rarely precipitates hemorrhage and frequently provides symptomatic relief for varying lengths of time. It is well recognized that shearing callus conditions are responsive to custom-made functional foot orthoses, whereas intractable plantar keratoma may require an alteration of the weight-bearing pressures of the responsible metatarsal, usually by surgery. Historically, proximal metatarsal osteotomies, metatarsal head resections, and plantar metatarsal head condylectomy-type procedures were commonly touted as effective treatments until studies revealed biomechanical side effects and rather high rates of adjacent formation of intractable plantar keratoma (commonly referred to by podiatric surgeons as transfer lesions). Disappointingly, success rates based on objective, acceptable results reported by

Hatcher[9] only improved from 46 to 61 percent when newer distal metatarsal osteotomy procedures were introduced in the 1970s. This has lead some podiatric surgeons to re-evaluate the criteria for performing metatarsal osteotomies.

In light of these results, a search for other methods of treating hyperkeratotic conditions took place in the 1980s. It resulted in the introduction of injectable, purified bovine collagen, Keragen, introduced by Collagen Corporation specifically for use with the foot. After an antigen test dose, the crossed-linked fibrillar collagen is administered subdermally beneath the lesion via injection. Preliminary results at 6 months revealed significant reduction in pain and lesion size.[10] However, despite the promise of this new method, it has not stood the test of time. There are skeptics who argue that the results will, at best, be temporary because the underlying pressure points have not been addressed. Another well-advertised treatment modality is the carbon dioxide laser. Laser treatments have been advocated for many foot conditions; unfortunately unbiased analysis by experienced authorities reveals that lasers have limited benefits compared to more traditional procedures and raise questions regarding cost-effectiveness. Lasers should not be used in bone surgery because of their ability to devascularize bone and render it susceptible to osteomyelitis. Their primary indication is for destruction of benign soft tissue lesions.

Mechanical Foot Dysfunction

Biomechanical foot abnormalities, unrecognized and left untreated, frequently result in structural foot deformity in the elderly. The associated foot dysfunction can result in a loss of mobility and independence and a decline in physical and mental well-being. Early signs and symptoms of these abnormalities include metatarsalgia, plantar arch pain, subtalar pain, and other chronic, recurring symptoms associated with standing and walking. As a rule, with biomechanical dysfunctions, weight-bearing and gait examination findings and weight-bearing foot radiographs yield subtle diagnostic hints only to those who are discerning and knowledgeable of foot mechanics. Customary laboratory tests and nonweight-bearing examinations and radiographs more commonly provide data insufficient to make a diagnosis.

Treatment consists of specialized shoe modifications or, more commonly, custom-made foot orthoses. Surgery is rarely indicated unless it promises restoration of normal or near-normal foot function. Historically, diagnosis and treatment were dependent on the practitioner's skill in assessing shoe wear patterns, stance and gait, weight-bearing radiographs, and performing a range of motion examination with the aid of joint range of motion measuring devices such as tractographs and goniometers. Continually, the use of force plates, along with computerized gait analysis, is enhancing our knowledge of biomechanical dysfunction in the foot.[11] Improved, although not perfected, diagnostic aids have appeared, including the Phillips biometer, K-square, the Electrodynogram System, the EMED-F System, and the Biokinetics Dynamic Pedobarograph. The latter three systems attempt to measure pressures at weight-bearing sites on the sole of the foot.

Metatarsal Disorders

Metatarsal conditions can create significant impediments to both ambulation and shoe fitting, particularly in the elderly. The 5 metatarsals in each foot form the osseous support structure between the digits and the rearfoot and are subject to the abuses of ill-fitting shoes and the lifetime microtrauma of standing and walking on often unyielding surfaces. The more common conditions seen include hallux valgus, hallux limitus/rigidus, tailor's bunion, and metatarsalgia, secondary to prominent metatarsal heads.

Hallux Valgus

Hallux valgus (also referred to as hallux abductovalgus or bunion deformity) refers to a malposition at the first metatarsophalangeal joint exhibited by great toe deviation, with rotation and prominence and/or hypertrophy of the first metatarsal head. The etiology of this condition is still debated, with the consensus favoring abnor-

mal foot mechanics, which create instability of the foot's medial column that stresses the joint. Other less common etiologies include pedal manifestations of arthritis (in particular rheumatoid arthritis), trauma, certain neuromuscular diseases, and predisposing anatomy. In its early stages, accommodative foot gear and attempts at controlling abnormal foot mechanics are most often attempted. The success rate, however, has proven disappointing, with many cases progressing to advanced stages in which surgery may be indicated. Once common procedures, such as the McBride bunionectomy, are now less frequently performed because of the realization that hallux abductovalgus/bunion deformity is more complex than first thought. Current trends include more exacting determinations as to the etiology, level(s) of deformity, and attempts at restoring cosmesis and function. Practically, this translates into the assessment by the foot surgeon of the needs of each patient, including activities, activity levels, projected longevity, occupational influences, and concerns over cosmesis in selecting the procedure(s) needed. Currently, we are seeing more joint prostheses used, osteotomies of the foot bones to correct angular deformities, and reliance on internal fixation (i.e., screws and pins) to maintain the exacting corrections obtained through surgery. While performing these procedures on an ambulatory or short hospital stay basis is becoming mandated by third-party payors, the so-called minimal incision office surgery for these types of problems has resulted in some disappointing results.

Hallux Limitus/Rigidus

Hallux limitus/rigidus refers to degenerative osteoarthritis of the first metatarsophalangeal joint. Patients notice painful, limited motion at the great toe, sometimes accompanied by deformity and almost always aggravated by standing and walking. Radiographic changes show joint degeneration. Conservative treatment measures include rest for the acutely inflamed joint, oral anti-inflammatory medications, use of rigid-soled shoes to lessen ambulatory stresses at the great toe joint, and, rarely, intra-articular steroid injections. When these fail to provide adequate relief, surgery can prove beneficial, primarily relieving pain and restoring motion to the great toe. As with the bunionectomies, joint prosthesis use for this condition provides options not previously available.

Tailor's Bunion

Tailor's bunion is a condition that is analogous to the bunion deformity of the great toe that occurs at the fifth digit. With deviation of the digit and enlargement of the fifth metatarsal head, this commonly creates skin irritation and/or bursitis, with resultant shoe fit problems. Treatments are similar, but they obviously must take into account the differing function of the lateral column of the foot and the location of the deformity.

Metatarsalgia

Metatarsalgia is a general term that refers to pain in the metatarsal area. There are numerous causes, but one in particular seen commonly in the elderly is secondary to loss of intrinsic muscle tone to the toes, causing subluxation of the toes with associated migration of the plantar metatarsal fat pad. This sequence of events leads to prominence of the metatarsal heads, which must bear weight when one normally stands and walks. This condition is epitomized in patients with severe pedal rheumatoid arthritis. Patients describe pain under the metatarsal heads that is accentuated by walking. The skin under one or more of the metatarsal heads may develop tender callosities and is subject to pressure ulcerations, especially if the toes are positioned dorsally on the metatarsal heads. Initial management is achieved with extra-depth shoes and cushioned innersoles. Keragen, as noted in the foregoing discussion, may be indicated in treating this condition. In patients with more severe cases, such as those with severe rheumatoid arthritis, surgery to remove the prominent and usually deformed metatarsal heads provides dramatic relief from pain and nearly always improves ability to ambulate.

SUMMARY

Most of the chronic foot disorders in the elderly develop gradually as a result of lifetime use and abuse, trauma, and poor preventive care. Although they seldom cause mortality, foot disorders can cause significant morbidity and lead to pain, inactivity, decreased socialization, and overall physical decline. Diagnosing foot problems in the geriatric population can be a challenge, even without obstacles. However, much gratification awaits the practitioner who can alleviate foot pain, improve function, limit disability, and restore independent ambulation.

REFERENCES

1. Williamson J: Old people at home: their unreported needs. Lancet 1:1117, 1964.
2. Johns Hopkins Health Services Research and Development Center: Health care for foot problems in the USA: patterns of professional practice. Patient Utilization and Cost of Care. January 1985.
3. McCarthy D, Port M, Solomon C: The characteristics of podiatric care in the Veterans Administration. J Am Podiatr Med Assoc 70:8, 1980.
4. Mortenson LE, Baum HM: Economics of foot care. Washington, D.C., Elm Services Inc, 1985, p 8.
5. Sapico SL, Bessman AN: Foot infection in the elderly diabetic. Geriatr Med Today 5:3, 1986.
6. Helfand AE: At the foot of south mountain: a 5-year longitudinal study of foot problems and screening in an elderly population. J Am Podiatr Med Assoc 63:10, 1973.
7. Anderson DW: Griseofulvin: biology and clinical usefulness, a review. Ann Allergy 23:103, 1965.
8. Hägermark O, Berlin A, Wallin I, et al: Plasma concentration of griseofulvin in healthy volunteers and outpatients treated for onychomycosis. Acta Derm Venereol 56:289, 1976.
9. Hatcher RW, Goller WL, Weil LS, et al: Intractable plantar keratoses: a review of surgical corrections. J Am Podiatr Med Assoc 68:6, 1978.
10. Collagen Podiatric Investigation Group: Subdermal collagen injections for the treatment of hyperkeratotic lesions. J Am Podiatr Med Assoc 76:8, 1986.
11. Schoenhaus HO, Gold M, Hylinski J, et al: A preliminary report of computerized analysis of gait. J Am Podiatr Med Assoc 69:1, 1979.

CHAPTER 31

Musculoskeletal Diseases

William P. Arend
David H. Collier
Catherine E. Harmon

Just as old age is creeping on apace,
And clouds come o'er the sunset of our day,
They kindly leave us, though not quite alone,
But in good company—the gout or stone.

Byron, *Don Juan*

Diseases involving the musculoskeletal system are commonly seen in elderly populations. Joint or muscle pain may be the most common complaint in individuals over the age of 65. It is important to realize, however, that most musculoskeletal symptoms do not signify underlying arthritis. Many aches and pains are due to self-limited problems such as bursitis, tendinitis, muscle sprain, and viral illnesses. In a random survey of 557 residents of Washtenaw County, Michigan, who were age 55 or older, 57 percent indicated the presence of arthritis.[1] More significantly, 24 percent of these elderly individuals said that their arthritis interfered with daily activities in the home or at work. In the 1976 Health Information Survey, arthritis was reported as a problem by 44 percent of Americans aged 65 and older (prevalence of 436.6 per 1000).[2] The prevalence rate of complaints of arthritis was 116.7 per 1000 for all age groups combined, nearly 25 percent of the rate for the elderly group.

Precise prevalence figures for various forms of arthritis in the elderly are not available, but it is likely that a form of arthritis as a primary diagnosis may be present in 5 to 10 percent of individuals between the age of 60 or 65 and over. It is important to determine whether an elderly patient's musculoskeletal complaints are a result of arthritis and, if so, which form is present. Therapy should be directed to the specific type of arthritis and should be

implemented carefully because the elderly are more prone to experience untoward side effects from antiarthritic drugs.

The specific diseases causing musculoskeletal complaints in the elderly can be divided into two groups: (1) those diseases seen primarily in the elderly and (2) those diseases of which the elderly exhibit particular clinical characteristics (Table 31–1).

DISEASES SEEN PRIMARILY IN THE ELDERLY

Osteoarthritis

Osteoarthritis may be present by radiologic or clinical criteria in up to 90 percent of individuals aged 65 and older. The symptoms of pain and discomfort may be a more important cause of functional lim-

TABLE 31–1. Musculoskeletal Diseases in the Elderly

Diseases Seen Primarily in the Elderly
Osteoarthritis
Pseudogout
Hydroxyapatite crystal deposition disease
Diffuse idiopathic sclerosing hyperostosis
(DISH)
Osteoporosis
Paget's disease of bone
Polymyalgia rheumatica (PMR) and giant cell
arteritis (GCA)

**Diseases with Particular Characteristics in the
Elderly**
Rheumatoid arthritis
Systemic lupus erythematosus (SLE)
Sjögren's syndrome
Polymyositis
Progressive systemic sclerosis
Gout
Septic arthritis

itation than actual physical disability caused by the osteoarthritis.[3] Other causes of joint complaints need to be carefully excluded in these patients and the osteoarthritis treated appropriately. Osteoarthritis is commonly classified as primary (idiopathic) and secondary (resulting from previous joint trauma; predisposing inflammatory joint diseases; presence of mechanical or anatomic joint abnormalities; and presence of endocrine, metabolic, or neurologic diseases). This classification scheme has limited usefulness in diagnosis or understanding the clinical manifestations of osteoarthritis. Osteoarthritis can be separated into six different clinical syndromes that are based upon the involved joints and the clinical presentation and course (Table 31–2).[4]

CLINICAL FEATURES

Certain clinical characteristics are common to most patients with osteoarthritis. The joint manifestations generally occur after the age of 50, unless the patient has suffered joint damage from injury, mechanical factors, or severe inflammatory arthritis. The joints involved include the distal interphalangeal (DIP), proximal interphalangeal (PIP), first carpometacarpal, hips, knees, first tarsal-metatarsal, lumbosacral, and cervical spine. Early symptoms of osteoarthritis include pain and stiffness in the involved joints, particularly with use. The symptoms tend to be relieved by rest during the day, may be worse at the end of the day, and may awaken the patient from sleep at night. Morning stiffness may be present but, as opposed to rheumatoid arthritis, usually lasts less than 30 minutes. Soft tissue swelling, joint warmth, and synovial proliferation are not seen, but osteoarthritic joints may develop secondary bony hypertrophy. Later in the disease, joint deformities and instability may occur. Physical findings in osteoarthritis include tenderness along periarticular ligaments and tendons or over damaged joints, the presence of synovial effusions, and limited joint motion with pain at the extremes of motion. The synovial fluid is noninflammatory, exhibiting a high viscosity, normal glucose, negative culture, and up to 2000 cells per cubic mm with less than 25 percent neutrophils.

PATHOPHYSIOLOGY

Osteoarthritis represents a failure of joint function resulting from many different disease mechanisms. Mechanical, environmental, and biochemical factors all

TABLE 31–2. Clinical Patterns of Osteoarthritis

Pattern	Sites(s)	Special Diagnostic Features	Course
Generalized	DIP, PIP, CMC, knee, spine	—	Usually slowly progressive; often asymptomatic
Inflammatory small joint	DIP, PIP; less often CMC, MTP, knee	Erosive x-ray changes; prominent signs of inflammation	Rapid course; early deformity
Isolated nodule	DIP, PIP	Prominent family history	Abrupt onset; rapid course
Unifocal, large joint	Knee, hip, shoulder	Consider mechanical or anatomic disturbance, osteonecrosis, Paget's disease	Slowly progressive; disabling
Multifocal, large joint	Shoulder, knee, hip, wrist, MCP, ankle	Consider crystals—chondrocalcinosis on x-ray; rule out hemochromatosis, endocrine, neurologic	Variable—often progressive and disabling
Unifocal, small joint	DIP, PIP, MTP, CMC	Consider trauma or occupation; look for asymptomatic joints	Variable—often leads to chronic morbidity

CMC = carpometacarpal (joint); DIP = distal interphalangeal (joint); MTP = metatarsophalangeal (joint); PIP = proximal interphalangeal (joint)

may interact, possibly in a genetically predisposed individual, to produce the clinical syndrome called osteoarthritis. The primary damage is to the articular cartilage, which is made up of collagen that gives tensile strength, and proteoglycans, which are large and highly hydrated molecules that contribute elasticity. In idiopathic or primary osteoarthritis, an early biochemical change in cartilage is a decrease in proteoglycans, probably caused by degradation from enzymes released by activated chondrocytes. The water content initially increases in early osteoarthritis, then decreases with time and disease progression. The articular cartilage becomes less elastic and more prone to mechanical damage from normal or abnormal forces, with destruction of collagen. The chondrocyte attempts to compensate by synthesizing more proteoglycans and collagen. Eventually, the chondrocyte fails, and the cartilage first exhibits surface fibrillation, followed later by deep fissures. Growth of surrounding bone occurs. Changes in subchondral bone may occur secondarily to changes in cartilage.

There is some evidence for decreased hardness of subchondral bone in early osteoarthritis. Multiple studies have demonstrated an inverse correlation between bone density and the prevalence of osteoarthritis. In secondary forms of osteoarthritis, trauma, previous inflammatory joint diseases or the presence of metabolic disturbances damage the cartilage, leading to the same series of events. It is important to realize that normal aging does not, in itself, lead to osteoarthritis. The biochemical and structural changes in the joint that accompany aging are not the same as those seen in early osteoarthritis. Osteoarthritis is more common in the elderly, not because of aging-related changes, but because the involved pathophysiologic mechanisms require long periods of time to develop.

CLINICAL SYNDROMES

Osteoarthritis in the elderly may be classified by six different clinical syndromes (see Table 31–2). Generalized or polyarticular osteoarthritis is seen most often in females who present either insidiously or abruptly with pain in a single joint. Other joints are soon involved, usually limited to the hands, knees, and spine. Most of these patients exhibit a slow progression and have a good functional outcome. Inflammatory small joint osteoarthritis occurs primarily in the DIP and PIP joints of the hands with acute redness, swelling, and pain. This entity is also called erosive osteoarthritis, and up to 25 percent of patients with this disorder eventually may develop rheumatoid arthritis. Isolated nodal osteoarthritis includes the rather rapid appearance of bony hypertrophy of DIP and PIP joints, called Heberden's and Bouchard's nodes, respectively. This disease has a strong familial pattern, with evidence of transmission as a dominant trait in women and as a recessive trait in men. Other joint involvement may be seen with time.

Unifocal large joint osteoarthritis occurs commonly in the knees or hips, but an increased incidence of shoulder involvement occurs with aging. Causes of secondary osteoarthritis should be considered in these patients, such as avascular necrosis of bone, congenital hip disease, or Paget's disease. Mechanical abnormalities with increased local shear stress, however, are thought to be a major culprit. Many of these patients eventually may require a total joint replacement. Multifocal large joint osteoarthritis may involve both large and small joints and also may represent a form of secondary osteoarthritis. These patients should be evaluated for underlying calcium pyrophosphate deposition disease (CPPD, or pseudogout), hypothyroidism, hyperparathyroidism, acromegaly, or hemochromatosis. Unifocal small joint osteoarthritis may represent the result of local trauma from repetitive use of a particular joint or may be the presenting manifestation of more generalized osteoarthritis. Osteoarthritis of the first carpometacarpal joint is a common example of this sixth type.

LABORATORY

Laboratory data are generally not helpful. The usual rheumatologic work-up of a complete blood count, erythrocyte sedimentation rate (ESR), and rheumatoid factor are most likely normal. The synovial fluid is nonspecific, showing a moderate leukocytosis. Radiographic findings, however, are usually diagnostic. The findings of asymmetric narrowing of the joint space, dense sclerosis of subchondral bone, and presence of marginal osteophytes are relatively specific for osteoarthritis.

MANAGEMENT

Therapy of osteoarthritis in the elderly should be conservative and influenced by the type, extent, and severity of joint disease. All patients should be educated about the nature and prognosis of their particular disease and instructed in general principles of joint protection and physical therapy. Obese patients should lose weight, particularly those with hip and knee disease. Nonsteroidal, anti-inflammatory drugs should be employed in the lowest effective doses, prescribed by a physician who is aware of the possible problems of these drugs in elderly patients. As a rule of thumb, the patient is started on half the usual dose of a nonsteroidal, anti-inflammatory agent, and the dose is increased cautiously as effectiveness and tolerability are assessed. Added analgesic therapy should be limited to acetaminophen and, rarely, to codeine. Intra-articular injection of steroids may be effective in particular patients but should not be administered to a single joint more than three or four times a year. Some patients with osteoarthritis of the knee may benefit from arthroscopy with irrigation to remove particles of cartilage and fibrous tissue. Patients with destructive disease of the hip or knee experiencing severe pain and limitation of function may benefit dramatically from total joint replacement.

Calcium Pyrophosphate Dihydrate (CPPD) Deposition Disease or Pseudogout

It is clear that CPPD deposition disease, osteoarthritis, and aging are interrelated. There is an increasing frequency with aging of asymptomatic deposition of CPPD crystals in articular cartilage, called chondrocalcinosis. The disease usually becomes symptomatic after the age of 50. Many of these patients also have osteoarthritis and the crystal deposition probably occurs secondarily. Any patient with chondrocalcinosis should be evaluated for the possible presence of underlying hyperparathyroidism, hypothyroidism, or hemochromatosis. In some patients, the crystals are shed from the articular cartilage into the joint space, inducing inflammation by attracting neutrophils. This clinical syndrome of acute or chronic arthritis is called pseudogout, but not every patient with chondrocalcinosis develops pseudogout.

Six different clinical patterns of CPPD crystalline-induced arthropathy have been described (Table 31–3).[5] Acute to subacute attacks of pseudogout occur with an increased frequency in the setting of osteoarthritis, especially in the knee. In addition, CPPD disease may mimic osteoarthritis in exhibiting progressive degenerative changes, often with an inflammatory component. A clue to this diagnosis is the presence of changes of osteoarthritis in unusual sites, such as wrists, metacarpal phalangeal (MCP) joints, shoulders, and elbows, as well as in the usual sites (i.e., knees and hips). In a small minority of patients with pseudogout, the condition may mimic rheumatoid arthritis, often with a positive serologic test for rheumatoid factor. Diagnosis of CPPD disease is made by aspiration of joint fluid and identification of the typical rhomboid crystals as weakly negatively birefringent by polarized microscopy. A presumptive diagnosis can be made when the chondrocalcinosis is seen in the fibrocartilage of the symphysis pubis, wrist, knee meniscus, or annulus fibrosis or in the hyaline cartilage in the knees, hips, shoulders, or elbows. Treatment of CPPD disease should include correcting any underlying condition, if possible. For acute attacks and chronic synovitis, nonsteroidal, anti-inflammatory drugs are used. Oral and intravenous colchicine has been shown to help acute attacks of pseudogout, and intra-articular steroids can also be used.

Apatite-Associated Arthritis

Aggregates of material containing hydroxyapatite crystals have been described in the synovial fluid of up to 50 percent of patients with osteoarthritis.[6] These crystals also are found in the synovium and carti-

TABLE 31–3. Clinical Patterns of Calcium Pyrophosphate Dihydrate Deposition Disease (CPPD)

Type	CPPD (%)	Sex Ratio	Attack Characteristics	Major Joints	Miscellaneous Features
A, Pseudogout	25	M > F	Acute to subacute	50% knee cluster attacks	Chondrocalcinosis, 20% hyperuricemia, 5% gout
B, Pseudo-RA	5	F > M	Subacute attacks, AM stiffness	MCP, wrist	RF 10%
C, Pseudo-OA	25	F > M	Progressive degenerative joint disease (DJD), inflammatory episodes	Knee, wrist, MCP, hip, shoulder, elbow	Flexion contractures
D, Pseudo-OA	25	F > M	Progressive DJD, noninflammatory	Knee, wrist, MCP, hip, shoulder, elbow	Flexion contractures
E, Lanthanic	4 to 25	F > M	Asymptomatic; chondrocalcinosis on x-ray	—	—
F, Neuroarthropathic	Rare	—	CPPD crystals found in both neuropathic and pseudoneuropathic joints	—	—

lage. It is likely that their deposition may be secondary to joint damage, but these crystals may be primarily involved in a particular clinical syndrome. These patients are predominantly elderly females (f:m is 4:1) who develop a rather rapid destruction of a shoulder, hip, or knee with joint instability. The synovial fluids contain large amounts of hydroxyapatite crystals (which may or may not be visible under a light microscope as crystal aggregates), few inflammatory cells, blood, and high levels of proteolytic enzymes and collagens. Radiographic findings may include calcific tendinitis, calcific bursitis, calcific periarthritis, joint degeneration, erosions, and atypical features of osteoarthritis. Nonsteroidal, anti-inflammatory drugs and joint aspiration and injection are used. Owing to the extensive destruction encountered, however, these patients often receive total joint replacement.

Diffuse Idiopathic Sclerosing Hyperostosis (DISH)

Also known as ankylosing hyperostosis or Forestier's disease, DISH is a radiographic diagnosis. Characteristics of DISH include (1) flowing ligamentous calcification and ossification along the anterolateral aspect of 4 or more contiguous verte-

brae called syndesmophytes; (2) relative preservation of intervertebral disc height; (3) no significant apophyseal or sacroiliac involvement; (4) olecranon and calcaneal spurs; and (4) extraspinal ligamentous ossification such as the sacrotuberous ligament. DISH is very common, with worldwide distribution. It is usually found incidentally in asymptomatic middle-aged to elderly men, but it may be the cause of spinal stiffness and low back pain. DISH also may accompany other rheumatic diseases such as rheumatoid arthritis (RAD-ISH). Approximately 22 percent of DISH patients are diabetic. It should be emphasized that DISH is not a variant of osteoarthritis, but a separate entity that presents with ligamentous calcifications around the spine. The osteophytic spurs of osteoarthritis differ radiographically as being distinct bony outgrowths of the vertebrae, usually with malalignment resulting from loss of disc spaces.

Osteoporosis

Osteoporosis (see Chapter 29) is most common in postmenopausal females and is the cause of over 250,000 hip fractures and 530,000 vertebral fractures per year in the U.S. By 80 years of age, 40 percent of white women will have sustained hip fractures, and 50 percent will have sustained vertebral fractures. The mortality rate for hip fractures is 12 to 20 percent. All individuals experience variable degrees of age-related bone loss, but this process occurs more rapidly in patients who develop osteoporosis. The vertebral and wrist fractures are usually caused by a loss of trabecular bone, which occurs more rapidly within a few years of menopause. Fractures of the femoral neck are caused by cortical bone loss, which starts at menopause and proceeds more slowly but continuously. In addition to fractures, osteoporosis patients often experience bone and muscle pain that may be misinterpreted as joint disease.

Osteoporosis is a histologic diagnosis of decreased bone mass per unit volume below the normal limit of bone mass in young adults. The ratio of mineral to matrix remains normal. The proportion of the population falling into this osteoporotic range rises with age. By age 60, 30 percent of women have trabecular osteoporosis, and about 50 percent have cortical osteoporosis. By age 80, the incidence of osteoporosis is virtually 100 percent. Osteopenia refers to radiologic evidence of bone loss, with at least 30 to 50 percent loss being present before detection by x-ray. These patients may have osteoporosis or osteomalacia, which has a decreased bone mineralization rate accompanied by increased osteoid surface that results in an area of unmineralized bone. The diagnosis of osteoporosis is made more sensitive by the use of dual-photon absorptiometry of the spine, quantitative computerized tomography of the spine, or single-photon absorptiometry of the forearm, to quantify relative calcium content. However, the widespread clinical usefulness of these modalities has yet to be determined. They may primarily be of value to follow patients on therapy for osteoporosis by measuring a possible decrease in rate of bone loss.

The development of osteoporosis in white women is greatly enhanced by the presence of one or more risk factors (Table 31–4). Women at high risk may be diagnosed as osteopenic before development of symptoms. In addition to presenting with hip, wrist, or vertebral fractures, osteoporotic patients may experience continuous back pain. This is caused by lumbar

TABLE 31–4. Factors Contributing to the Development of Osteoporosis

Well Established
Increasing age
Premenopausal oophorectomy
Corticosteroid use
Extreme immobility
Genetic factors

Moderate Evidence
Alcohol consumption
Cigarette smoking
Low dietary calcium

Inconclusive Evidence
Parity
Diabetes
Use of thiazide diuretics
Progesterone deficiency
Use of caffeine

lordosis with paraspinous muscle spasm, and the back pain may persist even after the fractures have healed. Patients diagnosed as having osteoporosis should be evaluated for secondary causes, such as hyperparathyroidism, hyperthyroidism, Cushing's syndrome, hypogonadism, and chronic liver or renal disease.

The treatment of osteoporosis is not totally satisfactory, but it is intended to slow the rate of bone loss and possibly to stimulate bone formation. Estrogen therapy with cyclic use of a progestational agent should be administered for 10 to 15 years after menopause. Supplemental calcium intake in premenopausal women should be 1000 mg per day, increasing to 1500 mg per day in postmenopausal women, probably with some vitamin D supplementation. Calcitonin is FDA approved for use in osteoporosis. Many experimental therapies for osteoporosis are still being evaluated. These include high-dose fluoride, vitamin D metabolites, low-dose parathyroid hormone, cyclic therapy with diphosphonates, and anabolic steroids. All patients at risk for osteoporosis should undertake at least 3 to 4 hours per week of weight-bearing exercise.

Paget's Disease of Bone

Paget's disease (osteitis deformans) of bone is a chronic condition characterized by increased osteoclastic bone resorption and disorganized formation of new bone so that weak and immature woven bone replaces normal lamellar bone. The incidence is 1 percent in the fifth decade, rising to 10 percent in the ninth decade, and averaging 3 percent of the population over age 40. There may be a strong genetic factor, and the disease is more common in men. Ninety-five percent of patients are asymptomatic at the time of diagnosis, usually made radiographically in the evaluation of an elevated serum level of alkaline phosphatase. The x-ray in Paget's disease shows variable degrees of lytic lesions, mixed with areas of sclerosis or increased bone density. Other laboratory findings are elevated serum and urine hydroxyproline, probably related to increased bone remodeling.

Pain in the pelvis, hips, or back may be the presenting complaint in 5 percent of patients with Paget's disease. The most likely bones involved with osteolytic and/or osteosclerotic changes are the cranial vault, long bones, pelvis, and spine. The bone remodeling and overgrowth in Paget's disease may occasionally be extensive enough to lead to bony deformities (kyphosis and bowing of the long bones of the extremities), neurologic complications (muscle weakness, paralysis, and rectal and vesical incontinence, resulting from impingement on the spinal cord), osteogenic sarcoma, or cardiac disease including high-output congestive failure. Most patients are treated with nonsteroidal, anti-inflammatory drugs or analgesics. Some patients with extensive Paget's disease may require more specific therapy with calcitonin, diphosphonates, or mithramycin.

Polymyalgia Rheumatica and Giant Cell Arteritis

Polymyalgia rheumatica (PMR) and giant cell arteritis (GCA) are closely linked. Both diseases occur primarily in the elderly, have overlapping clinical features, and frequently occur together. Therefore, any discussion of PMR must also include GCA.

DEFINITIONS

Polymyalgia rheumatica is a clinical syndrome that occurs almost exclusively in people over the age of 50. It is characterized by severe aching and stiffness of the neck, the upper arms and shoulders, and/or the pelvic girdle and thighs, which is especially prominent upon awakening. Constitutional symptoms such as fever, malaise, and weight loss are common. The major laboratory abnormality is a markedly elevated Westergren ESR, with values usually greater than 50 mm per hour. A prompt, clinical response to small, daily doses of corticosteroids (10 to 20 mg per day) is also characteristic.

Giant cell arteritis is primarily a pathologic term to describe a necrotizing granulomatous arteritis affecting predominantly the aorta and its large to medium-sized branches in a patchy distribution. GCA usually occurs in the elderly, is characterized by a high ESR, and may lead to sudden blindness. Constitutional symptoms are common. The clinically more descriptive terms, temporal arteritis and cranial arteritis, are used interchangeably with GCA.

RELATIONSHIP OF PMR TO GCA

Several studies have reported that between 50 and 62 percent of patients with GCA will also have PMR at some time during the course of their illness.[8] Symptoms of PMR may precede, occur simultaneously with, or follow the development of GCA. Conversely, numerous series of patients with PMR have described the coexistence of GCA in anywhere from 6 to 78 percent of cases, the most accurate estimate probably being close to 50 percent.[9] Most PMR patients with GCA will have arthritic-type symptoms. However, in PMR patients without clinical signs or symptoms of GCA, approximately 10 to 15 percent will have a positive temporal artery biopsy.

On the basis of overlapping clinical features, age, predisposition, and frequent occurrence of PMR and GCA in the same person, many authors view PMR and GCA as part of a spectrum of disease with a common underlying arteritis. Hunder and coworkers, however, have recently advanced a new concept of the PMR-GCA relationship in an attempt to reconcile the observations that (1) although PMR and GCA frequently coexist, they also appear to occur separately; (2) over half of the patients with PMR have no evidence of an arteritis, despite extensive investigation; (3) PMR occurs two to three times more frequently than GCA; and (4) joint scans indicative of synovitis are frequently positive in PMR. According to this theory, PMR and GCA have a single common etiology but two different clinicopathologic expressions—either synovitis or arteritis.[9]

ETIOLOGY

The cause of PMR and GCA is unknown. Because of the striking propensity of these diseases to occur almost exclusively in the elderly, an etiologic role of aging is a logical consideration. Both PMR and GCA rarely occur in persons younger than 55 years of age, and there is a similar average age of onset (65 to 70 years) for both diseases. Nevertheless, whether and how aging is implicated in PMR-GCA is unclear.

The causes and pathophysiologic mechanisms of PMR-GCA remain unknown. Many cases have a history of preceding viral illness, which may be able to trigger an autoimmune process. There is some circumstantial evidence to suggest a role for humoral immunity. However, favoring a role for cell-mediated immunity in GCA is the presence of plasma cells and giant cell granulomas near the disrupted internal elastic lamina of the involved arteries. This observation, plus the rarity of involvement of arteries without an internal elastica lamina such as the intracranial vessels, suggests a possible, but unproven, antigenic role for elastin.[10]

CLINICAL MANIFESTATIONS

By a ratio of 2:1, the typical patient with PMR is more commonly a woman over the age of 50, with an average age of 65 (range, ages 31 to 83).[8] The onset of symptoms is insidious in more than two-thirds of patients. However, the onset may be so abrupt that healthy individuals may go to bed at night seemingly well only to awaken the following morning with such severe aching that they describe feelings of "being run over by a truck."

PMR is characterized by symmetric proximal aching of the shoulders, hips, neck, upper arms, and thighs. Morning stiffness is prominent and prolonged. The pain is severe and may be described as myalgic, but it is often poorly localized. Movement leads to a dramatic increase in pain. Muscle weakness is not a feature of PMR, although limitations caused by pain may be misinterpreted as weakness. Constitutional symptoms include malaise, anorexia, night sweats, and weight loss; a low-grade fever, rarely exceeding 103° F, occurs in 60 percent of patients. Transient, mild effusions, especially of the knee, may occur. Rare reports of synovial fluid examinations in PMR show white blood cell counts of 1000 to 8000 per cubic mm.

The median age of patients with GCA is 70 years (range, ages 23 to 90). Females are affected twice as often as males. In approximately two thirds of cases, the onset is insidious, and constitutional symptoms are common. A low-grade fever is present in 50 percent, and patients with GCA may present with a fever of undetermined origin. Night sweats are common, but shaking chills are absent.

GCA is a great mimic and may present in numerous ways, as demonstrated by the initial manifestations of 100 consecutive cases of biopsy-proven GCA at the Mayo Clinic listed in Table 31–5.[11] The major clinical manifestations are usually related to local arterial involvement or systemic complaints.

Headache, probably secondary to arterial inflammation, is the most common initial and subsequent complaint and is present in 44 to 98 percent of cases. The headache usually begins early in the course of the disease and is the presenting

TABLE 31–5. Initial Manifestations of Giant Cell Arteritis (GCA) in 100 Patients— Mayo Clinic

Manifestations	Number of Patients
Headache	32
Polymyalgia rheumatica (PMR)	25
Fever	15
Visual symptoms without loss	7
Malaise/fatigue	5
Arterial tenderness	3
Myalgias	4
Weight loss/anorexia	2
Jaw claudication	2
Permanent visual loss	1
Tongue claudication	1
Sore throat	1
Arteritic angiogram	1
Hand/wrist stiffness	1

symptom in 30 to 45 percent of patients. The headache may be a severe pain, localized to the scalp arteries, or an ill-defined, throbbing sensation. The onset of a headache in an older patient should alert one to the possibility of GCA, especially in the presence of a high ESR. On physical examination, scalp tenderness, with or without nodules, may be present. The temporal arteries may be pulseless and have the consistency of rope. On the other hand, the temporal arteries of patients with biopsy-proven GCA are often clinically normal. Approximately 50 percent of GCA patients will also have PMR, and it is the initial complaint in 20 to 40 percent of cases. Synovitis is present in some patients, usually in association with PMR.

Ischemic syndromes that have been associated with GCA are listed in Table 31–6. Jaw claudication, secondary to ischemia of the masseter muscles, has been reported in 30 to 50 percent of GCA cases and is considered characteristic of the disease. Ocular symptoms are common, with the most dreaded complication of GCA being partial or complete loss of vision that is almost always irreversible. Blindness is generally caused by ischemic optic neuritis secondary to arteritis of the ciliary vessels or ophthalmic artery. Occlusion of the central retinal artery occurs infrequently.

Klein and coworkers reported that 34 of 248 GCA patients, or 14 percent, had evidence of definite or possible large artery involvement manifested by intermittent claudication of an extremity, often with absent or decreased pulses and bruits, and occasionally with Raynaud's phenomenon.[12] In addition, three of the patients had a dissecting aortic aneurysm and died of aortic rupture. Angiography was helpful in favoring the diagnosis of arteritis over that of atherosclerosis on the basis of (1) long segments of smooth arterial stenosis, alternating with areas of normal caliber; (2) smooth-tapered occlusions of affected large arteries; (3) absence of irregular plaque and ulcerations; and (4) predilection for subclavian, axillary, and brachial arteries.

LABORATORY FINDINGS

The ESR is the most helpful laboratory aid in PMR-GCA. The Westergren ESR is characteristically greater than 40 mm in one hour and is usually greater than 50 mm per hour. Anemia occurs in 40 to 60 percent of patients with PMR-GCA and may be the primary manifestation of GCA. The anemia is usually normochromic or hypochromic, with hematocrit in the range of 27 to 35 percent. Rheumatoid factor and tests for antinuclear antibody are present in low titer in 5 to 10 percent of cases, the same frequency expected in an elderly population. Abnormal liver function tests may be present in 33 percent of patients. Muscle enzymes, electromyography, and muscle biopsies are normal.

DIAGNOSIS

A diagnosis of PMR-GCA should be considered in any elderly patient who presents with unexplained proximal aching, new onset of headaches and/or visual disturbances, or unexplained fever or anemia, especially when accompanied by a high ESR.

If GCA is suspected, a temporal artery biopsy should be performed. Routine bi-

TABLE 31–6. Ischemic Syndromes in Giant Cell Arteritis (GCA)

Arteritic Involvement	Manifestations
Temporal artery	Headache, scalp necrosis
Facial artery	Claudication of the jaw and/or tongue, odynophagia, gangrene of the tongue
Ocular arteries (ophthalmic, posterior ciliary, retinal)	Ptosis, diplopia, partial or complete loss of vision
Aorta and its major branches	Dissecting aortic aneurysm, aortic rupture, Raynaud's phenomenon, extremity claudication, bruits, absent pulses
Coronary artery	Angina, myocardial infarction
Renal artery	Glomerulitis, renal artery stenosis
Mesenteric arteries	Abdominal angina

opsy of the temporal arteries of patients with PMR without symptoms of GCA is controversial. It is clear, however, that in PMR patients with signs or symptoms of arteritis or with failure to respond clinically or serologically to therapy, temporal artery biopsy is recommended. The histologic findings in the temporal arteries of patients with GCA include an infiltration of mixed mononuclear cells and giant cells within the media of the vessel wall, in close proximity to the disrupted elastic laminae.

TREATMENT

Patients with pure PMR usually respond dramatically to 10 to 15 mg of prednisone per day, with clinical improvement occurring often within 12 to 36 hours and a return to a normal ESR in 2 to 4 weeks. Treatment of GCA consists of 40 to 60 mg of prednisone daily. If ocular symptoms or signs of potentially life-threatening complications such as an aortic arch syndrome are present, corticosteroid therapy should be begun immediately, followed promptly by temporal artery biopsy. Once the clinical features of the illness have subsided and the laboratory abnormalities reflecting systemic inflammation have returned to normal, attempts should be made to taper the steroid dosage to the lowest necessary maintenance level. Usually, the initial corticosteroid dose needs to be continued for at least 1 month before beginning a tapering dose schedule of 10 percent weekly reductions. Maintenance of 5 to 10 mg of prednisone daily usually is required for 1 to 3 years.

DISEASES WITH PARTICULAR CHARACTERISTICS IN THE ELDERLY

Rheumatoid Arthritis

Rheumatoid arthritis is a common form of inflammatory arthritis that occurs in 1 to 2 percent of the general population. The incidence of this disease is greatest in females in the third and fourth decades. However, rheumatoid arthritis can occur in members of both genders at any age. Two percent or more of patients with rheumatoid arthritis experience the onset after the age of 60, with an equal frequency in males and females. In individuals over 60 years of age, rheumatoid arthritis manifests a few different patterns and characteristics than in younger patients.

CRITERIA

Revised criteria for the classification of rheumatoid arthritis have recently been drawn up by a committee of the American Rheumatism Association (Table 31–7).[13] The clinical and laboratory manifestations of rheumatoid arthritis may develop over time, and all may not be present initially. Therefore, these criteria are useful for classification of patients at any point but may have limited application as diagnostic criteria for any individual patient with disease of recent onset. If a patient fulfills four of these seven criteria, the diagnosis of rheumatoid arthritis has a sensitivity of 91 to 94 percent and a specificity of 89 percent. It is important to note that criteria 1 through 4, that is, morning stiffness or clinical evidence of arthritis, must be present for at least 6 weeks, with joint findings observed by a physician.

PATHOPHYSIOLOGY

The pathophysiology of rheumatoid arthritis is not known, but it is felt to involve an abnormal or exaggerated immune response to an exogenous agent in a genetically predisposed host. Over 60 percent of white patients with rheumatoid arthritis are positive for HLA-DR4 as compared with 30 percent or less of the normal population. How this genetic marker is related to the acquisition of rheumatoid arthritis has not been established. Although infectious agents are suspected to be involved in the induction of the disease, none has yet been proven.

Rheumatoid arthritis begins as an inflammatory disease of the synovium, the lining layer of joints and tendon sheaths. The earliest histologic changes include an increase in the thickness of the synovial lining cells, representing an infiltration of monocytes from the blood that develop into synovial macrophages, and a local proliferation of fibroblasts. The subsynovium exhibits an infiltration of monocytes and lymphocytes, as well as new growth

TABLE 31–7. The 1987 Revised Criteria for the Classification of Rheumatoid Arthritis*

Criterion	Definition
1. Morning stiffness	Morning stiffness in and around the joints, lasting at least 1 hr before maximal improvement
2. Arthritis of 3 or more joint areas	At least 3 joint areas simultaneously have had soft tissue swelling or fluid (not bony overgrowth alone), observed by a physician. The 14 possible areas are right or left PIP, MCP, wrist, elbow, knee, ankle, and MTP joints
3. Arthritis of hand joints	At least 1 area swollen (as defined above) in wrist, MCP, or PIP joint
4. Symmetric arthritis	Simultaneous involvement of the same joint areas (as defined in 2) on both sides of the body. (Bilateral involvement of PIP, MCP, or MTP is acceptable without absolute symmetry.)
5. Rheumatoid nodules	Subcutaneous nodules over bony prominences or extensor surfaces or in juxta-articular regions, observed by a physician
6. Serum rheumatoid factor	Demonstration of abnormal amounts of serum rheumatoid factor by any method for which the result has been positive in < 5% of normal control subjects
7. Radiographic changes	Radiographic changes typical of rheumatoid arthritis on posteroanterior hand and wrist radiographs, which must include erosions or unequivocal bony decalcification localized in or most marked adjacent to the involved joints. (Osteoarthritis changes alone do not qualify.)

*For classification purposes, a patient shall be said to have rheumatoid arthritis if he/she has satisfied at least 4 of these 7 criteria. Criteria 1 through 4 must have been present for at least 6 weeks. Patients with 2 clinical diagnoses are not excluded. Designation as classic, definite, or probable rheumatoid arthritis is *not* to be made.

of blood vessels. The synovium becomes hyperproliferative and grows over the articular cartilage, called pannus, with destruction of the cartilage. This synovial tissue also invades the adjacent bone and periarticular connective tissue. The cellular events in the synovium responsible for these events include activation of T cells, with release of factors that stimulate macrophages. These cells, in turn, release interleukin-1 and other mediators that induce fibroblasts in the synovium and chondrocytes in the cartilage to release enzymes. These enzymes degrade proteoglycans, collagen, and other connective tissue constituents, leading eventually to joint destruction.

CLINICAL COURSE

The clinical presentation and cause of rheumatoid arthritis are highly variable. The majority of patients present insidiously with multiple joint involvement. However, a minority of patients may experience a rather abrupt onset of joint pain and swelling, representing the inflammatory synovitis. The course of rheumatoid arthritis is characterized by remissions and exacerbations with variable degrees of functional disability. Up to two thirds of patients will maintain good joint function and be able to carry out near-normal activities of daily living. The remaining one third or more of patients with rheumatoid arthritis, however, will experience sufficient joint destruction to impair function.

Serologic abnormalities in rheumatoid arthritis include a positive rheumatoid factor in 60 to 70 percent. This is an antibody to the Fc portion of IgG and may be responsible for amplifying the inflammatory response in the synovium. It should be noted that the prevalence of rheumatoid factors increases with aging, and a low titer in an older patient may not be significant. Although studies vary, about 20 percent of people over age 60 years will have a positive rheumatoid factor. In addition, rheumatoid factors occur in other diseases such as systemic lupus erythematosus, subacute bacterial endocarditis, chronic lung disease, and chronic liver disease. Other serologic abnormalities found in rheumatoid arthritis include a positive test for antinuclear antibodies in up to 50 percent, usually in a low titer with a homogeneous pattern. The ESR may be elevated, and the patient may have an anemia secondary to chronic inflammation or blood loss. The synovial fluid in patients with rheumatoid arthritis is inflammatory, with 2000 to 75,000 cells per cubic mm, greater than 50 percent neutrophils, negative cultures, and a glucose that is less than 50 mg percent lower than blood.

In addition to joint disease, up to one half of patients with rheumatoid arthritis will have extra-articular manifestations. These are seen more often in patients with established destructive joint disease who have a high titer of rheumatoid factors. The extra-articular manifestations of rheumatoid arthritis include peripheral nodules, lung disease with interstitial fibrosis or pleural effusions, pericardial effusions, Sjögren's syndrome (dry eyes and mouth), neutropenia (Felty's syndrome), carpal tunnel syndrome, and vasculitis.

THERAPY

The treatment of rheumatoid arthritis involves psychological, physical medicine, surgical, and medical modalities in a multidisciplinary approach. Patient education, psychological support, and appropriate forms of physical therapy are most important to implement in all patients. Surgical intervention includes prophylactic synovectomies and total joint replacements. All patients with rheumatoid arthritis should receive aspirin or another nonsteroidal, anti-inflammatory drug. Elderly patients may not tolerate higher doses of these drugs and should be monitored carefully for possible side effects. Disease-modifying drugs are added early in most patients and include gold (oral or IM), hydroxychloroquine, sulfasalazine, penicillamine, methotrexate, or azathioprine. All patients receiving these drugs must be watched closely for side effects. In patients poorly responsive to this therapeutic regimen, the addition of low-dose oral prednisone (5 to 7.5 mg a day) may offer considerable relief of pain and stiffness. Injection of steroids into selected joints also is efficacious.

Rheumatoid Arthritis in the Elderly

Up to 25 percent of patients aged 60 and older who develop rheumatoid arthritis have a very acute onset, but a benign course.[14] This subset of disease predominates in males, involves more large joints, exhibits wide fluctuations in course, and has a good prognosis, with a remission usually within 1 year. Many of these patients appear to respond dramatically to low-dose steroids and resemble PMR in this regard.

Healey has described three subsets of rheumatoid arthritis in the elderly (Table 31–8).[15] The first subset is typical rheumatoid arthritis as seen in younger patients with the presence of rheumatoid factor. The second subset of patients manifests signs and symptoms of Sjögren's syndrome, with limited joint disease of a benign nature. The third subset of rheumatoid arthritis in the elderly includes the patients described above, with a sudden onset, severe stiffness, large joint predominance, and response to low-dose steroids. In another study, rheumatoid arthritis with onset after age 60 was characterized by a shorter duration of disease, less rheumatoid factor positivity, more systemic symptoms, and greater functional disability compared with younger patients.[16] (The use of antirheumatic drugs in the elderly is discussed below.)

Systemic Lupus Erythematosus (SLE)

This is a multisystem autoimmune disease that occurs predominantly in women in the second and third decades. SLE is characterized by an array of autoantibodies, including antibodies to soluble nuclear

TABLE 31–8. Subsets of Rheumatoid Arthritis in the Elderly

Subset 1. Rheumatoid Factor Present
Predilection for smaller joints—wrist, hand, foot
Synovitis likely persistent, progressive, leading to joint damage
Nodules—frequent
Radiographic erosion—frequent

Subset 2. Rheumatoid Factor Present
Sjögren's syndrome
Synovitis limited to few joints, often wrist, hand
Responsive to anti-inflammatory drugs
Nodules—rare
Radiographic erosions—minimal

Subset 3. Rheumatoid Factor Absent
Predilection for large joints—shoulder, hip, knee
Marked stiffness
Synovitis very responsive to low-dose steroid treatment
Not progressive
Nodules—none
Radiographic erosions—none

antigens and to cell surface determinants. Although the etiology is not known, SLE is thought to represent the end result of multiple abnormalities in regulation of the immune response. The major immune dysfunctions may be an overactive antibody response and deficient suppressor T cell function.

SLE is characterized by multiple organ involvement, with different patterns of clinical manifestations seen in different subsets of patients. The classification criteria for SLE are listed in Table 31–9.[17] Patients exhibiting 4 of 11 criteria, either serially or simultaneously, can be classified as having SLE with a sensitivity of 96 percent and a specificity of 96 percent. However, the clinical picture of SLE may emerge in any patient over many years, requiring an elapse of time before the diagnosis can be made.

The cumulative clinical features of SLE are listed in Table 31–10.[18] Cutaneous manifestations are seen in 88 percent, musculoskeletal in 83 percent, serositis in 63 percent, neuropsychiatric in 55 percent, Raynaud's phenomenon in 44 percent, vasculitis in 43 percent, and nephritis in 31 percent. The cumulative laboratory findings in SLE (Table 31–11) indicate that a positive test for antinuclear antibodies (ANA) is found in 94 percent or greater. Those SLE patients lacking ANA positivity when the test is performed on animal tissue substrates may show positivity on a substrate of human cells and possess anti-SSA antibodies. The clinical course is highly variable and depends on the nature and severity of organ involvement. SLE patients with significant renal or CNS disease tend to have a poorer prognosis.

SLE in the Elderly

Up to 20 percent of SLE patients may not develop the disease until the age of 50 or above. These patients with late-onset SLE have less severe disease, with lower frequencies of nephritis, CNS involvement, and cutaneous vasculitis.[18] Clinical features that are more common in late-onset SLE include polyserositis, pulmonary disease with infiltrates, Sjögren's syndrome, peripheral neuropathy, and serologic positivity for antibodies both to SS-A (Ro) and to SS-B (La). In one recent study, serositis or musculoskeletal manifestations were the presenting symptoms in 88 percent of late-onset SLE.[19]

THERAPY

The treatment of SLE is dictated by the organ involvement in any particular patient. The use of nonsteroidal, anti-inflammatory drugs, hydroxychloroquine, or low-dose prednisone is indicated in patients with relatively mild disease. High-dose steroids or immunosuppressive drugs should be limited to those patients with life-threatening disease, particularly of the kidneys or CNS. Patients with late-onset SLE tend to have relatively benign disease, and up to 40 percent of elderly patients will develop significant side effects to steroid treatment. Therefore, elderly patients with SLE should be treated in a conservative fashion with as little corticosteroids as possible.

Drug-induced Lupus

A syndrome resembling SLE can develop in up to 10 percent of patients treated with procainamide or hydralazine. Drug-induced lupus also has been reported secondary to use of isoniazid, phenytoin, phenothiazines, and some of the β-blockers. The usual clinical manifestations of drug-induced lupus are fevers, myalgias, arthralgias, serositis, and rash. As opposed to SLE, renal and CNS disease do not occur. Laboratory testing reveals a positive test for ANA, with a particular pattern of anti-histone antibodies present. Most patients with drug-induced lupus will feel better immediately after stopping the offending drug. Some patients will benefit from the use of nonsteroidal, anti-inflammatory drugs or a short course of corticosteroids. Because many patients with drug-induced lupus are older, this disease may be confused with PMR.

Sjögren's Syndrome

Sjögren's syndrome (keratoconjunctivitis sicca) can occur as a primary disease or may be secondary to another autoimmune disease such as rheumatoid arthritis or SLE. The prevalence of this disorder in

TABLE 31-9. The 1982 Revised Criteria For Classification of Systemic Lupus Erythematosus (SLE)*

Criterion	Definition
Malar rash	Fixed erythema, flat or raised, over the malar eminences, tending to spare the nasolabial folds
Discoid rash	Erythematous raised patches with adherent keratotic sealing and follicular plugging; atrophic scarring may occur in older lesions
Photosensitivity	Skin rash as a result of unusual reaction to sunlight, by patient history or physician observation
Oral ulcers	Oral or nasopharyngeal ulceration, usually painless, observed by a physician
Arthritis	Nonerosive arthritis involving 2 or more peripheral joints, characterized by tenderness, swelling, or effusion
Serositis	Pleuritis—convincing history of pleuritic pain or rub heard by a physician or evidence of pleural effusion *or* Pericarditis—documentation by ECG or rub or evidence of pericardial effusion
Renal disorder	Persistent proteinuria greater than 0.5 gm/day or greater than 3+, if quantitation not performed *or* Cellular casts—may be red cell, hemoglobin, granular, tubular, or mixed
Neurologic disorder	Seizures in the absence of offending drugs or known metabolic derangements; e.g., uremia, ketoacidosis, or electrolyte imbalance *or* Psychosis in the absence of offending drugs or known metabolic derangements; e.g., uremia, ketoacidosis, or electrolyte imbalance
Hematologic disorder	Hemolytic anemia—with reticulocytosis *or* Leukopenia—less than 4000/mm³ total on 2 or more occasions *or* Lymphopenia—less than 1500/mm³ on 2 or more occasions *or* Thrombocytopenia—less than 100,000/mm³ in the absence of offending drugs
Immunologic disorder	Positive LE cell preparation *or* Anti-DNA: antibody to native DNA in abnormal titer *or* Anti-Sm: presence of antibody to Sm nuclear antigen *or* False positive serologic test for syphilis (BFP-STS) known to be positive for at least 6 months and confirmed by *Treponema pallidum* immobilization or fluorescent treponemal antibody absorption test
Antinuclear antibody	An abnormal titer of antinuclear antibody (ANA) by immunofluorescence or an equivalent assay at any point in time and in the absence of drugs known to be associated with "drug-induced lupus" syndrome

*The proposed classification is based on 11 criteria. For the purposes of identifying patients in clinical studies, a person shall be said to have systemic lupus erythematosus if any 4 or more of the 11 criteria are present, serially or simultaneously, during any interval of observation.

the general population has been estimated to be from 0.05 percent to 0.44 percent.[20] However, screening of a female population with an average age of 81 (range, age 63 to 92) indicated that complaints of dry eyes or dry mouth were present in 39 percent. Definite Sjögren's syndrome was present in only 2 percent, however, with a possible diagnosis made in 12 percent. The major cause of dry eyes and dry mouth in this population was the use of medications that have these side effects. Primary Sjögren's syndrome in the elderly

tends to be a benign disease with fewer extraglandular features. It has been noted above that secondary Sjögren's syndrome frequently is seen in elderly patients with rheumatoid arthritis or SLE. Treatment is symptomatic, with the use of natural tear eyedrops, lubricant to place in the eye at night, and good oral hygiene.

Dermatomyositis

Polymyositis and dermatomyositis are autoimmune diseases of muscle character-

TABLE 31–10. Cumulative Clinical Features in 150 Patients with Systemic Lupus Erythematosus (SLE)

Manifestation	No. (%)	Manifestation	No. (%)
Cutaneous	132 (88)	Neuropsychiatric	83 (55)
Malar rash	91 (61)	Central nervous system	59 (39)
Alopecia	68 (45)	Peripheral neuropathy	32 (21)
Photosensitivity	68 (45)	Organic psychosis	24 (16)
Mucosal ulcers	35 (23)	Seizures	20 (13)
Discoid rash	22 (15)	Raynaud's phenomenon	66 (44)
Nodules	18 (12)		
Musculoskeletal	124 (83)	Vasculitis	65 (43)
Arthritis	114 (76)	Cutaneous	40 (27)
Ischemic necrosis	36 (24)	Mesenteric	19 (13)
Myositis	7 (5)	Digital ulcers	14 (9)
		Leg ulcers	9 (6)
Serositis	95 (63)	Nephritis	46 (31)
Pleurisy	85 (57)	Nephrotic syndrome	20 (13)
Pericarditis	35 (23)	Chronic renal failure	5 (3)
Peritonitis	12 (8)	Cardiopulmonary	8 (5)

ized by the presence of lymphocytic infiltrations on muscle biopsy and EMG changes of inflammatory myositis. The clinical manifestations include the rapid or insidious onset of proximal muscle weakness and atrophy, with a typical skin rash present in 41 percent.[21] The skin rash can vary from a heliotropic (purplish) discoloration of the upper eyelid, to an erythematous rash on the face, upper extremities, or trunk that can be indurated, to papules over the metacarpophalangeal joints. The major feature of dermatomyositis that is relative to elderly patients is an association with malignancy. In one study, the frequency of malignancy in dermatomyositis was 8.5 percent in all patients, with figures of 19.2 percent and 17.9 percent in males and females, respectively, over 50 years of age.[21] The average age for patients with malignancy was 62 years, compared with 47 years for all patients with dermatomyositis. In 70 percent of patients, the malignancy preceded the appearance of myositis by an average of 1.9 years. In the remaining 30 percent, myositis preceded malignancy by an average of 2.8 years. The most common tumors are carcinomas of the breast, lung, stomach, or ovary.[22] Patients with myositis and malignancy tend to respond poorly to steroid treatment, but the muscle disease may regress once the tumor is treated successfully. Treatment with high-dose corticosteroids may lead to steroid myopathy or the rapid development of osteoporosis in the elderly. Immunosuppressive drugs have been recommended to take the place of corticosteroids, but little evidence supports their advantage. Survival is significantly reduced in polymyositis patients over age 50, particularly those with dysphagia, high degree of muscle weakness, and pulmonary infiltration.

TABLE 31–11. Cumulative Laboratory Features in 150 Patients With Systemic Lupus Erythematosus (SLE)

Manifestation	No. (%)
Hematologic	
Anemia	86 (57)
Leukopenia	62 (41)
Thrombocytopenia	45 (30)
Direct Coombs' positive	40 (27)
Immunologic	
Hypocomplementemia	89 (59)
Rheumatoid factor	45 (34)
Hyperglobulinemia	45 (30)
Chronic BFP-STS	34 (26)
Antinuclear antibodies	141 (94)
Anti-ssDNA	134 (89)
LE cells	67 (71)
Anti-nRNP	51 (34)
Anti-Sm	26 (17)
Anti-nDNA	42 (28)
Anti-Ro (SS-A)	48 (32)
Anti-La (SS-B)	18 (12)

Progressive Systemic Sclerosis (Scleroderma)

This disease is characterized by variable degrees of progressive fibrosis of the skin and internal organs. The etiology is unknown, but fibroblasts in patients with scleroderma produce an excessive amount of collagen, possibly in response to microvascular injury. The prognosis in scleroderma is worse in patients who develop involvement of the lung, kidneys, or heart. Elderly patients with scleroderma have a poorer cumulative survival than do younger patients.[23] In those patients without lung, kidney, or heart disease, factors associated with reduced survival include older age, anemia, elevated ESR, and heavy use of alcohol or cigarettes.

Gout

Gout is an acute and chronic inflammatory arthritis caused by the formation of sodium urate crystals in synovial fluid, with subsequent neutrophil accumulation. Initial onset usually involves one joint, the metatarsophalangeal joint of the large toe in 60 percent of cases, followed by involvement of the instep, ankle, knee, wrist, fingers, and elbow, respectively. The characteristic attack is acute in onset, with maximal pain in hours commonly occurring at night or early morning and resolving within 1 day to 1 week. Chronic gout occurs if treatment of the hyperuricemia is neglected and can be manifested by tophi and multiple joint involvement. Gout has an overall male:female ratio of 3 to 6:1, but patients developing gout over the age of 60 are equally distributed between the genders.[24] Peak incidence is 50 years old.

A polyarticular onset is more common in gout in the elderly, usually involving the hands in females. Gout is caused by hyperuricemia secondary to either an overproduction of uric acid or an underexcretion of uric acid. A reduction in uric acid clearance probably contributes to hyperuricemia in 75 percent of patients with gout. A major cause of elevated levels of serum uric acid in elderly women with gout is the use of diuretics.[24] However, other secondary causes in the elderly must be considered, including other drugs, polycythemia, leukemia, and myeloproliferative disorders. Obesity is also associated with gout in some studies. The diagnosis of gout is made when intracellular uric acid crystals are seen in synovial fluid. The finding of hyperuricemia and arthritis does not necessarily give a diagnosis of gout. Older patients are at greater risk of being inappropriately diagnosed as having

gout, and the most common cause of pain in the first MTP is osteoarthritis.

The treatment of acute gout is with nonsteroidal, anti-inflammatory drugs or with colchicine. Attacks of gout can be prevented or abated by maintenance on nonsteroidal, anti-inflammatory drugs or colchicine. However, recurrent attacks or chronic gout should be treated by reducing the patient's serum uric acid level. Thiazide diuretics should be stopped, if possible. If no renal disease or tophi are present and renal excretion is less than 600 mg per 24 hours on a purine-free diet or less than 800 mg per 24 hours on a regular diet, a uricosuric drug (i.e., probenecid or sulfinpyrazone) can be used. Otherwise, a drug that inhibits uric acid synthesis (allopurinol) should be initiated.

Septic Arthritis

Infected joints once were considered a disease of children and adolescents but are now seen more often in adults, especially the elderly.[25] In a review of infectious arthritis of 113 unselected patients, 27 percent were over the age of 50.[26] If the cases of gonorrhea are excluded, almost half of the patients with septic joints are over 50 years of age. Risk factors for the development of infected joints include immunosuppressive drugs such as corticosteroids, malignancies, diabetes, liver disease, underlying damaged joints such as from rheumatoid arthritis, and prosthetic joints. The elderly are more likely to have these risk factors and, thus, an increased incidence of septic joints. Although *Staphylococcus aureus* is the most common organism cultured, there is an increased incidence of B-hemolytic streptococcus and gram negative organisms in the elderly as compared with the adult population as a whole.

A septic joint is a medical emergency. One must have a high index of suspicion to properly diagnose septic arthritis. The symptoms may at first be subtle, with fever present in only one third of cases. Usually, the joint is warm and swollen. Typically, the patient has pain with active or passive movement. In nongonococcal arthritis, the synovial fluid Gram stain demonstrates organisms between 25 and 75 percent of the time, and synovial fluid culture is positive in 60 to 100 percent. Blood cultures are important because in 10 percent of the cases, the organism is only grown from the blood. Crystals in joint fluid may be seen concomitantly with an infection. A neglected septic joint may cause rapid destruction and deterioration of the joint; thus, the more rapidly treatment is begun, the better the prognosis.

An increasing number of joint replacements are being performed in elderly patients, and up to 1 percent of these arthroplasties will become infected.[27] Risk factors include underlying rheumatoid arthritis, revision arthroplasties, and metal-to-metal prostheses. Infected prostheses may develop acutely in the immediate postoperative period or insidiously up to 1 to 2 years after surgery. The symptoms may be indolent. The major symptoms suggestive of a developing infection of a prosthetic joint is pain on weight-bearing, which is often in the absence of any local or systemic evidence of infection. Radiographs may show loosening and/or periosteal reaction. Organisms most commonly cultured are *Staphylococcus epidermidis* and *Staphylococcus aureus*. Infected prostheses usually need to be removed before the sepsis will respond completely to appropriate antibiotics. There are, however, some patients whose risk of surgery is so great that antibiotics are given indefinitely.

ANTIARTHRITIC THERAPY IN THE ELDERLY

Medications used to treat various forms of arthritis all have side effects, and elderly patients are particularly susceptible to certain drug toxicities.[28] Elderly patients may develop salicylate toxicity at lower drug doses than younger patients.[29] CNS side effects to salicylates are common in the elderly, particularly tinnitus, decreased hearing, or a depressed sensorium. The pharmacokinetics of nonsteroidal, anti-inflammatory drugs are altered in elderly patients with a decrease in binding to serum proteins, decreased renal clearance, and altered distribution volumes.[30] However, the increased prevalence of hematologic and gastrointestinal side effects to these medications seen in the elderly is more likely a result of an increased sensitivity to local stomach toxicity. Finally, elderly patients with underlying kidney

disease are at a higher risk for developing renal side effects from nonsteroidal, anti-inflammatory drugs. These medications should be instituted judiciously in elderly patients and maintained at the lowest effective dose with careful monitoring.

Other antiarthritic medications also should be used cautiously in elderly patients. Disease-modifying drugs for rheumatoid arthritis can be used in older patients, but serious hematologic and renal toxicity from gold may occur, rashes and taste disturbance from penicillamine are more common, and retinal toxicity from hydroxychloroquine may be more prevalent.[28] Low serum albumin concentrations in elderly patients increase the risk of side effects from the therapeutic use of corticosteroids.

REFERENCES

1. Barney JL, Neukom JE: Use of arthritis care by the elderly. Gerontologist 19:548, 1979.
2. Jack SS: Current estimates from the National Health Interview Survey, United States 1979. Vital and Health Statistics, Series 10, No 136 (DHHS Pub No PHS 81-1564). Washington, DC: US GPO 1981.
3. Baron M, Dutil E, Berkson L, et al: Hand function in the elderly: relation to osteoarthritis. J Rheumatol 14:815, 1987.
4. Cooke TDV, Dwosh IL: Clinical features of osteoarthritis in the elderly. Clin Rheum Dis 12:155, 1986.
5. McCarty DJ: Calcium pyrophosphate dihydrate crystal deposition disease (pseudogout syndrome): clinical aspects. Clin Rheum Dis 3:61, 1977.
6. Doherty M, Dieppe P: Crystal deposition disease in the elderly. Clin Rheum Dis 12:97, 1986.
7. Peck WA, Riggs BL, Bell NH, et al: Research directions in osteoporosis. Am J Med 84:275, 1988.
8. Hunder GG, Allen GL: Giant cell arteritis: a review. Bull Rheum Dis 29:980, 1976–1979 series.
9. Ettlinger RE, Hunder GG, Ward LE: Polymyalgia rheumatica and giant cell arteritis. Annu Rev Med 29:15, 1978.
10. Healey LA, Wilske KR: Manifestations of giant cell arteritis. Med Clin North Am 61:261, 1977.
11. Calamia KT, Hunder GG: Clinical manifestations of giant cell (temporal) arteritis. Clin Rheum Dis 6:389, 1980.
12. Klein RG, Hunder GG, Stanson AW, et al: Large artery involvement in giant cell (temporal) arthritis. Ann Intern Med 83:806, 1975.
13. Arnett FC, Edworthy SM, Block DA, et al: The American Rheumatism Association 1987 revised criteria for the classification of rheumatoid arthritis. Arthritis Rheum 31:315, 1988.
14. Corrigan AB, Robinson RG, Terenty TR, et al: Benign rheumatoid arthritis of the aged. Br Med J 1:444, 1974.

15. Healey LA: Rheumatoid arthritis in the elderly. Clin Rheum Dis 12:173, 1986.

16. Terkeltaub R, Esdaile J, Decary F, et al: A clinical study of older age rheumatoid arthritis with comparison to a younger onset group. J Rheumatol 10:418, 1983.

17. Tan EM, Cohen AS, Fries JF, et al: The 1982 revised criteria for the classification of systemic lupus erythematosus. Arthritis Rheum 25:1271, 1982.

18. Hochberg MC, Boyd RE, Abram JM, et al: Systemic lupus erythematosus: a review of clinico-laboratory features and immunogenetic markers in 150 patients with emphasis on demographic subsets. Medicine 64:285, 1985.

19. Johnson H, Nived O, Sturfelt G: The effect of age on clinical and serological manifestations in unselected patients with systemic lupus erythematosus. J Rheumatol 15:505, 1988.

20. Strickland RW, Tesar JT, Berne BH, et al: The frequency of sicca syndrome in an elderly female population. J Rheumatol 14:766, 1987.

21. Bohan A, Peter JB, Bowman RL, et al: A computer-assisted analysis of 153 patients with polymyositis and dermatomyositis. Medicine 56:255, 1977.

22. Barnes BE: Dermatomyositis and malignancy: a review of the literature. Ann Intern Med 84:68, 1976.

23. Medsger TA Jr, Masi AT: Survival with scleroderma. II: a life-table analysis of clinical and demographic factors in 358 male U.S. veteran patients. J Chronic Dis 26:647, 1973.

24. Ter Borg EJ, Rasker JJ: Gout in the elderly, a separate entity? Ann Rheum Dis 46:72, 1987.

25. Newman JH: The differential diagnosis of septic arthritis in the elderly. Comp Therapy 10:29, 1984.

26. Sharp JT, Lidsky MD, Duffy J, et al: Infectious arthritis. Arch Intern Med 139:1125, 1979.

27. Inman RD, Gallegos KV, Brause BD, et al: Clinical and microbial features of prosthetic joint infection. Am J Med 77:47, 1984.

28. Brooks PM, Kean WF, Kassam Y, et al: Problems of antiarthritic therapy in the elderly. J Am Geriatr Soc 32:229, 1984.

29. Grigor RR, Spitz PW, Furst DE: Salicylate toxicity in elderly patients with rheumatoid arthritis. J Rheumatol 14:60, 1987.

30. Woodhouse KW, Wynne H: The pharmacokinetics of non-steroidal anti-inflammatory drugs in the elderly. Clin Pharmacokinet 12:111, 1987.

CHAPTER 32

Mobility, Exercise, Muscular Problems, and Rehabilitation

Robert H. Meier, III

*Not by physical force, not by bodily swiftness and
agility, are great things accomplished, but by delib-
eration, authority, and judgment; qualities with
which old age is abundantly provided.*
CICERO, *De Senectute XIV*

The process of aging imposes the loss
of certain abilities on those who experience
the physiologic changes that accompany
advancing years. Therefore, everyone who
grows old will be faced with the reality of
disability to a greater or lesser extent. The
challenge for health care professionals for
this maturing population is not so much
curative, but emphasizes the restoration
and maintenance of ability. Meeting this
challenge is the essence of rehabilitative
diagnosis, therapeutic goal setting, and
treatment interventions. The medical
model of rehabilitation focuses on delaying the inevitable loss of mobility and
function or, when these are altered, instituting a multidisciplinary plan to restore
or maintain them. When mobility or function cannot be restored, rehabilitative care
can assist with the emotional and physical
transition of coping productively with the
disability. The demand for rehabilitation
is expanding as the number of elderly
citizens increases as a percentage of the
population. As the U.S. population grays,
the prevalence of disability and its associated problems will grow.

The medical issues associated with aging, which most commonly are related to
the extent of disability, are well known.
They include poor nutrition, inactivity,
diminished muscle mass, atrophy of the
skin, altered cardiovascular and pulmo-

nary function, diminished vision and hearing, and altered sexual function. These
issues directly affect the level of function
and expected ability. These medical
changes must be considered in the broader
context of the psychosocial milieu that
envelops the elderly person. Repeated loss
and changes in the support group,
whether spouse, family, or friends, often
occur with changes in vocation, avocational interests, living setting, and geographic location. These lifestyle changes,
in addition to altered physiology and function, are often devastating and make motivators for a continued productive life
difficult to find for many older individuals.

STROKE

Cerebrovascular disease is the third
most frequent cause of death in the U.S.,
but there has been a decreased incidence
of stroke in recent years. Although more
persons are surviving the initial onset,
they are living with the neurologic sequelae. The typical disability seen with involvement of the middle cerebral artery is
hemiplegia of the opposite side from the
pathology. The motor impairment that occurs is one in which the arm is more
paralyzed than the leg, so that although
many of these stroke victims may be able
to walk, there is often little functional use
of the affected arm, especially the hand.
Sensory deficits are frequently seen and
may decrease the person's awareness of
the affected side. This agnosia makes it
difficult for the person to compensate for

the impaired use of that side of the body. The sensory deficits are also often accompanied by a diminished visual field on the paralyzed side so that vision is compromised. The ability to swallow and communicate is also often impaired and can affect nutritional status, airway protection and communication with others.

Stroke rehabilitation in the acute care patient is based on a careful assessment of the neuromuscular, communicative, and cognitive deficits. The most important early problem is an impaired swallowing mechanism, which may compromise airway protection. The initial evaluation should assess the patient's ability to swallow without aspiration. If the airway is at risk, limiting fluid intake by mouth and changing to a firmer food consistency may help protect the airway. If the airway is at significant risk, a small nasogastric feeding tube should be used to ensure that adequate nutrition and fluids are consumed.

Early attempts to mobilize the patient from bed (i.e., 3 days after neurologic changes have stabilized) should only be done after careful assessment of the patient's skin, motor deficits, cognitive awareness, and sense of verticality. Often, the patient may not be aware of the vertical position and neglect the paralyzed side of the body as well. Trying to sit a patient in or out of bed makes little sense if the patient has poor sitting balance. Initial rehabilitation planning focuses on sitting balance and on what substitutions may be needed to assist with maintaining an upright, midline sitting position.

Passive range of motion exercise for the hemiplegic limbs should be provided twice daily. The hand can be immobilized in a functional position using a resting splint with the wrist slightly dorsiflexed. The foot should be maintained in a posterior splint, which keeps the ankle at neutral in order to prevent a plantar flexion contracture that may interfere with gait at a later time.

Most commonly, the hip and knee musculature of the plegic limb show the earliest voluntary recovery. Especially important for walking are the hip extensors, abductors, and flexors and the knee extensors. The hip flexors help to move the lower limb forward, and the hip and knee extensors stabilize the knee during weight-bearing. The hip abductors stabilize the pelvis and upper body during the stance phase of gait. Often voluntary motor function of the foot dorsiflexors does not return or is weak, but the foot can be supported for toe clearance while walking with an ankle-foot orthosis (short leg brace).

An attempt to stand a hemiplegic patient should not be attempted until adequate sitting balance, a sense of verticality, and adequate hip and knee control have been established with the supervision of a physical therapist. Once these elements of standing have been achieved, standing and walking inside the parallel bars can be attempted. If significant neglect of the affected limbs or impaired judgment continues, wheelchair mobility is the safest means of ambulation. Walking outside of the parallel bars should be tried when the patient can consistently transfer weight to the paretic leg without buckling of the knee. Often, a gait aid such as a hemi-walker or quad cane is necessary to help support the body while standing on the paretic limb.

The hemiplegic arm is often useless for bimanual function. In order to support the glenohumeral joint and prevent it from subluxation, an arm sling is provided to keep the weight of the arm, forearm, and hand from pulling on the glenohumeral capsule, muscles, and ligaments. Glenohumeral subluxation has been cited as a frequent cause of chronic shoulder pain in hemiplegic patients.

Activities of daily living (ADL), which include eating, hygiene skills, and dressing, should be explored in the early weeks following the onset of stroke. Self-feeding should not be started before an assessment of swallowing function; however, self-feeding and hygiene management are important achievements for the stroke victim. Dressing is usually more energy-consuming and requires the ability to plan and sequence motor activities. Substituting for the weak or paralyzed limbs requires more energy, problem-solving skills, and body balance. Therefore, dressing activities, like standing, should be started only after sitting balance has been achieved and there is adequate cognitive ability to plan and sequence motor activities. In addition, because dressing requires more effort, adequate cardiopulmonary reserve must be available to withstand the additional stress imposed on these systems.

Communication problems are most frequently seen in patients with left-sided hemisphere involvement. The extent of the aphasia or dysphasia should be assessed by a speech and language pathologist so that early intervention can be instituted. Speech therapy may need to continue for many months in the severely aphasic patient to achieve the most effective communication ability. Often, in the beginning, these patients respond best to gestures, single questions, simple commands, or pictures.

Cognitive assessment is also important in the early phase because the ability to understand and follow commands is an essential part of rehabilitative therapy. Persons who cannot learn or remember what they have recently learned will require a much longer period of rehabilitation or may not benefit much from any prolonged rehabilitation intervention.

The majority of stroke victims, however, experience enough return of function in the paretic leg to walk with or without a gait aid. Most stroke victims who are unable to walk safely can propel themselves in an appropriate wheelchair if placed in a barrier-free environment. These wheelchair users can usually transfer independently or with a slight assist from the wheelchair to the same surface level as a bed, commode, tub, or car.

PERIPHERAL VASCULAR DISEASE

The incidence of problems related to arterial occlusion or venous stasis increases with advancing age. Atherosclerosis of the major leg arteries may initially be ameliorated by angioplasty or vascular bypass surgery. A number of persons in the sixth and seventh decades, however, will require an amputation because of arterial disease. With improved vascular surgical interventions, most leg amputations can now be performed below the knee, whereas 20 years ago they were usually done above the knee. Salvaging the human knee mechanism is important because it requires much less energy to walk with a below-knee prosthesis than with an above-knee prosthesis. Because many patients who have undergone amputation also have myocardial and pulmonary disease with decreased reserves, the energy required to walk with an above-knee prosthesis may not be tolerable, condemning them to life in a wheelchair.

Modern amputation surgery should not be approached as mutilating or destructive but viewed as a reconstructive procedure that provides an ideal residual limb on which to place a functional prosthesis. The distal end of the residual amputated limb should be covered, using a myofascial closure over the smooth ends of the bone. Myofascial closure fixes the soft tissues over the ends of the bone of the limb, which then can be used as a more forceful level arm in the prosthesis.

After the amputation surgery, healing can be facilitated and pain decreased by placing the residual limb in a rigid dressing applied by the surgeon or prosthetist. Stump shaping can be achieved by applying a rigid dressing, Unna paste dressing, or Ace wrapping. In the acute postoperative period, the rehabilitation emphasis is placed on positioning and muscle strengthening to facilitate hip and knee (if present) extension. Also, assuming flexion postures by lying supine in bed or sitting in a wheelchair are avoided. Early ambulation with a walker or crutches should be initiated once arm and trunk muscles have adequate strength to support the patient in the standing position. Emphasis must also be placed on cardiopulmonary evaluation and, whenever possible, a conditioning program begun because prosthetic ambulation requires more energy than normal bipedal walking.

Once the amputation incision has healed and the stump has been shaped and compressed, a prosthetic prescription should be decided on by the rehabilitation team (i.e., the patient, physician, therapist, and prosthetist). Usually, the prosthesis can be fabricated in 2 to 3 weeks and prosthetic ambulation therapy can be instituted. If prosthetic fitting proceeds smoothly, most patients with below-knee amputations can accomplish initial walking training in about 2 weeks and those with above-knee amputations can be trained in 3 to 4 weeks. Most persons with below-knee prostheses can be trained as outpatients, but some patients with above-knee prostheses may need to be hospitalized for gait training, especially if significant cardiopulmonary pathology coexists.

Some elderly amputation patients may find the prosthesis useful only for transfers or short-distance ambulation on level surfaces. Others may not be prosthetic candidates. These groups of patients should be custom fitted for an amputee wheelchair to use as their primary means of locomotion.

ARTHRITIS

The relentless progression of inflammation, pain, erosion, destruction, biomechanical changes, and resulting dysfunction are the hallmarks of arthritides seen in the elderly. In osteoarthritis, the most commonly affected joint is the knee, but involvement of the hip and shoulder is also frequently seen.

While anti-inflammatory medications may decrease the inflammation and pain, they may not prevent the eventual changes in joint and bone architecture that result in dysfunction. During acute periods of inflammation, the joints need to be rested in a position that will allow maximum function when put to later use. In the legs, this position is extension at the hips and knees with the ankle at neutral. In the upper limb, the elbow should be in flexion, the wrist in slight dorsiflexion, and the metacarpal and interphalangeal joints in slight flexion.

In order to maintain muscle strength during the period of acute inflammation, gentle isometric exercises should be performed in the antigravity muscles of the legs, especially the quadriceps, hamstrings, and gluteals. As soon as inflammation begins to subside, active assistive range of motion exercise should be done twice daily to begin to restore full joint motion. When the inflammation has disappeared, active and active-resistive exercises should be added to functional training. As joint deformity occurs, brace support for weak or degenerating joints has not been shown to prevent further deformity. However, splints and functional orthoses may help support a joint and provide better function from weakened muscles and ligaments.

In rheumatoid arthritis, joint-protecting use of the hands and energy-conservation techniques can be very useful in permitting essential daily activities. Assistive devices for activities of daily living in the kitchen and bathroom can allow independence not otherwise possible.

In the patient with an arthritic foot, appropriately conforming footwear must be provided. The insole should conform to the foot deformities rather than attempt to correct them. The toe box may need to be high and wide to accommodate toe deformities. If there is significant metatarsal deformity or pain, a metatarsal pad or rocker bar on the sole can help decrease pain on walking.

Hip pain can be reduced by using a cane in the opposite hand, which will decrease the forces applied to the involved hip joint. The cane handle should be placed at the height of the level of the greater trochanter, allowing the elbow to be flexed about 30°. Wrist pain can be reduced by supporting the wrist with a volar splint while the hand is being actively used.

During the acute period, inflammation and pain can be decreased with a variety of heating modalities including whirlpool, ultrasound, or paraffin. Occasionally, heat may increase the swelling, thus increasing pain. In these instances, the use of cold may diminish the pain.

When ambulation is significantly impaired, a manual or motorized wheelchair should be prescribed and custom-measured. The use of a three-wheeled motorized scooter has had wide acceptance as a means of aiding function by making mobility easier.

PARKINSONISM

With Parkinson's disease, the inexorable process of increasing rigidity is complicated by the natural law of gravity. As the gait slows down, there is increased thoracic kyphosis. Gravity pulls the upper body forward, and the festinating gait increases in cadence or the patient falls forward.

In order to counteract the imbalance of forces, rehabilitation efforts should focus on maintaining an erect posture. The process requires education of the patient in neck, back, and hip extension exercises. The erector spinal muscles must be emphasized and strengthened. Prone lying to promote back and hip extension should also be monitored. Prolonged, flexed positions such as supine lying in bed or sitting should be avoided. Assisted stretching exercises for any joints becoming tight in a flexed attitude should be performed three times daily.

PHYSIOLOGIC CHANGES OF AGING

There are a number of physiologic changes that naturally occur in the geriatric population, directly affecting the rehabilitation process when a disabling illness occurs. The degree of involvement in these physiologic states often determines the time required to achieve maximal rehabilitation. These areas include (1) nutritional state, (2) skin integrity, (3) premorbid muscle mass, (4) level of activity, (5) cardiopulmonary reserve, (6) urinary and bowel continence, (7) visual and hearing acuity, (8) intact cognition, and (9) normal cutaneous sensation. If any one of these areas is impaired and then coupled with disabling pathophysiology, the rehabilitation process is greatly lengthened and functional outcome may be less than otherwise expected.

Nutritional State

Obviously, muscle energy expenditure can be achieved only with adequate caloric intake and energy stores. Adequate vitamin levels also are essential for maximum neurologic functions. Protein intake is essential to maintain optimal muscle mass. If adequate oral intake cannot be maintained, nasogastric, gastrostomy, or parenteral nutrition should be considered to restore adequate fluid, calorie, protein, and vitamin intake.

Skin

Elements of the skin atrophy, and the skin and subcutaneous tissues become more fragile. There is an increased risk of skin breakdown with decubitus ulcer formation. Patients at bedrest for significant periods need to be repositioned frequently on a soft surface. An eggcrate mattress placed over the hospital bed mattress often helps protect the skin if the patient is turned every 2 hours.

Shearing forces and direct pressure can quickly cause pressure necrosis of the skin. A patient whose skin is at risk should not be allowed to sit upright in bed for more than 20 to 30 minutes at a time because of the chance that shearing forces will lead to a presacral ulcer. If a patient wishes to be in an upright position, he or she should sit in a chair with a soft pressure-distributing seating surface.

Muscle Mass

Although the muscle mass decreases with age, muscle strength can be increased by regular exercise in the geriatric patient. (See discussion on exercise in the elderly.)

Level of Activity

Persons confined to a wheelchair for months because of gangrene of the leg cannot be expected to walk immediately after an amputation with prosthetic restoration. Not only is strength affected by inactivity, but endurance to sustain an activity is also greatly affected in a disease state. Often, while strength may return soon after increasing the level of activity and with improved health, endurance takes much longer to regain.

Cardiopulmonary Reserve

The process of aging often is accompanied by a lessened reserve of the myocardium and the ability of the lungs to adequately provide oxygen for energy demands. Therefore, an increase in energy consumption may not be tolerated, thus the level of function is limited by the amount of myocardial work possible and the ability of the body to distribute oxygen to meet muscle demands.

Urinary and Bowel Continence

A variety of lower urinary tract and/or neurologic problems may lead to urinary incontinence. In the bowel, diverticulosis, neurologic impairment, or poor motility may lead to continence problems. For the sake of social acceptance and safeguarding the integrity of the perineal and gluteal skin, fecal and urinary soiling must be minimized.

The cause of the urinary incontinence should be evaluated, which often requires neurourologic testing. Intermittent self-catheterization or an indwelling or external catheter should be utilized to prevent incontinence.

In bowel incontinence, a program should be established by carefully monitoring fluid intake, the amount of fiber in the diet, and the use of stool softeners, mild laxatives, and, if necessary, suppositories to develop a consistent time and frequency of bowel emptying.

Vision and Hearing Problems

The ability to see the environment and to hear surrounding sounds is essential to maximum function. If a significant motor disability occurs, it is much more difficult to learn to substitute or locomote safely if vision is diminished. Likewise, it is difficult to hear instructions or communicate with the environment if auditory abilities are significantly decreased.

At the onset of a rehabilitation program, visual and hearing acuity testing should be performed, and if there is any impairment, corrective lenses or amplification devices should be provided when appropriate.

Cognition

The ability to learn and retain new information in short-term memory and the ability to sequence and motor plan are essential for maximum function. Also, the demonstration of good judgment is important to the patient's relative safety.

Despite good motor abilities, the lack of judgment or the presence of impaired memory requires constant supervision for the disabled individual.

Sensation

Peripheral nerve sensory function often diminishes with aging. It becomes more difficult for elderly persons to know where their foot and knee are positioned in relation to the ground. Because of poor skin sensation, skin breakdown can occur and progress without the patient being aware of the problem. The skin of the foot needs to be protected with appropriate footwear. Lack of sensory feedback from the feet and legs may result in the need for gait aids or visual cues to ensure that the knees are locked before putting full body weight on the legs during the stance phase of gait.

WHEELCHAIRS AND GAIT AIDS

As the locomotor apparatus of the body begins to deteriorate, it may become necessary to provide external support to ensure continued safe ambulation. The addition of a cane in one hand may provide just enough support to permit walking a bit further. The cane may also decrease pain in the opposite leg. The use of crutches may be useful if a leg should not bear weight or is weak. Axillary crutches also add some stability to the trunk. If a crutch gait is too difficult to learn or if the patient is unsteady with crutches, a walker may permit continued mobility.

If walking becomes unsafe, too energy consuming, or too painful, a wheelchair, either manual or electric, becomes a useful functional alternative for mobility. The wheelchair should be individually prescribed according to the disability and needs of the individual. The wheelchair should also be custom measured to fit the patient and a wheelchair cushion prescribed to make sitting more comfortable and to protect the skin from breakdown.

In addition to these useful aids to promote mobility, other adaptive equipment may be liberating from the limitations of dysfunction imposed by the home environment. In the presence of extensor weakness in the legs, an elevated chair or commode seat can ease the effort of standing from the seated position. If it is difficult or unsafe to lower and raise oneself from a tub, a tub bench or a stool placed in the tub will allow bathing with the use of a hand-held shower. The installation of grab bars can assist in safe transfer into and out of the tub.

A reacher to obtain items that are above or below arm level is helpful. A button hook can assist with buttoning clothing when the fingers and joints of the hand lack the fine dexterity required to dress and undress. A rocker knife will allow cutting food when only one arm is available to use for feeding.

EXERCISE IN THE ELDERLY

Muscle mass, muscle strength, and aerobic capacity decrease after the age of 30 years. With exercise in elderly persons over age 70 years, training has shown an increase in fast twitch (type IIA) fibers. It is felt that the increased muscle strength in this age group is explained by both an increase in fiber size and in the recruitment of motor units on voluntary effort.[1]

DeVries studied the effects of exercise on 112 males between 52 and 87 years of age.[2] The most significant improvements were related to oxygen transport capacity. He also reported a decreased percentage of body fat, improvement in both systolic and diastolic blood pressures, and an increase in physical work capacity.

In the sedentary Framingham cohort studied by Kannel and Sorlie, overall morbidity and mortality resulting from cardiovascular and ischemic heart disease were inversely related to the level of physical activity for men.[3] For women, the effect of being sedentary on mortality was felt to be negligible.

Studies have shown that elderly persons can increase endurance through training.[4] Any exercise program in the older population should take into account musculoskeletal issues such as (1) cardiovascular reserve, (2) pulmonary reserve, (3) muscle strength, (4) endurance, (5) joint motion, and (6) bone density.

Generally, a conditioning program should consist of a warm up and stretching phase (10 to 15 minutes), low-impact aerobic exercise (lasting 20 to 40 minutes), and a cool down period (10 to 15 minutes). This program should be performed at least three times weekly, and positive results should be observed within 4 weeks of exercise.

Wenger indicates that with a decrease in aerobic capacity with aging, the energy cost of walking becomes an effective means of physical conditioning because it constitutes a larger percentage of total aerobic capacity.[5] Leon and Blackburn suggest activities such as brisk walking, jogging, stationary or distance cycling, swimming, and calisthenics are good forms of aerobic exercise.[6] These forms of exercise involve rhythmic, repetitive movements of large muscle groups of the legs and arms. A target heart rate of 70 to 85 percent of the maximal rate is necessary to significantly improve the maximal VO_2.

Maintaining cardiovascular fitness in the elderly not only improves physiologic performance, but the correct exercise prescription can improve the ability to function and the quality of life.

VOCATION AND AVOCATION INTERESTS

Most elderly persons have experienced the joy and satisfaction gained from work and play. Although a disability has occurred, it should not be assumed that because individuals are close to retirement age, they do not wish to return to work after physical rehabilitation of the disability. Vocational interests and plans should be inventoried and implemented wherever feasible. Avocational interests provide an enormous quality to life for many of us. Often, through avocational interests, the rehabilitation therapy program can be made more relevant to the patient. Avocational pursuits can also assist the patient's reintegration into the home and community.

SEXUAL FUNCTION

Despite the physiologic changes in sexual function with aging, a sexual history should be obtained so that any alteration in sexual function secondary to the disability can be explained to the patient. In addition, if needed because of the disability, alternative means of sexual pleasuring should be discussed with the patient and partner.

PSYCHOSOCIAL DETERMINANTS—THE ART OF SUBSTITUTION

No doubt the most important determinants of rehabilitation outcome are related to psychosocial issues. Studies of the outcome of stroke rehabilitation have often pointed to these issues as being of paramount importance to the quality of life for the disabled geriatric patient. The care, concern, and comfort that only a loving spouse, a faithful family, and supportive friends can give add greatly to the disabled person's motivation to improve. All the doctors, nurses, therapists, social workers, and clergy in the world cannot ensure the best functional outcome unless the patient can look forward to a meaningful quality of life. Perhaps that quality is not so much whether a leg or an arm can move, but whether there is a meaningful person who can help to pick up the pieces of the previous lifestyle. Only if there is someone or something to look forward to is it possible to identify motivators to encourage the patient to go through the day-to-day struggles of existence with a body that does not function properly.

Rehabilitation for the elderly is really the fine art of finding substitutes for the natural changes that occur with the aging process and for the changes in function from disability. Whether it is substituting one muscle for another, substituting an eggcrate mattress for the loss of subcutaneous tissue, or substituting a wheelchair for weakened legs, the art of rehabilitation in geriatric persons should always focus on the perceived needs of individuals and how they define their quality of life as the years advance. Hopefully, through rehabilitation we can find meaningful substitutes that match our patients' desires.

REFERENCES

1. Grimby G: Physical activity and muscle training in the elderly. Acta Med Scand Suppl 711:233, 1986.
2. DeVries HA: Physiological effects of an exercise training regimen upon men aged 52 to 88. Gerontol 25:325, 1970.
3. Kannel WB, Sorlie P: Some health benefits of physical activity. Arch Intern Med 139:857, 1979.
4. Benestad AM: Trainability of old men. Act Med Scand 178:321, 1965.
5. Wenger NK: Rehabilitation of the elderly cardiac patient. Cardiovasc Clin 12:221, 1981.
6. Leon AS, Blackburn H: Exercise rehabilitation of the coronary heart disease patient. Geriatrics 32:66, 1977.

IMMUNOLOGIC, HEMATOLOGIC, ONCOLOGIC, AND INFECTIOUS DISEASE PROBLEMS

CHAPTER 33

Immunologic Problems

Marguerite M. B. Kay

A disease is farther on the road to being cured when it breaks forth from concealment and manifests its power.

Seneca, *Epistulœ ad Lucilium*

Aging is characterized by a decline in the ability of individuals to adapt to environmental stress. This decline is exemplified physiologically by an inability to maintain homeostasis. Consequently, elderly individuals are confronted with biomedically enforced curtailment of normal activities. The magnitude of this problem is reflected in the rising cost of nursing care and chronic medical care, which was minimally estimated to be about $51 billion in federal funds for individuals 80 years and older in 1984, the most recent year for which statistics are available. This is approximately $8500 per person 80 years and older. In 1950, only 12 percent of people aged 65 could expect to live to age 90. Today, more than 25 percent of 65-year-olds can expect to live that long. This problem, which was not as apparent less than two decades ago, is becoming more critical. A U.S. Bureau of the Census publication shows that the fastest growing sector in the American population has been and will continue to be the group of people aged 65 years and older, at least until the year 2020. Thus, although there were only 4 million people in the over 65-year-old group in our country in 1900, there are 24 million today. This group is expected to increase in size, reaching 32 million in the year 2000 and 45 million by 2020. Those individuals 80 years and older are expected to number 12 million by the year 2000. Comparable socioeconomic problems are being faced by most, if not all, countries throughout the world.

Clearly, methods must be found that can delay the onset or lessen the severity of the diseases associated with aging, thereby extending the *productive* life span. This challenge, as well as the fact that aging is one of the principal unsolved problems in cellular and molecular biology, is attracting many researchers into the discipline of geriatrics/gerontology.

The immune system is one of the most attractive systems for aging studies because (1) our understanding of its differentiation and developmental processes at the cellular, molecular, and genetic levels is more comprehensive than that of perhaps any other physiologic system; (2) age-related homeostatic perturbations permit dissection of certain features of the immune functions that are analogous to the developmental phase of life; (3) immune functions can be approached mechanistically and are amenable to restorative manipulations; and (4) alterations in age-related immune functions may contribute to our understanding of the pathogenesis of those diseases that show peak incidence late in life, including neoplasia, infectious diseases, and autoimmune and immune complex diseases.[1-5]

Many of the crucial studies in the immune system have been performed in mice because (1) the ready availability of syngeneic, genetically identical animals permits transplantation studies; (2) animals with specific immune deficiencies are available as inbred strains or can be generated, for example, by thymectomy and radiation treatment; and (3) use of mice allows the researcher to live longer than her or his experimental subjects. The mean life span of mice is 24 months at most institutions. Mouse and human immune systems are very similar.

AGE-RELATED CHANGES IN IMMUNE FUNCTIONS AND POSSIBLE MECHANISMS

The immune system protects the body in a highly specific manner against foreign invasion by viruses, bacteria, fungi, and possibly one's own somatic cells which undergo neoplastic changes by seeking out and destroying them. Obviously, any factor or event that can decrease the nor-

mal policing activity of the immune system can promote the growth of invasive antigens (e.g., bacteria and cancer cells), which can, in turn, disrupt various physiologic functions of the body. Hence, it should be apparent that the immune system plays a major role in the preservation of health and therefore in life sustenance.

The immune system is organismal because its cells and molecules are distributed throughout the body and circulate within the blood and lymph. The major lymphoid tissues are the thymus, lymph nodes, spleen, and bone marrow. The stem cells, found primarily in the bone marrow, can differentiate into either T cells, B cells, or macrophages. B cells and macrophages are generated in the bone marrow, but T cells originate from pre-T cells under the influence of the thymus.

Cellular Changes

STEM CELLS. Stable, intrinsic alterations in the pluripotent stem cells will affect the lymphocyte and macrophage populations and, ultimately, immune functions. Thus, there has been a continuing search for alterations in the stem cells.

The transplantation potential of adult stem cells is less than that of young cells.[6] Stem cells can self-replicate in situ throughout the natural life span of an individual.[7] However, both the ability of stem cells to expand clonally and their rate of division decrease with age,[8-11] as does their ability to repair x-ray–induced damage,[12] their ability to home into the thymus,[13, 14] and their rate of B cell formation.[15, 16] Cells from adult donors exhibit impaired regenerative capacity. Old stem cells can reconstitute *unstressed* recipient mice to the same levels as cells derived from young individuals. However, stem cell production does not maintain homeostasis when an individual is *stressed*. The results of this study together with those of kinetic studies indicate that the generation time of old stem cells, or the differentiation time of their progeny, or both, are increased.

The observed kinetic alterations could be due in part to changes in the stem cells caused by the cellular milieu because they are responsive to differentiation-homeostatic factors. Thus, for example, when attempts were made to reverse the age-related kinetic properties of old stem cells by enabling them to self-replicate in syngeneic young recipients for an extended period, they still behaved like old stem cells kinetically. However, when young stem cells were allowed to self-replicate in syngeneic old recipients for 1 month, they began to behave like old stem cells kinetically. These results suggest that once stem cells have undergone subtle, intrinsic kinetic alterations in the aging mouse, these changes cannot be reversed by transplanting the cells into a young syngeneic recipient. Another observation reflective of an alteration intrinsic to stem cells is the finding that old stem cells are inferior to young stem cells in their ability to repair x-ray–induced DNA damage, even when the cells were allowed to grow in young recipients.

The nature of the cellular milieu is not known. However, lymphokines from a subpopulation of T cells may be involved in a positive manner. Evidence for this is derived from animal studies that show that hematopoiesis in heavily irradiated recipients reconstituted with parental stem cells is augmented by injection of T cells, and that an antitheta-sensitive regulatory cell that is present in normal adult bone marrow, spleen, and thymus is required for the promotion of differentiation of hematopoietic stem cells into erythrocytes. Thus, alterations in certain T cell subpopulations with age might explain some of the extrinsic changes that adversely influence stem cell kinetics and predispose elderly individuals to anemia.

Age-related kinetic alterations of stem cells are likely to affect the immune capacity of old individuals. For example, immunologically immature young mice (≤2 months of age) and immunologically inadequate old mice develop autoantibodies to erythrocytes following viral infection (see Figure 33–3.) However, the young mice with autoantibodies do not become anemic, whereas the old mice do.[17–20] Thus, when stressed, as with an infection, old individuals may not be able to maintain homeostasis by increasing cellular production to compensate for increased cellular destruction. The kinetic limitations in stem cell reserve may also account for the clinical observation that elderly individuals with sepsis frequently do not have an elevated white cell count, although there may be a shift to less mature leukocytes in their peripheral blood smears. The "anemia of chronic disease" seen most often in the elderly reflects a limitation of stem cell reserve. This should be taken into account when the use of cytotoxic drugs or drugs affecting the stem cell compartment are considered in an elderly patient. The importance of young stem cells was also shown in an immunorestorative study, in which the grafting into old mice of newborn thymus together with young bone marrow was effective in elevating the immunologic responsiveness of the old mice for an extended period of time *provided* that young stem cells were present.[21]

Stem cells may contribute to age-related osteopenia as a result of changes intrinsic to bone marrow–derived cells that regulate bone marrow formation or remodeling. Evidence for this is derived from studies that show that femoral mineral mass decreased when marrow cells from old mice were transplanted into young or mature x-irradiated recipients and increased when young marrow cells were given to aging mice.[22]

Osteoclasts, which reabsorb bone, appear to be derived from hematopoietic stem cells,[23] presumably monocytes.[24] Thus, the osteopenia observed in the elderly may, at least in part, be due to a defect in hematopoietic stem cells rather than to disorders of mineral metabolism.

MACROPHAGES. Macrophages are derived from peripheral blood monocytes, which are derived from a bone marrow precursor cell. Macrophages cooperate with T and B cells in many immune responses and phagocytize bacteria, some viruses, and senescent and damaged cells. Because macrophages confront antigens before T and B cells, any defect in them could decrease immune function in spite of the absence of appreciable changes in the antigen-specific T and B cells. Studies show that neither the number of macrophages in the peritoneum[25] nor their handling of antigens during both the induction of immune responses and phagocytosis is adversely affected by age.[26–28] For example, the phagocytic activity of peritoneal macrophages in vitro from old mice is equal to or better than that of young mice;[26] and the activity of lysosomal enzymes in splenic and peritoneal macrophages increases rather than decreases with age.[29, 30] The latter property especially could reflect qualitative alterations in certain types of macrophages. The ability of antigen-laden peritoneal macrophages of old mice to initiate primary and secondary antibody responses in vitro is comparable to that of young mice.[26] The capacity of splenic macrophages and other adherent cells to cooperate with T and B cells in the initiation of antibody response in vitro is unaffected by age.[27] The ability of macrophages to support and regulate lymphocyte responses to mitogens and antigens is also unchanged with age.[28, 31]

When antigen-processing ability of macrophages is indirectly assessed by injecting young and old mice with varying doses of sheep red blood cells, it is found that the slope of the regression line of the antigen dose-antibody response curve was lower, and the minimum dose of antigen needed to generate a maximum response was significantly higher for old mice. Such results could be explained by assuming that the antigen-processing macrophages prevented antigen-sensitive T and B cells from responding maximally to limited doses of the antigen. It is possible that an age-associated increase in phagocytic efficiency[29] contributes to the decrease in antigen-processing efficiency. The reduced antigen-processing activity is reflected by the failure of antigens to localize in the follicles of lymphoid tissues of antigen-stimulated old mice.[32, 33] One clinical implication of these results is that the poor immune surveillance noted against low doses of certain syngeneic tumor cells[34] could be due in part to the failure of T and B cells in an aging individual to confront neoplastic cells during their clonal emergence because of the inability of macrophages to initially "process" the tumor antigens. It could also explain why the resistance to allogeneic tumor cell challenge can decline with age by more than 100-fold in mice that manifest only a fourfold decline in T cell–mediated cytolytic activity against the same tumor cells.[35]

B CELLS. B cells can be identified by the presence of immunoglobulin (Ig) on their surface. The Ig can be detected by electron microscopy or, more commonly, by immunofluorescent staining. Generally, B cells cannot produce antibody without the direction of T cells unless the antigens consist of repetitive subunits such as are found in most carbohydrates or polysaccharides. In general, B cell deficiencies tend to predispose to bacterial infections. Assays for B cell activity include responsiveness to certain mitogens such as lipopolysaccharide (LPS), antibody production in response to T cell–independent and –dependent antigens, and colony-forming ability.

The number of B cells in humans does not change appreciably with age. If anything, the number in the spleen and lymph nodes tends to increase slightly. Although the total number of B cells remains relatively stable, the size of certain subpopulations of B cells appears to change with age. Cross-sectional and longitudinal studies in humans show that serum IgG and IgA and benign monoclonal gammopathies tend to increase with age[36] (Tables 33–1 through 33–5). An increase in IgG_1 and IgG_3 subclasses is responsible for the elevated IgG level. An increasing frequency of homogeneous immunoglobulins in the sera of aging mice and humans without B cell malignancy has been observed repeatedly. This condition is most often designated as benign monoclonal gammopathy or idiopathic paraproteinemia (IP). In humans, there is a clear age-related increase from 0 percent in the third decade to 19 percent in the tenth decade of life. Most of the Ig belongs to the IgG class, that of the IgM and IgA classes being less frequent. The etiology, mechanisms, and significance of this particular form of immunoglobulin production have not yet been resolved. However, evidence suggests that IP is caused by impairment of intrinsic cellular factors rather than factors extrinsic to the immune system. Since the occurence of IP can be increased by neonatal and adult thymectomy in both IP-susceptible C57B1 and IP-resistant CBA mice, it appears that im-

TABLE 33–1. Age-Related Changes in Stem Cells

Stem cells exhibit a decline with age in each of the following:
1. Clonal expansion (proliferative capacity)
2. Rate of generating colonies
3. Repair of x-ray–induced DNA damage
4. Ability to home to the thymus
5. Transplantation potential

TABLE 33–2. Concentration of IgG in Human Sera During Aging*

Age (years)	N	IgG Geometric Mean Value (range ± 1.96 SD)		Difference†
		mg/ml	*IU*	
20–30	23	10.86 (7.20–16.37)	135 (90–204)	P < 0.02
41–50	40	11.09 (7.13–17.23)	138 (89–214)	P < 0.02
51–65	49	11.60 (7.66–17.57)	144 (95–219)	ns ‡
> 95	59	12.48 (7.64–20.40)	155 (95–253)	

*From Radl J, et al: Clin Exp Immunol 22:84, 1975.
†Significance of difference between the given age group and the over-95 years group.
‡ns = not significant

pairment of intrinsic cellular factors may reflect alterations in T cells. Thus, the data suggest that these changes in the humoral immune system may be secondary to those occurring in the thymus or T cell populations. Further, the number of colony-forming B cells in the peripheral blood of humans decreases with age.

The responsiveness of B cells to stimulation with certain T cell–dependent antigens decreases strikingly with age.[37, 38] The responses of young and old mice were systematically evaluated by limiting dilution and dose-response methods.[39, 40] These studies revealed that the decline in responsiveness is caused by (1) a decrease with age in the number of antigen-sensitive immunocompetent precursor units (IU), which are made up of two or more cell types in various ratios,[41] and (2) a decrease in the average number of antibody-forming functional cells generated by each immunocompetent—that is, the immunologic burst size (IBS). We do not know the cause(s) for the reduction with age in both the relative number of IU and the IBS. It could be due to an increase in the number of regulatory cells, which can inhibit the precursor cells making up the IU from interacting with each other as well as inhibiting the proliferation of B cells.

Studies show that bone marrow of young and old mice generate similar spectra of B cell clones with regard to antibody production.[42] Down-regulation of these B cells may be due to anti-idiotypic antibodies.[42–45]

Qualitative changes in B cells also appear to occur with age. For example, the ability of old B cells to respond to T cell–dependent antigens, even in the presence of young T cells, is impaired.[46, 47] The alteration may occur at the membrane surface level. Thus, studies of Fc receptor–mediated immunoregulation revealed that the decline in B cell regulation with age is in part intrinsic to the receptor-mediated signaling mechanism.[48] The rate of capping and shedding of cross-linked surface immunoglobulins by B cells was slower in old individuals than in young individuals, and this age-related kinetic alteration was associated with a decrease in the density of surface immunoglobulins.[49]

TABLE 33–3. Concentration of IgA in Human Sera During Aging*

Age (years)	N	IgA Geometric Mean Value (range ± 1.96 SD)		Difference†
		mg/ml	*IU*	
20–30	23	1.93 (1.18–3.23)	136 (84–227)	P < 0.01
41–50	40	1.45 (0.63–3.36)	102 (44–237)	P < 0.01
51–65	49	1.65 (0.76–3.56)	124 (57–269)	P < 0.001
> 95	59	2.54 (1.16–5.54)	179 (82–390)	

*From Radl J, et al: Clin Exp Immunol 22:84, 1975.
†Significance of difference between the given age group and the over-95 years group.

TABLE 33–4. Concentration of IgM In Human Sera During Aging*

Age (years)	N	IgM Geometric Mean Value (range ± 1.96 SD)		Difference†
		mg/ml	*IU*	
20–30	23	1.06 (0.61–3.23)	125 (72–215)	ns
41–50	40	1.13 (0.52–2.48)	134 (61–293)	ns
51–65	49	1.18 (0.61–2.30)	140 (72–272)	P < 0.001
> 95	59	1.05 (0.34–3.24)	124 (40–383)	

*From Radl J et al: Clin Exp Immunol 22:84, 1975.
†Significance of difference between the given age group and the over-95 years group.

Humoral Immunity. Normal B cell immune functions reflective of humoral immunity have been analyzed in terms of circulating levels of natural isoantibodies and heteroantibodies and in terms of antigen-induced antibody response. Circulating levels of natural antibodies have been assessed systematically in humans. The results show that natural antibodies decline with age, starting shortly after the thymus begins to involute and after the level of serum thymosin, a thymic hormone, begins to decline.

Studies of the effect of age on antigen-induced antibody response show that primary, but not secondary, antibody response decreases with age. The onset of the decline in antibody response can occur as early as the start of thymic involution. This suggests that aging is affecting the T cells that regulate antibody response and not necessarily the antigen-specific B cells. Clinically, the effect of age on the primary antibody response is seen in situations in which one wishes to immunize a patient with a new antigen. For example, influenza virus mutates and changes antigenic type. Since it behaves like a new antigen, the elderly individuals who are most vulnerable to influenza and its sequelae are the individuals who are most difficult to immunize. Septicemia and pneumonia are the third and fourth leading causes of death among patients over 70.[50] LaForce and Meiklejohn will address the clinical aspects in greater detail in their chapter on infection.

There is a decrease in high affinity antibodies with age. High affinity antibodies are probably more effective than low affinity antibodies in combating infections. Antibody titers in the elderly are elevated to persistent DNA but not RNA viruses.[51]

T CELLS. T cells are responsible for protecting the body against viruses, fungi, and certain types of bacteria; for preventing the growth of certain neoplasms; and for regulating B cell antibody production to a large number of antigens. Increased susceptibility to infections by opportunis-

TABLE 33–5. Comparison of IgG Subclass Levels Between Young Adult and Aged Persons*

	Young Adults—Geometric Mean Value (range ± 1.96 sd) (mg/ml)	Aged Persons (> 95) Geometric Mean Value (range ± 1.96 SD) (mg/ml)	Significance of Difference Between the Two Groups†
N	108	57	
IgG1	6.4 (3.8–10.7)	7.3 (3.4–15.4)	P < 0.02
IgG2	3.0 (1.5–6.0)	3.3 (1.2–9.4)	ns
IgG3	0.5 (0.2–1.3)	0.8 (0.2–3.1)	P < 0.001
IgG4	0.3 (0.04–2.1)	0.3 (0.04–3.5)	ns

*From Radl J, et al: Clin Exp Immunol 22:84, 1975.
†ns = not significant

tic pathogens and viral, fungal, and protozoal organisms tends to be associated with T cell deficiency.

Human T cells are identified morphologically by their ability to form rosettes with sheep red blood cells (RBC), and mouse T cells by the presence of the theta antigen on their surface. Assays for T cell activity include responsiveness to plant mitogenic lectins such as phytohemagglutinin (PHA), concanavalin A (Con A), participation in delayed-type hypersensitivity (i.e., skin test) reactions, ability to mount graft-versus-host (GVH) reactions, and ability to help or suppress the responses of other cells. As with B cells, all three possible changes that could cause a decline with age in T cell functions have been detected: loss in number, shift in subpopulations, and qualitative changes.

In humans, the number of circulating T cells has been reported either to decrease progressively after adulthood[52-54] or to remain the same.[55-57] However, the absolute number of colony-forming, circulating T cells in humans decreases with age to a level that is about 15 percent of that of young adults.[56]

The evidence for qualitative changes with age is increasing. At the membrane level, it would be anticipated that surface receptors would be scrutinized because cell-to-cell interactions in immune responses are mediated through surface receptors. Two observations support the view that surface receptors change with age, one indicating loss and the other an emergence of new receptors. Thus, the surface density of theta receptors on T cells decreased with age,[58] as judged by immunofluorescence, and further, the theta receptors, visualized as a continuous ring in young cells, appeared as patchy to faintly visible incomplete rings in old T cells.

Evidence for the emergence of new receptors comes from two observations. (1) Young mice can undergo a syngeneic graft-versus-host response when they are injected with syngeneic cells from old donors.[59] (2) Young mice can also undergo a syngeneic mixed lymphocyte reaction and synthesize cytotoxic antibodies when they are injected with syngeneic cells from old donors. These latter observations have obvious implications for certain diseases of human aging, particularly neoplasia and autoimmune-immune and immune complex diseases because it has been shown that continuous graft-versus-host–like reactions can increase the incidence of lymphoid tumor formation and autoimmunity.

Intracellular changes with aging have also been detected. At the cytoplasmic level, both morphologic and functional changes have been observed. Thus, electron microscopic observations show swollen mitochondria containing myelinlike structures with reduced numbers of cristae in sheep RBC-rosetting T cells of old but not young humans.[60] Functionally, there seems to be an imbalance in the level of cyclic adenosine 3', 5'-monophosphate and cyclic guanosine 3'–5'-monophosphate in resting and T cell-specific mitogen-stimulated cells in older mice.[61, 62] Because the adenyl and guanyl cyclases are activated by modulation of surface receptors,[63] these observations provide further evidence for defective signal reception and/or transmission from membrane to cytoplasm and nucleus in old T cells.

At the nuclear level, it has been demonstrated that the frequency of PHA-responsive hypodiploid T cells increases with age, loss of X and Y chromosomes being most prevalent. In addition, it has been observed that the old PHA-stimulated T cells are not as efficient as young PHA-stimulated T cells in their ability to bind actinomycin. This suggests that chromatin structures of PHA-responsive T cells are undergoing alteration with age. Old PHA-stimulated T cells also show a decrease in ability to incorporate acetate, indicating that their histone metabolism may be undergoing a change with age that can affect their nuclear activities. Finally, at the nuclear-cytoplasmic level, *clonable* circulating human T cells exhibit a delay in initiating division and decreased proliferation capacity. The mean cell cycle duration of circulating T cells of old humans is longer than that of young adults, and this is due to an extension of the G_1 phase of the cell cycle. Extension of the cell cycle duration due to an increase in the G_1 phase has also been detected in other cells undergoing rapid turnover, including the gut epithelium and fibroblasts aged in vitro and in situ. The cause of the diminished proliferative capacity of T cells and other rapidly turning-over cells remains unsolved. However, it has been possible to enhance the proliferative capacity of old T cells by mixing T cell–specific mitogens with 2-mercaptoethanol—i.e., the response to the mixture of stimulants is greater than that of the sum of the responses to the individual stimulants. This would indicate that the age-related qualitative changes responsible for the decline in the proliferative capacity of T cells with age can be reversed.

Unscheduled DNA repair by human lymphocytes has been reported both to decrease and to remain unchanged with age. However, the studies performed to date have looked at the "average" of all DNA repair. This is not an appropriate approach because some genes shut down during development and are not reactivated, whereas other crucial genes are utilized continually.

Subpopulations of T cells shift with age, as indicated by the following items:

1. The decrease in mitogenic response of mouse T cells with age does not appear to be caused by a decrease in the number of T cells with theta antigenic receptors, T cells with mitogen receptors, the number of mitogen receptors per T cell, or the mitogen receptor–binding affinities, nor to an altered cell cycle time. These observations suggest that the number of T cells that are not responsive to T cell–specific mitogen is increasing with age at the expense of those that are responsive.

2. Density distribution analysis shows that the frequency of less dense cells increases at the expense of the more dense cells. This suggests that there is a relative increase with age in immature T cells at the expense of mature T cells.

3. T cell–suppressor function appears to increase with age. The increase has been detected in terms of both Con A stimulated suppressor activity and the number of T cells with Fc receptors for IgG (T_{gamma}).[64–66] However, it appears that nonspecific and antigen-specific suppressor cell activity may age at different rates. However, an age-related decrease in Con A stimulated suppressor activity[67] has also been reported.

4. T helper function also declines with age. This has been demonstrated in animals and in assays performed both in vivo and in vitro;[39, 40, 47, 68, 69] for example, the decrease with age in the carrier-primed T cell populations that can collaborate with reference hapten (2,4,-dinitrophenol)-primed young B cells is dramatic.[47]

Cell-Mediated Immunity. Functional studies have shown an age-related decrease in the development of delayed hypersensitivity to skin test antigens to which an individual has not been previously sensitized such as dinitrochlorobenzene.[70] Dinitrochlorobenzene usually sensitizes an individual on first contact. On a subsequent challenge, 95 percent of subjects younger than 70 years old will show a contact sensitivity reaction, whereas only about 70 percent of those older than 70 will show this reaction.[71] There is also a decline with age in responsiveness to ubiquitous antigens (*Candida*, mumps, *Trichophyton*, tuberculin).[70, 51] Reactivity to the tuberculin skin test declines after age 70. Reactivation of tuberculosis is most common in this group.

The proliferative capacity of T cells of humans and rodents to the plant mitogens PHA and Con A decline with age.[20, 56, 70, 72–74] No differences in natural killer cell activity have been observed in elderly humans.[75]

The helper function of T cells declines with age. In humans, T cell–suppressor function is not well defined. Both a decrease and an increase in the number and activity of suppressor cells have been reported. An age-related decrease with age in Con A stimulated suppressor activity has been detected,[67] as has an increase in both Con A stimulated suppressor activity and the number of T cells with Fc receptors for IgG (T_{gamma}).[64–66]

Activation and maintenance of most cellular and humoral immune responses involve soluble factors called lymphokines. Lymphokine synthesis by aged T lymphocytes appears to be reduced.[76] One lymphokine, interleukin 2 (IL-2), is required for T cell proliferation, differentiation of cytolytic T lymphocytes, and B cell activation. IL-2 synthesis requires T cell activation by mitogens or antigen and a second signal delivered by macrophage-produced interleukin 1. Defects in IL-2 production or expression of the cellular receptor appear to play a role in the age-related decline in immune function, some autoimmune disorders, acquired immune deficiency syndrome, and leukemia.

OTHER CELLS. This category of cells

comprises those that are neither T cells, B cells, macrophages, nor stem cells. Such cells with regulatory functions appear to increase in number or activity with age.[77, 78] It is very likely that these cells are at some stage of maturation destined to become either T cells, B cells, or macrophages.

Thymus

Since the involution of the thymus, which occurs at about the time of sexual maturity, precedes the age-related decline in T cell–dependent immune responses, a "cause and effect" relationship has been suspected—i.e., that thymic involution is responsible for the decline. This suspicion is supported by the following observations:

1. Thymic involution is associated with loss of cortical lymphocytes[79–81] and atrophic changes in the epithelial tissue[82] that synthesizes thymic hormones.[83–86] Thymic hormone levels decline. Thymic involution begins at the time of sexual maturity in humans.

2. Long-lived mice attain peak thymus weight later in life and retain a greater thymus-to-body weight ratio later in life than do short-lived mice,[87] and these changes precede the change in serum levels of thymic hormones.[88]

3. Thymus terminal deoxynucleotidyl transferase, which has been postulated to be the intrinsic somatic mutagen for immunologic diversification, begins to decrease at adulthood in long-lived mice.

4. Kinetic assessment of T cells in young adult, T cell-deprived adult thymectomized, x-irradiated, and bone marrow reconstituted recipients of thymic lobes from syngeneic donor mice 1 day to 33 months old revealed that the ability of the thymus graft to influence the maturation of precursor T cells into functional T cells decreases with increasing age, starting as early as 1 month of age.[89, 90]

5. Movement of T cell precursors of PHA-responsive cells ceases prior to adolescence in mice. The cause for this age-dependent cell traffic phenomenon is not known, but it would appear, by a process of elimination, that an extra-thymic regulatory mechanism is operating. This is because these precursor T cells have the capacity to migrate into the thymus, and even a grafted involuting thymus is, under extraordinary conditions, capable of accepting precursor T cells, as suggested by other thymus graft experiments.

In any event, these results indicate that shortly after early adolescence (10 to 12 weeks of age), immature T cells in the thymus, and perhaps peripherally also, are the sole source of generators of functional T cells. This means that they must possess the capacity to self-replicate for a reasonable number of times, or otherwise a shift in the subpopulations of T cells would ensue with advancing age.

6. Adult thymectomy of autoimmune-susceptible and autoimmune-resistant mice accelerates the decline in T cell–dependent humoral and cell-mediated immune responses[32, 91–93] and decreases longevity.[94]

7. Dietary restriction that extends life expectancy in mice slows the rate of immunologic maturation and the subsequent decline in immunologic vigor,[95–98] and these functional alterations are associated with stunting of thymus growth—specifically, of the cortical tissue.[99]

8. Grafts of thymus from young mice into syngeneic old mice can offer partial immunologic restoration, as does in vivo treatment of old mice and humans with thymic hormones.

9. The life span of T cell–deficient hypopituitary dwarf mice can be extended from 4 to 12 months by injections of lymph node cells but not thymocytes or bone marrow cells. Comparable life prolongation was demonstrated by injection of growth factors and thyroxine in untreated, but not in thymectomized, dwarf mice. This fact suggests that the immune system is closely linked through the thymus with the endocrine system for the sustenance of life.

In view of these observations, the thymus has been implicated as the aging "clock" of T cells. Because of the ability of T cells to regulate hematopoiesis, as mentioned earlier, some of the observed age-related alterations in stem cells and B cells could be due to changes in the thymus. Alternatively, changes in thymic activity could change the cellular milieu, since the thymus can modulate hormone levels.[100–104] However, the mechanisms responsible for the changes in T cell function have not yet been elucidated, and therefore we do not know whether the changes are extrinsic or intrinsic to the thymus.[104] The most likely extrinsic cause is a regulatory breakdown in the hypothalamus-pituitary-neuroendocrine axis in relation to the thymus. The most likely intrinsic cause is alteration of the thymic epithelial tissue, although alteration of the lymphoid component of the thymus cannot be excluded.

Support of the former possibility comes from various observations demonstrating that stress and other psychological factors can affect the immune response, as measured by skin graft rejection and by primary and secondary antibody responses.[104] Moreover, lesions in the anterior basal hypothalamus, but not in the medial or posterior hypothalamus, were found to depress delayed-type hypersensitivity and reduce the severity of anaphylactic reactions.[104] Further, growth hormones and insulin have been shown to act preferentially on T cell–dependent immune functions, whereas thyroxine and sex hormones act on both T and B cell responses.[100, 105–108] Finally, a single injection of antihypophysis serum into mice 25 to 35 days of age results in the development of a wasting disease and thymus atrophy in some but not all injected mice.[108] The wasting disease observed in mice treated with antihypophysis serum resembles that seen after neonatal thymectomy.[108] However, hormonal replacement therapy was not provided in these chemically hypophysectomized mice, and therefore thymic atrophy could have occurred secondary to the inability to maintain homeostasis as a result of inadequate thyroxine, corticosterone, growth hormone, and so on. Interestingly, degranulation of acidophilic cells in the anterior lobe of the pituitary has been observed in neonatally thymectomized mice.[108] Thus, it would appear that the thymus can modulate hormone levels.[103] The finding that grafting of neonatal thymus into old recipients corrects their abnormal serum levels of triiodothyronine and insulin further supports this view.[110]

Three possible mechanisms can be proposed to account for aging of the thymus that can be triggered by intrinsic or extrinsic factors. One is clonal exhaustion—i.e., thymus cells have a genetically pro-grammed clock mechanism that causes them to self-destruct and die after undergoing a fixed number of divisions. The mechanism is similar to that of the Hayflick phenomenon, which is seen in fibroblasts in vitro. It would require that the thymus count the number of migratory thymocytes leaving it or the number of divisions undergone by thymocytes, or both. Another possible mechanism is an alteration of thymus cell DNA, either randomly or through viral infection. Various stable alterations of DNA can occur, including cross-linking and strand breaks. The third possible mechanism is a stable molecular alteration at the non-DNA level through a subtle error-accumulating mechanism.

AGE-RELATED CHANGES IN AUTOREACTIVITY

The phenomenon of autoimmunity presents an extremely interesting and challenging problem. Thus, in an apparent paradox, autoaggressive manifestations of autoimmunity are often seen in immunologically hyporesponsive individuals, whereas normal healthy elderly individuals possess circulating autoantibodies. For example, a relatively high frequency of normal individuals ≥ 55 years of age have autoantibodies against a variety of cellular components, yet they do not have clinical manifestations of autoimmune disease (Figs. 33–1 to 33–4). In addition, standard assays for detecting autoantibodies require serum dilutions of 10- to 40-fold for the detection of "significant" positives. When serum dilutions below those recommended are used, all individuals tested are positive. It would appear, therefore, that most individuals have low levels of circulating autoantibodies. The complexity of the problem is further increased by recent evidence that certain autoantibodies perform important physiologic roles—e.g., enabling macrophages to remove senescent and damaged cells. Thus, positive autoantibody tests in elderly individuals should be evaluated in relation to clinical findings.

Facultatively pathologic autoantibodies and physiologic autoantibodies will be discussed briefly, as will the possible influ-

Text continued on page 390

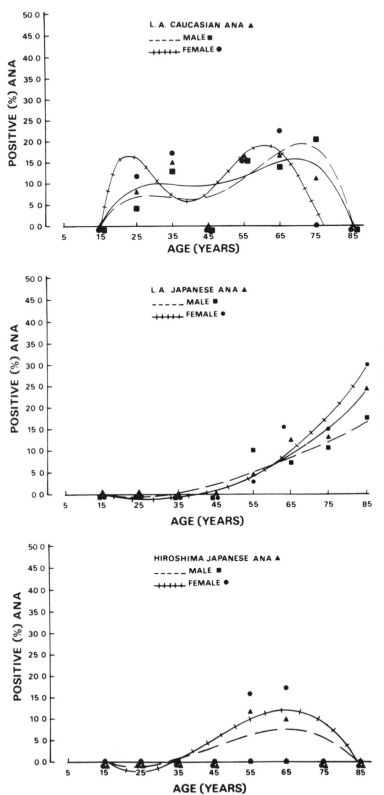

FIGURE 33–1. Age-related changes in the frequency of antinuclear antibodies (ANA) in asymptomatic Caucasians and Japanese living in Los Angeles. Positive ANA tests in different populations as a function of age. Sera were tested using cell monolayer cultures at a dilution of 1:20 in phosphate-buffered saline. Data were analyzed using the student T test.

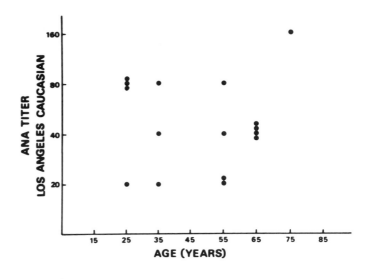

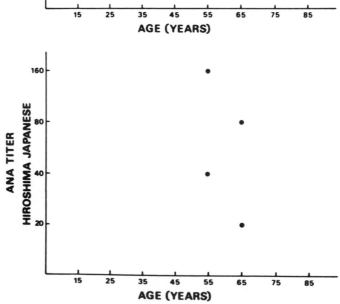

FIGURE 33–2. *Titers of ANA positive sera in different populations as a function of age. Positive sera were titered to a dilution of 1:160.*

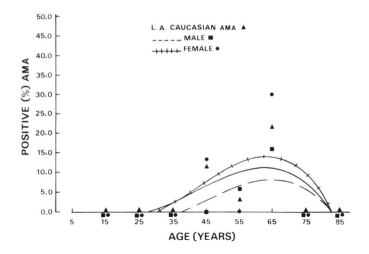

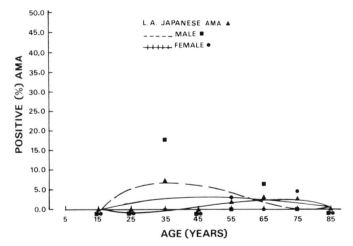

FIGURE 33–3. *Age-related changes in the frequency of antimitochondrial antibodies (AMA) in asymptomatic Caucasians and Japanese living in Los Angeles (15 to 17 percent positive at peak levels). Positive AMA tests in different populations as a function of age. Sera were tested at a dilution of 1·40 in phosphate-buffered saline.*

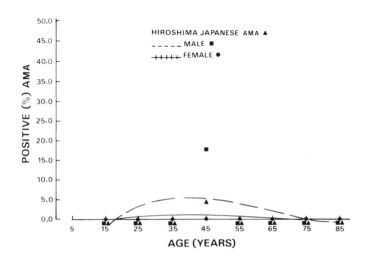

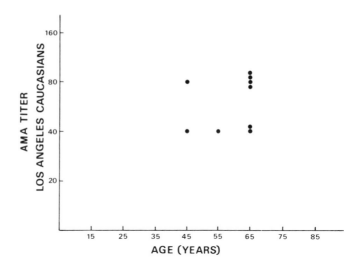

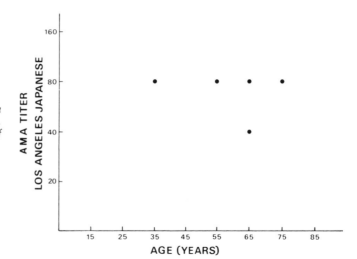

FIGURE 33–4. *Titers of AMA positive sera in different populations as a function of age. Positive sera were titered to a dilution of 1:160.*

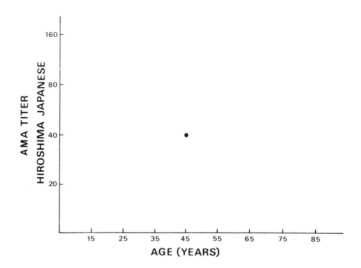

ences on them of age-associated changes in immunologic activities.

In recent years, improvements in immunoassays have allowed us to detect a relatively high frequency of normal older individuals with autoantibodies against a variety of cellular components (e.g., nuclei and mitochondria) but not more individuals with autoimmune disease.

Results of studies dealing with the incidence of autoantibodies in Caucasian and Japanese populations have revealed that the pattern of age-related changes varies with the geographic and ethnic group sampled (see Figs. 33–1 to 33–4). Regarding the influence of ethnic group and geographic location, we observed, for example, that the incidence of antinuclear antibodies (ANA) increased with age in Hiroshima Japanese living in Japan (J) and in Hiroshima Japanese living in Los Angeles (LA) starting at 55 years of age (peak incidence: LA $\simeq$ 23 percent positive; J $\simeq$ 8 percent positive), whereas a bimodal distribution with peaks at 35 and 60 years was observed in Caucasians living in Los Angeles (15 to 17 percent positive at peak levels). Several explanations can be offered for the observed age-related increase in autoantibodies in asymptomatic individuals. The concentration of autoantibodies may be below the threshold level necessary to trigger clinically detectable autoimmune disease, although this is unlikely because titers of 20 to 80 are observed in asymptomatic elderly individuals with a positive ANA test (Figs. 33–3 and 33–4). The type of autoantibody synthesized might not activate macrophages or antibody-dependent cytolytic cells (or both) or may not bind complement. Target antigens may not be normally accessible to sufficient quantities of autoantibodies, or autoantibodies may not have access to antigens in viable cells. These explanations, together with the evidence that autoimmune disease is most prevalent among individuals who are genetically predisposed and immunologically hypoactive,[111] suggest that facultatively pathologic manifestations become pathologic following an episode caused by extrinsic factors (e.g., viral infection), resulting in a sustained and elevated autoimmune response and sequestering of appropriate host cells. Viral infection has been shown to initiate autoimmune reactions in old

animals and those infected in utero. In humans, the rise in the incidence of autoantibodies to nuclei was observed to parallel the decline in titer of natural antibodies to *Salmonella* flagellin.[70, 112] The changes in immune function that may contribute to an age-related increase in autoimmune manifestations will be briefly reviewed.

T Cells

The role of T cells in the induction of facultatively pathologic autoantibodies is unclear at this time. As mentioned earlier, the helper function of T cells declines with age.[2, 5, 35, 113–123] The resulting decreased immune responsiveness could hinder or prevent eradication of microbes (e.g., viruses, mycoplasma) and allow them to circulate widely. Incorporation of microbial nucleic acids into the genome could result in the expression of microbial antigens on the surface of host cells. As a consequence, microbes or their products (enzymes or envelope glycoproteins) could alter membranes of host cells. For example, enzymes from these microbes could cleave molecules from cell surfaces, or viral envelope glycoproteins could fuse with cell membranes, thus exposing carbohydrate determinants to which B cells can make antibody. The microbe could alter specific groups of antigens that encode for "self" on cell surfaces such as the H-2 antigens in mice and HLA antigens in humans. Experiments in which cell-mediated cytotoxicity against cells infected with viruses such as vaccinia virus, Rous sarcoma virus, and mouse ectromelia virus indicate that matching of the K or D end of the major histocompatibility gene complex is required for efficient T cell killing.[124–130] Similar results are found when cells are modified by coupling with the trinitrophenyl (TNP) hapten.[131] For example, killer T cells sensitized to TNP-modified syngeneic cells have been observed to lyse unmodified syngeneic cells, indicating that TNP modification of self antigens can induce the breakage of tolerance. On the other hand, the altered cells could destroy normal cells.[132]

Support for the possibility that new antigens appear on cell surfaces with age comes from the work of Gozes et al, who showed that young mice can undergo a graft-versus-host response when injected with cells from syngeneic old donors. Young mice injected with syngeneic cells from old donors respond in a syngeneic mixed lymphocyte reaction and synthesize cytotoxic antibodies.[59, 133]

Parainfluenza virus infection of immunologically immature and immunodeficient aging mice, but not adult mice, resulted in autoimmune disease, as evidenced by Coombs' positive autoimmune hemolytic anemia and immune complex glomerular nephritis and antibasement membrane antibodies.[18] Viral-like particles were detected with transmission electron microscopy in cells from the spleen and peripheral blood of immunodeficient mice.[18]

The popular notion that age-related increase in the incidence of autoantibodies results from a decrease in suppressor T cell activity stems from the earlier evidence that suppressor T cell activity declines with age in short-lived, autoimmune disease-prone mice (e.g., NZB mice).[64, 104] Even though suppressor cell activity decreases with age in these short-lived mice, it is doubtful that this is the causative factor or etiology of this disease. Evidence indicates that B cell hyperactivity begins early in NZB mice and suggests the presence of defects intrinsic to B cells in addition to T cell defects.[134–136] In addition, virus infection plays a major role in the pathogenesis of the disease of NZB mice.

As mentioned earlier, suppressor T cell activity as determined by Con A–stimulated suppressor activity has been reported to increase and decrease with age.[64–67]

The response of T cells that are cytotoxic to B cells in the autologous mixed lymphocyte reaction (AMLR) decreases with age.[137] The AMLR is absent in systemic lupus erythematosus and chronic lymphocytic leukemia. It has been suggested that the AMLR protects individuals from aberrant or neoplastic clones of B cells. The age-related decrease in AMLR T cells might result in increased autoantibody production or B cell neoplasia through decreased regulation of B cell proliferation and activity. Natural killer cell activity does not decline in healthy elderly persons.[138] This suggests that T cell recognition of subtle membrane changes is adversely affected with aging, whereas larger differences represented by allogeneic cells are still recognized. Another interpretation would be that the cytotoxic T cells involved in the AMLR and natural killer assays are different effector populations or are controlled by different regulator cells.

Escherichia coli lipopolysaccharide (LPS), a polyclonal activator produced by gram-negative bacteria (e.g., those present in the gastrointestinal tract), stimulates more mouse red blood cell autoantibody-producing B cells from old than from young mice.[139] There are two probable explanations for this phenomenon. One is that environmental factors influence self-recognition by modifying self antigens. Another is that LPS carries carbohydrate moieties, or specific sugar configurations, that are also present on molecules in red blood cell membranes. Thus, antibodies to haptenic sugars (e.g., fucose, mannose) on the LPS molecule would cross-react with the same moieties present on cellular molecules.

In summary, the age-related increase in facultatively pathologic and perhaps pathologic autoantibodies appears to be due to aberrant immunoregulation, causing an imbalance between regulatory cells and antibody-producing cells. The data suggest that B cells acquire a certain degree of autonomy with age. This autonomy is not attributable merely to a decrease in suppressor cell activity, since suppressor cell activity has been generally reported to increase with age. Membrane changes affecting cellular signal reception or environmentally induced changes in the membrane antigens encoding for self are possible explanations.

Physiologic Autoimmunity

The concept of self-tolerance is a basic tenet of immunology. Ehrlich used the term horror autotoxicus to describe autoimmune disease that was felt to result from a breakdown in internal regulation that prevented reactions against self. The demonstrated existence of physiologic autoantibodies requires a revision of this view. Indeed, it is quite probable that immune cells recognize self rather than "non-self." Thus, for example, histocompatibility antigens present on cell surfaces identify a self cell to the immune cells that carry the same antigens. Non-self would simply be any cell or organism that does not carry self antigens.

Autoantibodies that participate in the removal of senescent and damaged cells will be used as an example of a physiologic autoantibody because to date this is the only such autoantibody for which a homeostatic function has been demonstrated and a mechanism of action has in part been elucidated.[138, 140–142]

Macrophages can distinguish mature self from dying and senescent self cells, as reflected by their ability to phagocytize damaged cells and cells that have reached the end of their functional life span, while sparing the mature cells. For example, macrophages of the liver and spleen remove syngeneic lymphocytes as well as antibody-coated erythrocytes.[143–146] Studies on the fate of aged erythrocytes indicate that they are eliminated intracellularly by macrophages rather than by osmotic lysis, both in vivo and in situ.[141, 143] Thus, macrophages appear to be performing an essential homeostatic role by permitting the presumably more efficient mature cells to carry out their functions without hindrance from the less efficient senescent cells.[146, 147]

A "neo-antigen" appears on the surface of senescent cells, leading to IgG binding and cellular removal.[146–148] This neo-antigen is recognized by the antigen-binding (Fab) region of a specific immunoglobulin (IgG) autoantibody in serum, which attaches to it and initiates the removal of cells by macrophages. IgG is present on senescent, damaged, and stored red cells. In addition, several laboratories have presented evidence that IgG binding is also involved in the removal of red cells in diseases such as sickle cell anemia, and IgG has also been implicated in the removal of aging platelets.

The neo-antigen on senescent red cells is called senescent cell antigen.[149] Senescent cell antigen is a glycosylated polypeptide that appears to be derived from band 3, the major protein involved in acid-base balance. Survival studies performed in vivo have shown an association between the presence of a senescent cell antigen and cellular removal.[14, 149–156] We have discovered human mutations of band 3 that result in a lengthened or shortened cellular life span.

Although senescent cell antigen was first demonstrated on the surface of senescent human erythrocytes, it has since been demonstrated on the surface of lymphocytes, polymorphonuclear leukocytes, platelets, embryonic kidney cells, and adult liver cells. A molecule immunologically related to band 3, the molecule from which senescent cell antigen is derived, has been found on all cells examined including neurons.

Thus, as cells age, new receptors are exposed on their surface membrane, enabling pre-existing IgG autoantibodies to attach immunologically to these receptors. This provides the necessary signal for macrophages to phagocytize senescent cells selectively. Thus, it appears that certain autoantibodies are contributing to the maintenance of immunologic homeostasis by removing senescent and damaged cells. Autoantibodies of this type have been identified as physiologic. Recent studies indicate that senescent cell antigen appears prematurely (i.e., on younger cells) in older individuals. The extent to which this physiologic autoantibody protects against the formation of pathologic autoantibodies that could arise as a consequence of death and decay of senescent cells within the organism is not yet known.

Besides the physiologic autoantibody described above, for which a homeostatic function has been demonstrated and a mechanism of action has in part been elucidated, other autoantibodies are being found with increasing frequency in normal, healthy individuals.[157–160]

Autoantibodies against endogenous biologic molecules have been described. For example, normal mice possess autoantigen-sensitive cells capable of producing anti-single-stranded DNA.[158] An IgG autoantibody to spermine, a polyamine, has recently been found in normal rabbits.[161] Autoantibodies to spectrin, a major structural protein of red blood cells, has been detected in the IgG fractions of autologous human serum.[76] The function of these autoreactive immunoglobulins has not been elucidated. They might be involved in the regulation and removal of macromolecules from the circulation following tissue damage from trauma or necrosis.

Auto-anti-idiotype antibodies are another example of a physiologic autoantibody. Idiotypic determinants of Ig are located on the Fab portion of the IgG molecule. Idiotypic determinants elicit specific anti-idiotypic antibodies in the same individual that synthesized the idiotype[162, 163] as well as in isologous and heterologous species.

Jerne hypothesized that the quantitative expression of antibodies or idiotypes may be regulated by the production of anti-idiotype antibodies, or idiotypes may be regulated by the production of anti-idiotype antibodies within the same individual. Regulation of antibody synthesis by autologous anti-idiotype responses has since been demonstrated. For example, a decrease in the plaque-forming cell response to *Pneumococcus* R36A vaccine and a subsequent increase in the number of anti-idiotype–specific plaque-forming cells have been demonstrated.[164, 165] Auto-anti-idiotypic antibody present in immune sera can block secretion of anti-trinitrophenyl antibody by plaque-forming cells in vitro. Thus, it appears that auto-anti-idiotypic antibody regulates antibody secretion, at least in vitro. In this regard, antibodies to the Fab fragments of human IgG are found in human sera.[166]

Szewczuk and Campbell[43] showed that the auto-anti-idiotypic response as determined by the hapten-augmentable plaque-forming response increases with age. Others have confirmed this finding.[44, 45] An increase in auto-anti-idiotypic response with age could contribute to the decreased immune responsiveness observed with "down-regulation" of the immune system. The antigenic experience of a lifetime that is stored in the idiotypic-anti-idiotypic repertoire of the immune system could contribute to age-related immunodeficiency by the accumulation of immunosuppressive recognition of B cell idiotypes.[141]

Antisperm autoantibodies have been detected in more than 60 percent of normal healthy males. Following vasectomy, the incidence of antisperm antibodies increases. Autoantibodies to other antigens such as nuclei, mitochondria, and smooth muscle do not develop after vasectomy.

Essentially 100 percent of the young healthy individuals tested in this laboratory have low levels of antibodies to thyroglobulin. Injection of the polyclonal activator lipopolysaccharide into mice results in production of IgG antibodies that are specific for mouse IgG.[160] Immunogen injection has the same effect.[160] Plaque-forming cells producing IgM anti-IgG autoantibody have been demonstrated.[160]

It appears that physiologic autoantibodies are capable of both modulating and terminating cellular processes. A physiologic autoantibody that initiates cellular or metabolic processes has yet to be discovered. It is known, however, that anti-Fab antibodies can induce lymphocyte DNA synthesis and cell division in vitro.[48, 56] However, the anti-Fab antibodies used to date have been xenogeneic and thus may not represent a physiologic situation.

The existence of physiologic autoantibodies indicates that there are B cells that produce autoantibody with regulatory functions that are fundamental to an individual's survival. Hence, these B cell clones must be part of the normal immune response. The effect of age on physiologic autoantibodies and the role physiologic autoantibodies may play in protecting against facultatively pathologic or pathologic autoimmune manifestations, and possibly neoplasia, have yet to be investigated.

CONCLUDING REMARKS

Normal immune functions can begin to decline as early as the time of sexual maturity. The decline is due to changes in the immune cells and their milieu. Cell loss, shift in the proportion of subpopulations, and qualitative cellular changes—the three possible types of changes that can cause the decline—have all been detected. The most visible cellular target of aging appears to be the T cells, changes in their regulatory subpopulations being most prominent. Since the changes are closely linked to the involution and atrophy of the thymus, an understanding of thymic changes could be the key to understanding immunosenescence.

Aging appears to disrupt the intercellular and intracellular communication that is essential for normal antigen-driven differentiation processes. Current studies are expanding into the more complex homeostatic network systems of regulatory autoantibodies.

As our knowledge of the aging immune system increases through further studies, it is anticipated that we may be able to develop methods for predicting, delaying, and minimizing the debilitative processes associated with immunologic aging.

REFERENCES

1. Good RA, Yunis EJ: Association of autoimmunity, immunodeficiency and aging in man, rabbits, and mice. Fed Proc Fed Am Soc Exp Biol 33:2040–2050, 1974.
2. Gross L: Immunologic defect in aged population and its relation to cancer. Cancer 18:201–204, 1965.
3. MacKay IR, Whittingham SF, Mathews JD: Ageing and immunological function in man. Gerontologia 18:285–304, 1972.
4. MacKay IR, Whittingham SF, Mathews JD, et al: The immunoepidemiology of aging. In Makinodian, T. Yunis E eds: Immunity and Aging. New York, Plenum Press, 1977.
5. Gardner ID, Remington JS: Age-related decline in the resistance to infection with intracellular pathogens. Infect Immun 16:593–598, 1977.
6. Ogden DA, Micklem HS: The fate of marrow cell populations from young and old donors. Transplantation 12:287–293, 1976.
7. Harrison DE: Normal function of transplanted marrow cell lines from aged mice. J Gerontol 30:279–285, 1975.
8. Kay MMB, Mendoza J, Divin J, et al: Age-related changes in immune system of mice of 8 medium and long-lived strains and hybrids. I. Weight, cellular, and activity changes. Mech Ageing Devel 11:295–346, 1979.
9. Micklem HS, Ogden DA, Payne AC, et al: Haemopoietic Stem Cells. Ciba Foundation Symp. 13. Amsterdam, Excerpta Medica, 1973, p 285.
10. Albright J, Makinodan T: Decline in the growth potential of spleen-colonizing bone marrow stem cells of long-lived aging mice. J Exp Med 144:1204–1214, 1976.
11. Chen MG: Age-related changes in hematopoietic stem cell populations of a long-lived hybrid mouse. J Cell Physiol 78:225–232, 1971.
12. Chen MG: Impaired Elkind recovery in hematopoietic colony-forming cells of aged mice. Proc Soc Exp Biol Med 145:1181–1186, 1974.
13. Kay MMB: Effect of age on T cell differentiation. Fed Proc 37:1241–1244, 1978.
14. Kay MMB: Immunologic aspects of aging: Early changes in thymic activity. Mech Ageing Devel 28:193–218, 1984.
15. Farrar JJ, Loughman BE, Nordin AA, et al: Lymphopoietic potential of bone marrow cells from aged mice: Comparison of the cellular constituents of bone marrow from young and aged mice. J Immunol 112:1244–1249, 1974.
16. Kishimoto S, Takahama T, Mizumachi H, et al: In vitro immune response to the 2,4,6-trinitrophenyl determinant in aged C57BL/6J mice: Changes in the humoral response to, avidity for the TNP determinant and responsiveness to LPS effect with aging. J Immunol 116:294–300, 1976.
17. Kay MMB: Immunologic aging patterns: Effect of parainfluenza type 1 virus on aging mice of 8 strains and hybrids. In Bergsma D, Harrison D, eds: Genetic Effects of Aging. New York, Alan R. Liss, 1978, pp. 213–240.
18. Kay MMB: Parainfluenza infection of aged mice results in autoimmune disease. Clin Immunol Immunopathol 12:301–315, 1979.
19. Kay MMB: Long term subclinical effects of parainfluenza (Sendai) infection on immune cells of aging mice. Proc Soc Exp Biol Med 158:326–331, 1978.
20. Kay MMB, Mendoza J, Hausman S, et al: Age-related changes in the immune system of mice of 8 medium and long-lived strains and hybrids. II. Short and long-term effects of natural infection with parainfluenza type 1 virus (Sendai). Mech Ageing Devel 11:347–362, 1979.
21. Hirokawa K, Albright JW, Makinodan T, et al: Restoration of impaired immune functions in aging animals. I. Effect of syngeneic thymus and bone marrow grafts. Clin Immunol Immunopathol 5:371–376, 1976.
22. Tyan ML: Femur mass: Modulation by marrow cells from young and old donors. Proc Soc Exp Biol Med 164:89–92, 1980.
23. Ash P, Loutit JF, Townsend KMS, et al: Osteoclasts derived from haematopoietic stem cells. Nature (London) 283:669–670, 1980.
24. Mundy GR, Varani J, Orr W, et al: Resorbing bone is chemotactic for monocytes. Nature (London) 275:132–135, 1978.
25. Shelton E, Davis S, Hemmer R, et al: Quantitation of strain BALB/c mouse peritoneal cells. Science 168:1232–1234, 1970.
26. Perkins EH: Phagocytic activity of aged mice. J Reticuloendothel Soc 9:642–643, 1971.
27. Heidrick ML, Makinodan T: Presence of impairment of humoral immunity of nonadherent spleen cells of old mice. J Immunol 111:1502–1506, 1973.
28. Callard RE: Immune function in aged mice. III. Role of macrophages and effect of 2-mercaptoethanol in the response of spleen cells from old mice to phytohemagglutinin, lipopolysaccharide and allogeneic cells. Eur J Immunol 8:697–705, 1978.
29. Heidrick ML: Age-related changes in hydrolase activity of peritoneal macrophages. Gerontologist 12:28, 1972.
30. Platt D, Pauli H: Effect of alpha-naphthylisothiocyanate on lysosomal enzymes and ^{14}C-leucine-incorporation of liver and spleen of young and old rats. Acta Gerontol 2:415–429, 1972.
31. Rosenberg J, Gilman S, Feldman J, et al: Effects of aging on cell cooperation and lymphocyte responsiveness to cytokines. J Immunol 130:1754–1758, 1983.
32. Metcalf D, Moulds R, Pike B, et al: Influence of the spleen and thymus on immune responses in ageing mice. Clin Exp Immunol 2:109–120, 1966.
33. Legge JS, Austin CM: Antigen localization and the immune response as a function of age. Aust J Exp Biol Med Sci 46:361–365, 1968.
34. Penn I, Starzl TE: Malignant tumors arising de novo in immunosuppressed organ transplant recipients. Transplantation 14:407–417, 1972.
35. Goodman SA, Makinodan T: Effect of age on cell-mediated immunity in long-lived mice. Clin Exp Immunol 19:533–542, 1975.
36. Radl J, Sepers JM, Skvaril F, et al: Immunoglob-

ulin patterns in humans over 95 years of age. Clin Exp Immunol 22:84, 1975.

37. Makinodan T, Peterson WJ: Relative antibody-forming capacity of spleen cells as a function of age. Proc Natl Acad Sci 48:234–238, 1962.

38. Makinodan T, Chino F, Lever WE, et al: The immune systems of mice reared in clean and in dirty conventional laboratory farms. II. Primary antibody-forming activity of young and old mice with long life spans. J Gerontol 26:508–514, 1971a.

39. Price GB, Makinodan T: Immunologic deficiencies in senescence. I. Characterization of intrinsic deficiencies. J Immunol 108:403–412, 1972a.

40. Price GB, Makinodan T: Immunologic deficiencies in senescence. II. Characterization of extrinsic deficiencies. J Immunol 108:413–417, 1972b.

41. Groves DL, Lever WE, Makinodan T, et al: A model for the interaction of cell types in the generation of hemolytic plaque-forming cells. J Immunol 104:148–165, 1970.

42. Tsuda T, Kim YT, Siskind GW, et al: Old mice recover the ability to produce IgG and high-avidity antibody following irradiation with partial bone marrow shielding. Proc Natl Acad Sci USA 85:1169–1173, 1988.

43. Szewczuk M, Campbell R: Differential effect of aging on the heterogeneity of the immune response to a T-dependent antigen in systemic and mucosal-associated lymphoid tissues. J Immunol 126:472–477, 1981.

44. Goidl E, Thorbecke G, Weksler M, et al: Production of auto-antiidiotypic antibody during the normal immune response: Changes in the auto-antiidiotypic antibody response and the idiotype repertoire associated with aging. Proc Natl Acad Sci USA 77:6788–6792, 1980.

45. Klinman N: Antibody-specific immunoregulation and the immunodeficiency of aging. J Exp Med 154:547–551, 1981.

46. Freidman D, Globerson A: The cellular basis of immune deficiency during aging. Isr J Med Sci 12:1957, 1976.

47. Callard RE, Basten A: Immune function in aged mice. IV. Loss of T cell and B cell function in thymus-dependent antibody responses. Eur J Immunol 8:552–558, 1978.

48. Scribner DJ, Weiner HL, Moorhead JW, et al: Anti-immunoglobulin stimulation of murine lymphocytes. V. Age-related decline in Fc receptor-mediated immunoregulation. J Immunol 121:377–382, 1978.

49. Woda BA, Feldman JD: Density of surface immunoglobulin and capping on rat B lymphocytes. I. Changes with aging. J Exp Med 149:416–423, 1979.

50. Smith IM: Infections in the elderly. Hosp Prac 7 (or July):69–77, 1982.

51. Dworsky R, Paganini-Hill A, Arthur M, et al: Immune responses of healthy humans 83–104 years of age. J Nat Cancer Institute 71:265–268, 1983.

52. Carosella ED, Monchanko, K, Braun M, et al: Rosette-forming T cells in human peripheral blood at different ages. Cell Immunol 12:323–325, 1974.

53. Foad B, Adams L, Yamauchi Y, et al: Phytomitogen responses of peripheral blood lymphocytes in young and old subjects. Clin Exp Immunol 17:657, 1974.

54. Smith MA, Evans J, Steel CM, et al: Age-related variation in proportion of circulating T cells. Lancet 2:922–924, 1974.

55. Weksler ME, Hutteroth TH: Impaired lymphocyte function in aged humans. J Clin Invest 53:99–104, 1974.

56. Kay MMB: Effect of age on human immunological parameters including T and B cell colony formation. In Orimo H, Shimada K, Iriki M, et al, eds: Recent Advances in Gerontology. Amsterdam, Excerpta Medica, 1979, pp 442–443.

57. Inkeles B, Innes J, Kuntz M, et al: Immunological studies of aging. III. Cytokinetic basis for the impaired response of lymphocytes from aged humans to plant lectins. J Exp Med 145:1176–1187, 1977.

58. Brennan PC, Jaroslow BN: Age-associated decline in theta antigen on spleen thymus-derived lymphocytes of B6CF1 mice. Cell Immunol 15:51–56, 1975.

59. Gozes Y, Umiel T, Meshorer A, et al: Syngeneic GVH induced in popliteal lymph nodes by spleen cells of old C57B1/6 mice. J Immunol 121:2199–2204, 1978.

60. Beregi E: Proceedings of the 6th European Symposium on Gerontologic Research, Munich, Germany, 1979.

61. Heidrick ML: Imbalanced cyclic-AMP and cyclic-GMP levels in concanavalin A stimulated spleen cells from aged mice. J Cell Biol 57:139a, 1973.

62. Tam CF, Walford RL: Cyclic nucleotide levels in resting and mitogen-stimulated spleen cell suspensions from young and old mice. Mech Ageing Devel 7:309–320, 1978.

63. Earp HS, Utsinger PD, Yount WJ, et al: Lymphocyte surface modulation and cyclic nucleotides. I. Topographic correlation of cyclic adenosine 3:5-monophosphate and immunoglobulin immunofluorescence during lymphocyte capping. J Exp Med 145:1087–1092, 1977.

64. Antel JP, Weinrich M, Aranson BGW, et al: Circulating suppressor cells in man as a function of age. Clin Immunol Immunopathol 9:134–141, 1978.

65. Kishimoto S, Tomino S, Inomata K, et al: Age-related changes in the subsets and functions of human T lymphocytes. J Immunol 121:1773–1780, 1978.

66. Gupta S, Good RA: Subpopulations of human T lymphocytes. X. Alterations in T, B, third population cells, and T cell with receptors for immunoglobulin M (Tmu) or G (Tgamma) in aging humans. J Immunol 122:1214–1219, 1979.

67. Hallgren HM, Yunis EJ: Suppressor lymphocytes in young and aged humans. J Immunol 118:2004–2008, 1977.

68. Segre D, Segre M: Humoral immunity in aged mice. I. Age-related decline in the secondary response to DNP of spleen cells propagated in diffusion chambers. J Immunol 116:731–734, 1976.

69. Krogsrud RL, Perkins EH: Age-related changes in T cell function. J Immunol 118:1607–1611, 1977.

70. Roberts-Thomson I, Whittingham S, Youngchaiyud U, et al: Ageing, immune response, and mortality. Lancet ii: 368, 1974.

71. Weksler ME: The senescence of the immune system. Hosp Prac 10:53–64, 1981.

72. Kay MMB: The thymus: Clock for immunologic aging? J Invest Dermatol 73:29–38, 1979.

73. Murasko D, Weiner P, Kaye D, et al: Decline in mitogen induced proliferation of lymphocytes with increasing age. Clin Exp Immunol 70:440–448, 1987.

74. Lutz HU, Kay MMB: An age specific cell antigen is present on senescent human red cell membranes. Mech Ageing Devel 15:65–75, 1981.

75. Good R, West A, Fernandes G, et al: Nutritional modulation of immune responses. Fed Proc 39:3098–3103, 1980.

76. Thoman ML: Role of interleukin-2 in the age-related impairment of immune function. J Am Ger Soc 33:781–787, 1985.

77. Roder JC, Bell DA, Singhal SK, et al: T cell activation and cellular cooperation in autoimmune NZB/NZW F$_1$ hybrid mice. J Immunol 115:466–472, 1975.

78. Michalski JP, McCombs CC, Talal N, et al: Suppressor cells and immunodeficiency in (NZB × NZW)F$_1$ hybrid mice. Eur J Immunol 9:440–446, 1979.

79. Boyd E: The weight of the thymus gland in health and in disease. Am J Dis Child 43:1162–1214, 1932.

80. Andrew W: Cellular Changes with Age. Springfield, IL, Charles C Thomas, 1952.

81. Santisteban GA: The growth and involution of lymphatic tissue and its interrelationships to aging and to the growth of the adrenal glands and sex organs in CBA mice. Anat Rec 136:117–126, 1960.

82. Hirokawa K: The thymus and aging. In Makinodan T, Yunis E, eds: Immunology and Aging. New York, Plenum Press, 1977, pp 51–72.

83. Hoshino T: Electron microscopic studies of the epithelial reticular cells of the mouse thymus. Z Zellforsch Mikrosk Anat 59:513–529, 1963.

84. Clark SL, Jr: In Wolstenholm GEW, Porter R, eds: Thymus: Experimental and Clinical Studies. London, Churchill, 1966, p 3.

85. Dardenne M, Bach JF, Salomon JC, et al: Studies on thymus products. III. Epithelial origin of the serum thymic factor. Immunology 27:299–304, 1974.

86. Goldstein AL, Hooper JA, Schulof RS, et al: Thymosin and the immunopathology of aging. Fed Proc, 33:2053–2056, 1974.

87. Yunis EJ, Fernandes G, Smith J, et al: Involution of the thymus dependent lymphoid system. In Jankovic BD, Isakovic K, eds: Microenvironmental Aspects of Immunity. New York, Plenum Press, 1973, pp 301–306.

88. Bach JF, Dardenne M, Pleau JM, et al: Isolation of biochemical characteristics, and biological activity of a circulating thymic hormone in the mouse and in the human. Ann NY Acad Sci 249:186–210, 1975.

89. Hirokawa K, Makinodan T: Thymic involution: Effect on T cell differentiation. J Immunol 114:1659–1664, 1975.

90. Hirokawa K, Sado T: Early decline of thymic effect on T cell differentiation. Mech Ageing Devel 7:89–95, 1978.

91. Miller JFAP: Effect of thymectomy in adult mice on immunological responsiveness. Nature (London) 208:1337–1338, 1965.

92. Taylor RB: Decay of immunological responsiveness after thymectomy in adult life. Nature (London) 208:1334–1335, 1965.

93. Pachciarz JA, Teague PO: Age-associated involution of cellular immune function. I. Accelerated decline of mitogen reactivity of spleen cells in adult thymectomized mice. J Immunol 116:982–988, 1976.

94. Jeejeebhoy MF: Decreased longevity of mice following thymectomy in adult life. Transplantation 12:525–526, 1971.

95. Jose DG, Good RA: Quantitative effects of nutritional protein and calorie deficiency upon immune response to tumors in mice. Cancer Res 33:807–812, 1973.

96. Walford RL: The immunologic theory of aging: current status. Fed Proc 33:2020–2027, 1974.

97. Bell RG, Hazell LA: Influence of dietary protein restriction on immune competence. I. Effect on the capacity of cells from various lymphoid organs to induce graft-vs-host reactions. J Exp Med 141:127–137, 1975.

98. Gerbase-Delima M, Meredith P, Walford R, et al: Age-related changes, including synergy and suppression, in the mixed lymphocyte reaction in long-lived mice. Fed Proc 34:159–161, 1975.

99. Weindruch R, Kristie J, Cheney K, et al: Influence of controlled dietary restriction on immunologic function and aging. Fed Proc 38:2007–2016, 1979.

100. Fabris N: Hormones and aging. In Makinodan T, Yunis E, eds: Immunology and Aging. New York, Plenum Press, 1977, p 73.

101. Piantanelli L, Fabris N: Contributions of hypopituitary dwarf and athymic nude mice to the study of the relationships among thymus, hormones and aging. In Harrison D, ed: Genetic Effects on Aging. New York, Alan R. Liss, 1977, pp 315–333.

102. Fabris N, Pierpaoli W, Sorkin E, et al: Lymphocytes, hormones and ageing. Nature 240:557–559, 1972.

103. Besedovsky H, Sorkin E: Changes in blood hormone levels during the immune response. Proc Soc Exp Biol Med 150:466–470, 1975.

104. Kay MMB: Immunological aspects of aging: Frontiers. Gerontology 31, 1985.

105. Stein M, Schiavi RC, Camerino, M, et al: Influence of brain and behavior on the immune system. Science 191:435–440, 1976.

106. Fabris N, Piantanelli L: Contributions of hypopituitary dwarf and athymic nude mice to the study of the relationships among thymus, hormones, and aging. In Bergsma D, Harrison D, eds: Genetic Effects on Aging. New York, Alan R. Liss, 1978, pp 313–333.

107. Grossman CJ: Interactions between the gonadal steroids and the immune system. Science 227:257–261, 1985.

108. Kay MMB, Makinodan T, eds: CRC Handbook of Immunology in Aging. Boca Raton, Fla, CRC Press, 1981.

109. Pierpaoli W, Sorkin E: Relationship between thymus and hypophysis. Nature (London) 215:834–837, 1967.

110. Piantanelli L, Basso A, Muzzioli, M, et al: Thymus-dependent reversibility of physiological and isoproterenol evoked age-related parameters in athymic (nude) and old normal mice. Mech Ageing Devel 7:171–182, 1978.

111. Fudenberg HH: Genetically determined immune deficiency as the predisposing cause of "autoimmunity" and lymphoid neoplasia. Am J Med 51:295, 1971.

112. Kay MMB: Immunodeficiency in old age. In Chandra RK, ed: Immunodeficiency Disorders. Edinburgh, Churchill-Livingstone, 1983, pp 165–186.

113. Krohn PL: Review lectures in senescence. II. Heterochromic transplantation in the study of aging. Proc R Soc Ser B 157:128–147, 1962.

114. Baer H, Bowser RT: Antibody production and development of contact skin sensitivity in guinea pigs of various ages. Science 140:1211–1212, 1963.

115. Stjernsward J: Age-dependent tumor-host barrier and effect of carcinogen-initiated immunodepression on rejection of isografted methylcholanthrene-induced sarcoma cells. J Natl Cancer Inst 37:505–512, 1966.

116. Stutman O, Yunis EJ, Good RA, et al: Deficient immunologic functions of NZB mice. Proc Soc Exp Biol Med 127:1204–1207, 1968.

117. Teague PO, Yunis EJ, Rodey G, et al: Autoimmune phenomena and renal disease in mice. Role of thymectomy, aging, and involution of immunologic capacity. Lab Invest 22:121–130, 1970.

118. Pazmino NH, Yuhas JM: Senescent loss of resistance to murine sarcoma virus (moloney) in the mouse. Cancer Res 33:2668–2672, 1973.

119. Menon M, Jaroslow RN, Koesterer R, et al: The decline of cell-mediated immunity in aging mice. J Gerontol 29:499–505, 1974.

120. Nielson HE: The effect of age on the response of rat lymphocytes in mixed leukocyte culture, to PHA, and in the graft-vs-host reaction. J Immunol 112:1194–1200, 1974.

121. Stutman O: Cell mediated immunity and aging. Fed Proc 33:2028–2032, 1974.

122. Girard JP, Paychere M, Cuevas M, et al: Cell-mediated immunity in an ageing population. Clin Exp Immunol 27:85–91, 1977.

123. Perkins EH, Cacheiro LH: A multiple-parameter comparison of immunocompetence and tumor resistance in aged BALB/c mice. Mech Ageing Devel 6:15–24, 1977.

124. Barthold DR, Kysela S, Steinberg AD, et al: Decline in suppressor T cell function with age in female NZB mice. J Immunol 112:9–16, 1974.

125. Gerber NL, Hardin JA, Chused TM, et al: Loss with age in NZB/W mice of thymic suppressor cells in the graft-vs-host reaction. J Immunol 113:1618–1625, 1974.

126. Koszinowski U, Ertl H: Lysis mediated by T cells and restricted H-2 antigen of target cells infected with vaccinia virus. Nature (London) 255:552–554, 1975.

127. Doherty P, Zinkernagel R: H-2 compatibility is required for T-cell-mediated lysis of target cells infected with lymphocytic choriomeningitis virus. J Exp Med 141:502–597, 1975.

128. Wainberg M, Markson Y, Weiss DW, et al: Cellular immunity against Rous sarcomas of chickens. Preferential reactivity against autochthonous target cells as determined by lymphocyte adherence and cytotoxicity tests in vitro. Proc Nat Acad Sci USA 71:3565–3569, 1974.

129. Dennert G: Thymus derived killer cells: specificity of function and antigen recognition. Transplant Rev 29:59–88, 1976.

130. Zinkernagel RM, Doherty PC: Immunological surveillance against altered self components by sensitized T lymphocytes in lymphocytic choriomeningitis. Nature 251:547–548, 1974.

131. Shearer GM: Cell-mediated cytotoxicity to trinitrophenyl-modified syngeneic lymphocytes. Eur J Immunol 4:527–533, 1974.

132. Proffitt MR, Hirsch MS, Black PH, et al: Murine leukemia: a virus-induced autoimmune disease? Science 182:821–823, 1973.

133. Callard RE, Basten A, Blanden RV, et al: Loss of immune competence with age may be due to a qualitative abnormality in lymphocyte membranes. Nature (London) 281:218–220, 1979.

134. DeHeer DH, Edgington TS: Aberrant maturational characteristics of the immune responses of NZB mice to autologous and heterologous erythrocyte antigens. Cell Immunol 19:183–193, 1975.

135. DeHeer DH, Edgington TS: Evidence for B lymphocyte defect underlying the anti-X–anti-erythrocyte autoantibody response to NZB mice. J Immunol 118:1858–1863, 1977.

136. Taurog JD, Moutsopoulos HM, Rosenberg YJ, et al: CBA/N X-linked B-cell defect prevents NZB B-cell hyperactivity in F_1 mice. Z Exp Med 150:31–43, 1979.

137. Fernandez LA, MacSween JM: Decreased autologous mixed lymphocyte reaction with aging. Mech Ageing Devel 12:245–248, 1980.

138. Bennett GD, Kay MMB: Homeostatic removal of senescent murine erythrocytes by splenic macrophages. Exp Hematol 9:297–307, 1981.

139. Meredith PJ, Kristie JA, Walford RL, et al: Aging increases expression of LPS-induced autoantibody-secreting B cells. Immunol 123:87–91, 1979.

140. Kay MMB: Mechanism of macrophage recognition of senescent red cells. Gerontologist 14(5):Part II 33, 1974.

141. Kay MMB: Mechanism of removal of senescent cells by human macrophages in situ. Proc Natl Acad Sci USA 72:3521–3525, 1975.

142. Kay MMB: Role of physiologic autoantibody in the removal of senescent human red cells. J Supramol Struct 9:555–557, 1978.

143. Jenkin CR, Karthigasu K: Elimination hepatiques de erythrocytes age et alters chez le rat. Compt Rend Soc Biol 161:1006–1007, 1967.

144. Klauser MA, Hirsch LJ, Leblond PF, et al: Contrasting splenic mechanisms in the blood clearance of red blood cells and colloidal particles. Blood 46:965–976, 1975.

145. Silobrcic V, Vitale B, Sunjic M, et al: Acute graft-versus-host reaction in mice. 3. Organ distribution of injected 51-chromium labeled lymphocytes. Exp Hematal 4:103–113, 1976.

146. Kay MMB: Aging of cell membrane molecules leads to appearance of an aging antigen and removal of senescent cells. Gerontology 31:215–235, 1985.

147. Kay MMB: Immune system: Expression and regulation of cellular aging. In Bergener M, Ermimi M, Stahelin HB, eds: Thresholds in Aging (the 1984 Sandoz Lectures in Gerontology). London, Academic Press, 1985, pp 59–82.

148. Kay MMB: Surface characteristics of Hodgkins cell. Lancet 2:459–460, 1975.

149. Kay MMB: An overview of immune aging. Mech Ageing Devel 9:35–59, 1979.

150. Kay MMB: Isolation of the phagocytosis-inducing IgG-binding antigen on senescent somatic cells. Nature 289:491–494, 1981.

151. Kay MMB: Molecular aging: A termination antigen appears on senescent cells. In Peeters H,

ed: Protides of the Biological Fluids 29, Oxford, Pergamon Press, 1982, pp 325–328.

152. Kay MMB, Goodman SR, Sorenson K, et al: The senescent cell antigen is immunologically related to band 3. Proc Natl Acad Sci USA 80:1631–1635, 1983.

153. Kay MMB, Tracey CM, Goodman JR, et al: Polypeptides immunologically related to erythrocyte band 3 are present in nucleated somatic cells. Proc Natl Acad Sci USA 80:6882–6886, 1983.

154. Kay MMB: Band 3, the predominant transmembrane polypeptide, undergoes proteolytic degradation as cells age. Monogr Devel Biol 17:245–253, 1984.

155. Kay MMB: Localization of senescent cell antigen on band 3. Proc Natl Acad Sci USA 81:5753–5757, 1984.

156. Cinader BH, Kay MMB: Differentiation of regulatory cell interactions in aging. Gerontology, 32:340–348, 1986.

157. Martin WJ, Martin SE: Thymus reactive IgM autoantibodies in normal mouse sera. Nature (London) 254:716–718, 1975.

158. Roder, JC, Bell DA, Singhal SK, et al: Regulation of the autoimmune plaque-forming cell response to single-stranded DNA (sDNA) in vitro. J Immunol 121:38–43, 1978.

159. Dresser DW, Popham AM: Induction of an IgM anti-(bovine)-IgG response in mice by bacterial lipopolysaccharide. Nature 264:552–554, 1976.

160. Dresser DW: Most IgM-producing cells in the mouse secrete autoantibodies (rheumatoid factor). Nature (London) 274:480–482, 1978.

161. Bartos D, Bartos F, Campbell RA, et al: Antibody to spermine: A natural biological constituent. Science 208:1178–1180, 1980.

162. Rodkey LS: Studies of idiotypic antibodies. Production and characterization of auto-antiidiotypic antisera. J Exp Med 139:712, 1974.

163. Brown JC, Rodkey LS: Autoregulation of an antibody response via network-induced auto-anti-idiotype. J Exp Med 150:67–85, 1979.

164. Kluskens L, Kohler H: Regulation of immune response by autogenous antibody against receptor. Proc Natl Acad Sci USA 71:5083, 1974.

165. Cosenza H: Detection of anti-idiotype reactive cells in the response to phosphorylcholine. Eur J Immunol 6:114, 1976.

166. Vos GH: Anti-Fab' antibodies in human sera. I. A study of their distribution in health and disease. Vox Sag 33:16–20, 1977.

CHAPTER 34

Hematologic and Oncologic Problems

Paul A. Seligman

There are some remedies worse than the disease.
(Graviora quadam sunt remedia periculis.)
> PUBLILIUS SYRUS, *Sententiœ*

The biologic processes of aging are associated with a number of changes in the hematologic system. Aging may also lead to a higher incidence of neoplasia. However, in discussing hematologic and oncologic problems it is difficult to separate biology from the socioeconomic conditions complicating the lives of the elderly, and it is necessary to include both of these factors when evaluating patients and considering treatment. For example, older persons tend to be relatively more anemic than young adults, a circumstance that may be related to the effects of aging on bone marrow reserve (see below). However, older persons with higher intelligence, periodic health examinations, and adequate health care who live at home and retain social activity tend to have higher hemoglobin levels,[1] indicating that socioeconomic conditions play an important role in influencing hemoglobin levels in the elderly. Similarly, various effects of aging can increase neoplastic potential (see below), but socioeconomic factors such as neglect and poor nutritional status may further complicate the diagnosis and treatment of neoplastic disease in the elderly. Therefore, since so many factors are involved, it is imperative that each elderly patient be considered as an individual in determining how and to what extent a hematologic or oncologic problem will be investigated and treated.

THE BIOLOGIC EFFECTS OF AGING ON HEMATOLOGIC FUNCTION

Although some hematologic values such as the hemoglobin level (see below) appear to be decreased in the elderly, there is controversy about whether these decreases are due to the effects of aging on diminished bone marrow proliferative capacity. It has been hypothesized that the bone marrow precursors for red cells, granulocytes, and platelets (noncommitted stem cells) have a limited proliferative capacity and thus diminish as the patient gets older. This concept is supported by studies demonstrating that the extent of the hematopoietic bone marrow and percentage of active bone marrow at any one site steadily shrink with age.[2] However, these studies show great individual variation from patient to patient, and the average bone marrow cellularity in the anterior iliac crest drops only 33 percent during adult life (from about 60 percent at age 20 to about 40 percent at age 70).[2] Since bone marrow reserves are probably not decreased in the elderly, and aplastic anemia is not common in the aged,[3] it can be suggested that effects of aging on bone marrow proliferative capacity may occur but do not have clinical significance within the existing human life span. This controversy notwithstanding, however, there are some poorly defined factors associated with the aging process that must be considered when evaluating hematologic laboratory data in elderly patients.

Although there have been conflicting reports,[4] a number of studies have indicated that hemoglobin level decreases as a function of age.[5, 6] However, as shown in Table 34–1 this average decline is not marked. The studies that show a drop in hemoglobin level in apparently physically "well" individuals still may not account for mild nutritional deficiency or other treatable causes for the anemia other than the mere biologic process of aging.

The total leukocyte count is decreased in elderly patients (Table 34–1), but the absolute number of granulocytes does not appear to change significantly in the elderly. Although older patients on the whole maintain an "adequate" leukocyte response to infection,[7] reports have indicated that compared to young adults patients over the age of 70 have a diminished leukocyte response to bacterial pyrogen[8] and that patients over the age of 55 have a smaller neutrophilic leukocytosis after the oral administration of prednisolone; certain responses of neutrophils such as production of superoxide may also be deficient.[9] Other studies indicate that a leukocyte response in the elderly person with infection often results in an increase in the number of immature forms rather than an increase in the leukocyte count itself.[10] Although the exact cause has not been explained, these studies indicate that the elderly have a mildly diminished granulocyte response to stress.

The slight decrease in the leukocyte count seen in persons over the age of 65 is mainly due to a decrease in the lymphocyte count, specifically a decrease in T lymphocytes.[11] Therefore, it is not surprising that lymphocytes from elderly subjects have shown significantly less mitogenic response to plant mitogens and growth factors.[12] B lymphocytes are normal in number in the peripheral blood, but lower immunoglobulin levels are seen in elderly subjects. The IgG antibody response to specific antigens is depressed, although this abnormality may be due to immunoregulatory T cell dysfunction.[13] The exact mechanisms for the decrease in T lymphocytes and altered immunoglobulin response seen in elderly patients are unexplained.

No age-related changes in the platelet count have been seen,[14] and there are no reports of platelet function abnormalities in the elderly. Although the elderly have a number of diseases including atherosclerosis that are associated with increased thrombotic phenomena, there is no definitive data available that indicate that the elderly have an acquired abnormality of the clotting system that would result in an increase in thrombus formation.

Although not necessarily a "hematologic value," it should be mentioned that the erythrocyte sedimentation rate (ESR) shows a progressive increase with age, and that there is a decrease in the percentage of elderly subjects who have ESRs that fall within the normal range.[15] Thus, apparently healthy persons over the age of 70 can have Westergren ESRs as high as 50 mm/hr. The cause for the increase in the ESR is presently unknown, although it is possible that a number of these elderly patients have preclinical diseases associated with a rise in the sedimentation rate.

ANEMIA IN THE ELDERLY

Anemia is probably the most common hematologic problem encountered in the

TABLE 34–1. Hematologic Values in the Elderly

	Hemoglobin (gm%) Mean (range ± 2SD)	Hematocrit (%) Mean (range ± 2SD)	Leukocyte Count/mm³ Mean (range ± 2SD)	Lymphocyte Count/mm³ Mean (range ± 2SD)
"Normal" adult values	m*—15.5 (13.3–17.7)† w*—13.7 (11.7–15.7)†	m—46.0 (39.8–52.2)† w—40.9 (34.9–46.9)†	m—7250 (3900–10,600)† w—7280 (3900–11,000)†	m and w—2500 (1000–4800)†
Over age 65	m—12.9 (9.9–15.9)‡	m—38.6 (29.8–47.4)‡	m and w—5280 (3130–8910)**	m and w—1520 (600–3500)**

*m = men; w = women
†"Normals" taken from Williams WJ: Peripheral blood. In Williams WJ ed: Hematology, New York, McGraw-Hill, 1981, pp 10–19.
‡Smith J, Whitelow DM: Hemoglobin levels in aged men. Conn Med Assoc J 105:816, 1971. (Most studies indicate hemoglobin levels are similar for both sexes over age 65.)
**Caird FI, Andrews GR, Gallie TB: The leukocyte count in old age. Age Aging 1:239, 1972.

elderly. Although as shown in Table 34–1, a mild decrease in hemoglobin might be expected in elderly patients, far too often mild and even moderate anemia (Hgb below 10 gm/100 ml) is ascribed to "the biologic effects of aging," and a correctable cause for the anemia is not investigated. Particularly in patients with cardiac or pulmonary disorders, which lead to decreased tissue oxygen tension, raising the hemoglobin level (i.e., from 11 to 13 gm/100 ml) may lead to a significant improvement in both physical and mental function in the elderly. Although it is possible that a "below normal" hemoglobin level may be caused by poorly defined factors such as lack of bone marrow reserve (see above) or lack of activity in an elderly patient, it is important that a sudden change in hemoglobin level of more than 1 gm/100 ml or a hemoglobin level below 11.5 gm/100 ml be investigated extensively for a correctable cause.

The following section on anemia in the elderly will be organized so that common specific causes for anemia will be considered. However, since more than one factor is often implicated as a cause of anemia in the elderly, at various points in this section the approach to and treatment of the elderly with "multifactorial" anemia will be considered.

Nutritional Anemias in the Elderly

As in other age groups, iron deficiency anemia is the most common cause of nutritional anemia in the elderly. In young adults menstruating females have a much higher incidence of iron deficiency than males, but there is almost an equal distribution of males and females with iron deficiency in the elderly population.[16]

Several reports have indicated that even with normal iron stores, serum iron and total iron-binding capacity (serum transferrin) are decreased in elderly patients.[17] Whether these decreases are the result of the mild decrease in erythropoiesis seen in the elderly or are caused by factors such as chronic inflammation (see below), the values indicate that for the elderly patient, on average, adequate iron is available for red cell production. Elderly patients also tend to have poorer diets than younger adults (normal diets contain 6 mg of iron/

1000 cal) and may not take in the approximately 10 mg of dietary iron that is required to absorb the 1 mg of iron needed daily by postmenopausal women and adult men.[1] Iron absorption itself may be compromised in elderly patients because many aged patients have achlorhydria that will inhibit the absorption of the ferric form of iron found mainly in plant products.

Even though any of the above factors may complicate iron deficiency anemia in the aged, particularly in females who have decreased iron stores, the most common major cause for iron deficiency in the elderly individual, as in all other adult patients, is blood loss. Although acute blood loss from a duodenal ulcer, hemorrhoids, and postmenopausal bleeding may be obvious, chronic intermittent blood loss may be difficult to diagnose and may cause significant iron deficiency anemia. It should be kept in mind that even small losses of blood can result in significant loss of iron. For example, if 1 ml of packed red cells contains approximately 1 mg of iron, an average loss of 6 ml of packed red cells a day (12 ml of blood) will result in a net loss of 5 mg of iron (i.e., 6 mg loss to 1 mg absorbed) a day if the patient is on a normal diet. Thus a subject who loses this amount of blood can deplete even the normal 1 gm of iron stores and manifest iron deficiency anemia within a year of the initiation of blood loss. The gastrointestinal tract is by far the most common site of chronic blood loss in the elderly patient.[16] Examples of gastrointestinal sites of chronic intermittent blood loss in the elderly patient include bleeding from internal hemorrhoids, colonic carcinoma, diverticula, and atrophic gastritis. Chronic aspirin ingestion, a situation often encountered in the elderly patient, can result in significant enough blood loss to cause iron deficiency anemia.[18]

It may be difficult to make the diagnosis of iron deficiency anemia in elderly patients. It is important to remember that the classic hypochromic microcytic red cell indices are not generally seen unless the hemoglobin level is below 10 gm/100 ml, although an examination of the peripheral smear may show a population of hypochromic microcytic cells much earlier in the course of the anemia. Also, since elderly people tend to have lower transferrin levels in serum and often have associated chronic diseases causing anemia, the transferrin saturation and serum ferritin levels may not be diagnostic for iron deficiency. The anemia of chronic disorders is characterized by normal iron stores, low or normal serum transferrin, and high serum ferritin.[19, 20] However, all of these disorders are associated with a low serum iron, resulting in iron deficiency and diminished erythropoiesis.[19] Diseases encountered in the elderly that are associated with this rather poorly characterized abnormality include collagen vascular disease, chronic infections, and neoplasia. Although anemia from these conditions is usually not severe, it may be complicated by iron deficiency. Therefore, a bone marrow biopsy or clot section must often be performed in order to diagnose iron deficiency in the elderly patient. Absent bone marrow iron stores indicate that iron deficiency exists and necessitate a trial of iron therapy.

Oral iron therapy generally requires that the patient take 60 mg of elemental iron in the form of either ferrous sulfate or ferrous fumerate three times a day. On this regimen persons with moderate anemia (Hgb 8 to 10 gm/100 ml) should normalize their hemoglobin level after 2 months of therapy. Reasons for failure to respond completely to oral iron therapy include poor compliance in taking the medication, poor iron absorption, or continued bleeding. In these patients a trial of intravenous iron as iron dextran is warranted,[21] with appropriate precautions taken to minimize the frequency and extent of the associated hypersensitivity reactions.[21] If a patient does not respond to intravenous iron therapy and does not have obvious active bleeding, another cause for the anemia should be considered, particularly if the patient has a chronic disorder.

In conclusion, it cannot be overemphasized that a search for a site of blood loss be conducted in every elderly patient with iron deficiency anemia because the most important treatment for most patients is correcting the cause of the bleeding.

Cobalamin (vitamin B_{12}) is a nutrient that is synthesized by microorganisms and is found in trace amounts in humans.[22] Although cobalamin acts as a coenzyme in at least two mammalian enzyme systems, it is still not known exactly how cobalamin deficiency causes megaloblastic anemia and neurologic abnormalities. The megaloblastic anemia is characterized by a hypercellular bone marrow associated with macrocytic anemia, pancytopenia, and abnormal neutrophil morphology (hypersegmented neutrophils). The neurologic disease is generally associated with abnormalities of the posterior spinal columns but can be manifest clinically as any abnormality including dementia and psychiatric problems.[23] Pernicious anemia is a disease caused by a lack of intrinsic factor, the cobalamin-binding protein found in the stomach, whose presence is essential for cobalamin absorption.[24] The lack of intrinsic factor is associated with gastric atrophy and achlorhydria. In patients with pernicious anemia a Schilling test demonstrates poor absorption of free cobalamin but normal absorption of cobalamin when intrinsic factor is added. The incidence of pernicious anemia increases markedly after the age of 50 years and parallels the incidence of atrophic gastritis seen in the elderly population. An immunologic mechanism has been proposed for pernicious anemia because the disease is associated with serum antibodies directed against intrinsic factor and the gastric parietal cell and, in some cases, against thyroid cells.[25]

Although the incidence of pernicious anemia associated with gastric atrophy, megaloblastic anemia, and neurologic diseases is relatively rare, a number of individuals with reduced intrinsic factor secretion and persistent low serum cobalamin levels but without anemia or central nervous system disorders have been described as having "latent pernicious anemia." One study has indicated that about 15 percent of nonanemic individuals over the age of 65 have below normal serum cobalamin levels.[26] With the advent of more sensitive measurements of cobalamin deficiency, achieved by measuring physiologic substances such as methylmalonic acid and homocystine in serum,[27] the percentage of elderly cobalamin-deficient subjects may increase even more. Elderly patients who are cobalamin deficient but are not anemic should still be treated with cobalamin because their red cell production may be diminished in response to a stress such as bleeding. In some patients, poorly defined abnormalities in neurologic function including memory loss may be improved even if the patient has no anemia.

Other causes for cobalamin deficiency can be seen in elderly patients. Achlorhydria associated with partial gastrectomy or atrophic gastritis with adequate amounts of intrinsic factor may be associated with cobalamin deficiency. The mechanism for cobalamin deficiency in these patients is related to the necessity for free acid in the stomach to release cobalamin from food so that it can be bound to intrinsic factor and absorbed. It takes these patients 10 years or longer to become cobalamin deficient. This time interval is long compared to the 3 to 5 years it takes for deficiency to develop in patients who lack intrinsic factor and cannot absorb any endogenous cobalamin found in the gut. Usually these patients with achlorhydria have a normal Schilling test because free cobalamin is easily absorbed. However, if the Schilling test is done with cobalamin bound to proteins (such as egg white protein) poor absorption is seen both with and without added intrinsic factor.[28] These patients should be treated with cobalamin (i.e., 100 μg IM biweekly until values normalize, then a maintenance dose of 100 μg IM/month) in the same manner as patients with classic pernicious anemia. A response to cobalamin treatment is usually associated with a brisk reticulocytosis that peaks about 4 days after the initiation of therapy. As erythropoiesis normalizes, the serum lactic dehydrogenase will fall within the normal range, and, more importantly, there may be a sudden drop in serum potassium to below normal levels.[29] This latter complication may be particularly dangerous in elderly patients who have coexistent heart disease. Improvement of the neurologic disease often takes much longer than a hematologic response, and in some cases neurologic abnormalities never completely normalize.

Folic acid (pteroylmonoglutamic acid) is the parent compound of a large number of related compounds that act as coenzymes in a number of metabolic systems in animal cells including purine and pyrimidine synthesis.[30] Folic acid deficiency causes megaloblastic anemia and pancytopenia that is indistinguishable from the clinical presentation of cobalamin deficiency. However, unlike cobalamin deficiency, folic acid deficiency by itself does not result in neurologic disease. Since the amount of folic acid in the diet is not greatly in excess of the nutritional requirement and since body folate stores are relatively low, folic acid deficiency will develop within 2 to 3 months in persons taking an inadequate diet.[31] This short time necessary to develop a deficient state is in contrast to the much longer time it takes to become cobalamin deficient (see above). Because elderly persons' diets are frequently inadequate and often do not contain fresh vegetables or fruits, which have the highest amounts of folic acid, it is not surprising that they develop nutritional deficiency of folates. Malabsorption caused by intestinal disease or alcohol intake that interferes with the metabolism of folic acid[32] may also complicate folic acid deficiency in the elderly.

Folic acid deficiency is demonstrated by the finding of a low serum folate value in a patient with macrocytic anemia. If the patient's diet is inadequate nutritionally, it may be helpful to determine the red cell folate level, an assay that is said to provide a better assessment of tissue folic acid stores.[33] Although patients require only about 50 μg of folic acid a day, treatment for folate deficiency generally consists of 1 or 2 mg of folic acid given orally daily. Persons who have megaloblastic anemia due to folate deficiency respond with a peak reticulocytosis about 4 days after the institution of therapy. It should be noted that patients who have megaloblastic anemia and are cobalamin deficient or who have mixed deficiencies (see below) will exhibit a hematologic response to milligram doses of folic acid; however, the folic acid therapy will not benefit neurologic disease. In fact, there have been reports that demonstrate that neurologic disease due to cobalamin deficiency may be severely exacerbated when treatment with folic acid is instituted.[34]

Since elderly patients may have a number of problems that will result in nutritional deficiency, it is not uncommon for these patients to have *combined* nutritional deficiency resulting in anemia. As would be expected, anemia caused by combined nutritional deficiencies may be difficult to characterize and often leads to a "trial and error" diagnostic and therapeutic approach.

Cobalamin and folic acid deficiency not only are difficult to distinguish from each other but often appear concurrently. This situation may occur in a patient with long-standing cobalamin deficiency who either does not take in enough folic acid in the diet or has megaloblastic changes in the gastrointestinal tract that lead to malabsorption of folic acid. When waiting for results of the serum assays for cobalamin and folic acid, it is best to institute therapy with both nutrients since, as indicated above, folic acid given alone in a cobalamin-deficient patient may exacerbate neurologic disease. Therapeutic trials with physiologic amounts of cobalamin and folic acid as a diagnostic test for a specific deficiency are no longer in vogue because serum radiodilution assays can be performed much more rapidly than in the past.

Folic acid or cobalamin deficiency may be complicated by iron deficiency. As an example, a patient may have macrocytic anemia, a low serum folate, and a normal serum iron. This patient may respond partially to folate but will remain anemic, although the macrocytic indices are not seen. Often a repeat serum iron determination will be lower than the initial value,[35] presumably because the iron is utilized for erythropoiesis when folic acid therapy is initiated. This patient may then show an increase in hemoglobin when treated with iron therapy. As with other patients who have iron deficiency, these patients should be investigated for blood loss. Conversely, other patients with obvious iron deficiency and hypochromic microcytic anemia who are folic acid or cobalamin deficient should be treated accordingly. Sometimes a clue to this form of mixed nutritional deficiency is the finding of many hypersegmented neutrophils on the peripheral smear, although there is still some controversy as to whether iron deficiency alone can cause this abnormality.[36]

Other Causes of Anemia Seen in the Elderly

Although hemolytic anemia is not a relatively common finding in elderly patients, there are some specific considerations when hemolysis occurs in old age. First, since hemolysis may coexist with nutritional deficiency, an elderly patient may not show the same degree of compensatory erythropoiesis as a younger patient with hemolysis, and thus the reticulocyte count may be lower than expected. Also, when hemolytic anemia is suspected in an elderly patient, associated diseases that produce hemolysis should be considered (see below).

Although idiopathic autoimmune hemolytic anemia of the "warm" antibody type is not more prevalent in the elderly, secondary causes for this form of immune hemolysis are significantly increased in people over the age of 45 years.[37] Drug-induced immune hemolytic anemia is commonly seen in the elderly, particularly that associated with alpha-methyldopa (Aldomet) and penicillinlike drugs. Autoimmune hemolysis secondary to a lymphoproliferative neoplasia or collagen vascular disease should always be considered in the elderly, especially because hemolysis may be the first clinical presentation of these diseases.

"Cold" antibodies (generally IgM) causing "cold agglutinin disease" are particularly common in the seventh and eighth decades of life. Although hemolytic anemia is not usually clinically significant when cold agglutinins are present, sometimes it can be extremely severe,[38] and, as with "warm" antibody hemolysis, the patient may have an associated disease such as a malignancy.

Hereditary hemolytic anemias due to hemoglobinopathies or enzyme deficiencies are rarely diagnosed for the first time in an elderly patient. Hereditary spherocytosis, on the other hand, is not uncommonly diagnosed in older patients.[39] Sometimes these patients present with gallbladder disease (bilirubin stones) and have mild hemolytic anemia, spherocytes on peripheral smear, and slight splenomegaly.

An ill-defined form of anemia classified as "refractory or sideroblastic anemia" is not uncommonly seen in older persons. The anemia is defined as refractory because specific therapy such as nutritional supplementation does not result in improvement. Frequently these patients have macrocytic anemia and varying degrees of leukopenia and thrombocytopenia associated with a hypercellular bone marrow.[40] Although familial or drug-induced sideroblastic anemia can be seen in persons of all ages, primary acquired idiopathic sideroblastic anemia is seen most frequently in patients over 50 years of age[41] and clinically resembles refractory macrocytic anemia except that ringed sideroblasts are seen in the bone marrow.[41] Sometimes patients with refractory anemia, particularly the sideroblastic variety, will respond to pharmacologic doses of folate or pyridoxine. Most often, however, elderly patients with refractory anemia will require maintenance transfusion therapy (see below). A variable number of these patients eventually develop acute granulocytic or monocytic leukemia (see below).

GENERAL CONSIDERATIONS

Table 34–2 contains a review of some general considerations that should be made in approaching the diagnosis and treatment of anemia in an elderly patient. Although there are a number of differences in elderly patients as opposed to the young adult population, it should be stressed that there are more similarities than differences, and a patient's old age should in no way negate the consideration of a reasonable investigation for a treatable cause for the anemia.

Patients who have refractory anemia, or severe anemia associated with nutritional deficiency or bleeding, may require transfusion therapy. Considerations for transfusion therapy are the same in the elderly

as in younger adults. However, since the elderly often have severe cardiac or pulmonary disease, individual patients may require hemoglobin levels greater than the 10 or 11 gm/100 ml that are anecdotally suggested as maintenance levels for patients receiving transfusion therapy. The appropriate level of hemoglobin in a patient should be assessed individually according to the symptomatology. Since many elderly patients have relative difficulty in accepting a fluid load, transfusions in aged patients should be carefully maintained. Specifically, patients with pernicious anemia often have low hemoglobin levels (less than 5 gm/100 ml), volume overload, high output cardiac failure, and underlying cardiac disease. Once the appropriate studies are done and the patient is started on cobalamin therapy, the patient may be slowly transfused with packed blood cells with careful observation for volume overload. However, most of these patients are well compensated, and although the level of the anemia may be worrisome, they do not require transfusion therapy because they begin to respond to cobalamin within a few days (see above).

MALIGNANCIES IN THE ELDERLY

THE BIOLOGIC EFFECTS OF AGING RELATING TO NEOPLASIA. Statistics clearly show that there is an increased prevalence of hematologic malignancies in

TABLE 34–2. Anemia in the Elderly (General Considerations)

Hyperproliferative Anemia		Hypoproliferative Anemia
With effective erythropoiesis (high reticulocyte count)	With ineffective erythropoiesis (normal or low reticulocyte count)	(With low reticulocyte count)
Hemolytic anemia	Nutritional deficiency	Iron deficiency (almost always
immune hemolysis	Cobalamin	due to blood loss)
secondary to:	Folic acid	Anemia of chronic disorders
Drugs	Refractory macrocytic anemia	Chronic infections
Neoplasia	(sideroblastic anemia)	Collagen vascular disease
Infections		Neoplasia
Collagen vascular disease		Anemia of chronic renal disease
Hereditary spherocytosis		Aplastic anemia
Hypersplenism		Idiopathic
secondary to:		Secondary to toxic substances
Infections		Miscellaneous
Collagen vascular disease		Hypothyroidism
Neoplasia		Pure red cell aplasia
Bleeding (acute)		

the aged population (see below). Although the term cancer represents a wide spectrum of disease and the etiologic factors causing cancer in any age group are still not well understood, there are a number of factors associated with the aging process that help to explain the higher incidence of cancer in the elderly.

DNA repair is a process that may be defective in the elderly.[42] Although these abnormalities in DNA repair cannot be directly linked to an etiology for hematologic malignancies in the elderly, it is known that certain chromosomal rearrangements are associated with both lymphomas and leukemias.

In caring for elderly patients, there is generally no problem with lack of appreciation for the higher incidence of neoplasia, but problems relating to the attitudes of the physician and other persons participating in the care of individual patients do exist.

Although it is sometimes appropriate, a sense of nihilism occurs far too often: "He doesn't need a work-up for cancer; he's too old for us to do anything about it anyway," or "He's too old to tolerate any type of cancer therapy—why don't you send him home." Although there are numerous written and anecdotal reports about the poor tolerance of the elderly for chemotherapy (see below), a number of treatment regimens are specifically available for elderly patients that may not be "curative" but do improve both the quality and quantity of life. These treatment regimens consist not only of traditional therapeutic modalities such as surgery, chemotherapy, and radiation therapy but also include nutritional and emotional support. Specific forms of therapy will be considered later under the description of individual neoplasias. As with any disease in the elderly, it must be emphasized that each patient must be treated on an individual basis.

Besides the individualization of specific therapy in elderly patients with cancer, it should be emphasized that the judicious use of various agents to maximize symptom control in this population should have a high priority. A better understanding of pain control and the more recent availability of drugs such as long-acting oral morphine should allow the physician to treat cancer pain effectively in elderly pa-tients. Thus, the physician should at least understand that when using oral morphine the very high doses that are required at times do not indicate addiction but are necessary to control pain. Also, the use of antinausea and anticonstipation medications is very helpful in combating some of the side effects of morphinelike drugs.

Hematologic Neoplasia in the Elderly

Hematologic malignancies are generally divided into two main categories: diseases affecting the lymphoid organs (lymphoproliferative neoplasias) and neoplastic proliferation of cells that are found in the bone marrow (myeloid neoplasms). Any of the hematologic malignancies can occur at any age, but a number of these diseases are much more prevalent in the elderly and will therefore be considered more extensively in the following section.

LYMPHOPROLIFERATIVE NEOPLASMS. Immune dysfunctions seen in the elderly (see above) not only may cause lymphoproliferative neoplasia but also may be profoundly affected by some of these diseases.[43] There are a number of classifications for lymphoid neoplasms, particularly lymphomas. Newer classifications including that of Lukes and Collins[44] specifically categorize lymphoid tumors according to B and T cell characteristics. This may be an important distinction in diseases of the elderly because the highly prevalent lymphoid tumors appear to be mainly of B cell origin including nodular lymphomas, chronic lymphocytic leukemia, Waldenström's macroglobulinemia, and multiple myeloma. In discussing these diseases, however, the older terminology will be used, particularly in categorizing non-Hodgkin's lymphomas, for which the presently more familiar Rappaport classification will be used as well as prognostic criteria best summarized as low-, intermediate-, or high-grade lymphomas.[47]

Lymphomas consist of neoplastic lymphoid cells that initially infiltrate the lymphoid organs. The non-Hodgkin's lymphomas comprise a wide spectrum of disease states in which specific entities are classified according to histologic patterns and staged according to clinical involvement in individual patients. The histologic classification and clinical staging aid in determining prognostic factors and therapy in individual patients, but these predictors are not as clear-cut as they are in the evaluation of Hodgkin's disease.

The most common lymphomas seen in the elderly population are those of follicular origin, indicating that they are derived from B cells. In the Rappaport classification these mostly low-grade lymphomas include all histologic types in the nodular category, although the most common form of nodular lymphoma is composed of poorly differentiated lymphocytes (nodular—PDLL). Nodular lymphomas generally pursue an indolent course compared with other lymphomas, particularly those seen in younger adults. In some contradiction to the clinical course of these diseases, careful staging procedures have shown that at presentation nodular lymphomas are frequently widespread, involving bone marrow and other organs in addition to the lymphoid tissues.[46] Although these forms of lymphoma respond to cytotoxic chemotherapy, at this point there is no evidence that aggressive therapy for the disease leads to prolonged survival.[47] Therefore, these patients are generally treated with intermittent therapy (such as an alkylating agent) when they develop symptoms from "bulk" disease, display constitutional symptoms, or exhibit pancytopenia due to bone marrow involvement. After a number of years, some patients with nodular lymphomas develop more aggressive disease, which may change to a more malignant histologic picture with an intermediate or high-grade appearance. At that time more aggressive therapy might be considered and should be individualized according to the patient.

Chronic lymphocytic leukemia (CLL), Waldenström's macroglobulinemia, and multiple myeloma comprise a spectrum of lymphoproliferative diseases that involve small B lymphocytes. Chronic lymphocytic leukemia has a markedly increased incidence in patients over 50[48] and is by far the most common form of leukemia seen in the elderly. The abnormality is characterized by proliferation of relatively long lived small lymphocytes that infiltrate organs and produce the major signs of the disease: enlarged lymph nodes, splenomegaly, and abnormal lymphocytes in the circulating blood. As the disease progresses, other organs are infiltrated, particularly the bone marrow. Bone marrow involvement results in anemia and eventually pancytopenia. Although the neoplastic B lymphocytes appear to be immunoincompetent,[48] certain immunologic phenomena may be observed, including monoclonal serum proteins (usually of the IgM variety) and autoimmune phenomena that often result in anemia or thrombocytopenia. An even more common occurrence is hypogammaglobulinemia, which is characteristically present in the late stages of the disease.[49] As with the nodular lymphomas, patients with CLL are treated with intermittent cytotoxic and steroid therapy if they become symptomatic or if marrow involvement leads to decreased peripheral blood counts. The hypogammaglobulinemia does not appear to be ameliorated by therapy, and these patients often die of infection. Eventually, after many years and in some cases decades, most patients with CLL become resistant to any form of therapy and die of progressive disease.

Macroglobulinemia is a disease that is similar to CLL, but the B lymphocytes are able to differentiate into larger lymphocytes or immature plasma cells that secrete a monoclonal IgM paraprotein. Clinically, macroglobulinemia may appear as CLL or an indolent lymphoma in which there is infiltration of lymphoid organs and the bone marrow. Often, however, the main symptoms are due to the presence of large amounts of the IgM paraprotein in the intravascular space, producing a hyperviscosity syndrome. Symptoms of hyperviscosity include weakness, headache, coma, retinal hemorrhages (with diagnostic segmentation of the retinal and conjunctival veins), hypervolemia, which may cause cardiac failure in compromised patients, and a bleeding diathesis that is related to platelet dysfunction due to adherent paraprotein.[50] Treatment with alkylating agents and steroids will destroy the neoplastic cells and result in a decrease in paraprotein production. However, if the patient has hyperviscosity syndrome, plasmapheresis should be instituted immediately to remove the paraprotein rapidly.[51]

Plasma cell myeloma (multiple myeloma) is an abnormality caused by neoplastic proliferation of both immature and mature plasma cells that are usually localized in "spotty areas" of the bone marrow. The plasma cells in more than 99 percent of cases secrete an immunoglobulin that appears in the serum as a monoclonal immunoglobulin or in the urine as immunoglobulin light chains. The intact immunoglobulin is usually of the IgG class, but IgA, IgD, and IgE monoclonal proteins have also been identified.[52] More than 50 percent of cases of myeloma occur in patients over 70 years old, and the etiology for the disease may be related to the immunologic dysfunction found in elderly patients. Other than this association and the rare cases in which the monoclonal protein is directed against a specific antigen,[53] the cause for the seemingly unrestrained neoplastic proliferation of plasma cells is unknown.

There is marked variation in the clinical manifestations of myeloma. A number of patients, particularly the elderly, are asymptomatic and have a monoclonal immunoglobulin in their serum (usually less than 3 gm/100 ml). This condition is termed benign monoclonal gammopathy, and although it usually remains asymptomatic, a number of these patients eventually develop symptomatic plasma cell myeloma.[54] Although the absolute level of the protein in serum is sometimes helpful, probably the best way of distinguishing benign monoclonal gammopathy from plasma cell myeloma is to demonstrate a rise in paraprotein level in the latter with time. Patients with definite plasma cell myeloma may have bone disease including osteoporosis and osteolytic lesions, mild to severe anemia with or without pancytopenia, and renal abnormalities that may be manifest on a spectrum from mild abnormalities such as proteinuria due to urinary excretion of light chains to severe renal failure due to a number of causes including tubular dysfunction, amyloidosis, or urate nephropathy. A bone marrow examination in a patient with myeloma will almost always show areas of increased plasma cells (greater than 15 percent of the cells) and usually areas where there are sheets of bizarre multinucleated plasma cells.[54] Treatment for plasma cell myeloma consists of intermittent melphalan and prednisone therapy. At the present time more aggressive ther-

apy has not been shown to be more effective.[55] However, recent studies indicate that elderly patients with myeloma treated with traditional chemotherapy have response and survival rates equivalent to those of younger patients.[58] The patient should be followed symptomatically while he or she is on therapy. The best criterion for an objective response is a decrease in the paraprotein level. About 50 percent of patients treated in this manner will respond to therapy; poor prognostic features include a high pretreatment tumor burden (as calculated by immunoglobulin synthetic rate[59]) or significant renal failure. Most patients that initially respond to therapy will become resistant within several years and manifest progressive disease. At that time the patient may respond to other chemotherapeutic agents such as BCNU, Adriamycin, and vincristine.[57] If the patient cannot tolerate chemotherapy or remains unresponsive, palliative measures can sometimes add to both the quality and quantity of life. These measures include low-dose radiation to areas of bone pain, medical management of renal disease, and treatment of hypercalcemia. Hypercalcemia is a common end-stage complication and should be assessed by measuring ionizable serum calcium levels because some paraproteins bind calcium and raise the total serum calcium level.[58] Patients with end-stage myeloma usually have decreased levels of normal immunoglobulins and therefore are prone to bacterial infections. If bone disease is prominent patients may suffer from excruciating pain, and it is important that the physician provide enough medication and emotional support to achieve pain control.

Hodgkin's disease, although thought to be primarily a disease of young and middle age, has a "bimodal" incidence and a second peak of prevalence in persons over the age of 50.[59] Compared with the disease found in young adults, Hodgkin's disease tends to be more aggressive in both histologic type and stage when it is diagnosed in elderly individuals.[43, 60] Usually these elderly patients are treated with combination chemotherapy (nitrogen mustard, vincristine, prednisone, procarbazine [MOPP]),[62] but a number of factors such as aggressive disease, nutritional deficiency, and other diseases found in the elderly generally lead to poor tolerance for chemotherapy and rather dismal survival rates.[43, 60]

Some relatively rare lymphomas seen in the elderly have a T cell origin and usually involve the skin (including mycosis fungoides and the "Sezary syndrome"). The aggressive T cell lymphomas seen in childhood are extremely rare in the elderly, as is Burkitt's lymphoma, an aggressive disease thought to be of B cell origin. Cases of acute lymphoblastic leukemia, which appear to have a "bimodal" incidence, have also been described in the elderly, but a number of these cases may represent the progressive stage of certain lymphomas and do not behave biologically like "classic" childhood acute lymphocytic leukemia (ALL).

Myeloid Neoplasms

Acute myelocytic leukemia (AML) and its morphologic variants increase in prevalence with age. Greater than 50 percent of the cases occur in patients over age 60. Although most cases of AML are diagnosed at clinical presentation, many patients with this disease have a preceding history of poorly defined hematologic abnormalities such as anemia or granulocytopenia. A number of patients, particularly the elderly, have a well-documented previous history of refractory macrocytic anemia (see above). Added to these cases are an increasing number of patients who develop leukemia several years after institution of cytotoxic therapy for lymphomas, myeloma, and some solid tumors.[55, 61] Many patients who have had previous hematologic problems or have received cytotoxic therapy have acute leukemia associated with a relatively hypocellular marrow and peripheral pancytopenia. It is for these patients that the designation "smoldering" leukemia seems appropriate. This form of AML is generally associated with a clinically indolent course and exhibits a poor response to chemotherapy. Therefore, it is suggested that these patients be treated symptomatically with blood transfusions, nutritional supplementation, and occasionally low doses of chemotherapeutic agents. However, most of the elderly patients with AML present with a markedly hypercellular bone marrow filled with myeloblasts and severe symptomatology due to pancytopenia. Although there is little disagreement that these patients appear clinically the same as young adults with AML, controversy does exist about how these patients should be treated. Currently accepted treatment for AML necessitates the use of high-dose cytotoxic agents so that bone marrow aplasia is achieved. This type of therapy (generally including an anthracycline antibiotic and cytosine arabinoside)[62] will result in a 50 to 70 percent complete remission rate in adults with AML. However, a number of reports[63, 64] have indicated that persons over the age of 60 have a response rate that is much lower. These studies suggest that most elderly patients do not respond because of early deaths due to complications caused by chemotherapy. In fact, it is these data that are most often cited and best support the hypothesis that the elderly cancer patient tolerates chemotherapy poorly. However, there is at least one other study that indicates that some patients who are elderly will have the same response rate as younger patients when treated with intensive antileukemic regimens.[65] This study indicates that it should be possible for the clinician to select elderly patients who might tolerate intensive therapy. A more recent study goes farther in indicating that intensive chemotherapy is the treatment of choice for elderly patients with ALL.[66] This recommendation is somewhat tempered by a large study recently reported from MD Anderson Hospital indicating that patients 70 years old or older with acute leukemia had an overall complete remission rate of 35 percent, a value lower than that reported for younger patients.[67] This latter study did indicate that patients without identifiable infection, liver enlargement, or elevated liver enzyme serum tests constituted a more favorable subgroup that might do well with intensive chemotherapy, although age greater than 75 years or previous hematologic conditions were independently associated with dismal remission rates.

Obviously, when considering therapy both the patient and his or her family should be included in the decision-making process. For those patients with unaggressive disease who are not given intensive chemotherapy, palliation can often be achieved with transfusions, prompt anticipation of infectious complications, and a trial of therapy with relatively nontoxic drugs such as vincristine and prednisone.

Although classic Philadelphia chromosome–positive chronic myelogenous leukemia has its peak incidence in young and middle-aged adults, other myeloproliferative diseases are common in the elderly. Polycythemia vera increases in incidence markedly after the age of 50. The disease is characterized by high hematocrit with increased red cell mass, trilineal hyperplasia in the bone marrow, and splenomegaly. Symptoms are characterized by hyperviscosity due to a high hematocrit and clotting and bleeding problems (sometimes occurring concurrently in the same patient) due to thrombocytosis with associated qualitative defects in platelet function.[68] In any patient with suspected polycythemia vera a red cell mass should be obtained to exclude spurious polycythemia on the basis of a decreased plasma volume. Also, patients should be investigated for secondary causes of polycythemia due to decreased tissue oxygen tension (i.e., pulmonary disease) and ectopic erythropoietin production due to a tumor (i.e., renal neoplasms). The treatment of polycythemia vera generally begins with phlebotomy therapy to decrease the hematocrit and allopurinol if a high uric acid level exists. When red cell production increases to the point that phlebotomies are no longer feasible or thrombocytosis becomes a problem, patients are treated with cytotoxic therapy. Radioactive phosphorus or oral alklyating agents are the usual treatment choice. Radioactive phosphorus has come into disrepute because of past reports that demonstrated a high incidence of development of acute leukemia in patients so treated.[69] However, reports have indicated that alkylating agents may have a similar leukemogenic potential.[70] If radioactive phosphorus is given judiciously it has the advantage of single dose therapy, and a slow decrease in the red count occurs over a 2- to 3-month period. After a number of years or even decades, most patients with polycythemia vera (who live long enough) enter a "burned out" phase in which myelofibrosis develops and extramedullary hematopoiesis results in massive splenomegaly and hepatomegaly. These patients become resistant to therapy and frequently die of problems related to pancytopenia.

Although less common than polycythemia vera, other myeloproliferative diseases are frequently seen in the elderly. These diseases include idiopathic myelofibrosis, which is sometimes difficult to separate from burned out polycythemia vera if no previous history is known. The peripheral blood picture of myelofibrosis may appear the same as that of chronic myelogenous leukemia with leukocytosis, anemia, and (often) thrombocytosis. The disease is generally difficult to treat, particularly the thrombocytosis, since the use of cytotoxic agents may result in severe granulocytopenia or anemia in these patients, who have a poor bone marrow reserve.

Nonhematologic Neoplasms in the Elderly

Nonhematologic neoplasms, particularly the more common cancers, have a higher prevalence in the elderly population. In fact, autopsy series have indicated that an astoundingly high rate of 32.5 percent of patients over 65 years have one or more forms of cancer.[71] This number overestimates the clinical picture of cancer in the elderly because there are a large number of "in situ" cancers, and other tumors have a low degree of invasiveness. However, as evidenced by the statistics cited at the beginning of this section, neoplasia causes significant clinical disease in the elderly. Some basic principles concerning cancer in the aged patient should be considered.

First, for most forms of malignancy in the elderly, as in other patients, early diagnosis is beneficial from a therapeutic standpoint. However, unlike younger patients, elderly persons, who often have coexisting diseases, are less apt to be taken seriously when they complain about subtle symptoms that might indicate early neoplasms. For example, a change in bowel habits in an older person may indicate a colonic tumor but is apt to be "written off" as simple constipation. Nocturia in an older male may represent changes due to senility, mild prostatism, or early prostatic carcinoma. Realistically, these kinds of symptoms should always be taken seriously by the elderly patient and his physician, but they usually do not indicate a neoplasm. Related to this problem is the question of performing screening tests on the elderly, particularly when the tests are uncomfortable or expensive. Screening tests will be discussed with each individual neoplasm (see below).

Another aspect of neoplastic disease that must be considered in the elderly is appreciation for the biology of an individual neoplasm. For example, an elderly patient with heart disease who has a prostatic tumor with pelvic spread should not receive extensive radiation treatment if it is felt that the heart disease will kill him before the anticipated spread of the cancer becomes lethal. Very elderly women with metastatic breast cancer to bone may require only local radiation and other palliative measures such as hormonal manipulation rather than intensive chemotherapy, since individual patients with breast cancer and bone metastases can survive for a number of years without aggressive treatment.

As has been previously stated, treatment for a specific neoplasia is not standardized and should be individualized, especially in the elderly patient. Less aggressive chemotherapy, nutritional supplementation, adequate pain control, and emotional support add to the quality of a cancer patient's life. A patient with cancer who lives 6 months relatively pain free, with just a few days in the hospital during that period, is certainly better off than a patient who lives a year but is hospitalized for half of that time because of side effects from chemotherapy. However, in other cases elderly patients should be given aggressive chemotherapy. In these cases it is important that to present the alternatives in a reasonable fashion to the patient so that he can participate in the decision-making process.

Following are the high incidence non-hematologic neoplasms that occur in the elderly.

PROSTATIC CARCINOMA. Prostatic carcinoma is almost never seen in men under the age of 40 but increases steadily in incidence so that it is the most common tumor in males over 80 years old. The clinical significance of prostatic carcinoma may be somewhat overestimated because reports of the high incidence are often taken from autopsy studies in which in situ carcinoma is found. On the other hand, prostatic carcinoma is the third most common cause of death from cancer in men, and unfortunately, by the time it causes clinical symptoms only about 50 percent of patients have limited and potentially curable disease.[72] Symptoms of prostatic carcinoma are similar to those associated with benign prostatic hypertrophy and include frequency of urination, hesitancy, and frank obstruction of urine flow.[72] When a lesion that is clinically suspicious for carcinoma is diagnosed histologically by needle biopsy, various staging procedures should be performed. A persistently elevated acid phosphatase concentration (two determinations) indicates that the patient has either extensive bulky disease in the pelvis or metastatic disease. A bone scan should be performed on all patients because this test is more sensitive for metastatic disease than routine x-rays,[73] and about 40 percent of patients with bony metastasis have normal serum acid phosphatase levels.[72] Lymphangiography is done in many centers to assess the extent of pelvic disease in those without bone metastasis. Hopefully, newer radioimmunoassays specific for serum prostatic acid phosphatase[74] not only may better assess the extent of disease in individual patients but also may be used as a screening test in males for occult prostatic neoplasms.

In patients with latent prostatic carcinoma (stage A) or clinically palpable carcinomas localized within the prostatic capsule (stage B), radical prostatectomy is generally performed, although radiation therapy can be used, usually with the same efficacy, especially in patients that are poor surgical risks.[72] There are a number of treatment alternatives for patients with large prostatic tumors or pelvic lymph node disease including the use of aggressive surgery followed by radiation therapy. However, it appears that most of these patients, particularly those with lymph node metastasis, eventually develop bony metastasis within 5 years.[72] There are at present no highly effective chemotherapy regimens for the treatment of metastatic prostatic carcinoma. However, endocrine manipulation is often helpful in patients with bony disease or large pelvic masses. About 80 percent of patients experience both subjective and objective remissions.[75] Generally, hormonal manipulation is not instituted until the patient is symptomatic. The usual initial treatment is 1 to 3 mg daily of diethylstilbestrol (DES), a dose that is effective in controlling disease but causes less toxicity than higher doses. Newer agents such as gonadotropin-releasing analogues (leuprolide) appear to show the same therapeutic effect as estrogens with fewer side effects.[76] When patients become refractory to hormonal therapy, orchiectomy has some chance of producing a remission.[75] With the use of hormonal manipulation as many as one-fifth of patients with metastatic disease from prostatic carcinoma will live 5 years.[75] This statistic should be kept in mind when dealing with these patients, since a diagnosis of metastatic cancer sometimes leads to overprescribed and potentially addictive pain medications, and some physicians perpetuate a nihilistic attitude toward the treatment of associated medical conditions.

BREAST CANCER. The incidence of breast cancer increases considerably at age 40 and then shows a slight but progressive increase in incidence up to and through the age of 80.[74] Breast cancer in men behaves biologically much like the tumor in women but is extremely rare and comprises only 1 percent of the total cases. Because older women have atrophic breasts it is often easier to palpate a tumor, making it imperative that every elderly woman have her breasts examined when seeking medical attention for even an unrelated problem. The prognosis for breast cancer is best related to the extent of disease at the time of diagnosis. Thus, all patients should not only have their breasts examined when seen by a doctor but should also be taught self-examination at home. As a general rule, the use of mammography as a screening test in elderly patients is not indicated because the lesions are usually easily identifiable, and predisposing conditions such as fibrocystic disease are not found in the elderly. In most centers, a modified radical mastectomy still remains the surgical treatment of choice for breast cancer. Although there are alternatives to this procedure (see below), past studies of patients operated on in this manner have indicated that an important prognostic finding in carcinoma of the breast is the presence of positive regional lymph nodes. Thus, a patient

with negative lymph nodes will have about an 80 percent chance of a 5-year survival, whereas survival for those with positive nodes is approximately half this figure.[77] Other factors, including the size of the tumor and estrogen receptor status (see below), may provide an index for the prognosis. Sometimes elderly women patients are first seen with a large inflamed breast mass. These patients with "inflammatory" breast carcinoma are felt to have a poor prognosis and often present with obvious metastatic disease. For many of these patients it is best to do a simple mastectomy, mainly to remove a potential source of infection, and provide palliative therapy.

Historical data, which documented the poor prognosis of patients with positive regional lymph nodes, prompted the initiation of postsurgical adjuvant chemotherapy protocols in which patients with positive nodes but no evidence for "macroscopic" metastasis were treated with either single agent therapy[78] or combination chemotherapy including Cytoxan, methotrexate, and 5-fluorouracil (CMF).[79] Although the adjuvant chemotherapy trials are continuing and new studies are being developed, most of the long-term follow-up studies indicate that postmenopausal patients treated in this fashion show a delay in onset of metastatic disease but no change in survival compared with untreated control groups.[80] Postmenopausal patients may not do as well as premenopausal patients in these studies because older patients receive less than "adequate" chemotherapy due to enhanced toxicity,[80] or they may have a slightly biologically different disease that results in drug resistance. Presently, a number of newer adjuvant studies, including adding hormonal therapy, are in progress. Although the final studies have not been published at the time this chapter was written, a recent National Cancer Institute bulletin indicated that all patients with breast cancer, including node negative cancer, should receive adjuvant therapy. Specifically, the bulletin proposes that all postmenopausal patients should receive at least adjuvant tamoxifen. Also, women with breast cancer, including older patients, are choosing to forego the traditional radical mastectomy and are requesting procedures such as tumor removal and radioactive implants[82] for a better cosmetic result with fewer surgical complications. So far this form of therapy is associated with a survival similar to that for radical mastectomy, and if axillary nodes are sampled and estrogen receptor levels measured, decisions concerning adjuvant chemotherapy studies can still be made.

The treatment of metastatic breast carcinoma utilizes both hormonal manipulation and cytotoxic therapy. Assays for estrogen receptors (and in some cases progesterone receptors) are readily available and accurate if the tissue is handled properly: the breast tissue should not be placed in fixative but put on ice immediately after removal. Studies have shown[83] that patients who are positive for estrogen receptors have a greater than two-thirds chance of responding to the appropriate hormonal manipulation, whereas receptor-negative patients have only a 10 percent response rate with the same therapy. Hormonal therapy in postmenopausal patients is generally begun with the antiestrogen agent tamoxifen, a drug that has similar efficacy but fewer side effects than estrogen.[84] Estrogen receptor–negative patients and receptor–positive patients who do not respond to hormonal manipulation are generally treated with chemotherapy. Chemotherapy includes CMF (Cytoxan, methotrexate, 5-fluorouracil) or other drug combinations containing Adriamycin.[85] There is controversy about whether estrogen-negative or estrogen-positive patients respond better to chemotherapy, but overall about 50 percent of patients will show either a complete or partial response. Unfortunately, even though patients with metastatic disease who respond to therapy may remain in remission for a number of years, almost all patients with metastatic breast cancer will eventually relapse.

CARCINOMA OF THE COLON AND RECTUM. Adenocarcinoma of the large bowel and rectum is another common tumor that increases in prevalence after the age of 60. Classically, about two-thirds of the lesions occur in the sigmoid colon and below, indicating that routine sigmoidoscopy of elderly patients as a screening test may be helpful, although this practice has not been widely used. Certainly a rectal examination is an easily performed screening procedure, and at least one study has shown that stool examinations for occult blood in the elderly population may be useful.[86] Left-sided colon lesions generally cause more symptomatology than lesions in the right colon, where bleeding may be the only manifestation.

The initial treatment of adenocarcinoma of the colon and rectum is surgical. Superficial lesions (Dukes A) have a better prognosis than lesions through the muscle of the bowel wall (Dukes B), which in turn has about twice the 5-year survival rate as lesions involving the regional lymph nodes (Dukes C). Although one report has shown that postsurgical adjuvant chemotherapy is effective for invasive but not metastatic lesions,[87] other studies have shown no advantage when postoperative chemotherapy is used.[88] It is often suggested that elderly patients with localized adenocarcinoma cannot tolerate curative surgery, and thus palliative procedures should be done. However, at least one study has shown that in selected patients over the age of 70 there is only a slight increase in mortality when curative surgery is performed, even when rectal carcinoma is present and necessitates an abdominal-perineal repair.[89] Even more important, the same study indicated that elderly patients had similar 5-year survival rates compared with the younger group of patients. Also, new surgical techniques indicate that for about two-thirds of patients with rectal cancer, anastamosis is now possible as opposed to colostomy.[90]

Metastatic adenocarcinoma of the colon and rectum generally involves the pelvis, liver, and lung. When metastatic disease is suspected, a biopsy may not be necessary if the patient exhibits an increase in the level of carcinoembryonic antigen (CEA) compared with values obtained immediately after surgery. About a third of patients with metastatic colon carcinoma exhibit a partial response to treatment with 5-flurouracil and have an associated increase in survival compared with nonresponders.[91] Combination chemotherapy[92] or hepatic artery infusion of chemotherapy for liver metastases shows some increase in response rate, but survival does not appear to be appreciably lengthened.[92]

LUNG CARCINOMA. Because there is a longer exposure to the carcinogen, lung cancer increases in elderly persons who smoke. Except for the small percentage of persons in whom surgical resection is possible, the treatment of non–small cell carcinoma of the lung is rather dismal, especially because many of the elderly patients who have a long smoking history have associated pulmonary disease. Often, prophylactic radiation therapy to areas where obstruction may occur and radiotherapy to relieve pain are the most appropriate forms of treatment.

Small cell carcinoma, although almost universally widespread at the time of diagnosis,[93] has a much higher response rate to chemotherapy, and various regimens such as the one used in a large study in Denmark[93] may be given a trial. Generally, if no response is seen after two courses of chemotherapy, or even if the patient shows a slight objective response but appears *subjectively* to be getting worse (with increased weakness and weight loss), therapy should be stopped.

ENDOMETRIAL CARCINOMA. This neoplasm is common in elderly women and often presents as postmenopausal bleeding. Hysterectomy is curative for the less invasive forms of endometrial carcinoma. A surgical series has shown that in at least selected patients over the age of 75 the procedure is tolerated as well as it is in a control group of patients under 60.[94] Metastatic endometrial carcinoma is relatively resistant to therapy, but recent statistics suggest that better patient and physician education has increased the percentage of patients treated surgically at an early and potentially curable stage of their disease.[95]

REFERENCES

1. Talley L: In Centovoli O, Patrick M, eds: Nursing Management for the Elderly. Philadelphia, JB Lippincott, 1979, p 85.
2. Hartsock RJ, et al: Normal variation with aging of the amount of hematopoietic tissue in bone marrow from the anterior iliac crest. Am J Clin Pathol 43:325–331, 1965.
3. Young N: Aplastic anemia: Research themes, clinical issues. In Brown EB, ed: Progress in Hematology X, Vol 11. New York, Grune & Statton, 1981, pp 1–42.
4. Purcell Y, Brozonic B: Red cell 2,3-diphosphoglycerate concentration in man decreases with age. Nature 251:511, 1974.
5. Smith JS, Whitelow DM: Hemoglobin levels in the elderly. Can Med Assoc J 105:816, 1971.
6. McLennan WJ, Andrews GR, MacLeod C, et al: Anemia in the elderly. Q J Med 42:1, 1973.
7. Sorso RD, Hammer, EA, Moore, DL: Leukocyte and neutrophil counts in acute appendicitis. Am J Surg 120:563, 1970.
8. Timaffy M: A comparative study of bone marrow function in young and old individuals. Gerontology Clin (Basel) 4:13, 1962.
9. Nagel JE, Pyle RS, Chrest JF, Adler WH: Oxidative metabolism and bactericidal capacity of polymorphonuclear leukocytes from normal young and aged adults. J Gerontol 37:529, 1982.
10. Thorbjarharson B, Loehr WJ: Acute appendicitis in patients over the age of sixty. Surg Gynecol Obstet 125:1277, 1967.
11. Diaz-Jonanen E, Strickland RG, Williams RC: Studies of human lymphocytes in the newborn and the aged. Am J Med 58:620, 1975.
12. Gillis S, Kozak R, Durante M, et al: Immunologic studies of aging. J Clin Invest 67:937–942, 1981.
13. Pahwa SG, Pahwa RN, Good R: Decreased in vitro humoral immune responses in aged humans. J Clin Invest 67:1094–1102, 1981.
14. Shapleigh JB, Mayes S, Moore CV: Hematologic values in the aged. J Gerontol 7:207, 1952.
15. Sharland DE: Erythrocyte sedimentation rate: The normal range in the elderly. J Am Geriatr Soc 28:346, 1980.
16. Council on Foods and Nutrition: Iron deficiency in the United States. JAMA 203:407–411, 1968.
17. Powell DEB, Thomas JH: The iron-binding capacity of serum in elderly hospital patients. Gerontol Clin (Basel) 11:36, 1969.
18. Roth WA, Waldes-Dapener A, Pieses P, et al: Topical action of salicylates in gastrointestinal erosion and hemorrhage. Gastroenterology 44:146, 1963.
19. Cartwright GE: The anemia of chronic disorders. Semin Hematol 3:351, 1966.
20. Lipschitz DA, Cook JP, Finch CA: A clinical evaluation of serum ferritin as an index of iron stores. N Engl J Med 290:1213, 1974.
21. Hamstra RD, Block M, Schocket A: Intravenous iron dextran in clinical medicine. JAMA 243:1726–1731, 1980.
22. Allen RH: The plasma transport of vitamin B_{12}. Br J Haematol 33:161–171, 1976.
23. Shulman R: Psychiatric aspects of pernicious anemia. Br Med J 3:366, 1967.
24. Castle WB: Current concepts of pernicious anemia. Am J Med 48:541–548, 1970.
25. Doniach D, Reitt IM: An evaluation of gastric and thyroid autoimmunity in relation to hematologic disorders. Semin Hematol 1:313, 1964.
26. Elwood PC, Shinton NK, Wilson CID, et al: Haemoglobin, vitamin B_{12}, and folate levels in the elderly. Br J Haematol 21:557, 1971.
27. Stabler SP, Marcell PD, Podell ER, et al: Elevation of total homocysteine in the serum of patients with cobalamin or folate deficiency detected by capillary gas chromatography–mass spectrometry. J Clin Invest 81:466–474.
28. Doscherholman A, Swaim WR: Impaired assimilation of egg Co^{57}-vitamin B_{12} in patients with hypochlorhydria and achlorhydria and after gastric resection. Gastroenterology 64:913–919, 1973.
29. Lawson DH: Early mortality in the megaloblastic anemias. Q J Med 41:1, 1972.
30. Huennekens FM: Folic acid coenzymes in the biosynthesis of purines and pyrimidines. Vitam Horm 26:375–386, 1968.
31. Herbert V: Minimal daily adult folate requirement. Arch Intern Med 110:649–659, 1962.

32. Sullivan LW, Herbert V: Suppression of hematopoiesis by ethanol. J Clin Invest 43:2048, 1964.
33. Schreiber C, Waxman S: Measurement of red cell folate level by ³H-pteroylglutamic acid radioassay. Br J Hematol 27:551, 1974.
34. Israels MCG, Wilkinson JF: Risk of neurological complications in pernicous anemia treated with folic acid. Br Med J 2:1072, 1949.
35. Hawkins CF: Value of serum iron levels in assessing effect of hematinics in the macrocytic anemias. Br Med J 1:383, 1955.
36. Beard ME, Weintraub LR: Hypersegmented granulocytes in iron deficiency anemia. Br J Hematol 16:161, 1969.
37. Dacie JV, Worlledge SM: Autoimmune hemolytic anemias. Prog Hematol 6:82, 1965.
38. Schubothe H: The cold hemagglutinin disease. Semin Hematol 3:27, 1966.
39. Race RR: On the inheritance and linkage relations of alcoholic jaundice. Ann Eugen 11:365–373, 1942.
40. Vilter RW, Janold T, Will JJ, et al: Refractory anemia with hyperplastic bone marrow. Blood 15:1, 1960.
41. Kuscher JP, Lee, GR, Wintrobe MM, et al: Idiopathic refractory sideroblastic anemia. Medicine 50:139, 1971.
42. Ringburg U, Lambert B, Swanbeck, G: DNA repair in conditions associated with malignancy. In Nieburgs H, ed: Prevention and Detection of Cancer, Vol. 1. New York, Marcel Dekker, 1977.
43. Fernandez G, Schwartz J: Immune responsiveness and hematologic malignancy in the elderly. Med Clin North Am 60:1253–1271, 1976.
44. Lukes RJ, Collins RD: Immunologic characterization of human malignant lymphomas. Cancer 34:1488, 1974.
45. Rappaport H: Tumors of the Hematopoietic System. In Atlas of Tumor Pathology, Sec. III, Fasc. 8. Armed Forces Institute of Pathology, Washington, DC, 1966.
46. Banks PM, Berard CW: Histopathology of the malignant lymphomas. In Williams WJ, ed: Hematology. New York, McGraw-Hill, 1977, p 1031.
47. Portlock CS, Rosenberg SA, Glatstein E, et al: Treatment of abnormal non-Hodgkin's lymphomas with favorable histologies: preliminary results of a prospective trial. Blood 47:747–756, 1976.
48. Doneshek W: Chronic lymphocytic leukemia—an accumulative disease of immunologically incompetent lymphocytes. Blood 29:566–578, 1967.
49. Jim RTS: Serum gamma globulin levels in chronic lymphocytic leukemia. Am J Med Sci 234:44, 1957.
50. Pachter MR, Johnson SA, Neblett TR, et al: Bleeding, platelets, and macroglobulinemia. Am J Clin Pathol 31:467–472, 1959.
51. MacKenzie MR, Fudenberg HH: Macroglobulinemia: An analysis of forty patients. Blood 39:874–886, 1972.
52. Kyle RA: Multiple myeloma: Review of 869 cases. Mayo Clin Proc 50:29, 1975.
53. Isoke T, Osserman EF: Pathologic conditions associated with plasma cell dyscrasias: A study of 806 cases. Ann NY Acad Sci 190:507, 1971.
54. Waldenstrom JG: Benign monoclonal gammopathies. In Azur HA, Rotter M, eds: Multiple Myeloma and Related Disorders, Vol. 1. Hagerstown, MD, Harper & Row, 1973, p 247.
55. Bergsagel DE, Bailey AJ, Langley GR, et al: The chemotherapy of plasma-cell myeloma and the incidence of acute leukemia. N Engl J Med 301:743–748, 1979.
56. Crawford J, Cohen HJ: An approach to monoclonal gammopathies in the elderly. Geriatrics 37:97, 1982.
57. Salmon S: Immunoglobulin synthesis and tumor kinetics of multiple myeloma. Semin Hematol 10:125–142, 1973.
58. Jaffe JP, Mosher DF: Calcium binding by a myeloma protein. Am J Med 67:343–346, 1979.
59. Greco RS, Acheson RM, Foote FM: Hodgkin's disease in Connecticut from 1935 to 1962. Arch Intern Med 134:1039, 1974.
60. Peterson BA, Pajak TF, Cooper MR: Effect of age on therapeutic response and survival in advanced Hodgkin's disease. Cancer Treat Rep 66:889, 1982.
61. Kaslow RA, Wisch N, Class JL: Acute leukemia following cytotoxic therapy. JAMA 219:75, 1972.
62. Rai KR, Holland JF, Glidwell O: Improvement in remission induction therapy of acute myelocytic leukemia. Proc AACR/ASCO 16:265, 1975.
63. Berard CW, Gallo RC, Jaffe ES, et al: Current concepts of leukemia and lymphoma: etiology, pathogenesis, and therapy. Ann Intern Med 85:351–366, 1976.
64. Hoagland HC: Acute leukemia and its complications. Mayo Clin Proc 53:260–262, 1978.
65. Reiffers J, Raynal F, and Broustet A: Acute myeloblastic leukemia in elderly patients. Cancer 45:2816–2820, 1980.
66. Foon KA, Zighelboim J, Yale C, et al: Intensive chemotherapy is the treatment of choice for elderly patients with acute myelogenous leukemia. Blood 58:467–470, 1981.
67. Walters RS, Kantarjian HM, Keating MJ, et al: Intensive treatment of acute leukemia in adults 70 years of age and older. Cancer 60:149–155, 1987.
68. Berger S, Aledort LM, Gilbert HS, et al: Abnormalities of platelet function in patients with polycythemia vera. Cancer Res 33:2683–2688, 1973.
69. Lawrence JH, Winchell HS, Donald WC: Leukemia in polycythemia vera: Relationship to splenic myeloid metaplasia and therapeutic radiation dose. Ann Intern Med 70:763, 1969.
70. Landow SA: Acute leukemia in polycythemia vera. Semin Hematol 13:33, 1976.
71. Suen KC, Law LL, Yermakov V: Cancer and old age. An autopsy study of 3535 patients over 65 years old. Cancer 33:1164–1168, 1979.
72. Pistenma DA, Bagshaw MA: Prostatic adenocarcinoma. Postgrad Med 67:135–145, 1980.
73. Pistenma DA, McDougall IR, Kriss JP: Screening for bone metastasis: Are only scans necessary? JAMA 231:46–50, 1975.
74. Cooper JF, Fot A, Herschman HH, et al: A solid phase radioimmunoassay for prostatic acid phosphatase. J Urol 119:388–391, 1978.
75. Prout GR: Prostate gland. In Holland JF, Frei E, eds: Cancer Medicine. Philadelphia, Lea & Febiger, 1974, pp 1680–1694.
76. The Leuprolide Study Group: Leuprolide versus diethylstilbestrol for metastatic prostate cancer. N Engl J Med 311:1281–1286, 1984.
77. Seidmann H: Cancer of the breast: statistical and epidemiological data. Cancer 24:1355–1350, 1969.
78. Fisher B, et al: L-phenylalamine mustard in the

management of primary breast cancer. N Engl J Med 292:117–123, 1975.

79. Bonnadonna G et al: Combination chemotherapy as an adjuvant treatment in operable breast cancer. N Engl J Med 294:405–409, 1976.
80. Bonnadonna G et al: Dose response effect of adjuvant chemotherapy of breast cancer. N Engl J Med 304:10–17, 1981.
81. Carter SK, et al: Adjuvant chemotherapy of breast cancer. N Engl J Med 303:831–832, 1980.
82. Hellman S, Harvis JR, Levene MB: Radiation therapy of early carcinoma of the breast without mastectomy. Cancer 46:988–994, 1980.
83. McGuire WL, et al: Progesterone and estrogen receptors. Adv Intern Med 24:127–143, 1979.
84. Stewart HJ, Forrest APM, Gunn JM: The tamoxifen trial. In Mouridsen HT, Palshof T, eds: Breast Cancer—Experimental and Clinical Aspects. Oxford, Pergamon Press, 1980, pp 83–88.
85. Javes SE, Durie BGM, Salmon SD: Combination chemotherapy with adriamycin and cyclophosphamide for advanced breast cancer. Cancer 36:90–97, 1975.
86. Greegor DA: Occult blood testing for detection of asymptomatic colon cancer. Cancer 28:131–134, 1971.
87. Li MC, Ross ST: Chemoprophylaxis for patients with colorectal cancer. JAMA 235:2825–2828, 1976.
88. Mauligit C, et al: Adjuvant immunotherapy and chemo-immunotherapy in colorectal cancer. Cancer 40:2726–2730, 1977.
89. Kragelund E, Baklev I, Bardram L, et al: Resectability, operative mortality, and survival of patients in old age with carcinoma of the colon and rectum. Dis Col Rect 17:617–621, 1975.
90. Goligher JC: Current trends in the use of sphincter-saving excision in the treatment of carcinoma of the rectum. Cancer 50:2627–2632, 1982.
91. Hahn RG, Moertel CG, Schutt AJ, et al: A double blind comparison of intensive course 5-fluorouracil by oral versus intravenous route in the treatment of colorectal carcinoma. Cancer 35:1031–1035, 1975.
92. Moertel CG: Chemotherapy of gastrointestinal carcinoma. N Engl J Med 299:1049–1052, 1978.
93. Hanson M, Hansen HH, Dowbersowsky P: Long-term survival in small cell carcinoma of the lung. JAMA 244:247–250, 1980.
94. Pierson RL, Fijge PK, Buchsbawa HJ: Surgery for gynecologic malignancy in the aged. Obstet Gynecol 46:523–527, 1975.
95. American Cancer Society: Uterine cancer. In Cancer Facts and Figures. New York, American Cancer Society, 1980, p 16.

CHAPTER 35

Infections, Chemoprophylaxis, and Immunoprophylaxis

F. Marc LaForce
Gordon Meiklejohn

A person's age is not dependent upon the number of years that have passed over his head, but upon the number of colds that have passed through it.

Dr. Woods Hutchinson,
Dr. Shirley W. Wynne, quoted

GENERAL CONCEPTS

Infectious diseases cause 30 percent of deaths in a geriatric population and are the most frequent cause of hospitalization in the institutionalized elderly.[1] Several factors account for the importance of infectious problems in the elderly. First and most important is the presence of associated illnesses such as chronic pulmonary disease and obstructive uropathy that can interfere with the host's ability to deal with infectious challenges. In addition, host defenses become somewhat compromised with age.[2] Antibody production is not as vigorous, and waning cell-mediated immunity has been well documented in the elderly.

Host response to infectious agents is less vigorous with age. For example, elderly patients with pneumococcal bacteremia are less likely to be febrile compared to younger bacteremic patients with severe infection. An important generalization is to suspect infection when faced with an obscure illness in an elderly patient and to draw a blood culture in such a situation.

For the most part, infections in the elderly are similar to those seen in younger patients, although some infections, such as herpes zoster and tuberculosis, are more common in the elderly. The most important factor that differentiates infectious diseases in the young from those seen in the old is the presence of underlying disease. Confused, demented patients aspirate oral secretions and if pneumonia develops are more likely to have a clinical course complicated by superinfection. Correction or amelioration of metabolic and anatomic abnormalities can play a pivotal role in the successful management of such patients.

ANTIBIOTIC USE

The correct choice of antibiotics in an individual clinical situation requires assessment of the patient, knowledge of the pathogens likely to cause the infection, and local sensitivity patterns. It is generally best to rely, if possible, on narrow spectrum agents that are less likely to alter normal flora. Although several infectious disease experts have advocated the use of bactericidal agents in the elderly on the presumption that such patients frequently have depressed host defenses, the data supporting such a contention are meager.

By age 90 glomerular filtration rate, renal plasma flow, and tubular secretory capacity are about half the values noted in the second decade of life.[3] Quite naturally, this phenomenon will result in higher blood levels of penicillins and cephalosporins, agents that are filtered and secreted. Aminoglycosides are primarily excreted by glomerular filtration and will reach higher than expected levels in the elderly. Since these agents can be ototoxic and nephrotoxic at high serum concentrations, it is important that aminoglycoside levels be measured in these patients.

Of course, the usual caveats associated with prudent antimicrobial therapy such as obtaining smears of potentially infectious material, Gram stain interpretation of such smears, proper cultures, and local bacterial sensitivity patterns and costs must always be considered whenever an appropriate antibiotic regimen is being considered.

One tendency that should be resisted is the tendency to broaden antimicrobial coverage progressively when a patient is not doing as well as might be hoped. There are several reasons for apparent antibiotic failure, not the least of which is the presence of an undrained focus of infection or the fact that the diagnosis may be wrong. It is usually quite safe to discontinue antimicrobial therapy in order to reevaluate a patient. These patients are under observation, and antimicrobial therapy can be restarted quickly if necessary. All too frequently the broadening of antimicrobial coverage serves to comfort the physician with the notion that the patient is "covered" but delays the performance of diagnostic tests that might otherwise be done.

IMMUNIZATIONS

Routine immunizations which are appropriate for all elderly patients are summarized in Table 35–1.

Pneumococcal Vaccine

Pneumococcal vaccine contains purified capsular materials of the 23 types of *Streptococcus pneumoniae* that are responsible for 87 percent of recent bacteremic pneumococcal disease in the United States. Interest in this vaccine has been stimulated because mortality from pneumococcal bacteremia in the first 24 hours is unaffected by antibiotics and because pneumococcal strains resistant to penicillin and other antibiotics have been identified.

Pneumococcal vaccine is recommended for all persons over 65 years and for those patients with chronic cardiac, pulmonary, or other diseases who are expected to suffer a disproportionate amount of pneumococcal infections. However, the question of its efficacy in high-risk patients is being hotly debated. There is no question that pneumococcal vaccine was effective when tested in South African gold miners, a group of young men with extraordinarily high attack rates of pneumococcal pneumonia. However, U.S. vaccine efficacy studies have yielded conflicting results. Three cohort studies done in the United States during the last 10 years have all been negative including a randomized double-blind controlled study in high-risk U.S. veterans. The results of these studies have been debated vigorously, and the only sure resolution to this question would be to do a randomized controlled study using cases of pneumococcal bacteremia as endpoints. Such a study would require more than 100,000 participants over 60 years of age and is likely never to be done in the United States.

Epidemiologists at the Centers for Disease Control (CDC) have proposed a novel method for measuring the efficacy of pneumococcal vaccine based on the assumption that vaccinated patients should suffer fewer pneumococcal infections due to serotypes contained in the vaccine compared to serotype distribution in patients who were not immunized. The advantage of this technique is that it allows a calculation of vaccine efficacy when only the serotype distribution is known in vaccinated and unvaccinated persons. Their analysis suggests that the vaccine is effective in about 60 percent of presumably immunocompetent recipients. However, the CDC data on efficacy in high-risk pa-

TABLE 35–1. Routine Immunizations Recommended in Adults over 65 Years

Vaccine	Frequency
Tetanus/diphtheria	Primary series, then every 10 years
Pneumococcal	Single dose after age 65
Influenza	Yearly in the fall

tients, the group for whom the vaccine is being promoted, are meager.[4]

Given these conflicting data, what recommendations should be made on the use of pneumococcal vaccine? It is impossible to give a confident answer at present. Fortunately, pneumococcal vaccine is very safe and to the best of our knowledge needs only to be given once. We favor the recommendation that all persons over 65 years of age receive a single dose of pneumococcal vaccine, but we feel equally strongly that a large randomized trial of pneumococcal vaccine should be done.[5]

Influenza Vaccine

Current influenza vaccines are preparations of formalin-inactivated virus grown in the allantoic fluid of chick embryos. The vaccines are trivalent, containing equal amounts of the hemagglutinin (15 μg) of each of the three types of influenza that have been prevalent for the last 10 years. These are two subtypes of influenza A (A/H3N2 and A/H1N1) and influenza B. The vaccines are highly purified, and most of the pyrogenic components that plagued the earlier influenza vaccines have been removed.

The antigens contained in the vaccines are changed frequently to accommodate the continuing antigenic drift, particularly of the influenza A/H3N2 type. This virus, and to a lesser extent influenza B, account for most of the excess mortality that is associated with influenza in the elderly. The influenza A/H1N1 subtype has little impact on the elderly population, despite repeated outbreaks during the last 10 years in young individuals.

Vaccine should be given annually to all individuals over 65 years of age, particularly to those with pulmonary or cardiac disease, who run a high risk from influenza. The amount of protection provided by the vaccines will vary with the fit between the vaccine virus and the epidemic strain. There is evidence that, even though the person may not be completely protected against influenza, the rates of pneumonia and deaths are lower in people who have been vaccinated than in those who have not.[6]

In most years vaccination should be done in the early fall. However, individuals who have not been vaccinated should receive vaccine along with amantadine if influenza A appears at any time during the winter. This is particularly important in closed populations such as nursing homes or for individuals who are at particularly high risk who have close contact with persons with influenza. Amantadine should be continued for 2 weeks, by which time the individual should have developed sufficient immunity to be protected.

Reactions to the vaccine in the elderly are infrequent and minor and consist mainly of low-grade fever and a few hours of malaise, which can usually be controlled with analgesic preparations. Vaccine should not be given to individuals who have a definite history of allergy to eggs. Current vaccines are useful but are still far from optimal. Research continues on adjuvants that might enhance the antibody response and lengthen the duration of immunity and on live vaccines that might be more effective.

Tetanus and Diphtheria Toxoids

Tetanus is an unusual disease with a high mortality rate and when not fatal is associated with a great deal of morbidity. Because of comprehensive immunization programs that have been in place in the United States for several decades, tetanus cases are now predominantly seen in the elderly. Serologic studies have demonstrated that about half of all persons over 60 years old have protective levels of tetanus antitoxin. Cases of tetanus in the elderly have been associated with a variety of wounds such as diabetic ulcers, which are usually not considered tetanus-prone.

The disease is completely preventable with immunization, and tetanus toxoid is one of the most potent vaccines available to clinicians. Thus, the status of tetanus immunity should be reviewed in all patients. Persons who have not received a primary series should be immunized, and boosters should be provided every 10 years. To facilitate record keeping the CDC has recommended that mid-decade birthdays (65, 75, and 85) be used as convenient reminders for tetanus toxoid boosters.

Diphtheria is an uncommon disease in the elderly, but its toxoid is included in tetanus vaccines, and the use of Td (tetanus and diphtheria toxoid vaccine) is recommended on the grounds of clinical prudence.

CHEMOPROPHYLAXIS

Infective Endocarditis

Infective endocarditis can be a devastating illness and, like most diseases, is particularly severe in the elderly. Implantation of bacteria onto a damaged or prosthetic valve is the initial step in the pathogenesis of endocarditis; hence it has been argued that transient bacteremia can place certain patients at risk from implantation of bacteria onto valvular tissue. Although no randomized controlled studies have shown the efficacy of antimicrobial prophylaxis to prevent infective endocarditis, the anecdotal association of recent dental and urologic procedures with streptococcal endocarditis is persuasive enough to warrant prophylaxis.

Durack has developed a useful way of approaching the issue of antimicrobial prophylaxis by assessing the risk of developing endocarditis by the type of procedure being done (Table 35–2) and the underlying heart disease (Table 35–3). Many elderly patients with calcific valvular disease or prosthetic valves belong into the category of patients who need pharmacologic prophylaxis when invasive urologic or

TABLE 35–2. Risk of Endocarditis on the Basis of the Procedure Likely to Cause Bacteremia*

Significant risk
  Dental procedures likely to cause bleeding
    (scaling, extractions, or oral surgery)
  Urinary catheterization, passage of urethral
    dilators, cystoscopy, and prostatectomy
    (particularly in the presence of infected urine)
  Drainage of abscesses
Very low risk
  Cardiac catheterization
  Insertion of cardiac pacemaker
  Endotracheal intubation
  Diagnostic procedures
    Endoscopy of upper and lower gastrointestinal
      tract
    Barium enema
    Liver biopsy
    Fiberoptic bronchoscopy

*Modified from Durack DT: In Mandell GL, Douglas RG, Bennett JE, eds: Principles and Practices in Infectious Diseases, 2nd ed. New York, John Wiley, 1985.

TABLE 35–3. Risk of Endocarditis as Related to Underlying Heart Disease*

High risk
  Prosthetic valves
  Aortic valve disease
  Previous endocarditis
  Mitral stenosis or insufficiency
  Intra-atrial alimentation catheters
Moderate risk
  Tricuspid and pulmonary valve disease
Low risk
  Coronary artery disease
  Cardiac pacemakers
  Postcoronary artery bypass (no
    prosthetic implants)

*Modified from Durack DT: In Mandell GL, Douglas RG, Bennett JE, eds: Principles and Practice of Infectious Diseases, 2nd ed. New York, John Wiley, 1985.

dental procedures are being done. We agree with the recommendations for prophylaxis as proposed by Durack (Table 35–4).[7]

Influenza: Amantadine/ Rimantadine

Several properly designed controlled studies have shown that amantadine and rimantadine are effective chemoprophylactic agents that prevent influenza A. These drugs do not interfere with the antibody response to influenza vaccine and, as stated above, a recommended approach for dealing with a high-risk unprotected population during an epidemic is to vaccinate and treat persons with amantadine or rimantadine for 2 weeks, by which time protective antibody titers would be present.

These agents may have troublesome side effects. Rimantadine appears to be less toxic. These agents ought not to be thought of as substitutes for routine influenza immunization because they have no activity against influenza B, are more expensive than influenza vaccine, and have important side effects. We strongly favor routine immunization but use amantadine or rimantadine as prophylactic agents when influenza A/H3N2 subtype is prevalent in populations in which a significant number of elderly patients have not been protected. We do not recommend amantadine or rimantadine for influenza A H1N1 epidemics because this virus has not caused a significant amount of illness in elderly persons.

TABLE 35–4. Recommendations for the Prophylaxis of Endocarditis*

Procedure	Regimen
Dental procedures	Penicillin V 2 gm orally 1 h before, then 1 gm 6 h later
	Erythromycin 1 gm orally 1 h before, then 0.5 gm 6 h later
Minor gastrointestinal or genitourinary procedures	Amoxicillin 3 gm orally 1 h before, then 1.5 gm 6 h later
High-risk patients	Ampicillin 2 gm IM or IV plus gentamicin 1.5 mg/kg IM or IV 0.5 h before gastrointestinal or genitourinary procedures

*Modified from Durack DT: In Mandell GL, Douglas RG, Bennett JE, eds: Principles and Practice of Infectious Diseases, 2nd ed. New York, John Wiley, 1985.

ECTED INFECTIONS

umonia

Pneumonia is an important cause of morbidity and mortality in the elderly. About half of all hospital admissions for pneumonia are for persons over 65 years, and mortality from pneumonia increases sharply with age. Some series report mortality of greater than 30 percent in persons over 70 years of age.

Most elderly patients with lower respiratory tract infections complain of fever, shortness of breath, cough, and increased sputum production. The clinical approach to such patients is straightforward. If obtainable, a sputum sample should be smeared and Gram-stained. Particular attention should be paid to the cytologic characteristics of the sample, and if buccal epithelial cells are numerous, the smear should not be interpreted and the culture discarded. If polymorphonuclear leukocytes are the predominant cells, a careful review of the slide is appropriate, since initial therapy can be based on the flora seen on the smear. Consultation with trained laboratory technicians is often of great value.

The causative agents of pneumonia in the elderly include common pathogens such as the pneumococcus and *Haemophilus influenzae*. However, the probability of pneumonia due to coliforms is more real if the patient is admitted from an institutionalized setting, since oropharyngeal colonization with enteric gram-negative bacilli occurs more frequently in such populations. Treatment should be based on results of a sputum Gram stain if possible. In the absence of such information, we favor empiric therapy with ampicillin in areas where ampicillin-resistant *H. influenzae* is not a problem. In areas with ampicillin resistance therapy with a second-generation cephalosporin such as cefamandole is appropriate. It should be emphasized that there is no correct regimen but that local antimicrobial resistance patterns are important considerations. Staphylococcal coverage may be more important during an influenza epidemic.

Herpes Zoster

Herpes zoster is an important disease in the elderly because its incidence increases with each decade of life and because the frequency of post-herpetic pain is more troublesome with advancing age.[8] The disease is caused by varicella zoster virus (VZV) and represents a reactivation of a latent virus acquired in childhood. The virus resides in sensory neurons, most often in the thoracolumbar area of the cord or in the fifth nerve, particularly the ophthalmic branch. The disease is characterized by a vesicular rash in a dermatomal distribution. The rash is often preceded by a burning or painful sensation. The rash usually appears 2 to 5 days after the beginning of pain and is unilateral. It does not cross the midline. The lesions resemble those of chickenpox and go through a rapid evolution from papules to vesicles to crusted lesions during a period of approximately a week. Pain in the affected dermatome often persists for 1 to 6 months, longer in more elderly individuals. A number of varicelliform lesions may be seen on other parts of the body, and occasionally a full-blown rash resembling varicella may occur.

Second attacks of zoster are relatively infrequent. When they occur in the ophthalmic branch of the fifth nerve, consideration should be given to the possibility of a zosteriform type of herpes simplex infection. The latter is important because it may lead to serious damage to the eye.

Before the appearance of the rash, the diagnosis of herpes zoster may be confused with many other causes of pain, such as pleurisy, appendicitis, or a collapsed intervertebral disc; these mistakes occasionally result in unnecessary surgery. After the rash appears, the diagnosis is almost always obvious. Confirmation of the diagnosis may be made by Tzanck smear, virus isolation, or one of a number of serologic tests for VZV.

Post-herpetic neuralgia can often be relieved by analgesics. Patients with only a small number of varicelliform lesions that are distant from the affected dermatome usually recover uneventfully. Those with extensive rashes may have visceral involvement and should be treated with acyclovir. This drug is highly effective in preventing viral multiplication. Steroids given during the early eruptive phase have been reported to reduce the incidence and severity of post-herpetic neuralgia. They should not be given to immunocompromized patients because of the danger of dissemination. Patients with VZV infection of the eye should be seen by an ophthalmologist.

Tuberculosis

The elderly are an important reservoir of tuberculous infection because many were infected decades earlier at a time when tuberculous infection was far more common than it is today. Cellular immunity wanes with age, and it is not surprising that some latent infections become active as persons become older. Recent epidemiologic studies of outbreaks of tuberculosis in nursing homes have also suggested that the elderly are susceptible to reinfection.

Tuberculosis in the elderly is a less dramatic illness when compared to disease in younger patients. In a recent series only one-third of elderly patients with active pulmonary tuberculosis complained of fever and weight loss.[9] Chest x-rays often suggest the diagnosis, and positive Ziehl-Neelsen smears are diagnostic in the appropriate setting. Occasionally the diagnosis is delayed when infiltrates on chest x-ray are felt to be due to old disease. The

most important step in the diagnosis of tuberculosis is suspecting its presence.

Short-term (9-month) therapy with isoniazid and rifampin has revolutionized the treatment of tuberculosis. There is ample clinical data to suggest that such a regimen is fully effective in the elderly.

The discovery of a patient with tuberculosis should trigger a report to state health authorities and an epidemiologic investigation. This is particularly true the infectious patient has been bedded a closed setting. All exposed patients staff should be skin tested, and if to be new converters they shoul fered isoniazid chemoprophyla year.

Some epidemiologists have that all patients admitted homes be skin tested and that tho to be positive should be given iso prophylaxis regardless of their chest x ay findings. Such a recommendation is controversial, and we favor a more conservative approach whereby patients above age 65 are offered isoniazid chemoprophylaxis when they have both positive skin test and a second risk factor such as recen PPD conversion or gastrectomy.

Urinary Tract Infections

Asymptomatic bacteriuria is a freque finding in the elderly and is associated with a significant reduction in survival not related to an increased incidence of fatal genitourinary infections. The exact meaning of this interesting but puzzling observation is unclear. Controlled studies have shown that routine bacteriologic screening of asymptomatic elderly with treatment of bacteriuric episodes has not decreased morbidity or mortality, and routine culturing of urine is not recommended.

Prostatic hypertrophy and renal stones predispose patients to more frequent and more serious urinary tract infections. An episode of urosepsis in a male patient ought to suggest the presence of obstruction or a prostatic source and necessitates evaluation.

The use of indwelling bladder catheters is far more common in the elderly. Over a period of time chronic bladder colonization with enterics is the rule in such pa-

25. Chernoff R, Mitchell CO, Lipschitz DA: Assessment of the nutritional status of the geriatric patient. Geriatr Med Today 3(5):129–141, 1984.
26. Chumlea WC, Steinbaugh ML, Roche AF, et al: Nutritional anthropometric assessment in elderly persons 65 to 90 years of age. J Nutr Elderly 4:39, 1985.
27. Lynch SR, Finch CA, Monson ER, et al: Iron status of elderly Americans. Am J Clin Nutr 36:1032–1045, 1982.
28. Lipschitz DA, Mitchell CO: The correctability of the nutritional, immune, and hematopoietic manifestations of protein calorie malnutrition in the elderly. J Am Coll Nutr 1:17–25, 1982.

CHAPTER 37

Management of Constipation and Diarrhea

John W. Singleton

I am profoundly grateful to old age, which has increased my eagerness for conversation and taken away that for food and drink. (Habeoque senectuti magnam gratiam, quæ mihi sermonis aviditatem auxit, potionis et cibi sustulit.)

CICERO, *De Senectute*

CONSTIPATION

Definition

Constipation is a symptom, and therefore each patient defines the word for himself or herself. Bowel frequency is one element of the definition. A survey of an apparently healthy North Carolina adult population revealed that 95 percent had three or more bowel movements per week.[1] A stool frequency of less than this could be considered constipation. A second element is stool consistency; hard, scybalous stools would be considered a characteristic of constipation by many patients. A third element is ease of passage. The necessity of straining in order to pass a stool of whatever character would be interpreted by many patients as constipation. Certainly the discovery of fecal impaction makes the diagnosis of constipation.

Popular mythology assigns constipation as one of the ills of old age. However, there are few objective data to substantiate this conception.[2] As a practical matter, constipation in an older person raises the same differential diagnosis and requires the same careful attention as it does in a younger patient.

Work-up

As with every other gastrointestinal complaint, work-up of constipation begins with a careful, detailed history. Bowel function, diet, medication, prior or current illness, and prior surgery deserve special attention. Medications that may cause constipation are listed in Table 37–1.

Diseases associated with constipation are listed in Table 37–2. The patient's history or physical findings may suggest one of these diseases. For example, a woman who has had a mastectomy for breast carcinoma and has bone pain might be constipated as a result of hypercalcemia.

A general physical examination should be performed, keeping in mind the conditions listed in Table 37–2. Abdominal examination may reveal hard feces in the descending or sigmoid colon, an abdominal tumor, or evidence of prior surgery. A digital rectal examination and test of the stool for occult blood should *always* be performed. Evidence of abnormal sphincter tone, anal tenderness suggesting an anal fissure or distal proctitis, or a perianal fistula should lead to a proctoscopic examination. A finding of fecal impaction requires disimpaction (see below) and consideration of its cause. Gross or occult

TABLE 37–1. Medications That May Cause Constipation

Opiate analgesics
Antacids, especially those not containing Magnesium
Anticholinergic agents
Anticonvulsants
Anti-Parkinson agents
Ganglionic blockers
Diuretics
Iron
Antihypertensive agents
Psychotherapeutic drugs
Contraceptive steroids
Monoamine oxidase inhibitors

TABLE 37–2. Diseases That May Be Complicated by Constipation

Metabolic and endocrine diseases
  Diabetes mellitus
  Porphyria
  Lead poisoning
  Hypokalemia
  Hypothyroidism
  Hypercalcemia
Neuromuscular disorders
  Chagas' disease
  Autonomic neuropathy
  Cauda equina tumor
  Trauma to the lumbosacral cord
  Paraplegia
  Tabes dorsalis
  Multiple sclerosis
  Myotonic dystrophy
  Systemic sclerosis
  Dermatomyositis
  Parkinson's disease
  Cerebrovascular disease
  Intracranial tumor
Colonic diseases
  Tumors
  Volvulus
  Hernias, internal and external
  Intussusception
  Inflammatory strictures
    Diverticular disease
    Lymphogranuloma venereum
    Syphilis
    Tuberculosis
    Crohn's disease
    Ischemic disease
    Endometriosis
  Ulcerative proctitis
  Diverticular disease
Anorectal diseases
  Rectocele
  Anal stenosis
  Anal fissure
  Perianal abscess
  Rectal prolapse
  Hemorrhoids

blood in the stool dictates a search for the bleeding lesion that may be the cause of the constipation.

Further work-up will depend on the findings thus far. If the history of constipation is short (i.e., under 1 week), the possibility of intestinal obstruction should be excluded by abdominal x-ray films taken both flat and upright, looking for air-fluid levels and bowel distention. If the problem is of longer duration, the physical examination is unrevealing, and none of the listed extraintestinal conditions that predispose to constipation is present, a colonic disorder should be sought by means of a double contrast barium enema and sigmoidoscopic examination.

Diagnosis

Several organic diseases of the colon can result in chronic constipation. Most important for the elderly patient is carcinoma. Carcinomas of the left colon cause partial obstruction and symptoms of pain and constipation relatively early in their course, in contrast to right-sided carcinomas, which more commonly present with occult bleeding and anemia or melena. Diverticular disease of the left colon may similarly present with constipation. Similarly, ischemic damage to the colon can be localized and may result in stricture. Idiopathic chronic ulcerative colitis is usually extensive when it presents in an elderly person, but it can affect only the distal rectum, where it causes constipation accompanied by passage of bloody purulent mucus concomitant with or independently of firm stool.

Recent years have seen some advances in our understanding of colonic motor disorders leading to constipation.[3] Two distinct mechanisms now appear to underlie most cases of severe idiopathic constipation: slowed colonic transit and failure of rectal expulsion. These can be elucidated by relatively simple physiologic studies. Slowed transit can be documented by studying the pattern of elimination of radiopaque markers by means of serial flat abdominal x-rays.[4] Failure of rectal expulsion is diagnosed at anal manometry by observing the patient's ability to expel a water-filled tethered balloon introduced into the rectum.[5] These rare but objectively demonstrable abnormalities of colonic motor function explain some cases of constipation that are refractory to conventional management.

Management

Certainly the most common cause of constipation in Americans, young and old, is the fiber-poor diet traditional in this society. Three simple modifications of patients' daily routine address this problem: (1) add 5 to 15 gm of dietary fiber to the daily diet, (2) ensure a fluid intake of at least 2 liters daily, more in hot weather, and (3) establish a daily routine for bowel evacuation—usually soon after breakfast or supper, when the gastroileocolic reflex will assist in stimulating colonic motility. Adding fluid and fiber to the diet can eliminate the need for laxatives in more than 90 percent of elderly persons with simple constipation, according to one recent study.[6]

Fecal impaction can present as diarrhea—thus the importance of the digital rectal examination in every patient. Occasionally stool may become impacted in the sigmoid colon, where it can be seen on abdominal x-ray. If impaction is present, it must be removed before investigation and subsequent bowel retraining can be accomplished. This is best done by administration of an oil-retention enema followed by manual disimpaction. Enemas made by dissolving 1 to 2 gm of dioctyl sodium sulfosuccinate in a quart of warm tapwater may also be useful. Once the impaction is cleared, a cathartic such as magnesium citrate 200 ml or bisacodyl 1 tablet each hour for three to five doses should be administered to clean the proximal colon. The patient should then be given a high-fiber intake plus 200 mg of dioctyl sodium sulfosuccinate and a fluid intake of 2 liters daily to prevent reimpaction. Bowel training should be pursued by establishing a regular daily time for bowel action. A glycerine suppository may be administered if no stool appears for 2 days, and if none is passed by the third day, a saline enema may be administered. Some patients with chronic constipation are benefited by daily administration of lactulose, 30 to 60 gm in two doses. Lactulose is poorly absorbed, and its metabolism by fecal bacteria gives rise to short-chain fatty acids that are osmotically active and stimulate water and sodium secretion by the colon.

So-called irritant laxatives (phenolphthalein, senna, cascara, anthraquinones, bisacodyl) should be avoided because dependence on them leads to permanent changes in colonic motility—the laxative colon. It is usually very difficult to wean such a dependent patient and colon from these drugs.

Colonic Pseudo-obstruction

Marked dilatation of the colon, to cecal diameters in excess of 10 cm, occurs in a wide variety of acute settings and, more rarely, as a chronic condition. In the acute situation attention should be directed to correction of the underlying metabolic, infectious, or circulatory abnormality, and colonoscopic decompression should be considered when cecal caliber reaches 10 to 12 cm in order to avoid cecal perforation.[7] Chronic colonic pseudo-obstruction is much rarer. Abnormalities of colonic myenteric nerves have been found in some cases, and ileostomy is sometimes required for treatment.[8]

DIARRHEA

Definition

Like constipation, diarrhea is a symptom. Its definition in any individual case depends largely on the patient's perceptions. It is always necessary to ascertain exactly what the patient means by diarrhea. Often it will be an increase in number of formed stools, incontinence, or laxative-induced loose stool. However, some objective standards are available. Daily output of stool by weight in normal individuals on a standard American diet rarely exceeds 200 gm; daily stool weights in excess of 200 gm constitute diarrhea.[9]

In evaluating a patient's complaint of diarrhea, it is very useful for the physician to inspect the patient's stool. What the patient regards as diarrhea may turn out to be formed stool passed in several small movements daily. Further, presence of mucus, pus, blood, foul odor, fat droplets, and pale foamy stool are characteristics that are helpful in diagnosing the cause of the diarrhea. Mucus, pus, or bright blood suggests a distal colonic ulcerating lesion. Foul odor and foamy, greasy stool suggest small bowel malabsorption. Fat droplets suggest pancreatic insufficiency.

Work-up

ACUTE DIARRHEA. It is helpful to divide diarrhea into acute and chronic forms, the dividing line between the two being a duration of 2 weeks since onset. As with constipation, a careful detailed history is the most helpful diagnostic technique. A history of similar cases in the immediate environment, recent travel, unusual exposure, or new medication will often provide a presumptive diagnosis of acute diarrhea. A history of antibiotic administration within 2 weeks of the time of onset should bring *Clostridium difficile* to mind.

Acute diarrhea of only a few days' duration is best managed symptomatically, with diagnostic studies postponed in anticipation of its spontaneous resolution. Most cases will turn out to be self-limited and infectious in etiology. When fever and toxicity are present, however, the stool should be examined for fecal leukocytes, stool culture, and ova and parasites. A history of antibiotic administration should lead to a search for the toxin of *C. difficile* in the stool. If an enteric pathogen is found, specific treatment is usually indicated (see below). If no pathogen is found and diarrhea persists, sigmoidoscopy and further work-up as for chronic diarrhea are indicated.

CHRONIC DIARRHEA. The approach to diarrhea of more than 2 weeks' duration is somewhat different because it cannot be anticipated that it will clear spontaneously. Here again, a careful history is all important. Circumstances surrounding the onset of the diarrhea are particularly revealing; inquire about a new living arrangement, new medication, abdominal surgery, travel, or other unusual exposure. The temporal and symptomatic pattern of the diarrhea is significant. Small bowel diarrhea is characteristically infrequent (three to five times daily), and each stool is large in volume and may be accompanied by periumbilical crampy pain and bloating. Diarrhea due to disease of the distal colon produces frequent stools (10 to 30/day) that are small in volume ("little squirts"), contain blood, mucus or pus, and are accompanied by tenesmus.

The majority of patients seeking care for chronic diarrhea have so-called functional symptoms. This is probably true of geriatric patients as well as younger people. It is important to be able to recognize the pattern of such symptoms. A long history, perhaps life-long, of bowel dysfunction suggests that the present symptoms have a functional basis. Alternating diarrhea and constipation, often complicated by intermittent laxative use, is a characteristic pattern of functional bowel disorder. Presence or absence of nocturnal diarrhea is

a useful diagnostic clue. Diarrhea that comes only during the waking hours is often functional. Diarrhea that wakes the patient from sleep is more likely to have an organic cause. The new onset of chronic diarrhea in a geriatric patient with previously normal bowel habit should precipitate a thorough diagnostic work-up.

A complete physical examination, always including a digital rectal examination, may reveal the cause of chronic diarrhea in the old person to be congestive heart failure, an abdominal tumor, fecal impaction, or a rectal tumor. Complete blood count, chemistries, and urinalysis should be done to uncover anemia, diabetes, or uremia.

If the history and visual inspection of the stool verify that the patient does have diarrhea, culture and examination for ova and parasites on a liquid stool should be done. Several of the organisms that cause acute diarrhea can persist to cause chronic diarrhea as well: *Entamoeba histolytica, Campylobacter jejunii, Salmonella, Yersinia,* and *Giardia,* among others.

Flexible sigmoidoscopy may be performed at the same time as the stool examination or certainly following a negative report of the stool examination. It is best performed with no prior preparation other than a recent bowel movement, especially if the changes of mild ulcerative colitis are to be appreciated. Idiopathic or infectious proctosigmoiditis, ischemic colitis, diverticulitis, and colon cancer in the inspected segment can thus be diagnosed or ruled out. Biopsy of abnormal-appearing mucosa should be done to exclude collagenous or microscopic colitis.[10]

If the results of the flexible sigmoidoscopic examination are negative, a double contrast barium enema x-ray should be done. This sequence is especially appropriate for geriatric patients because of the high prevalence of colon cancer, diverticular disease, and ischemic colitis in such patients. If the colon is normal on barium examination, consideration should be given to the possibility of gastric, pancreatic, or small bowel disease causing secretory, inflammatory, or malabsorptive diarrhea.

Secretory diarrhea is characterized by persistence of diarrhea in spite of withdrawal of all oral intake (with support by intravenous fluid administration) for 72

TABLE 37–3. Causes of Secretory Diarrhea

Laxative abuse
Pancreatic islet cell tumor
Medullary carcinoma of thyroid
Gastrin-secreting tumor or hyperplasia
(Zollinger-Ellison syndrome)
Malignant carcinoid syndrome
Secreting villous adenoma
Idiopathic secretory diarrhea
Congenital chloridorrhea

hours. Known causes of secretory diarrhea are listed in Table 37–3. Special attention must be given to the possibility of factitious diarrhea due to laxative abuse. Secretory diarrhea caused by abnormal peptide secretion (gastrin, vasoactive intestinal peptide, and so on) is rare.

Malabsorptive diarrhea characteristically ceases when oral intake is stopped. The most common cause of malabsorptive diarrhea is lactose intolerance due to intestinal mucosal lactase deficiency. Lactase deficiency is characteristic of persons of Asian or black ancestry and should always be sought by history. Withdrawal of all lactose-containing milk products (hard cheese and butter contain little lactose and need not be withdrawn) is often useful as a therapeutic trial early in the work-up of chronic diarrhea. Other causes of malabsorptive diarrhea are given in Table 37–4. Curiously enough, many of the conditions listed in Table 37–4 present in middle age or later and so must be considered in chronic malabsorptive diarrhea. The most useful screening test for steatorrhea is the ^{14}C-triolein breath test. More accurate but much more expensive and cumbersome is a 72 hour stool collection analyzed for fat.

TABLE 37–4. Causes of Malabsorptive Diarrhea

Lactose intolerance (lactase deficiency)
Nontropical sprue (adult celiac disease)
Fructose malabsorption
Mannitol or sorbitol ingestion (in "sugarless" chewing gum)
Poorly absorbed salts: Mg^{++}, phosphate, citrate, sulfate
Whipple's disease
Extensive Crohn's disease
Radiation damage to small bowel mucosa
Chemotherapeutic agent damage to small bowel mucosa
Hypogammaglobulinemia
Intestinal lymphoma
Intestinal amyloidosis
Intestinal lymphangiectasia
Carcinomatosis

Microscopic examination of a single stool sample for fat is so inaccurate as to be useless. If ^{14}C-triolein or stool fat test results indicate steatorrhea, further work-up should aim to distinguish pancreatic insufficiency from primary small bowel disease. Results of the D-xylose absorption test are normal in pancreatic insufficiency but abnormal in small bowel mucosal disease. An abnormal D-xylose test result would lead to a small bowel barium x-ray, small bowel biopsy, and perhaps small bowel culture. A normal D-xylose test result in spite of steatorrhea focuses attention on the pancreas. Plain abdominal films may show pancreatic calcification, and diabetes may be present; there may be a history of pain, alcoholism, or weight loss to further support the diagnosis of chronic pancreatitis with pancreatic insufficiency.

Management of Diarrhea

Acute diarrhea without systemic symptoms of fever or leukocytosis is usually self-limited and requires only that dehydration be avoided. Glucose-containing electrolyte solution should be given by mouth and other food and fluids withheld until diarrhea subsides (Table 37–5). Loperamide, 2 mg two to four times daily, may improve the patient's comfort. This drug is preferred to diphenoxylate because it is nonaddicting and has little effect on the sensorium. If an infectious agent is identified on stool examination, specific therapy should be prescribed as indicated in Table 37–6.

Treatment of chronic diarrhea is much more complicated. If the work-up reveals a cause or pathophysiologic condition that underlies the symptom, treatment decisions may be easy. There will always be

TABLE 37–5. Glucose-Electrolyte Solution (Cholera Solution) for Oral Treatment of Dehydrating Diarrhea

4 tablespoons table sugar (sucrose) or glucose
½ teaspoon baking soda (sodium bicarbonate)
¼ teaspoon table salt (sodium chloride)
¼ teaspoon "Adolph's Salt Substitute" (potassium chloride)

Dissolve above ingredients in 1 quart of potable drinking water. It may be flavored with citric acid crystals or lemon juice.

TABLE 37–6. Specific Therapy for Infectious Diarrhea

Amebiasis	Metronidazole, 750 mg P.O. tid × 5–10 days
	plus
	Diiodohydroxyquin, 650 mg tid × 20 days
Giardiasis	Metronidazole, 250 mg P.O. tid × 10 days
Campylobacter jejunii	Erythromycin, 250 mg qid × 5 days
Shigella	Trimethoprim-sulfamethoxazole, 1 "double-strength" tablet qid × 5 days
	or
	Tetracycline, 2.4 gm in a single oral dose
Salmonella	Antibiotic therapy of acute diarrhea prolongs the carrier state and is contraindicated.
Clostridium difficile	Vancomycin, 250 mg P.O. tid × 10 days

patients, however, in whom no specific organic cause for diarrhea can be found. Most such patients will be thought to have a disorder of gastrointestinal motility[11] or a manifestation of irritable bowel syndrome. For such patients trials of psyllium to give form to the stool, loperamide to slow colonic transit and increase colonic fluid absorption, or cholestyramine to bind bile salts in the intestinal lumen may yield useful results.

References

1. Drossman DA, Sander RS, McKee DC, et al: Bowel patterns among subjects not seeking health care. Gastroenterology 83:529, 1982.
2. Kallman H: Constipation in the elderly. Am Fam Physician 27:179, 1983.
3. Read NW, Timms JM: Defecation and the pathophysiology of constipation. Clin Gastroenterol 15:937, 1986.
4. Hinton JM, Lennard-Jones JE, Young AC, et al: A new method for studying gut transit times using radio-opaque markers. Gut 10:842, 1969.
5. Turnbull GK, Lennard-Jones JE, Bartram CI, et al: Failure of rectal expulsion as a cause of constipation: why fibre and laxatives sometimes fail. Lancet 1:767, 1986.
6. Hope AK, Down EC: Dietary fibre and fluid in the control of constipation in a nursing home population. Med J Aust 144:306, 1986.
7. Fausel CS, Goff JS: Nonoperative management of acute idiopathic colonic pseudo-obstruction (Ogilvie's syndrome). West J Med 143:50, 1985.
8. Anuras S, Shirazi SS: Colonic pseudoobstruction. Gastroenterology 79:525, 1984.
9. Krejs GJ, Fordtran JS: Diarrhea. *In* Sleisenger MH, Fordtran JS, eds: Gastrointestinal Disease, 3rd ed. Philadelphia, W.B. Saunders, 1983, p 257 ff.
10. Jessurun J, Yardley JH, Lee EL, et al: Microscopic and collagenous colitis: different names for the same condition? Gastroenterology 91:1583, 1986.
11. Fordtran JS, Santa Ana CA, Morawski SE, et al: Pathophysiology of chronic diarrhoea: insights derived from intestinal perfusion studies in 31 patients. Clin Gastroenterol 15:477, 1986.

CHAPTER 38

Hepatobiliary Disease

John M. Vierling

Let me play the fool:
With mirth and laughter let old wrinkles come,
And let my liver rather heat with wine
Than my heart cool with mortifying groans.
Why should a man, whose blood is warm within,
Sit like his grandsire cut in alabaster?
SHAKESPEARE, *The Merchant of Venice*

The liver and biliary tract perform a variety of functions that are integrally related to health. The liver is the principal site of synthesis for plasma proteins, glycoproteins, and lipoproteins as well as the site of uptake, conjugation, and excretion of bilirubin, the synthesis of cholesterol, and the elaboration of bile. The liver is also the principal site of alcohol metabolism, biotransformation of medications and xenobiotics, and metabolism of trace elements such as copper. An intact biliary tract is required for normal function of the hepatocytes as well as for delivery of bile to the intestine, where it is required for the digestion of fats and absorption of fat-soluble vitamins.

Despite increasing knowledge of normal hepatic physiologic function, the relationship between normal physiologic changes occurring with age and susceptibility to disease is poorly understood. Although none of the major hepatobiliary diseases afflicting elderly patients occurs uniquely in this age group, several diseases are particularly important because of their severity in the elderly or because of their increased incidence in this age group. The diseases discussed in this chapter are listed in Table 38–1.

LIVER

Alterations in Hepatic Physiology with Aging

Several alterations of hepatic physiologic function have been described in man and animals during aging. Despite these alterations, however, the large functional reserve of the human liver appears to protect the elderly from significant reductions in hepatic function. After the age of 50 both total body weight and liver weight decrease. The weight of the liver, which is approximately 2.5 percent of body weight prior to age 50, decreases to a mean of 1.6 percent by age 90.[1] The decrease in weight is associated with a decreased number of hepatic cells, increased binucleate cells, and increased nuclear volume. Histologically, the liver in elderly patients often shows enlarged hepatocytes, enlarged nuclei, multiple nucleoli, and deposition of lipofuscin pigment.[2, 3]

Despite diminished mass and altered morphology, levels of aminotransferase and bilirubin are unchanged by normal

TABLE 38–1. Hepatobiliary Topics Discussed

Liver
Viral hepatitis
Hepatotoxicity of medications
Chronic hepatitis
Primary biliary cirrhosis
Primary sclerosing cholangitis
Alpha-1-antitrypsin deficiency
Hemochromatosis
Alcoholic liver disease
Cirrhosis and complications
  Ascites and edema
  Bacterial peritonitis
  Coagulopathy and
    thrombocytopenia
  Variceal hemorrhage
Cardiac failure
Neoplasia
Transplantation
Gallbladder and Bile Ducts
Cholelithiasis
Acute cholecystitis
Chronic cholecystitis
Choledocholithiasis
Acute cholangitis
Carcinoma
  Gallbladder
  Extrahepatic bile ducts

aging. Hepatic synthesis of major serum proteins is substantially unaltered. However, serum albumin may be reduced in elderly patients who have decreased mobility.[4]

As cardiac output diminishes during aging, hepatic blood flow also decreases. Concurrently, the activity of microsomal oxidative enzymes also diminishes, and decreased metabolism of antipyrine, aminopyrine, chlorodiazapoxide, and meperidine is observed.[5, 6] Because of diminished blood flow and diminished activity of the microsomal oxidative enzymes, there is decreased clearance of drugs whose extraction ratio is low and whose metabolism depends on microsomal enzymes.[7] Aging, however, has little effect on the metabolism of drugs conjugated by glucuronidation.[8]

DISEASES OF THE LIVER

The incidence and prevalence of liver diseases in the elderly appear to be decreased compared to those in the entire population. This is the result of the morbidity and mortality of liver diseases among younger patients. However, the impact of a variety of liver diseases is severe in the elderly population. The major clinical manifestations leading to diagnostic evaluation of elderly patients for liver disease include jaundice, hepatomegaly, abnormal liver test results and coagulopathy. Manifestations of less severe liver disease often are nonspecific and are associated with vague symptoms of malaise, fatigability, diminished appetite, weight loss, nausea, or vomiting. Still other patients are entirely asymptomatic but are found to have abnormal liver test results on screening blood chemistries.

Assessment of Liver Function

Studies of standard laboratory tests reveal no abnormalities of bilirubin, aminotransferases, or albumin in healthy elderly persons. In contrast, great interest and controversy exist concerning age-related changes in alkaline phosphatase. Some studies indicate an increase in "normal"

alkaline phosphatase concentration during aging, whereas others report that alkaline phosphatase is unchanged.[9, 10] Interpretation of these data is difficult because patients with occult liver disease, Paget's disease, or metabolic bone disease may have been included in the study groups. In one study in which patients were selected on the basis of normal liver biopsy, alkaline phosphatase levels were normal.[10]

Several reports indicate that the uptake and excretion of sulfobromophthalein (BSP) is abnormal in the elderly, but other reports disagree.[11, 12] However, indocyanine green clearance may decrease as a result of diminished hepatic blood flow. Tests of true hepatic function such as aminopyrine clearance, galactose elimination, or caffeine clearance have not been systematically studied in this age group.

Viral Hepatitis

Viral hepatitis may be caused by the hepatitis A virus, hepatitis B virus, non-A, non-B viruses, hepatitis D (delta) virus in patients with hepatitis B, and, more rarely, by Epstein-Barr virus or cytomegalovirus. After 60 years of age, the incidence of hepatitis A decreases while that of hepatitis B and non-A, non-B increases.[13] The decrease in hepatitis A reflects the increased prevalence of immunity (antibody to hepatitis A), which reaches a peak after 50 years of age. The relative increase in hepatitis B and non-A, non-B hepatitis appears to be the consequence of increased blood transfusion in the aged.

Different types of viral hepatitis have similar clinical symptoms. Symptoms of typical viral hepatitis include malaise, anorexia, nausea, vomiting, diarrhea, and right upper quadrant discomfort. Urticarial rash, arthralgia, or arthritis may occur as a prodrome to hepatitis B. As jaundice develops, patients also note dark urine. When jaundice is minimal or absent, symptoms are often misdiagnosed as a flulike illness. It is noteworthy that some elderly patients may present with altered mental status or depression. On physical examination, the majority exhibit tender hepatomegaly and mild jaundice. Aminotransferase levels are usually elevated more than 10 times, whereas elevations of alkaline phosphatase and bilirubin are less striking. Although epidemiologic features and clinical findings may suggest the type of viral hepatitis, confirmation requires the performance of specific serologic tests (Table 38–2).

Viral hepatitis exhibits increased morbidity and mortality in individuals over the age of 40 years.[14] Elderly patients have more severe symptoms and a more prolonged course of biochemical abnormalities than younger patients. It is reasonable to consider hospitalization in all patients over 60 years of age with acute viral hepatitis because of the severity of illness, the potential for compromised hydration and nutrition, and the need for diagnostic evaluation to exclude biliary obstruction. Despite the potential for a fulminant or prolonged course, acute hepatitis A typically resolves within 1 to 3 months. There is no chronic disease potential. In contrast, chronic hepatitis and cirrhosis occur in approximately 3 to 5 percent of patients with hepatitis B and up to 55 percent of patients with non-A, non-B hepatitis related to transfusion.

There is no curative therapy for acute viral hepatitis. Bedrest is indicated in symptomatic patients but does not change the course of the illness. A well-balanced, normal calorie, high-protein diet should be encouraged. If nausea and anorexia are present, the majority of calories should be ingested at breakfast because these symptoms are minimal during the morning. If oral intake is inadequate or results in nausea and vomiting, intravenous hydration or hyperalimentation may be required. Sedatives and tranquilizers are contraindicated because they may precipitate hepatic encephalopathy. Corticosteroids have no place in the treatment of acute viral hepatitis regardless of its severity. Currently, studies are in progress to evaluate the efficacy of interferon in the treatment of acute viral hepatitis B.

Even though the majority of patients with acute viral hepatitis recover without sequelae, mortality is increased in patients over the age of 60 years compared with younger individuals. In this older age group, mortality ranges between 3 and 6 percent[14] compared with 0.1 to 1 percent in the younger population. The principal cause of death is hepatocellular failure. Clinically, this is associated with hepatic encephalopathy, diminishing liver size, prolongation of prothrombin time, stable or diminishing aminotransferase levels, and hypoglycemia.[15]

Hepatotoxicity of Medications

Elderly patients are at increased risk for hepatotoxic reactions because of the increased use of medications in this age group and because of the alterations in drug metabolism that occur in older people.[7] The severity of hepatotoxic drug reactions ranges from benign and reversible to fulminant and lethal. The possibility of liver injury caused by medications should

TABLE 38–2. Interpretation of Serologic Tests in Acute Liver Disease

HBsAg	IgM Anti-HBc	IgM Anti-HAV	IgM Anti-Delta	Interpretation
+	+	–	–	Acute hepatitis B
–	+	–	–	Acute hepatitis B
–	–	+	–	Acute hepatitis A
+	–	+	–	Acute hepatitis A in chronic hepatitis B carrier
+	–	–	+	Acute hepatitis D (delta) in chronic hepatitis B carrier
+	–	–	–	Acute non-A, non-B (NANB) or other injury in chronic hepatitis B carrier
–	–	–	–	Acute NANB or other injury

be considered in all elderly patients with liver disease or abnormal liver test results. In this setting, all but the most urgently required medications should be discontinued. For drugs that are urgently needed, alternative agents should be sought. In Table 38–3 are listed agents associated with lesions of chronic hepatitis. Discontinuation of the offending drug usually results in resolution of the hepatic abnormalities. With some agents, particularly isoniazid, increasing age predisposes the patient to an increased frequency of hepatotoxicity. For example, between the ages of 20 and 34 years, 0.3 percent of patients receiving isoniazid develop hepatic abnormalities. This figure increases to 1.2 percent between the ages of 35 and 49 years, and 2.3 percent after the age of 50.[16]

Chronic Hepatitis

Chronic hepatitis is defined as persistent inflammation of the liver for at least 6 months. Since morphologic features indistinguishable from chronic hepatitis may occur in resolving acute hepatitis, liver biopsy should not be performed until 6 months of disease has elapsed. Two types of chronic hepatitis are recognized histologically. Chronic persistent hepatitis is a benign disease characterized by portal tract inflammation with lymphocytes, minimal focal lobular necrosis, and absence of piecemeal necrosis of periportal hepatocytes or fibrosis. The disease does not progress and requires no treatment. In contrast, chronic active hepatitis is characterized by piecemeal necrosis of periportal hepatocytes and bridging necrosis or multilobular necrosis with collapse. The disease may progress to fibrosis, cirrhosis, and portal hypertension and may culminate in liver failure. The principal causes of chronic active hepatitis in the elderly population are hepatotoxicity and viral

hepatitis. Either hepatitis B or non-A, non-B hepatitis may result in chronic hepatitis. Patients with hepatitis B infection may become superinfected with hepatitis D (delta) virus, which can exacerbate clinical symptoms and accelerate histologic progression to chronic active hepatitis and cirrhosis.[17] As noted in Table 38–3, several hepatotoxic medications may result in chronic hepatitis. Autoimmune chronic hepatitis commonly affects females between the ages of 10 and 50 years. Although it is infrequent in the elderly, cases in postmenopausal women have been described.[18]

Clinically, patients with chronic persistent hepatitis are either asymptomatic or have nonspecific fatigue. The dominant biochemical abnormality is a moderate elevation of aminotransferases. Patients with chronic active hepatitis also may be asymptomatic or have symptoms of malaise, fatigue, anorexia, abdominal pain, or jaundice. Physical examination in patients with chronic persistent hepatitis may be entirely normal or may show mild hepatomegaly. Physical examination in patients with chronic active hepatitis generally shows hepatomegaly. When cirrhosis is present, patients may show signs of portal venous hypertension with splenomegaly, vascular spiders, palmar erythema, and gynecomastia. Disease progress is associated with chronic elevation of aminotransferases, increasing hyperbilirubinemia, decreased albumin, and prolongation of prothrombin time. In patients with autoimmune chronic active hepatitis, hypergammaglobulinemia increases with time. However, the course of chronic active hepatitis in individual patients is highly variable. Some patients remain asymptomatic for a substantial period, whereas others exhibit a more rapidly progressive course to cirrhosis and death.

Rational therapy requires identification of the etiologic agents and understanding of the pathophysiology. Corticosteroid

TABLE 38–3. Chronic Hepatitis Caused by Medications

Proven	Probable	Rare
Oxyphenisatin	Isoniazid	Aspirin
Nitrofurantoin	Acetaminophen	Sulfonamides
Alpha-methyldopa	Papaverine	Propylthiouracil
Dantrolene		Chlorpromazine
		Halothane

therapy should be reserved for symptomatic patients with autoimmune chronic active hepatitis. The use of corticosteroids in the elderly may exacerbate tendencies for osteoporosis, glucose intolerance, cataracts, or hypertension.[18] The dose of corticosteroids may be minimized by the addition of azathioprine. Corticosteroids have no role in the treatment of chronic hepatitis B, chronic hepatitis D (delta), or non-A, non-B hepatitis. Studies are in progress to evaluate the efficacy of antiviral agents in the treatment of younger patients with chronic hepatitis B, chronic hepatitis D (delta), and non-A, non-B hepatitis.

Differential Diagnosis of Chronic Hepatitis

The hepatic histologic picture of several liver diseases may be indistinguishable from that of chronic hepatitis and may result in diagnostic and therapeutic confusion. This is particularly true for primary biliary cirrhosis, primary sclerosing cholangitis, alpha-1 antitrypsin deficiency, and hemochromatosis.

Primary biliary cirrhosis (PBC) predominantly affects females (female/male ratio 11:1), with a peak age of onset between the fifth and sixth decades.[19] Patients may be entirely asymptomatic or may exhibit one or more symptoms of cholestasis. The most frequent symptoms and signs are fatigue, pruritus, jaundice, and hyperpigmentation of the skin. Most patients show hepatomegaly even in the absence of jaundice. PBC is frequently associated with "autoimmune" diseases such as scleroderma, Sjögren's syndrome, arthritis, and thyroiditis. Clinical hypothyroidism occurs insidiously in a majority of patients with PBC. Biochemical test results reveal a disproportionate elevation of alkaline phosphatase levels and mild to moderate elevations of aminotransferases. In the early phases of the disease, bilirubin may be normal; with progression, bilirubin rises. Antimitochondrial antibodies are present in over 90 percent of patients. The diagnostic evaluation requires a liver biopsy and demonstration of an unobstructed extrahepatic biliary tract. In the majority of patients obstruction can be excluded by ultrasonography. In difficult diagnostic situations an endoscopic retrograde cholangiogram should be performed.

Although a retrospective study indicated that asymptomatic patients with PBC may have a life expectancy comparable to that of age- and sex-matched controls,[20] a recent independent evaluation suggests that decreased life expectancy is characteristic of this group.[21] Among symptomatic patients, life expectancy is decreased. Prognosis is adverse among elderly patients with bilirubin levels of >5 mg/dl and biopsy-proven cirrhosis. Progression of disease results in decreased bile secretion, causing malnutrition and steatorrhea. Although there is no curative therapy for PBC, recent reports indicate that colchicine may retard progression or diminish mortality.[22] Symptomatic therapy consists of cholestyramine or phenobarbital for relief of pruritus, administration of fat-soluble vitamins parenterally on a monthly basis, and maintenance of adequate intake of calcium and vitamin D to retard hepatic osteodystrophy.[19]

Primary sclerosing cholangitis (PSC) predominantly affects males and is associated with inflammatory bowel disease in approximately 60 percent of cases.[23] PSC may be clinically and histologically indistinguishable from chronic hepatitis or PBC. Laboratory investigation shows cholestatic abnormalities and the absence of antimitochondrial antibodies. Liver biopsy is not diagnostic and often is misconstrued as showing chronic persistent hepatitis, chronic active hepatitis, or PBC. Diagnosis requires endoscopic retrograde cholangiography demonstrating strictures in the extra- or intrahepatic biliary tree. There is no proved curative therapy for this disease, but controlled trials are investigating the use of cyclosporine and methotrexate. Selected patients with loci of high-grade strictures may benefit from mechanical dilatation.[23]

Alpha-1 antitrypsin deficiency (A1ATD) induces chronic liver disease as a result of retention of abnormal antiprotease within hepatocytes. Production of A1AT is controlled by codominant genes, the normal phenotype being designated PiMM. The homozygous phenotype PiZZ results in <15 percent of the production of various inhibitor activity and is associated with early onset of liver disease or emphysema. However, heterozygote phenotypes such as PiMZ, SZ, or SS exhibit an intermediate concentration of serum protease inhibitor activity and an increased incidence of liver disease with advancing age.[24] In a prospective study, the prevalence of heterozygosity for A1AT deficiency in adults was 2.4 percent, but this figure was increased to 9.2 percent among patients with cirrhosis.[25] Similarly, the prevalence of PiMZ is significantly greater in patients with cryptogenic cirrhosis and HBsAg-negative chronic active hepatitis. Heterozygote patients with histologic diagnoses of chronic active hepatitis with cryptogenic cirrhosis are often elderly, and their prognosis is poor.[26] It is important, however, to recognize patients with A1AT deficiency because a higher than expected incidence of primary hepatocellular carcinoma or cholangiocarcinoma occurs, and therapy with corticosteroids is ineffective.

Hemochromatosis is an autosomal recessive disorder of iron metabolism that results in accumulation of iron and damage to multiple organs. Cirrhosis is the principal manifestation in patients who are middle-aged or older.[27] Patients may also exhibit diabetes mellitus, peripheral neuritis, arthritis, and testicular atrophy. Clinical manifestations generally occur in males over the age of 40 and in females after menopause because of the protective loss of iron during menstruation. Recent evidence that the frequency of heterozygotes in the general population is 1:9 to 1:13 makes this the most common inherited recessive disorder yet identified.[28] In all patients with chronic abnormalities of liver test results, serum iron, iron-binding capacity, and ferritin should be measured. Diagnosis is strongly suggested by a high serum iron concentration, high saturation of iron-binding protein, and an increased ferritin value. When these studies are abnormal, liver biopsy should be performed and a portion submitted for quantitation of hepatic iron. Treatment consists of phlebotomy to decrease iron stores. Alterations in the clinical state of patients, especially signs of decompensated cirrhosis, should suggest the development of hepatocellular carcinoma. This frequent complication of hemochromatosis shows an increased prevalence with age: in one study, 60 percent of patients older than 70 years had hepatocellular carcinoma.[29]

Alcoholic Liver Disease

The spectrum of alcoholic liver disease includes fatty liver, alcoholic hepatitis, and alcoholic cirrhosis.[30] Although it is generally agreed that alcoholic liver injury is the leading cause of hepatic morbidity and mortality in the United States, the prevalence of this disease in the elderly is undefined. Studies of patient survival, however, suggest that the prevalence of alcoholic hepatitis and cirrhosis in the elderly would be lower than that in the younger population. This follows from the fact that the 5-year survival for patients with biopsy-proven alcoholic hepatitis is approximately 60 percent from the time of recognition of the illness. Similarly, patients with alcoholic cirrhosis have an overall 5-year survival from the time of diagnosis of 41 percent if they continue to drink.[31] Thus, a minority of patients with severe alcoholic liver disease who continue to drink would be expected to survive past the age of 65 years.

In all elderly patients with abnormal liver test results, the quantity and duration of alcohol consumption should be ascertained. Clinical features that suggest the possibility of alcoholic hepatitis include anorexia, prominent jaundice, hepatomegaly, fever, and leukocytosis. The serum aminotransferases are usually moderately elevated, and the aspartate aminotransferase value characteristically is higher than that of alanine aminotransferase. Diagnosis is substantiated by liver biopsy showing the characteristic histologic features of hepatocellular necrosis, alcoholic hyaline, and a polymorphonuclear infiltrate. In some instances, however, the histologic picture is more subtle and requires scrutiny by a skilled hepatopathologist. In Table 38–4 are summarized prognostic factors in patients with alcoholic liver disease.

TABLE 38–4. Prognostic Factors in Alcoholic Liver Disease

Positive	Negative
Abstinence	Histology of alcoholic hepatitis and cirrhosis
	Ascites
	Encephalopathy
	Bilirubin > 20 mg/dl
	Prothrombin time > 8 sec over control

Studies indicate that the prognosis of alcoholic hepatitis and/or cirrhosis is significantly improved by abstinence. The majority of published controlled studies of corticosteroid use in patients with alcoholic hepatitis has shown no benefit.[32]

Cirrhosis and Its Complications

Cirrhosis, defined as diffuse scarring and regenerative nodules, reaches a peak prevalence between 45 and 65 years of age. As noted, a variety of diseases may culminate in cirrhosis. In cirrhotic patients, nonspecific symptoms such as fatigue, loss of appetite, weight loss, nausea, and abdominal discomfort predominate. In patients with established cirrhosis the most important adverse prognostic factors include (1) rapid rise of bilirubin level; (2) ascites that is resistant to diuretic therapy; (3) spontaneous hepatic encephalopathy; (4) recurrent variceal hemorrhage; (5) prothrombin time prolonged 8 seconds above control (without response to parenteral vitamin K); and (6) recurrent septicemia or spontaneous bacterial peritonitis.

ASCITES AND EDEMA. Fluid retention in cirrhosis is manifested by ascites and peripheral edema and less often by ascites alone. With new onset ascites, diagnostic paracentesis is necessary to evaluate the possibility of malignancy, bacterial peritonitis, and chylous ascites. If results of these studies are negative, the clinician should also consider the possibility that hepatocellular carcinoma has developed within the cirrhotic liver. This theory can be evaluated by measuring the alpha-fetoprotein level and performing an imaging study of the liver with either ultrasound or computerized tomography. For symptomatic relief, sodium restriction (2 to 4 gm/day) and water restriction (if the serum sodium level is <130 mEq/liter) should be ordered. Diuresis[33] should be initiated with spironolactone in a dose of 25 mg bid. Subsequent increments in dosage can be prescribed every third day as necessary to a dose of 400 mg/day. Response is best judged by daily weights; the goal is a loss of 0.5 to 1.5 lbs/day, which corresponds to the maximum mobilization of ascites fluid of 700 to 900 ml/day. In patients who are unresponsive to

this regimen, furosemide may be added. In patients unresponsive to diuretics, therapeutic paracentesis (removal of 1000 to 2000 ml) may be beneficial.[34] In patients treated with a sequential regimen, true refractory ascites is rare. For such patients, peritoneal-venous (LeVeen) shunt may be considered if liver function is stable.

BACTERIAL PERITONITIS. Prospective studies have documented that the prevalence of infected ascites fluid on admission to the hospital is 10 to 27 percent.[35] Most patients reported have had alcoholic hepatitis and cirrhosis. The clinical spectrum is diverse: some patients show clinical signs of peritonitis whereas others are asymptomatic. Thus, a high index of suspicion is required, and diagnostic paracentesis should be performed. In all patients, spontaneous bacterial peritonitis must be differentiated from secondary bacterial peritonitis due to a perforation of the bowel. Lateral or upright films of the abdomen to exclude free peritoneal air should be taken in each patient.

Spontaneous bacterial peritonitis is defined as positive results of an ascitic bacterial culture associated with an ascitic neutrophil count of $\geq 250/mm^3$ and an absence of an intra-abdominal source of infection. Spontaneous bacterial peritonitis is also frequently diagnosed in patients with similar neutrophil counts whose bacterial cultures show no growth. In such patients infection is probable if there has been no recent antibiotic therapy and there is no alternative explanation for an elevated polymorphonuclear white cell count in the ascitic fluid such as peritoneal carcinomatosis, pancreatitis, hemorrhage, or tuberculosis.[36] The prevalence of the culture-negative variant is related to the method of ascitic fluid culture. Inoculation of blood culture bottles at the bedside is more than twice as sensitive as conventional methods of detecting bacterial growth.[37] Therapy for suspected peritonitis should be instituted before obtaining culture results. A recent randomized controlled trial[38] indicates that cefotaxime is the most effective therapy. The choice of antibiotics can be subsequently modified on the basis of culture sensitivities.

COAGULOPATHY AND THROMBOCYTOPENIA. Coagulopathy is a frequent complication of cirrhosis and portal hypertension. Typically, both the prothrombin time and the partial thromboplastin time are abnormal. Prolongation of the prothrombin time is correlated with the severity of hepatocellular dysfunction. Isolated prolongation of the partial thromboplastin test suggests either a specific coagulation factor deficiency of the first stage of the intrinsic cascade or a circulating inhibitor. Evaluation of such a prolongation may require a quantitative assay of coagulation factors and special tests for anticoagulants. The latter are most frequently described in patients with autoimmune chronic active hepatitis. Thrombocytopenia is also frequent in patients with cirrhosis due to hypersplenism. Initially, all patients with a prolonged prothrombin time should receive a single injection of parenteral vitamin K. In patients who are actively bleeding or who require emergent surgery, the coagulopathy can be treated by administration of fresh frozen plasma. Because of the short half-lives of individual clotting factors, this therapy will require maintenance infusions at 4- to 6-hour intervals. Thrombocytopenia itself rarely requires treatment unless the bleeding time is abnormal. Such patients may require either platelet transfusion or administration of deaminase Δ-arginine vasopressin (dΔAVP, desmopressin) for treatment of von Willebrand's disorder.[39]

VARICEAL HEMORRHAGE. Hemorrhage from esophageal varices is a major complication of portal venous hypertension. It should be suspected in all patients with gastrointestinal hemorrhage who have cirrhosis or signs of chronic liver disease. Fiberoptic panendoscopy is mandatory for diagnosis, since up to 40 percent of patients with varices are found to be bleeding from another lesion such as gastritis, peptic ulcer, or Mallory-Weiss tear. In patients without cardiorespiratory contraindications, an intravenous infusion of vasopressin 0.2 to 0.4 unit/minute should be initiated. If variceal hemorrhage persists, several options are available. The first is insertion of a Sengstaken-Blakemore tube for direct tamponade. The second option is performance of therapeutic endoscopy for variceal sclerosis or direct variceal ligation. The third option, portosystemic shunting, is associated with an increased risk of postoperative encephalopathy and mortality in patients over 60 years of age. In one series, 63 percent of patients older than 60 years had encephalopathy within 6 months of shunting compared with 27 percent of younger patients.[40]

Hepatic Consequences of Congestive Heart Failure

Congestive heart failure is frequently associated with hepatic abnormalities. Ventricular failure results in elevated central venous pressure and chronic passive congestion of the centrilobular portion of the hepatic sinusoids. Atrophy of hepatocytes in this region results in elevated serum aminotransferase values that are less than 5 times the upper limit of normal and a serum bilirubin level that is generally ≤4 mg/dl. In contrast, left ventricular failure with reduction of cardiac output may cause true centrilobular necrosis of hepatocytes. Such patients often show more severe abnormalities of aminotransferase levels and hyperbilirubinemia of greater than 10 mg/dl. Resolution of the circulatory failure results in prompt amelioration of the liver injury.

Hepatic Neoplasia

The incidence of hepatocellular carcinoma (HCC) in North America is 1 to 3 × 10^5/year. The prevalence of HCC increases with age in North America, and cirrhosis is the most important etiologic association of HCC.[41] In contrast, the most important etiologic association in endemic areas is hepatitis B virus. In the United States 60 to 90 percent of patients with HCC have coexisting cirrhosis. HCC may occur in patients with cirrhosis due to hemochromatosis, postnecrotic cirrhosis, or alcoholic cirrhosis, or cirrhosis due to A1ATD. Quantitatively, alcoholic cirrhosis appears to be the most important etiologic association in North America. The risk of HCC occurring in a cirrhotic liver appears to be approximately 5 to 10 percent.

Clinically, HCC should be expected in patients with unexplained clinical deterioration of stable chronic liver disease or a perineoplastic syndrome such as hypoglycemia or polycythemia, and right upper quadrant pain. Patients with more advanced tumors may exhibit hepatic arterial bruits or a hepatic friction rub due to capsular invasion. The alpha-fetoprotein level is an effective screening test; 80 percent of patients with symptomatic HCC have levels greater than 500 ng/ml. Hepatic imaging can be performed by ultrasonography or computed tomography, both of which are more than 80 to 90 percent sensitive. Arteriography is usually reserved for patients in whom surgical resection is considered. Histologic confirmation requires percutaneous, laparoscopic, or open liver biopsy. Prognosis is worst in patients older than 45 years of age.[42] Since most HCC occurs as multiple tumors, resectability in the older age group is uncommon, and the prognosis is dismal.

Metastatic tumors that spread by the bloodstream commonly affect the liver. Patients may present with signs or symptoms due to either the primary tumor or the hepatic metastases. Symptoms related to hepatic metastases are nonspecific and include malaise, weight loss, decreased appetite, and abdominal pain. Hepatomegaly is generally present, and elevations of alkaline phosphatase and aminotransferases occur in the majority of patients. Ultrasonography or computed tomography usually reveals multiple filling defects. Histologic confirmation can be obtained by percutaneous or laparoscopic liver biopsy or by thin needle aspiration under ultrasound or computed tomographic guidance.

Hepatic Transplantation in the Elderly

Until recently, age over 55 years was considered a contraindication to liver transplantation. However, several centers have performed successful transplants in patients over 66 years of age, the oldest recipient being 76 years of age. All such transplants have been performed in patients with nonalcoholic cirrhosis. The possibility of transplantation therefore may be considered in selected elderly patients who otherwise meet standard inclusion criteria for transplantation.

DISEASES OF THE GALLBLADDER AND BILE DUCTS

Cholelithiasis

Prevalence of cholelithiasis increases with advancing age and is twice as common in females in almost all age groups. Between the ages of 80 and 89 years, gallstones were identified in 22 percent of males and in 38 percent of females. The prevalence increased to 31 percent in males over the age of 90 years.[43] In another study, the prevalence was more than 50 percent in the elderly.[44] The majority of gallstones in elderly patients are composed of cholesterol and result from formation of bile that is supersaturated with cholesterol. A minority of patients have calcium bilirubinate stones resulting from chronic hemolytic anemia or cirrhosis. Increasing age is associated with increasing lithogenicity of bile, apparently due to an increased secretion of biliary cholesterol. In addition to lithogenicity, factors such as gallbladder emptying and mucous production may affect the formation of cholesterol gallstones. With respect to gallbladder function, delayed filling has been reported in the elderly, but gallbladder emptying appears to be normal.

When cholelithiasis is suspected, the diagnostic test of choice is real-time ultrasonography. This test has a sensitivity of 95 to 99 percent and a specificity of 95 percent. In patients with compromised ultrasound examinations owing to excessive intestinal gas, obesity, or impediments to the optimal placement of the transducer, oral cholecystography (sensitivity 85 to 95 percent, specificity 80 to 90 percent) can be used. In a situation of high suspicion, a negative result with both of these tests indicates a greater than 95 percent chance that gallstones are absent. It must be emphasized, however, that both these tests are insensitive for choledocholithiasis. Persistent symptoms of biliary-type pain or abnormal liver test results may require endoscopic retrograde cholangiography (ERCP).

The majority of gallstones are asymptomatic. Asymptomatic cholelithiasis can be defined as gallstones in the absence of (1) biliary-type pain, (2) abnormal liver test results, (3) bilirubinuria, and (4) a history of cholecystitis, cholangitis, or pancreatitis. The natural history of asymptomatic cholelithiasis has been well defined in prospective and retrospective studies. In a 15-year follow-up of patients with an initial mean age of 54 years, only 18 percent developed symptoms of biliary pain.[45] After 10 to 20 years of follow-up, another study reported biliary pain in 19 percent and mild transient jaundice in 4.5 percent.[46] Adjustment of mortality statistics for elective cholecystectomy with or without common bile duct exploration for factors of age, sex, and anesthesia risk indicates that there is no advantage to prophylactic cholecystectomy compared with expectant management.[47] However, prophylactic cholecystectomy should be considered for certain specific patients. These include patients with diabetes mellitus because complications of cholecystitis tend to be more severe and more often fatal, patients with chronic hemolytic anemia, and patients who intend to travel or live for extended periods in remote regions where medical care is unavailable.

Acute Cholecystitis

The incidence of acute cholecystitis is increased in the elderly and is associated with substantially greater morbidity and mortality.[48] Recent studies indicate that the majority of deaths related to acute cholecystitis occur in patients older than age 65. In one series of 2401 cases of acute cholecystitis, 70 percent of deaths occurred in patients older than age 65, and the mortality in elderly patients was approximately 10 percent compared to less than 2 percent in patients younger than 65 years.[48]

Signs and symptoms of fever, right upper quadrant pain, tenderness to palpation, and leukocytosis may not be present in elderly, diabetic, or immunocompromised patients. When suspected, the diagnosis must be pursued aggressively because delay in surgical management results in increased morbidity and mortality. Real-time ultrasonography should be performed to detect gallstones because only 5 percent of acute cholecystitis is "acalculous." Cholelithiasis, however, does not necessarily imply acute cholecystitis. Thus, a radionuclide scan should be performed to detect obstruction of the cystic duct. Once cholecystitis is confirmed, surgery should be performed with minimal delay.[48] It is inappropriate to treat patients conservatively and operate only after resolution of the acute phase because this regimen is associated with a higher rate of infection and failure. The role of antimicrobials in the treatment of elderly patients with acute cholecystitis remains debatable; however, after age 60 years bacterial contamination of bile is more prevalent.[49]

Chronic Cholecystitis

Most patients with chronic cholecystitis relate a history of symptoms of postprandial dyspepsia or recurrent attacks of biliary pain with nausea and vomiting. In time, the wall of the gallbladder becomes chronically inflamed, stones are universally present, and the concentrating and emptying function is lost. The diagnostic test of choice is real-time ultrasonography. The therapy of choice is cholecystectomy, which carries a mortality rate of 0.5 percent in patients less than 50 years of age and 1 percent in patients over 50 years of age.[50] Dissolution therapy with chenodeoxycholic acid can be considered in symptomatic patients who are poor surgical risks, have radiolucent stones (cholesterol gallstones), and evidence of a functioning gallbladder on oral cholecystography. Unfortunately, this therapy is minimally efficacious and may result in diarrhea or abnormal liver test results. Extracorporeal shock-wave lithotripsy represents a promising new alternative to cholecystectomy and dissolution therapy, but it has not yet been evaluated in elderly patients.

Choledocholithiasis

Choledocholithiasis may be complicated by extrahepatic biliary obstruction, acute ascending cholangitis, hepatic abscess, and pancreatitis. Chronic obstruction of the extrahepatic biliary tree may progress to secondary biliary cirrhosis. Choledocholithiasis is noted in approximately 15 percent of patients undergoing cholecystectomy for chronic cholecystitis with stones.

The prevalence of common bile duct stones increases with age and correlates with an increased diameter of the common bile duct that accompanies aging.[51] Acutely, patients with choledocholithiasis may have abdominal pain, nausea, vomiting, fever, bilirubinuria, and jaundice. Evidence of dilatation of an obstructed bile duct should be sought by ultrasonography; however, acute obstruction may not result in immediate dilatation. Thus, ERCP is often required for definitive diagnosis. When ERCP reveals choledocholithiasis, a sphincterotomy should be performed to allow spontaneous passage of the stones, or endoscopic retrieval. This procedure is particularly appropriate for elderly patients who are poor surgical risks because of its rare mortality and acceptable complication rate (less than 5 percent). The principal disadvantage of this approach is that the diseased gallbladder, often containing additional stones, remains intact. Definitive therapy requires cholecystectomy and common duct exploration. Shock-wave lithotripsy has recently been performed on common duct stones but has not been evaluated in elderly patients.

Acute Cholangitis

Acute cholangitis can be subdivided into suppurative and nonsuppurative varieties on the basis of the presence or absence of pus in the extrahepatic biliary tree. Acute cholangitis has a poor prognosis, and its incidence is increased in elderly, diabetic, or immunocompromised patients. In such patients, the classic signs of acute cholangitis (fever, jaundice, and tender liver) may be absent. Instead, patients may show changes in mental status and may have gram-negative septicemia. A high index of suspicion is necessary for accurate diagnosis. Patients should be treated with antimicrobials directed against the organisms most likely to be present in the biliary tree such as *Escherichia coli*, *Klebsiella*, *Enterobacter*, and *Enterococcus*. Septic patients should undergo emergent decompression of the biliary tract after rehydration and administration of antimicrobials.

Carcinoma of the Gallbladder

Carcinoma of the gallbladder is a rare tumor. The risk factors are advancing age (75 percent of current patients are over 65 years old) and the chronic presence of gallstones (present in 80 percent). Gallbladder carcinoma is often an incidental finding at surgery performed for cholelithiasis. The overall prognosis is poor, with less than 5 percent survival after 5 years. In the majority of patients, the tumor is unresectable at diagnosis. In 10 to 25 percent of tumors, resection is possible and increases survival. Rarely, the tumor is confined to the submucosa, and resection may be curative.

Carcinoma of the Extrahepatic Biliary Tract

Cholangiocarcinoma increases in incidence after the age of 60 years; in patients with inflammatory bowel disease (most commonly chronic ulcerative colitis) it often presents at a younger age. Tumors infiltrate the wall of the bile ducts and induce a sclerotic process that can be difficult to distinguish from a benign stricture. The cholangiocarcinoma usually presents with obstructive jaundice and cholestatic abnormalities of liver tests. Chronic cholestasis results in pruritus and weight loss due to malabsorption. Percutaneous or endoscopic retrograde cholangiography is essential because therapy and prognosis are dictated by location of the tumor within the biliary tract. Tumors involving the proximal biliary tract (above the right and left hepatic ducts) are often unresectable. Even if resected, such patients have a very poor prognosis, with less than 5 percent survival at 1 year. Tumors localized at the middle third of the biliary tract are rare, and their prognosis is similar to tumors in the lower third of the biliary tract. The latter are potentially resectable with a Whipple procedure, and approximately 30 percent of patients survive for 5 years. The role of adjuvant chemotherapy or radiotherapy remains debatable. In patients with obstruction of the common bile duct who are not surgical candidates, biliary decompression appears to prolong life (median survival 6 to 16 months versus 1 to 3 months without biliary drainage) and to reduce the duration of hospitalization. Decompression can be achieved either surgically or by percutaneous insertion of transhepatic catheters. Decompression may be complicated by cholangitis, sepsis, leakage, or localized pain. The efficacy of combined chemotherapy and radiotherapy remains unproved.

REFERENCES

1. Calloway NO, Foley CF, Lagerbloom P: Uncertainties in geriatric data: II. Organ size. J Am Geriatr Soc 13:20, 1965.
2. Carr RD, Smith MJ, Keil PG: The liver in the aging process. Arch Pathol 70:1, 1960.
3. Andrew W: The Anatomy of Aging in Man and Animals. London, Heinemann, 1971, p 161.
4. Woodford-Williams E, Alvarez AS, Webster D, et al: Serum protein patterns in "normal" and pathological ageing. Gerontologia 10:86, 1964.
5. Schmucker DL: Age-related changes in drug disposition. Pharmacol Rev 30:445, 1979.
6. Gillette JR: Biotransformation of drugs during aging. Fed Proc 38:1900, 1979.
7. Gerber JG: In Schrier RW, ed: Clinical Internal Medicine in the Aged. Philadelphia, WB Saunders Co, 1982, p 51.
8. Kraus JW, Desmond PV, Marshall JP, et al: Effect of aging and liver disease on disposition of lorazepam. Clin Pharmacol Ther 24:411, 1978.
9. Leask RGS, Andrews GW, Caid FI, et al: Normal values for sixteen blood constituents in the elderly. Age Ageing 2:14, 1973.
10. Kampmann JP, Sinding J, Moller-Jorgensen I: Effect of age on liver function. Geriatrics 30:91, 1975.
11. Thompson EN, Williams R: Effect of age on liver function with particular reference to BSP excretion. Gut 6:266, 1965.
12. Koff RS, Garvey AJ, Burney SW, et al: Absence of an age effect on sulfobromophthalein retention in healthy men. Gastroenterology 65:300, 1973.
13. Dienstag JL: Non A, non B hepatitis. I. Recognition, epidemiology and clinical features. Gastroenterology 85:439, 1983.
14. Gibinski K: Hepatitis in the aged. Digestion 8:254, 1973.
15. Jones EA, Schafer DF: Hepatology. Philadelphia, WB Saunders Co, 1982, p 415.
16. Mitchell JR, et al: Isoniazid liver injury: Clinical spectrum, pathology and probable pathogenesis. Ann Intern Med 84:181, 1976.
17. Rizzetto M, Bonino F, Verme G: Hepatitis delta virus infection of the liver: Progress in virology, pathobiology, and diagnosis. Semin Liver Dis 8:350, 1988.
18. Lebovics E, Schaffner F, Klion FM, et al: Autoimmune chronic active hepatitis in post-menopausal women. Dig Dis Sci 30:824, 1985.
19. Vierling JM: Hepatology. In Schrier RW, ed: Clinical Internal Medicine in the Aged. Philadelphia, WB Saunders Co, 1982, p 825.
20. Roll J, Boyer JL, Barry D, et al: The prognostic importance of clinical and histological features in asymptomatic and symptomatic primary biliary cirrhosis. N Engl J Med 308:1, 1983.
21. Balasubramaniam K, Grambsch PM, Wiesner RH, et al: Asymptomatic primary biliary cirrhosis

(PBC): patients have a diminished survival (abstr). Hepatology 7:1025, 1987.
22. Kaplan MM, Alling DW, Zimmerman HJ, et al: A prospective trial of colchicine for primary biliary cirrhosis. N Engl J Med 315:1448, 1986.
23. Lindor KD, Wiesner RH, LaRusso NF: Recent advances in the management of primary sclerosing cholangitis. Semin Liver Dis 7:322, 1987.
24. Cox DW, Smyth S: Risk for liver disease in adults with alpha-1-antitrypsin deficiency. Am J Med 74:221, 1983.
25. Hodges JR, Millward-Sadler GH, Barbatis C, et al: Heterozygous MZ alpha-1-antitrypsin deficiency in adults with chronic active hepatitis and cryptogenic cirrhosis. N Engl J Med 304:557, 1981.
26. Vierling JM: Epidemiology and clinical course of liver diseases: identification of candidates for hepatic transplantation. Hepatology 4:84S, 1984.
27. Basset ML, Halliday JW, Powell LW: Genetic hemochromatosis. Semin Liver Dis 4:217, 1984.
28. Olsson KS, Ritter B, Rosén U, et al: Prevalence of iron overload in central Sweden. Acta Med Scand 213:145, 1983.
29. Finch SC, Finch CA: Idiopathic hemochromatosis, an iron storage disease. Medicine 34:381, 1955.
30. Lieber CS, Leo MA: Major Problems in Internal Medicine. Philadelphia, WB Saunders Co, 1982, p 259.
31. Alexander JF, Lischner MW, Galambos JT: Natural history of alcoholic hepatitis. II. The long-term prognosis. Am J Gastroenterol 56:515, 1971.
32. Schenker S: Alcoholic liver disease: Evaluation of natural history and prognostic factors. Hepatology 4:36S, 1984.
33. Linas SL, Anderson RJ, Miller PD, et al: In Epstein M, ed: The Kidney in Liver Disease. New York, Elsevier, North-Holland, 1978, p 313.
34. Simon DM, McCain JR, Bonkovsky HL, et al: Effects of therapeutic paracentesis on systemic and hepatic hemodynamics and on renal and hormonal function. Hepatology 7:423, 1987.
35. Runyon BA: Low-protein concentration ascitic fluid is predisposed to spontaneous bacterial peritonitis. Gastroenterology 91:1343, 1986.
36. Runyon BA, Hoefs JC: Culture negative neutrocytic ascites: A variant of spontaneous bacterial peritonitis. Hepatology 4:1209, 1984.
37. Runyon BA, Umland ET, Merlin T: Inoculation of blood culture bottles with ascitic fluid: Improved detection of spontaneous bacterial peritonitis. Arch Intern Med 147:73, 1987.
38. Felisart J, Rimola A, Arroyo V, et al: Cefotaxime is more effective than ampicillin-tobramycin in cirrhotics with severe infections. Hepatology 5:457, 1985.
39. de la Fuente B, Kasper CK, Rickles FR, et al: Response of patients with mild and moderate hemophilia A and von Willebrand's disease to treatment with desmopressin. Ann Intern Med 103:6, 1985.
40. Arnman R, Olsson R, Scherstein T: Survival after portacaval shunt: Who and how? Acta Med Scand 199:167, 1976.
41. Kew MC, Popper H: Relationship between hepatocellular carcinoma and cirrhosis. Semin Liver Dis 4:136, 1984.
42. Chlebowski RT, Tong M, Weissman J, et al:

Hepatocellular carcinoma: Diagnostic and prognostic features in North American patients. Cancer 53:2701, 1984.

43. Torvik A, Hoivik B: Gallstones in an autopsy series. Incidence, complications and correlations with carcinoma of the gallbladder. Acta Chir Scand 120:168, 1960.

44. Strohl EL, Diffenbaugh WG: Biliary tract surgery in the aged patient. Surg Gynecol Obstet 97:467, 1953.

45. Gracie WA, Ransohoff DF: The natural history of silent gallstones: The innocent gallstone is not a myth. N Engl J Med 307:798, 1982.

46. Comfort MW, Gray HK, Wilson JM, et al: The silent gallstone. A ten to twenty year follow-up study of 112 cases. Ann Surg 128:931, 1948.

47. Ransohoff DF, Gracie WA, Wolfenson LB, et al: Prophylactic cholecystectomy or expectant management for silent gallstones. Ann Intern Med 99:199, 1983.

48. Glenn F: Surgical management of acute cholecystitis in patients 65 years of age and older. Ann Surg 193:56, 1981.

49. Nielsen ML, Justesen T: Anaerobic and aerobic bacterial studies in biliary tract disease. Scand J Gastroenterol 11:437, 1976.

50. McSherry CK, Glenn F: The incidence and causes of death following surgery for nonmalignant biliary tract disease. Ann Surg 191:271, 1980.

51. Edholm P, Jonsson G: Bile duct stones related to age and duct width. Acta Chir Scand 124:75, 1962.

CHAPTER 39

Common Gastrointestinal Diseases

William R. Brown

I am very grateful to old age because it has increased my desire for conversation and lessened my desire for food and drink.

CICERO, *De Senectute XIV*

GENERAL COMMENTS

Diseases of the digestive system are among the most common diseases in the elderly. According to one study of elderly patients, 27 percent admitted to hospital as medical emergencies had major diseases of the digestive system, and 42 percent of those with chronic illness had important digestive disorders. Although no digestive disease is unique to the elderly, several of these diseases have more severe consequences in this age group or their frequency increases with advancing age.

Advancing age may bring changes in all the major functions of the digestive tract, but elderly patients' abdominal symptoms ordinarily should not be ascribed to age alone. In particular, symptoms that suggest the irritable bowel syndrome occurring for the first time in advanced age or changes in the pattern of bowel movements should not be dismissed as "functional" or psychosomatic in origin before a thorough search for organic illness has been conducted.

The rapidly increasing availability of endoscopy for the diagnosis and even for the treatment of digestive diseases now often requires the physician to choose between a radiographic examination and an endoscopic study for his patient. The latter study may be perceived as more difficult, hazardous, and costly. As fiberoptic instruments have improved, however, both esophagogastroduodenoscopy and colonoscopy have become quite safe even in the elderly,[1-3] and even more complex procedures such as retrograde cholangiopancreatography and endoscopic sphincterotomy of the sphincter of Oddi are being done more frequently without untoward consequences. Thus, the elderly should not be denied procedures on the basis of old age alone. Nevertheless, because complications (e.g., infection, hemorrhage, aspiration, and bowel perforation) that may attend endoscopic studies can be especially serious in the elderly, the procedures should be used with special caution and prudence in these patients.

It is to be hoped that in the future, endoscopy of the gastrointestinal tract will become less expensive. Even now, though, the cost of an endoscopic procedure may be offset by its greater diagnostic accuracy and therapeutic potential.

SWALLOWING DISORDERS

Presbyesophagus

The term presbyesophagus refers to an abnormal frequency of tertiary (nonperistaltic) contractions and inadequate relaxation of the lower esophageal sphincter in elderly persons.[4] Whether these changes are the result of aging per se, however, or of associated vascular, metabolic, or neurologic changes is debated. The symptom of dysphagia in the elderly should not be attributed to presbyesophagus until carcinoma of the esophagus and other structural conditions such as those cited below have been excluded.

Cricopharyngeal Achalasia

This problem, which is strongly associated with advanced age, may cause a sensation of a "lump in the throat" or high dysphagia, sometimes with nasopharyngeal regurgitation, on swallowing. It may be due to fibrosis of the cricopharyngeal muscle, leading to paradoxical contractions of the muscle or its failure to relax normally during the pharyngeal phase of swallowing. A Zenker's, or hypopharyngeal, diverticulum may be an associated finding. Cricopharyngeal achalasia may be treated by myotomy of the muscle, and the Zenker's diverticulum may be simultaneously extirpated surgically.

Hiatal Hernia and Esophageal Reflux

DIAGNOSTIC CONSIDERATIONS. As many as 50 to 70 percent of persons over age 70 may have a hiatal hernia compared to a prevalence of no more than 10 percent in persons under the age of 40. The hernia, however, often is unassociated with symptoms and deserves no attention. Weakness of the lower esophageal sphincter, not a hiatal hernia per se, is believed to be the critical determinant in whether reflux of gastric content into the esophagus will occur. Overeating, obesity, and cigarette smoking may contribute to the severity and frequency of esophageal reflux. The predominant symptom of esophageal reflux is heartburn, a burning retrosternal pain, which may be relieved by the ingestion of an antacid.

Some special features of esophageal reflux in the elderly may include very subtle symptoms; dysphasia, secondary to an inflammatory stricture in the distal esophagus, as the predominant symptom; aspiration of gastric contents, resulting in coughing, wheezing, morning hoarseness, sore throat, or pulmonary infection; frequent misinterpretation of the esophageal symptoms as pain of cardiac origin.

Distinguishing between chest pain of esophageal origin and that of cardiac origin may be as difficult as it is important.[5] Some of the differentiating characteristics are these: The pain due to esophageal reflux may be made worse by drinking coffee, tea, or acidic juices; it may be relieved by taking antacids or assuming an upright position; it usually is not exacerbated by exertion. The pain due to ischemic heart disease usually is unaffected by the composition of foods swallowed or by a change in position and is worsened by exertion. Making a definitive diagnosis of the cause of the chest pain may require an esophageal manometric study with acid perfusion (Bernstein test) or even a provocative challenge with ergonovine or a cholinergic agent during the manometric study. The challenge may induce coronary vasospasm, so it must be conducted cautiously with simultaneous cardiac monitoring. Esophageal abnormalities that may cause anginalike chest pain include diffuse esophageal spasm (repetitive, simultaneous, nonperistaltic esophageal contractions of prolonged duration interspersed with normal contractions), and "nutcracker" esophagus (peristaltic but high-amplitude contractions and no or incomplete relaxation of the lower esophageal sphincter).

Patients who have a brief and uncomplicated history of esophageal reflux may be treated symptomatically for a period of 2 to 4 weeks without prior diagnostic study. However, a more complicated history or an inadequate response to the therapeutic trial should prompt further evaluation.

Since the barium esophagogram is not sensitive in detecting mucosal abnormalities, esophagoscopy with biopsy of the mucosa is usually the most rewarding study in suspected reflux esophagitis. The patient's symptoms of reflux may be more severe than visual inspection of the esophagus would suggest, so the biopsy may be necessary in order to establish the presence of esophagitis.

TREATMENT. Initially, nonsurgical therapy, consisting of pharmacologic and nonpharmacologic measures, usually is effective. Basic (stage I) therapy involves the following[6]:

- Eat three small meals a day. Avoid between-meal snacks.
- Avoid foods that decrease lower esophageal sphincter pressure (alcohol, fats, chocolate, peppermint).
- Take nothing by mouth for 3 to 4 hours before retiring.

- Elevate the head of the bed 3 to 6 inches with bricks or blocks.
- Avoid stooping and straining.
- Lose weight if obese.
- Avoid drugs that decrease pressure in the lower esophageal sphincter (nicotine, progesterone, theophylline, anticholinergics, diazepam, beta-adrenergic agonists, calcium channel blockers).
- Take a liquid antacid 1 and 3 hours after meals and at bedtime.

Patients who do not respond to stage I medical therapy within 2 weeks should start stage II therapy: except for the HS antacid, stage I therapy is continued, and a histamine H_2-antagonist (e.g., ranitidine, 150 mg bid) is added. If symptoms persist beyond 2 weeks, drugs that increase pressure in the lower esophageal sphincter (e.g., bethanechol, 10 to 25 mg tid and HS, or metochlopramide, 10 mg tid and HS) may be added; both of these drugs may have severe side effects in the elderly and should be used with caution.

Bougienage is the primary therapy for most patients with benign esophageal stricture; it is successful in 75 to 80 percent of patients. When medical treatment of reflux esophagitis fails, the patient may be a candidate for an antireflux operation. Since this major surgery carries an increased risk in the elderly, it is not to be recommended until more conservative measures have been thoroughly tested and failed. A hiatal hernia with a benign, peptic stricture above it is illustrated in Figure 39–1.

DISEASES OF THE STOMACH AND DUODENUM

Peptic Ulcer

Even though gastric acid secretion tends to diminish with aging, peptic ulcers of both the stomach and duodenum remain common in the elderly. Indeed, ulcer disease may present initially in old age. The peak incidence of gastric ulcers occurs at about 55 to 65 years of age. Gastric and duodenal ulcers occur with about equal frequency in the elderly, whereas duodenal ulcers predominate in younger persons. Often the symptoms of peptic ulcer

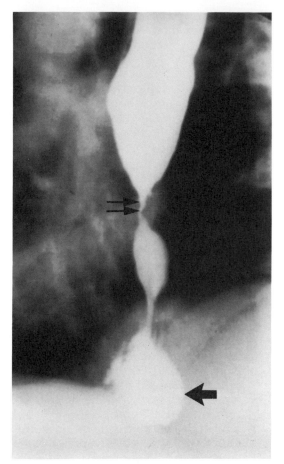

FIGURE 39–1. Barium esophagogram showing a sliding hiatal hernia (arrow) with a stricture above it (double arrow).

disease in elderly patients are atypical or nonspecific. Also, peptic ulcer disease in this age group may present with a major complication such as acute hemorrhage or perforation without antecedent symptoms. The symptoms of gastric versus duodenal ulcers may be indistinguishable, and so are the symptoms of benign versus malignant gastric ulcers. Vomiting within 30 minutes after food ingestion is, however, more frequent with a gastric ulcer. A benign gastric ulcer is not a premalignant condition. Aspirin, alcohol, and nonsteroidal anti-inflammatory drugs (NSAIDs) are considered risk factors for gastric ulcer because they break down some gastric mucosal defenses.

DIAGNOSIS AND MANAGEMENT OF GASTRIC ULCERS. In the past, most gastric ulcers were discovered on an upper gastrointestinal x-ray study done for patients' abdominal complaints. As fiberoptic endoscopy has become a more common initial examination, however, ulcers are being found increasingly often by this method. In the elderly, most gastric ulcers identified radiographically should also be examined endoscopically so that biopsies can be done and the lesions can be brushed for cytologic examination. The radiographic appearance of a large, benign gastric ulcer is illustrated in Figure 39–2. Although the risk of malignancy in a gastric ulcer is low (probably no more than 1 percent), making the diagnosis promptly is important in directing the patient's subsequent care.

Medical therapy for gastric ulcer consists of:

- An H$_2$-receptor antagonist such as cimetidine, 300 mg tid with meals and HS, or ranitidine, 150 mg bid. Sucralfate, 1 gm tid ½ hour before meals and HS, also may be effective.
- NSAIDs, aspirin, and alcohol should be discontinued. Alternatives to NSAIDs (gold therapy, salicylo-salicylic acid) should be used for patients whose diseases, e.g., rheumatoid arthritis, require them.
- The duration of treatment is determined by the patient's response. Most ulcers heal within 8 weeks, and therapy can be discontinued. Large ulcers may take longer to heal. If the ulcer has not shown substantial healing or complete healing within 8 to 10

weeks, a reassessment to determine whether it is a gastric malignancy should be conducted. Except for very large gastric ulcers (greater than 2.5 cm in diameter) that have demonstrated continued healing, surgery is recommended for ulcers that have not healed by 12 to 15 weeks.

DIAGNOSIS AND MANAGEMENT OF DUODENAL ULCERS. Duodenal ulcers may be diagnosed radiographically, but fiberoptic endoscopy is superior, especially for identifying small ulcers. Since duodenal ulcers have no malignant potential, they need not undergo biopsy, and endoscopic examination of a duodenal ulcer that has been seen radiographically ordinarily is not indicated. The following are key features of the medical therapy of duodenal ulcers:

- An H$_2$-receptor antagonist drug generally is the basic medication. Cimetidine, 300 mg tid and HS, 400 mg bid, or 900 mg HS; ranitidine, 150 mg bid or 300 mg HS; and famotidine, 40 mg HS, have all been shown to be 80 to 90 percent effective in healing uncomplicated duodenal ulcers within 6 weeks. Sucralfate, 1 gm qid before meals and HS, also is effective.
- An antacid 1 and 3 hours after meals and HS is effective but is less frequently prescribed because of poor patient compliance and diarrhea.

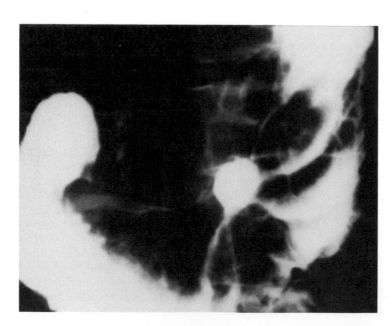

FIGURE 39–2. Upper gastrointestinal radiograph showing a large, benign gastric ulcer with mucosal folds radiating from the edge of the ulcer crater.

- Anticholinergics are not recommended for initial treatment of duodenal ulcer because of the frequency of untoward side effects, especially in the elderly.
- Strong gastric secretagogues (alcohol, coffee, broth) should be avoided.
- Salicylates, NSAIDs, and cigarette smoking should be avoided.
- Bedtime snacks, which stimulate nocturnal gastric acid secretion, should be avoided.
- About 75 percent of healed duodenal ulcers recur within 1 year after therapy is stopped. An HS dose of cimetidine (400 mg), ranitidine (150 mg), or famotidine (20 mg), or sucralfate, 1 gm bid, is about 80 percent effective in preventing recurrences and is indicated in patients who have frequent recurrences, complicated ulcers, or medical problems requiring the use of ulcerogenic drugs.
- Unresponsiveness of duodenal ulcers to routine medical treatment should prompt an evaluation for a gastric hypersecretory state (Zollinger-Ellison syndrome).
- Surgery for duodenal ulcer disease nowadays is reserved for complications of the ulcer (major hemorrhage, perforation, gastric outlet obstruction).

SPECIAL CONSIDERATIONS FOR MANAGING PEPTIC ULCERS IN THE ELDERLY. The side effects of medications used in ulcer therapy deserve special consideration in the elderly. Calcium-containing antacids may exacerbate constipation, magnesium-containing antacids may cause diarrhea, and aluminum-containing antacids must be used with caution in the presence of poor renal function. Generally, the complications caused by H_2-receptor antagonists and sucralfate are few. However, cimetidine can cause mental confusion in elderly persons[7] and may alter the metabolism of certain drugs (diazepam, warfarin, theophylline, propranolol, phenytoin, lidocaine). About 3 percent of patients taking ranitidine have headache, rash, or dizziness. Sucralfate may cause constipation.

Hemorrhage from either gastric or duodenal ulcer is less well tolerated in the elderly than in younger persons. Thus, special attention to making the diagnosis of bleeding early and instituting care promptly is important. Strict management of blood and fluid replacement in order to avoid either hypovolemia or blood-volume overload is essential. In general, increased age of the bleeding patient should prompt surgery earlier than in younger persons. A relatively low-risk operation (vagotomy and pyloroplasty) usually is preferred to more extensive ulcer surgery in elderly persons. Patients in this age group also may be candidates for endoscopic treatment, e.g., electrocoagulation or laser therapy, for their bleeding ulcer.

Chronic Gastritis and Nonulcer Dyspepsia

Atrophy of the gastric mucosa and associated decreased acid secretion (chronic atrophic gastritis) are features of old age. Chronic atrophic gastritis is believed to be an asymptomatic state, but it may lead to achlorhydrin and cobalamin deficiency and predispose to the development of gastric cancer.

Recently, attention has focused on chronic gastritis of the antrum (the type of gastritis sometimes called type B gastritis).[8] Renewed interest in this form of gastritis has been prompted by the discovery that a *Campylobacter*-like organism, now referred to as *Campylobacter pylori*, often is associated with the gastritis.[9] Histologically, this chronic, active antral gastritis has both acute and chronic inflammatory cells in the lamina propria and decreased numbers of mucus-secreting cells in the epithelium. Symptoms of upper abdominal pain, anorexia, nausea, and fullness may be associated. Both the frequency of such gastritis and the presence of *C. pylori* in the gastric mucosa increase strikingly with age, and the organisms are present in up to 90 percent of patients with this kind of gastritis. The dyspepsia that may be caused by such chronic, active antral gastritis responds poorly to H_2-receptor antagonists but has been improved by the use of bismuth compounds (Pepto-Bismol) or antibiotics that are effective against *C. pylori*. The recently appreciated association of *Campylobacter*-like organisms with gastritis is currently undergoing intensive investigation, and more definitive guidelines for management of the condition likely will be forthcoming soon. *C. pylori* is also associated with duodenal ulcer (in more than 90 percent of patients in some series), but the pathogenetic relationship to the ulcers is undefined.

DISEASES OF THE COLON

Diverticular Disease

DIAGNOSTIC CONSIDERATIONS. The prevalence of colonic diverticulosis increases with age and is estimated to be about 25 to 40 percent in people aged 65 to 74 years. Diverticular disease predominantly affects people in the Western world and has been attributed to the low fiber content of the usual Western diet. Most diverticula are diffusely distributed in the sigmoid colon, but they may be present anywhere in the colon and can vary in number from single to many in an individual patient. As the number of diverticula increases, the frequency of symptoms attributed to them also increases, but many symptoms, such as nonspecific abdominal pain, diarrhea, and constipation that may be associated with the diverticulosis may be due to other causes. About 80 percent of persons with colonic diverticula seem to remain symptom-free throughout life. The most common symptom that seems reliably correlated with the presence of diverticula is colicky or gripping pain in the left lower quadrant of the abdomen that is worse after meals. A cordlike loop of colon may be palpable in the left side of the false pelvis. The diverticula are best demonstrated radiographically, by barium enema.

TREATMENT OF UNCOMPLICATED DIVERTICULOSIS. The treatment of uncomplicated diverticulosis now usually includes an increased dietary intake of vegetable fiber, especially of cereal grains. The effectiveness of bran in the relief of symptoms of diverticular disease has been reported in most of the relevant controlled trials.[10] The rationale for using a high-fiber diet in the treatment of diverticular disease is based on observations that increased volume and weight of stool in the sigmoid colon will increase the radius of the bowel and concurrently decrease intraluminal pressure. Anticholinergic drugs often are tried in the treatment of diverticulosis, but

their efficacy is unestablished, and their use may be a factor in inducing pseudo-obstruction of the colon (Ogilvie's syndrome), which can be a serious complication in the elderly, as well as the more common side effects of dry mouth, blurred vision, and urinary retention.

COMPLICATIONS OF DIVERTICULOSIS. The principal complications of diverticulosis are diverticulitis, hemorrhage, and colonic obstruction.

DIVERTICULITIS. In most persons the course of diverticulitis is a benign one of self-limited episodes, but in others the disease may be severe and may even require surgical intervention. Patients with diverticulitis typically complain of left lower quadrant pain of increasing severity and have associated signs of abdominal infection (fever, leukocytosis, and peritoneal signs). In the aged, however, the signs of an acute inflammatory process may be muted and the severity of the patient's condition underestimated. Diagnostic evaluation of suspected diverticulitis should include a plain x-ray film of the abdomen for the presence of free air and sigmoidoscopy to search for other conditions such as rectal carcinoma. Careful sigmoidoscopy is safe even in the presence of acute diverticulitis with localized perforation. In most instances, barium enema should be deferred during the acute inflammatory process, but it should be done at some time during the work-up.

The treatment of diverticulitis usually includes broad spectrum antibiotics, nasogastric suction, and careful management of fluid requirements by intravenous infusion. In the average case, ampicillin or a cephalosporin will provide sufficient antibiotic coverage, but in patients with more severe sepsis, gentamicin or tobramycin together with clindamycin should be added to the regimen. Antibiotic treatment, once started, should be continued for not less than 7 to 10 days. Emergent resection of the colon (usually a staged operation requiring a temporary colostomy) is indicated if generalized peritonitis, persistent colonic obstruction, or signs of pericolic abscess are present.

HEMORRHAGE. Rectal bleeding in some form occurs in 10 to 25 percent of patients with known diverticular disease, and severe hemorrhage occurs in 3 to 5 percent, but the bleeding does not always originate in the diverticula. When bleeding is from a diverticulum, it is located in the right colon in about two-thirds of cases. The bleeding may be massive and may continue for several days.

Diagnostic evaluation of the patient with presumed hemorrhage from colonic diverticulosis should include efforts to exclude bleeding from an upper gastrointestinal source, by placement of a nasogastric tube, and searches for other causes of lower gastrointestinal bleeding (e.g., hemorrhoids, neoplasms, and inflammatory bowel diseases). Radionuclide imaging after injection of ^{99}Tc-labeled autologous erythrocytes often quickly gives the approximate location of the bleeding site. The more invasive selective mesenteric arteriographic studies also can be performed, and, if the bleeding rate exceeds 1 ml/minute, extravasation into the lumen may be demonstrated and a diverticulum may even be outlined. In the patient whose bleeding has stopped, colonoscopy can be undertaken, provided that the colon can be adequately prepared, as with an isosmotic electrolyte, polyethylene glycol-containing solution. Colonoscopy is a sensitive means of identifying angiodysplastic lesions, which in the elderly may be an even more common cause of massive colonic bleeding than diverticula.

The treatment of hemorrhage from colonic diverticular disease involves the usual measures of fluid and blood replacement, with special attention to the decreased tolerance for hypovolemia in the elderly and the associated diseases and medications that often characterize this age group. If hemorrhage continues, intraarterial infusion of vasopressin at the site of the bleeding vessel may effect cessation. Surgical excision of the affected segment of colon sometimes must be undertaken if hemorrhage continues despite the above measures.

Colorectal Neoplasms

Some aspects of colorectal cancer are discussed in Section VIII, Chapter 33. Here we will emphasize some special features of making the diagnosis and preventing colorectal neoplasms in the elderly.

THE PROBLEM. Cancer of the colon and rectum is second only to lung cancer as a cause of cancer-related deaths in the United States. The incidence of colorectal cancer increases dramatically after age 40, doubling every 10 years until it peaks at age 75.

Colorectal cancer should now be regarded as a preventable disease. The evidence permitting this sweeping statement is the fact that the majority of colonic carcinomas almost certainly are derived from adenomatous polyps, and removal of these premalignant lesions can result in a dramatic reduction in the frequency of development of colorectal cancer; a surveillance program using annual sigmoidoscopy and fulgeration of any visualized polyps in more than 21,000 patients resulted in a greater than 85 percent reduction in the subsequent development of rectosigmoid carcinoma.[11] Adenomatous polyps can be detected with a high percentage of accuracy by various combinations of techniques, including testing feces for the presence of occult blood and examining the colon by barium enema, flexible sigmoidoscopy, or colonoscopy (see below). Finally, most adenomatous polyps can be removed from the rectum or colon with a reasonable measure of safety. With colonoscopes and colonoscopists proliferating year by year, the main deterrent to the prevention of colorectal cancer is the occasional complication from the procedure and its expense.[12]

Other important considerations in the management of colorectal adenomas are the relationship between the size of the polyps and the likelihood of cancer being associated with them, and the duration required for progression of an adenoma to a carcinoma. In large series, the malignancy rate in adenomas of less than 1 cm in diameter has been about 1 percent, whereas in those greater than 2 cm it is nearly 50 percent.[13] The data on the interval between the detection of an adenoma and its progression to a carcinoma are fragmentary, but it probably is on the order of 5 to 15 years.[13] We conclude that balanced judgment is called for in screening for colonic adenomas and for their removal in the elderly. Although we generally favor surveillance for colonic neoplasms, the risk of performing a sigmoidoscopic or colonoscopic polypectomy may outweigh the risk of cancer developing from an adenoma, especially a small one, within the expected lifetime of a patient.

SCREENING FOR COLONIC NEO-PLASMS. When screening for colonic neoplasms is considered desirable, several methods are available. Testing for occult blood in the feces is a useful screening technique but is not ideal because patient compliance may be low, the tests are not specific for neoplastic disease, and they have both significant false-positive and false-negative rates. Hemoccult II (Smith-Kline Diagnostics, Sunnyvale, CA), which includes guaiac-impregnated paper, is now probably the most widely used test for fecal occult blood. In asymptomatic patients over the age of 40 the test results are positive in about 3 to 4 percent, and the predictive value for adenoma or carcinoma is about 45 percent; the false-positive rate is about 2 to 3 percent.[11] The positive predictive value increases to about 80 percent in persons over age 70. Food with a high peroxidase content (turnips, horseradish, broccoli, cauliflower) can cause the test results to be falsely positive, and drugs or chemicals that may cause gastrointestinal blood loss (nonsteroidal anti-inflammatory drugs, alcohol, aspirin) can cause a positive test result. Vitamin C can inhibit the oxidation reaction of the test, causing a false-negative result. Ordinarily, the patient should collect at least six fecal smears (on three Hemoccult II cards), and the slides should be tested within 4 days. A single positive test result for occult blood should be regarded as significant and its cause evaluated. It is important to remember that as many as 30 percent of patients with colonic carcinoma and 70 percent with adenomas will not have a positive test result for fecal occult blood; this lack of sensitivity of the test has prompted some workers to advocate routine proctosigmoidoscopy at 3- to 5-year intervals in persons over 50 years of age, or even an initial colonoscopy followed by periodic sigmoidoscopy.

Nowadays the flexible sigmoidoscope, which has a length of 60 cm, is greatly preferred to the rigid sigmoidoscope because of the greater safety and comfort for the patient as well as the much higher yield of significant lesions detected by the flexible instrument (Fig. 39–3). The choice of whether to use barium enema or colonoscopy for cancer screening is not easily made. Colonoscopy is definitely superior to the barium enema in detecting adeno-mas, especially small ones, but the barium enema is less expensive and may be safer (depending on the skill of the examiner). The risk of colonoscopy is largely that associated with the accompanying polypectomy, but of course, the ability to perform polypectomy by means of the colonoscope is a major asset of the instrument and helps to account for its increasing popularity. If barium enema is to be used for surveillance of colonic neoplasms, the air-contrast technique should be used because its yield is 40 to 60 percent greater than that of the single-contrast enema.

In Figure 39–4 is illustrated a schematic approach to the screening of an average-risk person over the age of 50 years for colonic neoplasms. More rigorous screening is required in high-risk persons: patients with inflammatory bowel disease, familial polyposis, previous colonic cancer, or adenomatous polyps.

Hemorrhoids and Anal Fissures

Anal fissures may cause a burning or tearing pain that is initiated by defecation and resolves soon after defecation. Nonthrombosed hemorrhoids are not painful and usually present as rectal bleeding or an anal mass that appears during defecation. Rectal bleeding should not be attributed to hemorrhoids without an examination to exclude inflammatory or neoplastic causes of the bleeding. Thrombosed hemorrhoids may cause severe, persistent anal pain and tenderness. Although the diagnosis of an anal fissure can be established by rectal examination alone, sigmoidoscopy should be performed to exclude inflammation or neoplastic lesions of the rectum, which can cause similar symptoms.

Medical management of nonthrombosed hemorrhoids includes sitz baths, stool softeners, topical anesthetics, and emollient suppositories. Several approaches are available for the therapy of nonthrombosed hemorrhoids that fail to respond to medical management. Rubber band ligation is appropriate for internal hemorrhoids that can be ligated 0.5 cm or more above the pectinate line; ligation of internal hemorrhoids below this point causes severe pain.

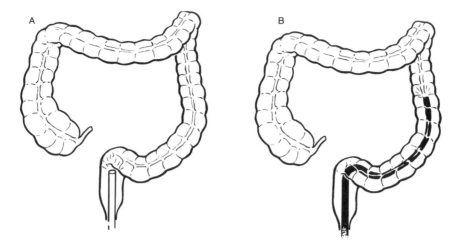

FIGURE 39–3. *Usual depth of insertion of rigid sigmoidoscope, A and flexible sigmoidoscope, B. (From Goff JS: Rigid vs flexible sigmoidoscopy. In Levine JS, ed: Decision Making in Gastroenterology. Toronto, BC Decker Inc, 1985, p 22.)*

A thrombosed external hemorrhoid may present as an acutely painful, hard anal mass that is tender to palpation, round, and bluish. It arises below the pectinate line and is covered by squamous epithelium. If symptoms are severe, become increasingly severe, or fail to respond to medical treatment (as above), the thrombosed vessel should be excised under local anesthesia. Prolapsed, thrombosed internal hemorrhoids can be differentiated from external hemorrhoids because the former are covered by red rectal mucosa.

COLORECTAL CANCER SCREENING PROGRAM

AVERAGE-RISK PATIENTS

```
                    ┌─────────────────────────┐
                    │  Individuals over  50   │
                    └─────────────────────────┘
                                 │
   ┌─────────────────┐      ┌─────────────────────────┐
   │ Digital Rectal  │◄─(−)─│  Fecal Occult Blood     │
   │  Examination    │      │     Test (annual)       │
   │    (annual)     │      └─────────────────────────┘
   │Proctosigmoidoscopy│                 │(+)
   │   (3-5 years)   │                   ▼
   └─────────────────┘      ┌─────────────────────────┐
          │(+)              │   Digital Rectal        │
                            │   Examination           │
                            │ Proctosigmoidoscopy     │
                            └─────────────────────────┘
                              (−)│        │(+)
                                 ▼        ▼
                     ┌─────────────────────────┐
                     │  Double-Contrast        │
                     │  Barium Enema           │
                     │  Colonoscopy            │
                     └─────────────────────────┘
                      (−)│              │(+)
   ┌─────────────────┐   ▼              ▼  ┌──────────────────┐
   │  Upper GI and   │◄─(+)─────────────── │ Diagnosis.Therapy│
   │Small Bowel Series│                    │    Follow-Up     │
   └─────────────────┘                     └──────────────────┘
```

FIGURE 39–4. *A schema for the surveillance of average-risk persons for colonic neoplasms.*

If medical treatment of the prolapsed hemorrhoid fails, injection of a mixture of an anesthetic with hyaluronidase may result in relief of pain and prompt reduction of the prolapsed hemorrhoid.

Single anal fissures usually occur in the posterior midline. The presence of multiple fissures or fissures not in the midline should prompt an inquiry for inflammatory bowel disease, infection, or anal cancer. An acute fissure is a superficial tear with a reddish base that bleeds easily. If the fissure is chronic, a sentinel pile may be evident as a swollen tag of skin at the anal verge, and gentle eversion of the anus reveals the fissure with the white transverse fibers of the internal sphincter exposed in the base. Simple fissures may be treated with sitz baths, stool softeners, topical anesthetics, and a high-fiber diet. Treatment of more severe or persistent symptoms may require sphincterotomy or anal dilatation.

REFERENCES

1. Stanley TC, Cockings JB: Upper gastrointestinal endoscopy in the elderly. Postgrad Med J 54:257, 1978.
2. Jacobsohn WZ, Levy A: Endoscopy of upper gastrointestinal tract is feasible and safe in elderly patients. Geriatrics 32:80, 1977.
3. Mann SK, Mann NS, Tsai MF, et al: A comparison of fiberoptic colonoscopy in older and younger patients. VA Practitioner 3:49–56, 1986.
4. Soergel KH, Zboralski FE, Amberg JR: Presbyesophagus: esophageal motility in nonagenarians. J Clin Invest 43:1472, 1964.

5. Benjamin SB, Castell DO: Chest pain of esophageal origin. Arch Intern Med 143:772, 1983.

6. Struthers JE, Jr: Reflux esophagitis. In Levine JS, ed: Decision Making in Gastroenterology. Toronto, BC Decker, 1985, pp 130–131.

7. Kimelblatt BJ, Cerra FB, Calleri G, et al: Dose and serum concentration relationships in cimetidine-associated mental confusion. Gastroenterology 78:791, 1980.

8. Strickland RG, Mackay IR: A reappraisal of the nature and significance of chronic atrophic gastritis. Digest Dis 18:426, 1973.

9. Blaser MJ, Brown WR: Campylobacter and gastroduodenal inflammation. Adv Intern Med. 34:21, 1989.

10. Almy TP: Some disorders of the alimentary tract. In Andres R, Bierman EL, Hazzard WR, eds: Principles of Geriatric Medicine. New York, McGraw-Hill, 1985, pp 662–681.

11. Sherlock P, Lipkin M, Winawer SJ: The prevention of colon cancer. Am J Med 68:917, 1980.

12. Welch CE: Polyps and cancer of the colon. Am J Surg 138:625, 1979.

13. Day DW, Morson BC: The adenoma-carcinoma sequence. Maj Prob Pathol 10:58, 1978.

14. Goff JS: Rigid vs flexible sigmoidoscopy. In Levine JS, ed: Decision Making in Gastroenterology. Toronto, BC Decker, 1985, pp 22–25.

CHAPTER 40

Diabetes Mellitus and Hyperlipidemic Disorders

Fred D. Hofeldt

One evil in old age is that, as your time is come, you think every little illness is the beginning of the end. When a man expects to be arrested, every knock at the door is an alarm.

SYDNEY SMITH, *Letter (1836)*

Diabetes mellitus is a common medical condition of the elderly[1-3] and is seen in nearly 20 percent of those over 70 years of age. The incidence of diabetes is six to eight times greater in the elderly than in young adults and is three times greater than in the general population. The prevalence of frank diabetes in the elderly over 65 years of age is approximately 10 percent, and an additional 10 percent will have diabetic results on oral glucose tolerance tests. The most common type of diabetes in the elderly is type II or non-insulin-dependent diabetes mellitus (NIDDM), which has a hereditary association, is aggravated by obesity and diabetogenic drugs, and often responds to diet or anti-hyperglycemic drug therapy. The presentation of type I or insulin-dependent diabetes mellitus (IDDM), however, is by no means rare in the elderly. Acute illness or stress may act to precipitate or aggravate pre-existing diabetes, and some patients present in an insulin-deficient state with diabetic ketoacidosis. Following resolution of this decompensated state, patients frequently can be managed with diet or oral agents. The elderly diabetic patient has more complicating coronary artery disease, cerebral vascular disease, peripheral vascular disease, neuropathy, blindness, and nephropathy than the nondiabetic elderly patient.

Associated with aging is an age-related deterioration in carbohydrate tolerance[6-9] that affects probably 20 percent of the

elderly and as much as 50 percent of those with physical inactivity or obesity. Hemoglobin A_{1C} increases with age, mainly as a reflection of elevated postprandial glucose levels as fasting glucose values change little with aging. Aging is associated with a change in body composition—an increase in adipose mass that may contribute to the carbohydrate intolerance of aging and the risk of diabetes mellitus. Upper body segment obesity with excessive adipose accumulation in the neck, shoulders, and abdomen has been associated with a higher risk of diabetes mellitus in males and females compared to lower body segment obesity involving the hips or thighs.[4, 5] For example, the risk of diabetes mellitus is increased approximately three times with obesity per se, but with upper segment obesity the risk increases ten times. Studies of this age-related deterioration in carbohydrate tolerance implicate an acquired state of insulin resistance. Studies in elderly humans have not showed decreased insulin secretion, in contrast to studies in aging animals, which suggest that there is decreased insulin secretion per beta cell. Hence, it is the peripheral changes in insulin metabolism and action that characterize the hyperglycemia of human aging. These changes include a decreased metabolic clearance rate of insulin and defective insulin action in promoting glucose transport in muscle and fat cells. The number of the insulin receptors on target tissues is not decreased; hepatic glucose production remains normal and is suppressed normally by insulin in elderly patients. Fink et al[10, 11] have shown decreased in vivo glucose uptake in elderly patients compared to nonelderly patients. This defect exists in elderly patients even when their carbohydrate tolerance is normal, suggesting that it may be an ubiquitous feature of aging per se. The carbohydrate intolerance of aging can be readily distinguished from diabetes mellitus. The criteria established by the National Diabetes Data Group for diabetes is so generous that it need not be modified for elderly patients.[12] Since there is very little change in fasting glucose values with aging, the finding of fasting glucose values of more than 140 mg/dl on two occasions establishes the diagnosis of diabetes mellitus in the elderly. Symptoms of hyperglycemia are usually present at this time. A glucose tolerance test rarely needs to be performed in elderly patients to establish the diagnosis of diabetes mellitus. Elderly patients with type II diabetes manifest the same metabolic defects as those seen in maturity-onset type II disease, namely, delayed but enhanced insulin secretion to an oral glucose stimulus, peripheral insulin resistance, and increased fasting hepatic glucose production.[13–15]

Diabetes mellitus and aging share certain similarities, and as such, diabetes mellitus is considered a model for premature aging.[16–17] With aging there is a progressive increase in capillary basement membrane thickening, which is also seen in patients with long-standing diabetes mellitus, especially if hyperglycemia is not controlled. Atherosclerotic complications occur commonly in elderly patients and prematurely in diabetic patients. Increasing collagen cross-linking and resistance to collagenase digestion is seen with aging and at a earlier age in patients with diabetes mellitus. Human skin fibroblasts, when maintained in tissue culture, have a finite in vitro life span. With increasing donor age of these fibroblasts, there is a decreased cell replication. A marked reduction in the replication life span of fibroblasts is seen in patients with diabetes mellitus. Hence, the combination of diabetes plus aging leads to a functional age greater than the chronologic age in the diabetic. It has been estimated that the chronologic age of the diabetic patient plus the years' duration of diabetes is an assessment of the "functional" or physiologic age.

Aging with its physiomental deterioration and changes in nutritional status[18, 19]

makes the elderly diabetic patient more difficult to manage. These changes include alterations in memory, hearing, and vision; muscle weakness and incoordination; arthritis; absent teeth or loose dentures. There may also be insufficient financial resources, lack of support systems, or an absent spouse. Older patients may be housebound, which is associated with reduced social contacts, reduced physical activity, and inadequate diet. Functional impairment is not too uncommon in the elderly. In a survey of institutionalized elderly patients,[20] mental impairment was seen in 32 percent, malnutrition in 39 percent, visual impairment in 23 percent, gait disturbances in 39 percent, and incontinence in 29 percent.

With aging there is a decrease in the metabolic rate,[21] which results in a reduced caloric requirement of approximately 500 kcal per day. This reduced metabolic rate is due to changes both in the resting or basal metabolic rate and in that due to physical activity. The major decrease in energy expenditure occurs because of reduced activity.[22] The principles of dietary management in elderly diabetic patients are the same as those in younger patients with important emphasis on avoiding hypoglycemia; if unrecognized, hypoglycemia may accelerate mental deterioration. Overweight patients are prescribed a 1200 to 1500 kcal diet. Many older diabetic patients are of ideal or less than ideal body weight and need approximately 25 kcal/kg body weight. Meals should be proportioned into three equal feedings, and snacks are advised for insulin-treated patients. Avoidance of a high-fat diet as advocated by the American Diabetes Association[23] addresses the issue of a coexisting lipid disorder. Increasing the dietary fiber content to 40 gm/day assists in digestive function and has a beneficial effect on carbohydrate intolerance and hyperlipidemia. Fructose can be used as a sugar substitute, realizing its caloric content.[24] The elderly diet is influenced by altered food preferences caused by aging, changes in taste and smell perception, difficulty in swallowing due to loss of salivary secretions, loose dentures or missing teeth, and altered gastrointestinal function with constipation, bloating, abdominal gas, and discomfort. There is a decreased appreciation of thirst, which makes the elderly person more prone to dehydration. Preparing foods is difficult because of diminished vision, incapacitating arthritis, tremor, and musculoskeletal weakness. Houseboundness and poor food selection contribute to a monotonous diet. The elderly comprise one of the poorer socioeconomic groups, 20 percent existing at or below the poverty level.

The majority of elderly diabetic patients will respond to oral hypoglycemics. The major class of drugs used to lower blood glucose in type II diabetic patients is the sulfonylureas. In 1956 the first agent, tolbutamide, was released for clinical use in the United States. In subsequent years additional oral hypoglycemic agents such as chlorpropamide, acetohexamide, and tolazamide were effectively used in the management of adults with diabetes. These agents have been called the first-generation sulfonylureas. The newer or second generation agents available in the United States are glyburide and glipizide (see Table 40–1). The choice of an oral agent depends on understanding its metabolic characteristics, such as its hepatic metabolism, the toxicity of its metabolic by-products, and their accumulation in patients with renal disease. Mild renal impairment occurs with aging—nearly a 30 percent decline in creatinine clearance may be seen in older subjects. Of the first-generation sulfonylurea agents, tolbutamide (Orinase) has been the agent of choice because of its short half-life, its hepatic metabolism to inactive compounds, and the safety associated with a wide dosage range from 0.25 to 3.0 gm daily.

The second-generation sulfonylureas are superior because of their nonionic binding to serum proteins and their less active or inactive metabolites. First-generation oral agents are characterized by ionic binding to serum proteins and can be displaced or can displace similar acidic drugs such as phenylbutazone, warfarin, and salicylates. This characteristic may increase the level of free sulfonylureas causing hypoglycemia, especially in ill patients whose food intake is limited and who may be ingesting other medications such as aspirin. The elderly are notorious for their polymedication, consuming a number of over-the-counter medications, shared medications, and self-prescribed medica-

tions. Fewer drug-drug interactions occur with the nonionic binding, second-generation sulfonylureas. The second-generation sulfonylureas are metabolized to less active compounds, especially glipizide, whose metabolites are inactive. They have a very potent effect in lowering blood glucose levels and should be prescribed to the elderly with mild diabetes at the lowest possible daily dose (e.g., 1.25 mg for glyburide or 2.5 mg for glipizide) with careful glucose monitoring prior to any dose increase. In Table 40–1 the various oral agents are listed as well as those preferred in elderly patients. With acute stress, a mild non-insulin-requiring elderly diabetic patient may experience sudden metabolic decompensation with progression to severe hyperglycemia, hyperosmolar dehydration or coma, or even diabetic ketoacidosis. The impaired thirst mechanisms accompanying aging contribute to the dehydration.[25–28] Hence, insulin therapy may be required for the acute illness.

Insulin treatment is required in symptomatic elderly patients. About 30 percent of insulin-requiring type II diabetic patients can be treated with one injection of intermediate-acting insulin a day, and this regimen may be sufficient for many elderly diabetic patients. A reasonable starting dose for insulin is 0.5 to 0.7 unit/kg. If short-acting insulin is needed, the premixed insulin preparations are ideal because they are easier for older patients to draw the correct dose. Obesity is associated with insulin resistance and increases insulin requirements, leading to more intensified insulin programs such as the split-mix use of NPH (*n*eutral *p*rotamine *H*agedorn) and regular insulin before breakfast and NPH and regular insulin before supper. With these split-mix regimens, two-thirds of the insulin dose is given in the morning before breakfast, and the remainder before supper. Usually 4 to 16 units of preprandial regular insulin are sufficient when the patient mixes insulin himself. Lente-regular insulin combinations should be avoided because mixing causes loss of the short-acting insulin activity. During acute illnesses that require hospitalization for infections or surgery, insulin infusions will ideally maintain normal plasma glucose levels.

A well-instituted home glucose monitoring (HGM) program improves compliance

TABLE 40–1. Comparison of Oral Hypoglycemic Agents

Drug	Daily Dose Range (mg)	Tablet Size (mg)	Administration	Metabolism
First-Generation				
Tolbutamide*	500–3000	250, 500	bid–qid	Liver to inactive metabolites; short half-life (4 hr)
Tolazamide	100–1000	100, 250, 500	qd–bid	Liver to metabolites with hypoglycemic activity; medium half-life (7 hr)
Acetohexamide	500–1500	250, 500	qd–bid	Short half-life (2 hr) but liver metabolites have 6-hr half-life
Chlorpropamide	100–750	100, 250	qd	Renal excretion of unmetabolized drug; long half-life (36 hr)
Second-Generation				
Glyburide*	1.25–20	1.25, 2.5, 5	qd–bid	Liver to weakly active metabolites; medium half-life (10 hr)
Glipizide*	2.5–40	5, 10	qd–bid	Liver to inactive metabolites; short half-life (4 hr)

*Most ideal agents for elderly patients.

and provides guidelines for altering therapy. A blood glucose measuring meter is very useful in elderly patients. Urine testing is rarely sufficient and should be discarded. Insulin-treated patients require more frequent HGM determinations, which are done by checking a fasting glucose value and a glucose profile (before the lunch, midday, and bedtime measurements) and should be done at least once during the week and once on the weekend. In patients treated with diet or oral agents, a fasting HGM value performed once on a weekday and once on the weekend may be sufficient. Many times it is difficult for these patients to test at more frequent intervals owing to the complexity of their life situation and physical impairment due to the aging process.

Exercise may be limited by the physical, mental, and neuromuscular deterioration accompanying aging and by the tendency toward inactivity and houseboundness. An exercise program depends on the functional capacity of the individual. In many elderly patients, it is important simply to promote ambulation or prescribe a walking exercise program.[22, 29] Attention must be given to household hazards that may lead to falls and injury.

The treatment goal is to relieve symptoms. These include polyuria, polydipsia, decreased visual acuity, fatigue, weight loss, general malaise, vaginitis, or recurring urinary tract infections. Lowering the blood glucose level to levels below the renal threshold is sufficient to relieve glycosuria and nocturia. With aging, the renal tubular glucose resorption threshold may increase from 180 to approximately 280 mg/dl, allowing the patient to be asymptomatic at higher glucose values. The accepted glucose profile in the elderly diabetic is maintenance of a fasting plasma glucose level at or below 150 mg/dl and a plasma glucose profile under 200 mg/dl.

Of special concern in elderly diabetic patients is hypoglycemia, which can go unrecognized. Hypoglycemia is potentiated by alcohol, malnutrition, and beta blockers. Approximately 4 to 8 percent of elderly patients are alcoholics.[30] Hypoglycemia is a myocardial stress and may unmask subclinical coronary artery disease or cerebral vascular insufficiency. Hypoglycemia is particularly dangerous in the patient with autonomic neuropathy, in whom there is a deficient counterregulatory hormonal response of glucagon and catecholamines to the hypoglycemia. Autonomic neuropathy may also cause a decrease in gastric emptying and gastrointestinal motility that affects the absorption of nutrients. The elderly patient with autonomic neuropathy also needs to be observed for hypoglycemic unawareness. Hypoglycemia may be associated with other medical illnesses such as disorders of the gastrointestinal tract, causing a failure of nutrient absorption, renal failure, chronic liver disease, hypopituitarism, hypothyroidism, and adrenal insufficiency. Hypothermia may be a clue to undiagnosed hypoglycemia. Because of the seriousness of hypoglycemia in elderly patients, the criteria for blood glucose control should be less strict, as previously discussed.

Diabetic patients undergoing surgical procedures need a very thorough preoperative assessment of the cardiopulmonary, hepatic, renal, and central nervous system functional reserve capacity. They need careful intraoperative and postoperative observation for complicating disorders of these vital organ systems, particularly infection or hypernatremia.[27, 28] The insulin-treated patient can be managed during surgery with the administration of one-half the usual NPH insulin dose given subcutaneously just prior to surgery with a saline 5 percent dextrose infusion at 125 ml/hr. The evening dose of NPH is held on the day before surgery. Even better intraoperative management is provided by a regular insulin infusion adjusted to maintain a blood glucose level of 150 to 180 mg/dl during the operative procedure attainable by varying the rate of the infusion from 1 to 3 units/hr. Postoperatively, the blood sugar level is measured at 6-hour intervals and treated with regular insulin doses until the patient has resumed oral feeding, at which time their previous insulin program can be reinstituted. With constant glucose solutions being infused, 4 to 16 units of regular insulin given every 6 hours, adjusted by glucose measurement, are usually required. Intraoperative hypoglycemia should be avoided at all costs.

Foot Care

Good foot care[31–33] is essential in all diabetic patients, particularly the elderly patient, in whom the aging process has led to poor foot sensation, foot deformities, and peripheral vascular insufficiency. In this setting, patients are prone to foot trauma, ulceration, and infection. The foot should be inspected at each office visit and also inspected daily by the patient to ensure the absence of any lesion. Patients should be taught to inspect their feet visually and to palpate the foot for pressure points, warm spots, or breaks in the skin. The feet should be kept dry and clean; they should be washed several times weekly to ensure good hygiene. Dry feet can best be treated by the application of a lanolin-containing preparation. Footware

should be supportive and comfortable. Ideally, patients should wear well-fitted leather shoes. Walking barefoot should be avoided. Toenails should be neatly trimmed transversely and the nail edges filed carefully. Pressure spots need to be evaluated for the need of a metatarsal bar. Foot ulcers are slow to heal because of atherosclerotic and microvascular diseases, and neuropathic-related complications. Penetrating ulcers should be aggressively treated with hospitalization and intravenous antibiotics. These infections are usually polymicrobial. Superficial ulcers can be treated at home with local foot care, debridement, and oral antibiotics. When infection is present, limited ambulation is advocated for proper healing. With proper attention to good foot care, quality of life is improved, morbidity is less, and amputation is avoided.

Atherosclerosis

Diabetic patients have more complicating atherosclerosis, comprising peripheral vascular disease, cerebral vascular disease, and arteriosclerotic coronary heart disease. These conditions are increased approximately two to three times in diabetic patients compared with the general population.

Atherosclerotic disease in these patients is poorly related to the duration or severity of the diabetes and represents an accelerated aging process that accompanies diabetes plus the presence of other risk factors for atherosclerosis.[34] Macrovascular atherosclerotic disease is multifactorial, and assessment requires consideration of the patient's family history for atherosclerotic disease. Likewise, smoking, hypertension, dyslipidemia, obesity, and renal disease with its accompanying hypertension and lipid disorder are all additive factors. Coronary atherosclerosis occurs prematurely and is more severe in diabetic patients than in age-matched controls;[35–38] a similar relationship exists in diabetic patients for cerebral vascular disease.[39, 40] Diabetic patients, besides having more overall coronary artery disease, have a more diffuse disease process, more collateralization, and more myocardial infarctions. They may experience silent (painless) myocardial infarction much the same as nondiabetics.[41] The fatality rate is one to two times higher in the older diabetic than in the nondiabetic patient.

Peripheral vascular disease of the lower extremities is likewise increased in the diabetic patient compared with the general population. As with coronary artery disease, duration of diabetes is less associated with the presence of peripheral vascular disease than age. Atherosclerotic peripheral vascular disease contributes to disability with claudications, foot ulcerations, ischemia, and amputations. Diabetic patients with peripheral vascular disease and an ischemic extremity should be evaluated for small vessel bypass surgery as a consideration for limb salvage. Cerebral vascular disease with stroke or transient ischemic attacks is more common in diabetic patients. When stroke does occur, the elderly diabetic patient is more likely to experience associated complications or death than the same event occurring in the nondiabetic. This result appears to be related to the presence of the underlying coronary artery disease.

Therapeutic approaches for these atherosclerotic manifestations are symptomatic. Aspirin, 325 mg per day, may play a preventive role. Vascular surgery for coronary, peripheral, and cerebral vascular disease merits the same consideration as in nondiabetics but carries additional risks in diabetic patients of any age, particularly the elderly, who may have compromised multisystem organ function or reserve. Intravenous dye contrast studies in diabetic patients need cautious consideration, and when performed, the patient should be well hydrated to avoid complications of renal insufficiency. Mannitol administration may also be preventive. Although cessation of smoking and lowering of the blood pressure in hypertensive patients are recommended, there is no proof that altering any of the risk factors for atherosclerosis is beneficial to the elderly diabetic patient with established macrovascular disease. However, recent evidence in younger patients suggests that normalizing serum lipid levels may reduce the incidence of coronary insufficiency and fatal myocardial infarction[42, 43] and possibly reverse the course of large vessel atherosclerosis.[44–47]

Retinopathy

Diabetic retinopathy is less common in elderly patients with type II diabetes than in patients with type I diabetes. However, diabetes continues to be the leading cause of blindness in the United States. In the elderly type II patient, visual loss may be due to vascular insufficiency of the macula rather than to proliferative retinopathy. Photocoagulation is useful in preventing progression to blindness in patients with proliferative retinopathy, which includes a moderate-to-severe neovascularization on or near the disc with or without vitreous hemorrhage, and focal photocoagulation is of value in nonproliferative diabetic retinopathy with macular edema. The efficacy of photocoagulation in the treatment of other background retinopathy has yet to be established. If loss of vision has occurred from a vitreous hemorrhage or retinal traction, vitrectomy may be helpful. Control of hypertension is recommended. Other preventive treatments of retinopathy are not well established.

Cataracts

There is an increased prevalence of cataracts in diabetic patients under the age of 70. In patients over age 70, cataracts are equally common in diabetic and nondiabetic patients. Patients with significant visual impairment from cataracts are surgical candidates if diabetic retinopathy is not severe enough to prevent useful vision.

Nephropathy

Again, diabetic nephropathy is more common in type I than type II diabetes but is the cause of end-stage renal disease in approximately 5 to 20 percent of type II diabetic patients. Nephropathy in most patients follows a slowly progressive course over many years, leading to mild renal insufficiency. However, an accelerated form of diabetic glomerulosclerosis may be superimposed, and this leads to renal failure. Proteinuria is the first manifestation of diabetic nephropathy and is detected by the finding of more than 15 μg/min of urinary microalbumin.[48] A sensitive radioimmunoassay is necessary to detect microalbuminuria (15 to 150 μg/min) because the dipstick for albumin will be negative when microalbuminuria is present; this condition is termed incipient nephropathy. Elderly patients with proteinuria or impaired renal function need to be evaluated for other forms of urinary tract disease such as obstructive uropathy, urinary tract infections, hypertensive nephropathy, and papillary necrosis. Diabetic nephropathy can be diagnosed clinically if there is persistent proteinuria, diabetic retinopathy, diabetes of more than 10 years' duration, and no clinical or laboratory evidence of kidney or renal tract disease other than diabetic glomerulosclerosis. In patients with declining renal function, control of hypertension and the use of low-protein diets (0.8 gm protein per kg body weight) may slow its progression. Aggressive control of blood glucose is more important in arresting the progression of complications before clinical nephropathy occurs—i.e., microalbuminuria. With end-stage renal disease, the choice between hemodialysis, peritoneal dialysis, or no dialysis must be based on the individual, the needs of the patient's family, community resources, and the medical team. Although renal transplantation has been performed in diabetic patients under age 60, this is a less viable option in the elderly diabetic patient. As renal failure advances, there is a decrease in the insulin requirement.

Neuropathy

The etiology of diabetic neuropathy is multifactorial; abnormal metabolism involving the sorbitol-myoinositol pathway may lead to axonal dysfunction or anatomic abnormalities with neural ischemia, and segmental demyelinization may occur. Neuropathy may affect the peripheral nervous system, isolated cranial or spinal nerves, or the autonomic nervous system or may be manifest as a specific neuropathic syndrome such as diabetic neuropathic cachexia or diabetic amyotrophy. The most common presentation is that of a symmetrical, bilateral peripheral neuropathy with pain or paresthesia of the extremities, loss of the Achilles reflex, and

alterations on sensory testing. Treatments for this disorder have been notoriously ineffective. Improved glycemic control is always advocated. Specific drug therapies have included supplemental B vitamins, oral pyridoxine, diphenylhydantoin, clonazepam, amitriptyline, imipramine, fluphenazine, and carbamazepine. The most effective combination is that of a tricyclic antidepressant and a phenothiazine; however, these drugs should be cautiously prescribed to the elderly patient because induced cardiac arrhythmias or oversedation can occur.

Diabetic neuropathic cachexia is a syndrome characteristically seen in depressed middle-aged to elderly males who have mild type II diabetes. The syndrome presents with profound weight loss, cachexia, and severe pain of the extremities with a bilateral symmetrical neuropathy. These patients frequently are evaluated for occult malignancy or radiculoneuropathy. Spontaneous recovery is the rule, but the course of the disease is shortened with amitriptyline 25 to 50 mg/HS and fluphenazine 1 mg bid or tid. Diabetic amyotrophy is a disorder characterized by progressive weakness and wasting of the pelvic girdle and thigh muscles and is associated with severe pain. There is little or no sensory involvement. This syndrome is also associated with mild diabetes and usually resolves spontaneously within a year.

Autonomic neuropathy has many manifestations in the elderly diabetic patient, including impotence, neurogenic bladder, disordered gastrointestinal motility, gastroparesis, orthostatic hypotension, or altered autonomic cardiac function. In evaluating the neurogenic bladder, one must exclude functional obstructive uropathy. Neurogenic bladder may improve with frequent voiding, application of suprapubic pressure, and bethanechol chloride, 10 to 50 mg tid or qid. Gastroparesis diabeticorum may respond to metoclopramide, 5 to 15 mg qid taken 30 minutes before each meal and at bedtime, frequent small feedings of liquid or semisolid food, and application of abdominal (stomach) pressure while upright. Diabetic diarrhea may be neuropathic or due to small bowel bacterial overgrowth or pancreatic insufficiency. Tetracycline 250 mg qid for 7 to 10 days may be helpful. Metoclopramide, 5 to 15 mg qid, or clonidine, 0.05 mg bid, can be tried. Patients with orthostatic hypotension should be evaluated for anemia and volume depletion. Sudden postural changes should be avoided. Orthostatic hypotension may respond to the wearing of elastic stockings, a high-sodium diet, 9-alpha-fluorohydrocortisone, 0.05 to 0.2 mg daily, or clonidine.[49] Cardiovascular autonomic neuropathy with cardiac denervation is manifest as a fixed tachycardia, loss of cardiac deceleration to deep breathing, loss of cardiac responsiveness to the Valsalva maneuver, and sudden death. When these autonomic cardiovascular reflexes are absent, the diabetic patient is at risk for sudden cardiopulmonary death following minor or major surgical procedures. Impotence occurs in 50 percent of diabetic men and has multiple etiologies such as deteriorating marital relationships with performance anxiety, associated endocrinopathy (e.g., hypogonadism, hypopituitarism, and hypothyroidism), vascular insufficiency, drug or alcohol usage, or diabetic autonomic neuropathy. Testosterone treatment is effective only in hypogonadal patients. Some neuropathic patients may respond to bethanechol chloride, 10 to 50 mg tid. Impotence may be precipitated by initiating antihypertensive therapy. If the condition is considered serious, a penile prosthesis may be required.

DYSLIPIDEMIAS

Sufficient evidence is available to implicate the dyslipidemias (disorders resulting in high cholesterol, high triglyceride, or low high-density lipoprotein (HDL) cholesterol) in promoting the atherosclerotic process,[42, 43, 50–53] which results in clinically significant coronary artery disease, cerebral vascular disease, and peripheral vascular disease. The association of dyslipidemia with atherosclerosis in the elderly is complex because there are always multiple other etiologies underlying atherosclerosis, including genetics, hypertension, smoking, hyperinsulinism, obesity, lack of physical activity, diabetes, and renal disease.[37, 38] Epidemiologic studies[50–54] consistently relate the incidence and complications of coronary artery disease positively to total cholesterol and low-density lipoprotein (LDL) cholesterol, with

a less positive association with hypertriglyceridemia. According to the Framingham Heart Study,[50] begun in 1949, in persons under the age of 50 years there is a linear relationship between total cholesterol level and risk for coronary artery disease; however, in persons over the age of 50, total cholesterol loses its value as a predictor in men and women unless the level exceeds 300 mg/dl. A negative risk correlation exists for the high-density lipoproteins. The ratio of total cholesterol to HDL cholesterol or LDL cholesterol to HDL cholesterol is positively correlated with coronary artery disease. According to family studies, an even better predictor of coronary artery disease is the Apo B100 to Apo A-1 ratio. In evaluating the dyslipidemic disorder, attention should be given to age-related lipid values.[55] Plasma cholesterol increases with age in both sexes until approximately age 60, when cholesterol values in men plateau or slightly decrease, whereas women show a later plateau or continued rise.[15, 56] Plasma triglyceride levels increase in both sexes with aging, values being higher in elderly men than in women. A plateau occurs in men at age 50 to 60, followed by a decline with further aging, whereas in elderly females the plateau may occur later with a fall in later years.[15, 56] Lipoprotein lipase activity is decreased with aging, which accounts for some of these changes in plasma triglyceride levels. Fasting free fatty acids are unaltered with aging. LDL degradation in peripheral tissue is decreased with aging. Tissue content of cholesterol and cholesterol ester increases with age. The activity of 3-hydroxy-3-methylglutaryl coenzyme-A reductase (the rate-limiting enzyme for cholesterol synthesis) is normal. Plasma total cholesterol levels in excess of 260 mg/dl and LDL cholesterol in excess of 190 mg/dl are abnormal in patients older than 65 years of age.[55]

The treatment of these dyslipidemic disorders must be approached from the standpoint of the multiple contributing factors to the atherosclerotic process such as obesity, smoking, and hypertension. Since atherosclerosis is a slow progressive disease,[57, 58] concern exists about its degree of prevention, stabilization, or reversibility. This question has long been debated, and the association of blood lipids with atherosclerosis (known as the lipid hypothesis) is well accepted. Currently, there is evidence supporting the treatment of hypercholesterolemia.[42, 43, 59, 60] The Lipid Research Clinic Coronary Primary Prevention Trials[42] report that cholesterol reduction reduces mortality and morbidity from coronary artery disease. For every 1 percent reduction in cholesterol, there was a 2 percent reduction in cardiovascular mortality. Likewise, the Framingham Study[50] showed that for a 1 percent rise in total cholesterol, there was a 2 to 3 percent rise in the rate of coronary heart disease. The Helsinki heart study[41] likewise supports the findings of the beneficial effect of cholesterol lowering on cardiovascular mortality and describes a major protective role of HDL cholesterol. Other studies[44-47] have shown that 1 to 2 years of treating a hyperlipidemic disorder causes stabilization of atherosclerotic plaque formation or its regression. Hence, it is prudent to screen elderly individuals for hypercholesterolemia and treat those individuals with hypercholesterolemia with diet. If diet is not successful in reducing blood cholesterol to less than 290 mg/dl or LDL cholesterol to less than 190 mg/dl, then drug therapy should be instituted in patients with established atherosclerosis.

Elderly patients with the chylomicronemia syndrome with severe hypertriglyceridemia (values exceeding 1000 mg/dl) will experience more morbidity and mortality from recurrent pancreatitis than younger patients—hence, the importance of treating this syndrome. The chylomicronemia syndrome is associated with eruptive xanthomas of the skin, lipemia retinalis, and pancreatitis. Peripheral neuropathy and dementia may also be seen. The syndrome usually results from the combination of a genetic disorder in very low density lipoprotein (VLDL) metabolism plus a secondary cause of hypertriglyceridemia or two secondary causes of hypertriglyceridemia occurring simultaneously.[61] In acute pancreatitis, the hypertriglyceridemia levels will resolve rapidly when the patient's oral lipid intake is restricted. Secondary causes such as hypothyroidism, diabetes mellitus, drugs, nephrotic syndrome, uremia, obesity, estrogens, glucocorticoid excess, hepatocellular liver disease, and alcoholism should be sought. If the secondary causes cannot be identified or effectively treated, then clofibrate, gemfibrozil, or nicotinic acid may be necessary (Table 40–2). Dietary approach to treating hypertriglyceride disorders consists of weight reduction, avoidance of alcohol, and progressive fat restriction (Table 40–3), especially if chylomicronemia is present. Fish oils are useful in treating hypertriglyceridemia[62] but may aggravate hyperglycemia in diabetic patients.[63]

Hypercholesterolemia in the elderly patient may occur on a genetic basis but is more likely to be sporadic and acquired. Hypercholesterolemia can occur in association with hypothyroidism, nephrotic syndrome, obstructive liver disease, and diabetes mellitus. Hypercholesterolemia in the elderly patient is significant when it is associated with a personal history of atherosclerotic disease. Exercise[64] and dietary modification are the first steps[65] in treatment; they consist of prescribing various stages of a prudent fat-restricted diet as

TABLE 40–2. Hypolipidemic Drugs

Generic	Trade Name(s)	Dose	Side Effects
Cholestyramine	Questran	16–24 gm/day	GI upset
Colestipol	Colestid	30 gm/day	Constipation, interferes with absorption of fat-soluble vitamins A, D, E, K, and other drugs
Nicotinic acid (Niacin)	Nicobid, Nico-400 Nicolar	2–6 gm/day	Flushing and pruritus, hyperuricemia, hyperglycemia, hepatitis, dermatitis
Probucol	Lorelco	1 gm/day	Few except minor GI symptoms
Clofibrate	Atromid-S	2 gm/day	Few except minor GI symptoms
Gemfibrozil	Lopid	1.2 gm/day	Few except minor GI symptoms
Lovastatin	Mevacor	10–80 mg/day	Few, cataracts (?) watch liver function tests, myalgias, myositis

TABLE 40–3. Dietary Treatment[80]

Dietary Component	Stage		
	I	II	III
Fat (as percent of calories)	30%	30%	20%
Saturated fat (as percent of calories)	10%	7%	7%
Carbohydrate (as percent of calories)	50%	50%	55–60%
Protein (as percent of calories)	20%	20%	20%
Cholesterol (mg/day)	300	200	100
P/S ratio*	>1	>1	>1

*Ratio of polyunsaturated fat to saturated fat. This usual value is about 0.3.

shown in Table 40–3. Use of the mono-unsaturated fats such as olive oil are effective in reducing cholesterol levels and preventing coronary artery disease.[66, 67] The use of soluble fiber-containing foods such as oatmeal and oat bran can be useful in treating the hyperlipidemias.[68] Diet modifications may lead to a 10 to 15 percent reduction in cholesterol levels and may normalize minimally elevated cholesterol values. Drugs[69–71] used for treating the hyperlipidemic disorders are shown in Table 40–2. The primary cholesterol-lowering agents are the bile absorption resins (cholestyramine, colestipol), nicotinic acid, probucol, and lovastatin. Nicotinic acid may worsen diabetic control. Gemfibrozil may also lower cholesterol levels.[41] In some elderly patients the cost of treating the lipid disorder may significantly interfere with effective management. Convenient dosage forms for the various agents are shown in Table 40–2 along with their major side effects. It is debatable at this time whether an isolated low HDL cholesterol value needs treatment. Certain drugs will elevate HDL levels (gemfibrozil), nicotinic acid, phenytoins, and estrogens).[72] The use of estrogens in postmenopausal females has been reported in several studies to have the beneficial effect of decreasing coronary artery disease and fatal myocardial infarction.[73–75]

The incidence of dyslipidemia approximates 70 percent in diabetic patients.[76, 77] In diabetic patients, elevated triglycerides may have an additive adverse effect on the progression of atherosclerosis, particularly peripheral vascular disease.[78] Improved diabetic control is advocated in treatment of diabetic dyslipidemias;[79] however, in most instances, both a more rigid lipid-lowering diet and drug therapy are required to treat the associated lipid disorder effectively.

Long-term studies are not available in elderly patients but are certainly needed to clarify the issue of aggressive management of dyslipidemia and to determine what impact modification of risk factors will have on atherosclerosis.

REFERENCES

1. Palumbo PJ: Diabetes mellitus: incidence, prevalence, survivorship and cause of death in Rochester, Minnesota 1945–1970. Diabetes 25:566, 1976.
2. Bennett PH: Diabetes in the elderly: diagnosis and epidemiology. Geriatrics 37:39, 1984.
3. Wilson PWF, Anderson KM, Kannel, WB: Epidemiology of diabetes in the elderly. Am J Med 80(5A):3–9, 1986.
4. Vague J: The degree of masculine differentiation of obesities. Am J Clin Nutr 4:20–39, 1956.
5. Ohlson LO, Larsson B, Svardsudd K, et al: The influence of body fat distribution on the incidence of diabetes mellitus. Diabetes 34:1055–1058, 1985.
6. Davidson MB: The effect of aging on carbohydrate metabolism. Metabolism 28:688–705, 1979.
7. DeFronzo RA: Glucose intolerance and aging. Diabetes Care 4:493–501, 1981.
8. Horwitz DL: Diabetes and aging. Am J Clin Nutr 36:803–808, 1982.
9. Raven GM, Raven EP: Age, glucose intolerance and NIDDM. J Am Geriatr Soc 33:286–290, 1985.
10. Fink RI, Kolterman OG, Griffin J, et al: Mechanism of insulin resistance in aging. J Clin Invest 71:1523–1535, 1983.
11. Fink RI, Kolterman OG, Kao M, et al. The role of the glucose transport system in the postreceptor defect in insulin action associated with human aging. J Clin Endocrinol Metab 58:721–725, 1984.
12. National Diabetes Data Group. Classification and diagnosis of diabetes mellitus and other categories of glucose intolerance. Diabetes 28:1039–1057, 1979.
13. Olefsky JM, Kolterman OG: Mechanisms of insulin resistance in obesity and non-insulin dependent (type II diabetes). Am J Med 70:151–168, 1981.
14. DeFronzo RA: New concepts in the pathogenesis and treatment of non-insulin-dependent diabetes mellitus. Am J Med 74(1A):52–81, 1983.
15. Truglia JA, Livingston JN, Lockwood DH: Insulin

resistance: receptor and post-binding defects in human obesity and non-insulin dependent diabetes mellitus. Am J Med 79(2B):13–22, 1985.

16. Kent S: Is diabetes a form of accelerated aging. Geriatrics 31:140–151, 1976.

17. Eckel RH, Hofeldt FD: Endocrinology and metabolism in the elderly. In Schrier RW, ed: Clinical Internal Medicine in the Aged. Philadelphia, WB Saunders Co, 1982, pp 222–255.

18. Morley JE: Nutritional status of the elderly. Am J Med 81:679–695, 1986.

19. Young EA: Nutrition, aging and the aged. Med Clin North Am 67:295–313, 1983.

20. Pinholt EM, Kroenke K, Hanley JF, et al: Functional assessment of the elderly. Arch Intern Med 147:484–488, 1987.

21. McGandy RB, Barrows CH, Spanias A, et al: Nutrient intake and energy expenditure in men of different age. J Gerontol 21:581–587, 1966.

22. Richter EA, Ruderman HB, Schneider SH: Diabetes and exercise. Am J Med 70:201–208, 1981.

23. Vinik AI, Franz SJ, Crapo PA, et al: Nutritional recommendation and principles for individuals. Diabetes Care 10:126–132, 1987.

24. Osei K, Falko J, Bossett BM, et al: Metabolic effects of fructose as a natural sweetener in the physiologic meals of ambulatory obese patients with type II diabetes. Am J Med 83:249–255, 1987.

25. Phillips PA, Rolls BJ, Ledingham JG, et al: Reduced thirst after water deprivation in healthy elderly men. N Engl J Med 311:753–759, 1984.

26. Miller PD, Krebs RA, Neal BJ, et al: Hypodipsia in geriatric patients. Am J Med 73:354–356, 1982.

27. Beck LH, Lavizzo-Mourey R: Geriatric hyponatremia. Ann Intern Med 107:768, 1987.

28. Snyder NA, Feigal DW, Arieft AI: Hypernatremia in elderly patients. Ann Intern Med 107:309–319, 1987.

29. Lane NE, Bloch DA, Wood PD, et al: Long-distance running and the development of musculoskeletal disability. Am J Med 82:772–781, 1987.

30. Hurt RD, Finlayson RE, Morse RM, et al: Alcoholism in elderly persons. Mayo Clin Proc 63:753–768, 1988.

31. Bessman AN, Kasim S: Managing foot infections in the older diabetic patient. Geriatrics 40:54–63, 1985.

32. Wheat LJ, Allen SD, Henry M, et al: Diabetic foot infections. Arch Intern Med 146:1935–1940, 1986.

33. Edmonds ME: The diabetic foot: pathophysiology and treatment. Clin Endocrinol Metab 15:889–916, 1986.

34. Pirat J: Diabetes mellitus and its degenerative complications. Diabetes Care 1:168–188, 1978.

35. Kannel WB: Lipids, diabetes and coronary heart disease. Am Heart J 110:1100–1107, 1985.

36. Minaker KL: Aging and diabetes mellitus as risk factors for vascular disease. Am J Med 82(Suppl 113):47–53, 1987.

37. Aronow WS, Starling L, Etienne F, et al: Risk factors for coronary artery disease in persons older than 62 years in a long-term health care facility. Am J Cardiol 57:518–520, 1986.

38. Criqui MH: Epidemiology of atherosclerosis: an update overview. Am J Cardiol 57:186–230, 1986.

39. Kuebler TW, Bendick PJ, Fineberg SE, et al. Diabetes mellitus and cerebrovascular disease: prevalence of carotid artery occlusive disease and associated risk factors in 482 adult diabetic patients. Diabetes Care 6:274–278, 1983.

40. Wolf PA, Kannel WB Veter J: Current status of risk factors for stroke. Neurol Clin 1:317–343, 1983.

41. Chipkin SR, Frid D, Alpert JS, et al: Frequency of painless myocardial ischemia during exercise tolerance testing in patients with and without diabetes mellitus. Am J Cardiol 59:61–65, 1987.

42. Lipid Research Clinics. Coronary primary prevention trial results. JAMA 251:351–374, 1984.

43. Frick MH, Elo O, Haapa K, et al: Helsinki heart study: primary prevention trial with gemfibrozil in middle-aged men with dyslipidemia. N Engl J Med 317:1237–1245, 1987.

44. Malinow NR: Regression of atherosclerosis in humans. Postgrad Med 73:232–242, 1983.

45. Duffield GM, Lewis B, Miller NE, et al: Treatment of hyperlipidemia retards progression of symptomatic femoral atherosclerosis. Lancet II:639–641, 1983.

46. Nikkila EA, Viikinkoski P, Valle M, et al: Prevention of progression of coronary atherosclerosis by treatment of hyperlipidemia. Br Med J 289:220–223, 1984.

47. Blankenhorn DH, Nessim SA, Johnson RL, et al: Beneficial effects of combined colestipol-niacin therapy on coronary atherosclerosis and coronary venous bypass grafts. JAMA 257:3233–3240, 1987.

48. Veberti G, Keen H: The patterns of proteinuria in diabetes mellitus. Diabetes 33:686–692, 1984.

49. Fedorak RN, Field M, Chang EB: Treatment of diabetic diarrhea with clonidine. Ann Intern Med 102:197–199, 1985.

50. Castelli WP, Garrison RJ, Wilson WF, et al: Incidence of coronary heart disease and lipoprotein cholesterol levels: the Framingham Study. JAMA 256:2835–2838, 1986.

51. Martin MH, Halley SB, Browner WS, et al: Serum cholesterol blood pressure and mortality: implications from a cohort of 361,662 men (MRFIT). Lancet II:933–936, 1986.

52. Stamler J, Wentworth D, Neaton JD: Is relationship between serum cholesterol and risk of premature death from coronary heart disease continuous and graded? (MRFIT). JAMA 256:2823–2828, 1986.

53. Grundy SM: Cholesterol and coronary heart disease. JAMA 256:2849–2859, 1986.

54. Kannel WB, Castelli WP, Gordon T, et al: Serum cholesterol, lipoproteins and the risk of coronary heart disease. Ann Intern Med 74:1–12, 1971.

55. Rifkind BM, Segal P: Lipid research clinics program references values for hyperlipidemia and hypolipidemia. JAMA 250:1869–1872, 1983.

56. Kreisberg RA, Kasim S: Cholesterol metabolism and aging. Am J Med 82 (Suppl B):54–60, 1987.

57. Enos WF, Holmes RH, Beyer J: Coronary disease amongst United States soldiers killed in action in Korea. JAMA 256:2859–2862, 1986.

58. Strong JP: Coronary atherosclerosis in soldiers. JAMA 256:2863–2866, 1986.

59. Detre KM: Secondary prevention and lipid lowering results and implications. Am Heart J 110:1123–1127, 1985.

60. Levy RI: Primary prevention of coronary heart disease by lowering lipids. Am Heart J 110:1116–1122, 1985.

61. Chait A, Brunzell JD: Severe hypertriglyceridemia: role of familial and acquired disorders. Metabolism 32:209–214, 1983.
62. VonSchacky C: Prophylaxis of atherosclerosis with marine omega-3 fatty acids. Ann Intern Med 107:890–899, 1987.
63. Glauber H, Wallace P, Griver K, et al: Adverse metabolic effects of omega-3 fatty acids in non-insulin-dependent diabetes mellitus. Ann Intern Med 108:663–668, 1988.
64. Seals DR, Hagberg JM, Hurley BF, et al: Effects of endocrine training on glucose tolerance and plasma lipid levels in older men and women. JAMA 252:645–649, 1984.
65. Kuske TT, Feldman EB: Hyperlipoproteinemia, atherosclerosis risk and dietary management. Arch Intern Med 147:357–360, 1987.
66. Grandy SM: Comparison of monounsaturate fatty acids and carbohydrates for lowering plasma cholesterol. N Engl J Med 314:745–748, 1986.
67. Mensink RP: Katan MB: Effect of monounsaturated fatty acids versus complex carbohydrates on high-density lipoproteins in healthy men and women. Lancet I:122–124, 1987.
68. Anderson JW, Story L, Sieling B, et al: Hypocholesterolemic effects of high-fiber diets rich in water soluble plant fibers: long term studies with oat-bran and bean-supplemental diets for hypercholesterolemic men. J Can Diet Assoc 45:120–129, 1984.
69. Hoeg JM, Gregg RE, Brewer HB: An approach to the management of hyperlipoproteinemia. JAMA 255:512–521, 1986.
70. Kashyap M: The clinical management of hyperlipidemia. Mod Med 55:62–112, 1987.
71. Naito HK: Reducing deaths with hypolipidemic drugs. Postgrad Med 82:102–112, 1987.
72. Glueck CJ: Nonpharmacologic and pharmacologic alterations of high density lipoprotein cholesterol: therapeutic approach to prevention of atherosclerosis. Am Heart J 110:1107–1115, 1985.
73. Ross RK, Paganini-Hill A, Mack TM, et al: Menopausal oestrogen therapy and protection from death from ischemic heart disease. Lancet I:858–860, 1981.
74. Bush TL, et al: Estrogen use and all cause mortality. JAMA 249:903–906, 1983.
75. Stampfer MJ, Willett WC, Colditz GA, et al: A prospective study of postmenopausal estrogen therapy and coronary heart disease. N Engl J Med 313:1044–1049, 1985.
76. Bunneg SC, Vajanamarhute C, Pasatrat S, et al: Lipid disorders in Thai diabetics. Tohoku J Exper Med 141(Suppl):605–609, 1983.
77. Chait A: Hyperlipidemia: forstalling complications in older diabetics. Geriatrics 40:71–78, 1985.
78. Vogelberg KH, Grimm K, Gries FA: Hypertriglyceridemia in insulin dependent diabetes with peripheral vascular disease. Horm Metab Res 15:90–94, 1985.
79. Dunn FL, Raskin P, Bilheimer DW, et al: The effect of diabetic control on very low-density lipoprotein-triglyceride metabolism in patients with type II diabetes mellitus and marked hypertriglyceridemia. Metabolism 33:117–123, 1984.
80. Report of the National Cholesterol Education Program, Expert Panel on Detection, Evaluation and Treatment of High Blood Cholesterol in Adults. Arch Intern Med 148:36–69, 1988.

CHAPTER 41

Pituitary, Thyroid, Adrenal, and Parathyroid Diseases in the Elderly

Leonard R. Sanders

The loss of youth is melancholy enough, but to enter into old age through the gate of infirmity most disheartening.
WALPOLE, *Letters: To George Montagu*

Aging is associated with anatomic and functional changes in the endocrine glands and the organ systems they affect. Anatomic changes include glandular atrophy and fibrosis, and nodular formation. Age-related functional alterations include changes in various hormone levels that result from reductions in basal metabolism and metabolic clearance rates. Altered glandular secretion, increased target tissue resistance, and reduced glandular sensitivity to negative feedback also contribute to altered hormone levels. Because the endocrine system has tremendous hormonal reserve, these changes rarely cause overt clinical disease. Nevertheless, elderly persons are susceptible to the spectrum of endocrine disorders. They also have a higher incidence of nonendocrine systemic disease that can alter endocrine function. Moreover, elderly patients often show atypical clinical presentations of endocrine disease, and symptoms of endocrinopathies may mimic symptoms of normal aging. Nonetheless, the basic approach to endocrine disorders in the elderly is similar to that in the young. This chapter will review the age-related changes of pitui-

tary, thyroid, adrenal, and parathyroid function that are important for diagnosis and treatment of endocrine disease. In addition, it will cover selected clinical examples of dysfunction in these glands.

GENERAL ASPECTS OF ENDOCRINE FUNCTION AND DYSFUNCTION

Physiology

Regulation of hormone production and pituitary–target-gland relationships is summarized in Figure 41–1. Central nervous system neurotransmitters, hypothalamic hormones, and target-gland hormones regulate pituitary function. The pituitary secretes regulatory (trophic) hormones that stimulate target glands to synthesize and secrete target-gland hormones. Thus, the hypothalamus and pituitary gland directly control other endocrine glands, including the thyroid, adrenals, ovaries, and testes. The hypothalamus and pituitary also control some functions of the kidneys, the mammary glands, the uterus, and intermediary metabolism. Target-gland hormones act on target cells to induce physiologic responses. This action depends on receptor number and receptor affinity for the hormone. Target-gland hormones also feed back at several levels on the CNS-hypothalamic-pituitary system to modulate subsequent target-gland secretion. Unlike most endocrine glands, the parathyroid glands have no hypothalamic-

The opinions or assertions contained herein are the private views of the author and are not to be construed as official or as reflecting the views of the Department of the Army or the Department of Defense.

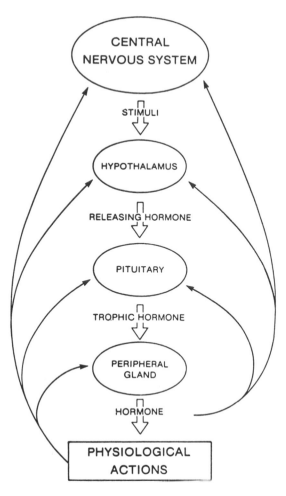

FIGURE 41–1. Organization and regulation of the endocrine system. (From Baxter JD: Principles of endocrinology. In Wyngaarden JB, Smith LH, Jr, eds: Cecil's Textbook of Medicine. Philadelphia, WB Saunders Co, 1985, p 1221; by permission.)

pituitary control. Calcium has direct negative feedback on the parathyroid glands and is the major regulator of parathyroid hormone (PTH) secretion.

Pathophysiology

Functional endocrine system disorders produce hypofunction or hyperfunction. The causes of altered endocrine function are summarized in Figure 41–2. Malignant disease is relatively common and more aggressive in the elderly and can cause glandular hypofunction by direct destruction of the gland. Defective conversion of prohormones to active forms also occurs with age. Other causes of hypofunction from direct glandular destruction include infection, hemorrhage, and autoimmune disease. Autoimmune disease can cause chronic cellular injury with mild hypofunction that may not present clinically

except during periods of stress. Additionally, antibodies can block hormonal action or access to target-organ receptors. Autoimmune diseases are not as common in the elderly as in the young. Other causes of impaired hormone production include deficiencies in target-cell enzymes, receptors, effectors, and response systems. In many cases receptor numbers decrease with age, causing less sensitivity to hormonal action.[1] This may cause adaptive increases in secretion of hormones necessary to maintain normal function.

Prevalence of glandular hyperfunction does not usually increase with age, but endocrine hyperfunction may have an atypical clinical presentation in elderly patients. Hyperfunction may result from tumor or hyperplasia within a gland or from ectopic hormone production. The latter occurs more often in elderly patients.[2] Hyperfunction may also result from antibodies that directly stimulate or damage glan-

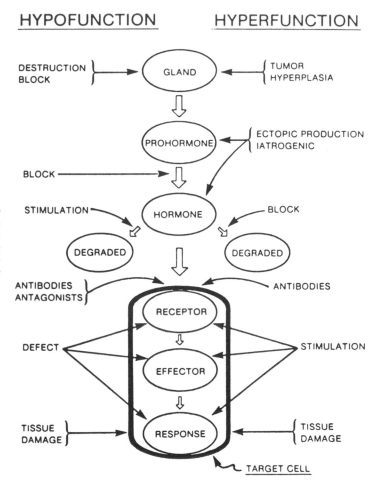

HYPOFUNCTION   HYPERFUNCTION

FIGURE 41–2. Causes of endocrine hypofunction or hyperfunction. (From Baxter JD: Principles of endocrinology. In Wyngaarden JB, Smith LH, Jr, eds: Cecil's Textbook of Medicine. Philadelphia, WB Saunders Co, 1985, p 1229; by permission.)

dular tissue, causing release of stored hormone.

Altered hormonal degradation may cause an excess or deficiency of various hormones. Metabolic clearance rates (MCR) decrease with age, causing increased hormonal reserves.[1] In the absence of endocrine disease, compensatory decreases in glandular secretion usually maintain normal hormone concentrations. However, in endocrine deficiency states, normal hormone replacement doses may cause hyperfunction. Thus, elderly patients with hormone deficiency may require lower replacement doses.

PITUITARY

Growth Hormone

CHANGES WITH AGE. Growth hormone (GH) is secreted by the anterior pituitary in response to GH-releasing hormone (GHRH) from the hypothalamus. Growth hormone stimulates the liver to release somatomedin-C (SM-C), which produces the main biologic effects. Aging impairs GH secretion and causes mild GH deficiency.[3, 4] This condition is correlated with reductions in SM-C and thus has biologic effects.[4] The most important effect of GH is growth. However, the physiologic actions of GH suggest that it has a role in maintenance of bone and muscle mass, which both decline with age. Therefore, age-related GH deficiency may contribute to the decreased lean body mass and osteoporosis seen in the elderly.[4] Nonetheless, current evidence does not show that GH deficiency causes clearly identifiable clinical sequelae in the aging population.

ACROMEGALY. Growth-hormone excess causes acromegaly, and diagnosis and treatment of this state in the elderly are similar to that in young patients. Symptoms include headache, increased sweating, enlargement of hands and feet, and reduced energy and potency. Baseline GH levels are greater than 10 ng/ml. Since stress can elevate GH levels in normal people, a GH-suppression test is necessary to diagnose acromegaly. This test requires measurement of GH levels 60 to 90 minutes after ingestion of 100 gm of glucose. Normal people suppress GH to less than 5 ng/ml. Failure to suppress signifies acromegaly, and the usual cause is a pituitary adenoma. Computed tomography (CT) or magnetic resonance imaging (MRI) scanning of the pituitary can usually determine the exact location and size of the adenoma. Surgical, radiation, or medical therapy is performed on an individual basis. Bromocriptine mesylate, at a dose of 10 to 60 mg/day, significantly lowers GH and improves symptoms in many acromegalic patients.[5] Thus, poor operative candidates or patients needing adjunctive therapy after radiation or surgery may benefit from this therapy. However, bromocriptine mesylate causes postural hypotension and nausea, which may be particularly distressing to the elderly. Slowly increasing the dose by 2.5 mg every 3 to 4 days may improve tolerance. A long-acting somatostatin analogue (octreotide acetate) is more potent in lowering GH levels and is better tolerated.[6] The drug was recently released and approved for control of symptoms caused by carcinoid and vasoactive intestinal polypeptide tumors. However, the drug remains investigational as a therapy for acromegaly, and administration requires two to three daily injections. In the future, octreotide acetate may replace bromocriptine mesylate as the standard therapy for acromegaly.

Prolactin

CHANGES WITH AGE. Age-related physiologic changes in prolactin levels have no clinical sequelae in the elderly. Levels may slightly decrease in women and increase in men.[7] After intravenous thyrotropin-releasing hormone (TRH), normal TRH-stimulated prolactin elevations may have a delayed peak response.[8] However, studies are not conclusive. Prolactin excess causes impotence, a common sexual dysfunction in elderly males. Thus, a baseline prolactin level is important in

the work-up of impotence. As with all suspected pituitary tumors, CT or MRI scanning may localize the tumor. Therapy with 2.5 mg of bromocriptine mesylate three times daily will usually decrease tumor size and improve optic nerve compression. Therefore, headache and visual field disturbances are not absolute contraindications to bromocriptine mesylate therapy.[9] However, patients who deteriorate or do not improve require neurosurgical consultation and usually transsphenoidal hypophysectomy.

Gonadotropins

FEMALE CHANGES WITH AGE. At about 45 to 50 years of life, ovarian follicular maturation ceases and ovarian estrogen production declines. The clinical consequences of these events are the menopause and the climacteric. The menopause is permanent cessation of menses. Menopause does not occur suddenly but follows a transition period of regular to irregular cycles. During this transition period, lower estradiol levels reduce negative feedback, and follicle-stimulating hormone (FSH) levels increase. High FSH levels cause intermittent ovulation due to episodic estradiol secretion from residual follicles.[10] Periods of anovulation cause unopposed estrogenic stimulation of the endometrium and dysfunctional uterine bleeding. Both of these conditions cause irregular vaginal bleeding. Eventually follicular development stops completely, causing permanent cessation of menses.

The climacteric defines a constellation of symptoms and signs that are endocrinologic, physiologic, and psychological in nature.[11] Estrogen deficiency causes most features of this syndrome. Vasomotor instability (hot flashes), genitourinary atrophy, and accelerated bone loss are the major problems of the climacteric.[12, 13] Vaginal atrophy is frequent and causes dryness, irritation, and dyspareunia. Infections of the vagina, urethra, and bladder are also common. The hot flash is the most common and annoying symptom of the climacteric and occurs in 65 to 76 percent of menopausal women.[12] A burning sensation in the head, upper chest, and back are cardinal features. Other features include headachelike pressure, palpitations, weakness, fatigue, faintness, vertigo, and profuse sweating. Women with nocturnal hot flashes have associated insomnia, sleep deprivation, and fatigue. Hot flashes are associated with central nervous system (CNS) changes causing gonadotropin-releasing hormone (GnRH) release and pulsatile elevations in luteinizing hormone (LH). These events and altered hypothalamic thermoregulation probably cause the hot flash.[11] Therapy for specific problems of the climacteric is outlined in Chapters 20 and 29.

MALE CHANGES WITH AGE. Although the normal male maintains gonadal function much longer than the female, male gonadal function declines with age.[14] Testosterone levels usually remain in the normal range, but there is progressive decline in total and free testosterone.[15, 16] The number of Leydig cells diminishes with age, accounting for the decline in testosterone. The remaining Leydig cells function normally.[14] Plasma LH and FSH levels increase continually with age and correlate with decreasing testosterone levels.[14, 15] Gonadotrophs in older men respond normally to stimulation. Thus the major abnormality in the pituitary-testicular axis is in the testes.[16] There is no clear relationship between these endocrinologic changes and the lower level of sexual activity observed in elderly males.

Antidiuretic Hormone

CHANGES WITH AGE. The posterior pituitary stores antidiuretic hormone (ADH) and oxytocin. However, only alterations in ADH (arginine vasopressin) are of clinical importance in the elderly. Antidiuretic hormone is synthesized in the paraventricular and supraoptic nuclei of the hypothalamus. The supraoptic nucleus serves as a conduit for the axons of both nuclei, which end in the posterior pituitary.[17] There is no identifiable ADH deficiency with normal aging. In fact, elderly patients have elevated baseline ADH levels and may have greater ADH output for any given osmotic stimulus.[18] These changes result from increased osmoreceptor sensitivity. Progressive renal resistance to ADH action also occurs with age and may precede and contribute to the en-

hanced osmostat sensitivity.[18] These two changes offset each other and maintain normal plasma osmolality.

SIADH. An excess of ADH causes water retention and the syndrome of inappropriate antidiuretic hormone secretion (SIADH). Primary water intoxication is uncommon in the elderly. However, secondary causes of elevated ADH and water retention are relatively common.[18] Pulmonary, neurologic, and malignant diseases occur more commonly in elderly patients and may be associated with excess ADH secretion. Enhanced osmoreceptor sensitivity may also predispose these patients to SIADH. Symptoms of hyponatremia include lethargy, apathy, agitation, disorientation, anorexia, nausea, and leg cramps. These symptoms occur commonly in the elderly but should not be attributed simply to normal aging. The above symptoms are also common manifestations of hypothyroidism and adrenal insufficiency. Patients with hyponatremia, normal volume status, and no evidence of thyroid or adrenal disease probably have SIADH. The additional finding of inappropriate concentration of the urine osmolality relative to plasma osmolality usually confirms the diagnosis. Water restriction and treatment of the underlying disease is the appropriate therapeutic approach to SIADH. However, if the predisposing condition is cancer, it is often not curable. In this case, 300 mg of demeclocycline two to four times daily may correct the hyponatremia.[19]

CHLORPROPAMIDE. Type II diabetes mellitus is common in elderly patients, and oral hypoglycemic agents are often necessary for treatment. One such agent, chlorpropamide, enhances ADH release and the effect of ADH on the kidneys. Therefore, this drug is a potential cause of ADH-induced hyponatremia. Elderly people often have poor mental function, physical disability, and indifference. These problems may contribute to hyponatremia and water intoxication. Thus, the second-generation oral-hypoglycemic agents (glipizide and glyburide), which have no water-retaining properties, are more appropriate for the elderly diabetic. These agents are also less likely to cause drug interactions.

DIABETES INSIPIDUS. A deficiency of ADH causes diabetes insipidus (DI) and associated polyuria. Since hypothalamic neurons function after isolated pituitary damage, hypothalamic damage is necessary for development of substantial central DI. Causes include trauma, infection, granulomas, autoimmunity, and idiopathic destruction of ADH-producing nuclei in the hypothalamus. Excessive thirst or dehydration and urine output greater than 3 liters per 24 hours suggest DI. Patients with these features, a relatively high plasma osmolality (>295 mOsm/kg), and a relatively low urine osmolality (<280 mOsm/kg) probably have DI. Partial nephrogenic DI is likely in the elderly because of age-related renal resistance to ADH.[18] Normally, work-up of suspected diabetes insipidus requires a water deprivation test or hypertonic saline infusion.[20] However, these tests are too dangerous for most elderly patients. Elderly patients are likely to develop stroke and thromboembolism from dehydration, and seizures and congestive failure from hypertonicity. DI is more safely diagnosed by comparing plasma ADH with urine osmolality or by a therapeutic trial of desmopressin acetate.[18, 20] The treatment of choice for central diabetes insipidus is desmopressin acetate. The usual dose is 5 to 10 μg intranasally twice daily. As with most drugs used in the elderly, the initial dose is low (5 μg at bedtime). Upward adjustments in dosage depend on the patient's electrolyte balance and symptoms of polyuria.

THYROID

Functional Alterations with Aging

Aging reduces the peripheral metabolism of thyroxine (T_4), which decreases the metabolic clearance rate of this hormone.[21] However, no reproducible age-related increases occur in T_4 concentration because of compensatory decreases in T_4 secretion. Reduced peripheral monodeiodination of T_4 to triiodothyronine (T_3) decreases T_3 levels with age.[22] Reported results of TRH testing vary in the elderly.[21, 22] Women usually have normal responses, but men may have blunted or normal responses. A blunted test response indicates no significant rise in thyroid-stimulating hormone (TSH) after administration of 500 μg of intravenous TRH. In both sexes, normal TRH testing insures normal functioning of the hypothalamic-pituitary-thyroid axis. An elderly female with a blunted test response has hyperthyroidism, hypothalamic disease, or pituitary disease. However, an elderly male with the same test results may be normal. Thyroid-binding globulin (TBG) levels remain normal with age.[21] Changes in TBG will alter the total but not the free levels of T_3 and T_4. TBG levels may decline in cirrhosis, hypoproteinemia, nephrotic syndrome, and other systemic illnesses. In these conditions, free T_4 gives a more accurate measure of metabolically active thyroid hormone. If free T_4 is not available, the free thyroxine index (FT_4I) estimates the relative concentration of free T_4. However, free T_4 and TSH remain the best measure of thyroid hormone status in the elderly and in the young.

Clinical Syndromes of Thyroid Dysfunction

HYPERTHYROIDISM. Elderly hyperthyroid patients have many of the symptoms and signs seen in young patients. They appear anxious and restless, have a fine tremor of the hands, and have a rapid pulse rate. However, elderly patients may also present with depression, profound weight loss, apathetic facies, lethargy, myopathy, hypokinesia, and supraventricular dysrhythmias. The hyperthyroid patient with these features has apathetic hyperthyroidism. Elderly patients with isolated atrial fibrillation commonly have hyperthyroidism. Hyperthyroidism caused by isolated elevation of T_3 (T_3 toxicosis) is also more common with age. If superimposed on chronic illness, hyperthyroidism may occur with isolated elevation of T_4 (T_4 toxicosis).

Diagnosis of hyperthyroidism requires measurement of T_3 by radioimmunoassay and free T_4. Diagnosis of thyrotoxicosis caused by silent thyroiditis requires performance of the thyroid radioactive iodine uptake (RAIU) test or fine needle aspiration (FNA). Patients with this condition have a low thyroid RAIU test result, and treatment is given primarily with beta blockers. Primary hyperthyroidism characteristically has high free T_4 and T_3 levels but low TSH. However, equivocal cases may require use of highly sensitive TSH assays or TRH testing. In hyperthyroidism, baseline TSH levels are very low (hyperthyroid range) with highly sensitive assays. TRH testing shows a blunted response in hyperthyroidism but is not reliable in elderly males.

Toxic multinodular goiter causes thyrotoxicosis in the elderly more commonly than does Graves' disease. Although therapeutic approaches to both conditions are similar, specific therapy requires consideration of each patient's unique clinical condition. Nonetheless, appropriate initial therapy for both conditions includes the thioamides propylthiouracil (100 mg three times daily) or methimazole (15 mg twice daily). However, serious hyperthyroidism may require higher doses of the thioamides and addition of a beta blocker to control tachycardia and dysrhythmias. Propranolol (10 to 20 mg three to four times daily) is most commonly used. However, because of beta-1 selectivity and less CNS penetration, atenolol (25 mg two to three times daily) may be better tolerated. Corticosteroids block peripheral conversion of T_4 to T_3 and may be efficacious in patients with severe hyperthyroidism. Dexamethasone (2 mg four times daily) is useful. However, if concomitant adrenal insufficiency is present, intravenous hydrocortisone (100 mg three times daily) is necessary to obtain the mineralocorticoid effect. Radioactive iodine is the usual definitive therapy for hyperthyroidism, and multinodular goiters require two to three times the dose required for Graves' disease. However, definitive therapy for large multinodular goiters with symptoms of compression is surgery. Either form of definitive therapy will damage the thyroid gland, and if done before depletion of stored hormone it may release thyroid hormone into the circulation. This may precipitate dysrhythmias or thyroid storm, and elderly patients are particularly susceptible to these complications. Therefore, definitive therapy is safe only after the patient becomes eumetabolic with medical therapy.

HYPOTHYROIDISM. Hypothyroidism has a 2 to 4 percent prevalence in the elderly, and TSH and free T_4 should be measured in patients with hypothyroid symptoms.[21] Common causes include autoimmune destruction of the thyroid, pre-

vious ^{131}I therapy, or thyroid surgery, and inadvertent discontinuation of thyroid hormone replacement therapy. Hypothyroid symptoms mimic those of normal aging, and diagnosis requires a high index of suspicion. Features are the same as those seen in young patients but are more severe. Symptoms include mental slowness, decreased energy, fatigability, poor memory, somnolence, slow speech, and a low-pitched voice. Signs include water retention, periorbital and peripheral edema, delayed reflexes, and hypothermia. A high TSH and low free T_4 confirm the diagnosis. Hypothyroid tissues are excessively responsive to thyroid hormone, and the elderly are predisposed to cardiovascular complications. Thus, elderly patients require cautious thyroid hormone replacement. Appropriate initial therapy is 25 to 50 µg per day of T_4 with an increase of 25 µg per day every 3 to 4 weeks. Repeat TSH and free T_4 levels guide further therapy. The normal 6- to 7-day half-life of T_4 increases with age. Therefore, it may take about 2 months to obtain steady-state levels of T_4 in elderly patients. For the same reason, elderly patients may require lower T_4 replacement doses.

Myxedema coma is an uncommon medical emergency that most often affects the elderly patient with chronic hypothyroidism. It develops progressively from fatigue, lethargy, stupor, coma, hypoventilation, hypoxia, hypothermia, hyponatremia, bradycardia, hypotension, and shock, to eventual death. Accurate temperature measurement requires a low-reading rectal thermometer. The combination of the above symptoms and signs with a low free T_4 and high TSH confirms the diagnosis. However, strong clinical suspicion is reason enough to begin treatment. Delay while awaiting thyroid-function test results before starting therapy may cause serious morbidity and possibly death. Treatment includes immediate intravenous infusion of 400 to 500 µg of T_4 followed by maintenance infusion of 50 to 100 µg daily. Development of dysrhythmias requires antidysrhythmic therapy or a lower dose of T_4.

Further management requires a thorough search for infection, adrenal insufficiency, and other medical problems. Cosyntropin-stimulated cortisol values will screen for adrenal insufficiency. Intravenous infusion of 100 mg of hydrocortisone three times daily is appropriate until cortisol results are available. If results do not show adrenal insufficiency, cortisol infusions are no longer required. Hypoventilation may require ventilatory support. Hyponatremia results from decreased free water clearance and if severe may increase mortality.[23] Plasma sodium levels of less than 120 mEq/liter require correction, but rapid correction with hypertonic saline alone may cause fluid overload. Thus, the combination of hypertonic saline and furosemide may prove most useful.[24] The optimal rate of correction remains controversial.[23–25] However, since myxedematous patients have chronic hyponatremia, steady continuous correction may prove more important than a rapid rate. Correcting the sodium level to 125 to 130 mEq/ liter at a rate of about 0.5 mEq/liter/hr is probably optimal.[25]

EUTHYROID SICK SYNDROME. Nonthyroidal systemic illnesses can cause changes in thyroid function tests that mimic hypothyroidism. The euthyroid sick syndrome refers to this condition.[26] Because elderly people are more susceptible to systemic illnesses, they are also more susceptible to this disorder. Laboratory studies in the euthyroid sick syndrome show a low T_3, high reverse T_3 (rT_3), low to normal T_4, and usually normal free T_4 and TSH levels. If the free T_4 is low, measurement of TSH and rT_3 will help differentiate hypothyroidism from the euthyroid sick syndrome. TSH values are almost always elevated in primary hypothyroidism. However, in elderly sick patients, TSH values may be relatively lower when primary hypothyroidism coexists. Furthermore, hypopituitarism and secondary hypothyroidism may occur in these patients with resulting low free T_4 and TSH values. As in healthy elderly males, TRH testing in euthyroid sick female patients may show blunting of TSH responses. Thus, TRH testing does not help with diagnosis and should not be routinely performed. Although normal free T_4 and TSH values usually exclude the euthyroid sick syndrome, thyroid function tests may remain equivocal in elderly sick patients. Clinical judgment must be used in the approach to these patients. Thyroxine therapy may exacerbate the underlying illness in euthyroid

sick patients. However, patients with highly suggestive symptoms and signs of hypothyroidism may require T_4 therapy. Critically ill patients with suspected secondary hypothyroidism also require screening and treatment for adrenal insufficiency.

THYROID NODULES. The major concern about thyroid nodules is cancer. The age-specific incidence of thyroid cancer increases only slightly with age.[21] However, thyroid cancer is likely to grow faster, metastasize earlier, and undergo anaplastic degeneration more often in the elderly. Thus, although thyroid cancer usually has a good prognosis, it is not as good in the elderly as it is in the young. In order of frequency, thyroid cancers include papillary, follicular, medullary, and anaplastic types. They usually present as a solitary thyroid nodule or as a cervical mass. Early FNA permits early diagnosis and removal of malignant lesions. The approach to suspicious lesions may require additional testing with thyroid scan and ultrasound. If these patients are poor surgical candidates or are at low risk for cancer, T_4 therapy may suffice. Although T_4 therapy is appropriate for benign lesions, some elderly patients develop cardiovascular or neurologic sequelae on this therapy. Furthermore, most benign thyroid nodules do not regress with T_4 therapy.[27] Therefore, benign lesions may require only periodic examinations (without T_4 therapy) in some elderly eumetabolic patients.

ADRENALS

Functional Alterations With Aging

The hypothalamic-pituitary-adrenal axis is essentially normal in the elderly.[28] However, there is some resistance to cortisol suppression by dexamethasone with aging.[29] Cortisol circulates 99 percent bound to corticosteroid-binding globulin (CBG). The elderly have impaired metabolic removal of cortisol, but a compensatory 25 to 30 percent reduction in cortisol secretion maintains normal plasma levels.[30] An age-related reduction in renal excretion of cortisol metabolites also occurs, but this normalizes when expressed as a function of glomerular filtration rate (GFR).[30]

The elderly have reduced renin secretion and secondarily reduced aldosterone secretion.[31] Because they also have progressive age-related loss of renal function, they are predisposed to problems of hyperkalemia. Accordingly, potassium supplements, potassium-sparing diuretics, and angiotensin-converting enzyme inhibitors are potentially hazardous.

Adrenal medullary function is usually normal in the elderly. However, plasma norepinephrine levels increase progressively with age,[32] due partially to reduced plasma clearance and increased spillover into the plasma.[32] Epinephrine levels are usually normal, but these levels may also be relatively higher in the elderly.[32] Cardiovascular responsiveness to beta-adrenergic stimulation decreases with age, but vascular responsiveness to alpha-adrenergic stimulation remains intact.[32] The exact mechanisms and clinical significance of these changes are unclear.

Clinical Syndromes of Adrenal Dysfunction

CUSHING'S SYNDROME. Hyperfunction of the adrenal cortex may be primary or secondary. Conditions that cause hyperfunction include bilateral adrenal hyperplasia due to excess adrenocorticotropin hormone (ACTH), adrenal adenoma or carcinoma, and bilateral adrenal nodular hyperplasia. The most common cause of biologic Cushing's syndrome is Cushing's disease, an ACTH-secreting microadenoma of the pituitary. Patients with Cushing's syndrome may have obesity, hirsutism, acne, wide violaceous striae, easy bruising, insomnia, impaired memory, depression, and emotional lability. Further evaluation shows thinning of the skin, hypertension, proximal muscular weakness, and back pain due to osteoporosis. The presence of the above features warrants a diagnostic work-up.[33]

The work-up of Cushing's syndrome begins by performing a 1-mg dexamethasone suppression test. The patient ingests 1 mg of dexamethasone at 11 P.M. Normally, the cortisol level the following morning is less than 5 µg/dl. A cortisol level greater than 5 µg/dl requires additional investigation. Initially, this includes collection of a 24-hour urine sample for measurement of free cortisol. If this value

is normal, Cushing's syndrome is not present and no additional work-up is necessary.[33] If it is abnormal, a low-dose dexamethasone suppression test is necessary. With this test, the patient receives 0.5 mg of dexamethasone orally every 6 hours for 2 days. Normally, serum cortisol decreases to less than 5 µg/dl and urinary free cortisol to less than 20 µg/24 hours. Cortisol values higher than these are diagnostic of Cushing's syndrome. This test is abnormal in 99 percent of patients with Cushing's syndrome. However, false-positive tests may occur in patients with alcoholism and depression. Localization of excess ACTH or cortisol production requires baseline ACTH measurement followed by high-dose dexamethasone testing. With the high-dose test the patient ingests 2 mg of dexamethasone four times daily for 2 days. Patients with ACTH-producing pituitary tumors suppress serum and urine cortisol values to less than 50 percent. Failure to suppress cortisol levels by 50 percent signifies cortisol excess from adrenal adenoma or carcinoma, or ectopic ACTH production. Baseline ACTH levels are low in patients with primary adrenal cortisol excess and are normal or high in Cushing's disease and ectopic ACTH production. Although ectopic ACTH levels are higher than ACTH levels in Cushing's disease, there is significant overlap.

Cushing's syndrome usually occurs in patients less than 50 years of age but can occur in patients older than 70 years.[33] Furthermore, 15 percent of cases are caused by ectopic ACTH production and occur most frequently in males older than 60 years.[30] These patients may not be obese. Instead, they present with weight loss, muscle wasting, hypokalemic alkalosis, edema, hypertension, impaired glucose tolerance, and increased pigmentation.[30] About 65 percent of these patients have ACTH levels greater than 200 pg/ml. Bronchial carcinoid tumors are the most common cause. If the chest x-ray is normal, tumor localization requires CT scanning of the chest or selective venous sampling. The treatment of choice for all forms of Cushing's syndrome caused by tumors is surgical removal of the tumor. If there are contraindications to surgery, cyproheptadine may be helpful in 30 to 50 percent of patients with pituitary Cushing's disease.[34] If surgical cure is not complete or if radiation therapy effects are slow, cyproheptadine may further lower cortisol levels. Medical therapy that blocks cortisol production is useful for nonresponders, patients with ectopic ACTH syndromes, and those with inoperable functioning adrenal carcinomas.[34] Drugs used include ortho-para-prime DDD, aminoglutethimide, and metyrapone. Most adrenal carcinomas in elderly patients are nonfunctional adrenal masses.[35]

ADRENAL INSUFFICIENCY. Adrenal insufficiency is an uncommon disease that usually occurs between the ages of 20 and 50 years. Because about 90 percent of the adrenals must be destroyed to result in adrenal insufficiency, the condition usually develops insidiously over months to years. Although adrenal insufficiency is unusual in the elderly, symptoms of such a condition are similar to those characteristic of old age. Therefore, this condition is an important consideration in elderly patients. Causes of adrenal insufficiency include autoimmune and granulomatous diseases, bacterial infections, metastatic disease, infiltrative disorders, and secondary failure from pituitary dysfunction. Autoimmune disease is most common, but tuberculosis remains a strong consideration in elderly patients.[36]

Symptoms of adrenal insufficiency include fatigability, weakness, weight loss, myalgias, arthralgias, anorexia, nausea, and general debility.[37] These patients look chronically ill and may be apathetic and confused. Patients with these symptoms and signs require screening for adrenal insufficiency with a short cosyntropin stimulation test. Normally, after 250 μg of intravenous cosyntropin, plasma cortisol increases by more than 7 μg/dl to a value greater than 18 μg/dl. Values lower than these (30 and 60 minutes after the injection) confirm the presence of adrenal insufficiency.

Patients with acute adrenal insufficiency require infusion of 5 percent dextrose in normal saline. Dextrose corrects or prevents hypoglycemia, and normal saline replenishes volume. These patients also require intravenous infusion of 100 mg of hydrocortisone three times daily. Lifelong cortisol replacement is usually necessary. Standard doses of oral hydrocortisone in younger patients are 20 mg in the morning and 10 mg in the evening. These doses

may require a reduction in elderly patients owing to decreased metabolic clearance of cortisol. Mineralocorticoid replacement with 0.05 mg of fludrocortisone daily may be necessary for volume and electrolyte maintenance. Because elderly patients are predisposed to congestive heart failure, the sodium retention with fludrocortisone requires extreme caution. If difficult breathing or edema develop, it may be necessary to taper or stop the drug. Many elderly patients require only additional dietary salt and hydrocortisone. However, salt craving, hyponatremia, and hyperkalemia suggest a need for additional fludrocortisone.

PARATHYROID

Functional Alterations With Aging

Parathyroid hormone (PTH), calcitonin, and vitamin D maintain normal calcium and phosphate balance. Several clinically important changes in parathyroid-calcium metabolism occur in elderly patients.[38, 39] Parathyroid hormone levels increase with age. This increase results from impairment in renal function, vitamin D production, and gastrointestinal calcium absorption. Reduced renal function causes retention of biologically inactive PTH fragments, increases plasma phosphate, and decreases 1,25-dihydroxyvitamin D production. The elderly are less exposed to the sun, with subsequent reduction in 25-hydroxyvitamin D production.[40] In addition to decreased vitamin D levels, there is an age-related defect in gut absorption of calcium. The net effect of these changes is a lower plasma ionized calcium level, which increases PTH. There is no agreement about the effect of age on calcitonin levels or the effects of calcitonin on mineral metabolism in the elderly.[41]

Clinical Syndromes of Parathyroid Dysfunction

Parathyroid dysfunction causes hypercalcemia or hypocalcemia. Hypocalcemia related to parathyroid problems is rare in elderly patients. The most important causes of hypercalcemia in elderly patients are hyperparathyroidism, cancerous involvement of bone, and the humoral hypercalcemia of malignancy. Elderly patients commonly take thiazide diuretics for treatment of hypertension. These medications decrease renal excretion of calcium and may elevate serum calcium levels and complicate underlying hyperparathyroidism. Paget's disease of bone is more common in elderly patients and, if coupled with immobilization, it may cause associated hypercalcemia. However, the majority of elderly patients with hypercalcemia have primary hyperparathyroidism. In fact, 17 to 20 percent of all cases of hyperparathyroidism occur in the elderly.[42, 43] The incidence in females is twice that in males, and female predominance correlates positively with age.

Symptoms and signs of hypercalcemia are similar to those in younger patients. Patients with chronic and mild hypercalcemia are usually asymptomatic, but often these patients admit to lack of energy and depression. Elevations of calcium above 12 to 13 mg/dl may cause anorexia, nausea, vomiting, constipation, polyuria, polydipsia, dehydration, hypertension, weakness, and fatigue. The clinician suspects hyperparathyroidism when an elevated calcium level occurs on routine screening tests. Diagnostic studies include measurement of fasting serum calcium, phosphate, and PTH levels. A positive correlation between serum PTH and calcium levels suggests primary hyperparathyroidism. The main differential diagnosis is the humoral hypercalcemia characteristic of malignancy. Some squamous cell tumors release PTH-like substances that have poor cross reactivity with immunoreactive PTH measured in standard assays. However, there is some cross reactivity, and PTH levels may be normal or mildly elevated. Although ectopic PTH production occurs most commonly in the elderly, most parathyroid disease in the elderly is primary hyperparathyroidism.[42, 43]

There is no consensus on how to approach asymptomatic patients with primary hyperparathyroidism and mild hypercalcemia.[44] Estrogen therapy in postmenopausal women will lower serum calcium levels and decrease bone resorption.[45] However, experience with this therapy is limited, and the estrogen dose required may cause complications. My approach to elderly patients with asymptomatic hyperparathyroidism is as follows. If the calcium level is elevated but is persistently less than 1 mg/dl above the upper normal limit and there are no complications from hypercalcemia, periodic observation is appropriate. Periodic observation includes a history and physical examination and determinations of serum and urine calcium and phosphorus, creatinine clearance, and bone density. The frequency of these observations will vary but should initially be once or twice per year. Evidence of unexplained depression, weakness, fatigue, osteopenia, excessive hypercalciuria, renal dysfunction, renal stones, hypertension, or peptic ulcer disease requires parathyroidectomy. Asymptomatic hyperparathyroidism that causes persistent fasting serum calcium levels of greater than 1 mg/dl above the upper normal limit also requires parathyroidectomy.

TABLE 41–1. Changes in Circulating Hormonal Levels Seen With Aging*

Hormone	Change
Pituitary related	
Growth hormone	N or ↓
Prolactin	N
Somatomedin-C	↓
Arginine vasopressin	↑
Thyroid	
Thyroxine	N
Triiodothyronine	↓
Adrenal	
Cortisol	N
Dehydroepiandrosterone	↓
Aldosterone	↓
Renin	↓
Norepinephrine	↑
Epinephrine	N
Gastrointestinal and pancreatic	
Insulin	↑
Glucagon	↑
Gastric inhibitory peptide	N
Pancreatic polypeptide	↑
Gonadal	
Testosterone (males)	↓
Luteinizing hormone	↑
Follicle-stimulating hormone	↑
Calcium regulatory	
Parathormone	↑
Calcitonin	↓
1,25-dihydroxyvitamin D	↓

*N = no change, ↓ = decrease, ↑ = increase.
From Morley JE, Korenman SG: Aging. In Bagdade JD, et al, eds: The Year Book of Endocrinology. Chicago, Year Book Medical Publishers, 1987, p. 107, by permission.

SUMMARY

The endocrine system undergoes many changes as a result of normal aging. Age-related changes in circulating hormonal levels are summarized in Table 41–1. Other changes with age include alterations in hormonal metabolism and secretion. However, adaptive responses usually prevent or delay the clinical expression of disease. Nevertheless, true endocrine disease often abolishes these adaptive responses, and the clinician must make appropriate adjustments in hormonal replacement therapy. Elderly patients commonly present with vague symptoms and signs related to normal aging that are similar to those associated with endocrine dysfunction. Elderly patients also present with altered manifestations of common endocrine disorders. Therefore, age-related changes may delay the diagnosis of true endocrine disease. For these reasons, an exceptionally high index of suspicion is necessary to make these diagnoses. Thorough evaluation and reevaluation with a good history and physical examination, standard laboratory tests, and endocrine function tests are necessary in elderly patients. These evaluations facilitate the diagnosis and treatment of endocrine diseases in the elderly patient.

REFERENCES

1. Korenman SG: Introduction. In Korenman SG, ed: Endocrine Aspects of Aging. New York, Elsevier Science Publishing, 1982, pp 1–7.
2. Orth DN: Ectopic hormone production. In Felig P, et al, eds: Endocrinology and Metabolism. New York, McGraw Hill, 1987, pp 1692–1735.
3. Lang I, Schernthaner G, Pietschmann P, et al: Effects of sex and age on growth hormone response to growth hormone-releasing hormone in healthy individuals. J Clin Endocrinol Metab 65:535–540, 1987.
4. Vermeulen A: Nyctohemeral growth hormone profiles in young and aged men: Correlation with somatomedin-C levels. J Clin Endocrinol Metab 64:884–888, 1987.
5. Besser GM, Wass JAH: The medical management of acromegaly. In Black PM, et al, eds: Secretory Tumors of the Pituitary Gland. New York, Raven Press, 1984, pp 155–168.
6. Baumann G: Acromegaly. Endocrin Metab Clin North Am 16:686–703, 1987.
7. Vekemans M, Robyn C: Influence of age on serum prolactin levels in women and men. Br Med J 4:738–739, 1975.
8. Yamaji T, Shimamoto K, Ishibashi M, et al: Effect of age and sex on circulating and pituitary prolactin levels in humans. Acta Endocrinol 83:711–719, 1976.
9. Molitch ME, Elton RL, Blackwell RE, et al: Bromocriptine as primary therapy for prolactin-secreting macroadenomas: results of a prospective multicenter study. J Clin Endocrinol Metab 60:698–705, 1985.
10. Sherman BM, West JH, Korenman SG: The menopausal transition: analysis of LH, FSH, estradiol, and progesterone concentrations during menstrual cycles of older women. J Clin Endocrinol Metab 42:629–636, 1976.
11. Judd HL, Korenman SG: Effects of aging on reproductive function in women. In Korenman SG, ed: Endocrine Aspects of Aging. New York, Elsevier Science Publishing, 1982, pp 163–197.
12. Jaffe RB: The menopause and perimenopausal period. In Yen SSC, Jaffe RB, eds: Reproductive Endocrinology: Physiology, Pathophysiology and Clinical Management. Philadelphia, WB Saunders, 1986, pp 406–423.
13. Lindsay R: Estrogens in prevention and treatment of osteoporosis. In Avioli LV, ed: The Osteoporotic Syndrome: Detection, Prevention and Treatment. Orlando, Grune & Stratton, 1987, pp 91–107.
14. Swerdloff RS, Heber D: Effects of aging on male reproductive function. In Korenman SG, ed: Endocrine Aspects of Aging. New York, Elsevier Science Publishing, 1982, pp 119–135.
15. Deslypere JP, Vermeulen A: Leydig cell function in normal men: Effect of age, life-style, residence, diet, and activity. J Clin Endocrinol Metab 59:955–962, 1984.
16. Tenover JS, Matsumoto AM, Plymate SR, et al: The effects of aging in normal men on bioavailable testosterone and luteinizing hormone secretion: response to clomiphene citrate. J Clin Endocrinol Metab 65:1118–1126, 1987.
17. Helderman JH: The impact of normal aging on the hypothalamic-neurohypophyseal-renal axis. In Korenman SG, ed: Endocrine Aspects of Aging. New York, Elsevier Science Publishing, 1982, pp 119–135.
18. Lye M: Electrolyte disorders in the elderly. Clin Endocrinol Metab 13:377–398, 1984.
19. Robinson AG: Disorders of antidiuretic hormone secretion. Clin Endocrinol Metab 14:55–88, 1985.
20. Baylis PH, Gill GV: The investigation of polyuria. Clin Endocrinol Metab 13:295–310, 1984.
21. Melmed S, Hershman J: The thyroid and aging. In Korenman SG, ed: Endocrine Aspects of Aging. New York, Elsevier Science Publishing, 1982, pp 33–53.
22. Harman SM, Wehmann RE, Blackman MR: Pituitary-thyroid hormone economy in healthy aging men: Basal indices of thyroid function and thyrotropin responses to constant infusions of thyrotropin releasing hormone. J Clin Endocrinol Metab 58:320–326, 1984.
23. Ayus JC, Krothapalli RK, Arieff AI: Treatment of symptomatic hyponatremia and its relation to brain damage: A prospective study. N Engl J Med 317:1190–1199, 1987.
24. Berl T, Schrier RW: Disorders of water metabolism. In Schrier RW, ed: Renal and Electrolyte Disorders. Boston, Little, Brown, 1986, pp 1–77.
25. Sterns RH: Severe symptomatic hyponatremia: Treatment and outcome. Ann Intern Med 107:656–664, 1987.

26. Wartofsky L, Burman KD: Alterations in thyroid function in patients with systemic illness: The "euthyroid sick syndrome." Endocrine Rev 3:164–217, 1982.

27. Gharib H, James EM, Charboneau JW, et al: Suppressive therapy with levothyroxine for solitary thyroid nodules: A double-blind controlled clinical study. N Engl J Med 317:70–75, 1987.

28. Sapolsky R, Armanini M, Packan D, et al: Stress and glucocorticoids in aging. Endocrinol Metab Clin North Am 16:965–980, 1987.

29. Oxenkrug GF, Pomara N, McIntyre IM, et al: Aging and cortisol resistance to suppression by dexamethasone: A positive correlation. Psychiat Res 10:125–130, 1983.

30. Wolfsen AR: Aging and the adrenals. In Korenman SG, ed: Endocrine Aspects of Aging. New York, Elsevier Science Publishing, 1982, pp 55–79.

31. Tsunoda K, Abe K, Goto T, et al: Effect of age on the renin-angiotensin-aldosterone system in normal subjects: Simultaneous measurement of active and inactive renin, renin substrate, and aldosterone in plasma. J Clin Endocrinol Metab 62:384–389, 1986.

32. Lakatta EG: Catecholamines and cardiovascular function in aging. Endocrinol Metab Clin North Am 16:877–891, 1987.

33. Aron DC, Findling JW, Tyrrell JB: Cushing's disease. Endocrinol Metab Clin North Am 16:705–730, 1987.

34. Krieger DT: The medical management of Cushing's disease. In Black PM, et al, eds: Secretory Tumors of the Pituitary Gland. New York, Raven Press, 1984, pp 273–285.

35. Huvos AG, Hajdu SI, Brasfield RD, et al: Adrenal cortical carcinoma. Clinicopathologic study of 34 cases. Cancer 25:354–361, 1970.

36. Nerup J: Addison's disease—clinical studies. A report of 108 cases. Acta Endocrinol (Copenh) 76:127–141, 1974.

37. Burke CW: Adrenocortical insufficiency. Clin Endocrinol Metab 14:947–976, 1985.

38. Insogna KL, Lewis AM, Lipinski BA, et al: Effect of age on serum immunoreactive parathyroid hormone and its biological effects. J Clin Endocrinol Metab 53:1072–1075, 1981.

39. Marcus R, Madvig P, Young G: Age-related changes in parathyroid hormone and parathyroid hormone action in normal humans. J Clin Endocrinol Metab 58:223–230, 1984.

40. Slovik DM: Vitamin D endocrine system, calcium metabolism, and osteoporosis. In Cohen MP, Foa PP, eds: Special Topics in Endocrinology and Metabolism, Vol 5. New York, Alan R Liss, 1983, pp 83–148.

41. Eastell R: Hormonal factors: PTH, vitamin D, and calcitonin. In Riggs BL, Mellton LJ III, eds: Osteoporosis: Etiology, Diagnosis, and Management. New York, Raven Press, 1988, pp 373–388.

42. Roof BS, Gordan GS: Hyperparathyroid disease in the aged. In Greenblat RB, ed: Geriatric Endocrinology. New York, Raven Press, 1978, pp 33–79.

43. Tibblin S, Palsson N, Rydberg J: Hyperparathyroidism in the elderly. Ann Surg 197:135–138, 1983.

44. Scholz DA, Purnell DC: Asymptomatic primary hyperparathyroidism. 10-year prospective study. Mayo Clin Proc 56:473–478, 1981.

45. Selby PL, Peacock M: Ethinyl estradiol and norethindrone in the treatment of primary hyperparathyroidism in postmenopausal women. N Engl J Med 314:1481–1485, 1986.

INDEX

Note: Page numbers in *italics* refer to illustrations; page numbers followed by t refer to tables.